Handbook on
Mental Health Policy
in the United States

Handbook on
MENTAL HEALTH POLICY IN THE UNITED STATES

EDITED BY
David A. Rochefort

FOREWORD BY
Senator Edward M. Kennedy

Greenwood Press
New York • Westport, Connecticut • London

Library of Congress Cataloging-in-Publication Data

Handbook on mental health policy in the United States.

Includes index.
1. Mental health policy—United States. I. Rochefort,
David A. [DNLM: 1. Health Policy—United States.
2. Mental Health Services—United States. WM 30 H2355]
RA790.6.H33 1989   362.2′0973   88–32052
ISBN 0–313–25009–X (lib. bdg. : alk. paper)

British Library Cataloguing in Publication Data is available.

Library of Congress Catalog Card Number: 88–32052
ISBN: 0–313–25009–X

First published in 1989

Greenwood Press, Inc.
88 Post Road West, Westport, Connecticut   06881

Printed in the United States of America

The paper used in this book complies with the
Permanent Paper Standard issued by the National
Information Standards Organization (Z39.48-1984).

10 9 8 7 6 5 4 3 2 1

5-14-90

To my Parents

Contents

Foreword
Senator Edward M. Kennedy   xi

Preface   xv

Part 1.   Introduction

1. Mental Illness and Mental Health as Public Policy Concerns
    David A. Rochefort   3

2. The Contemporary Mental Health System: Facilities,
    Services, Personnel, and Finances
    Frederic G. Reamer   21

Part 2.   Epidemiologic Analysis of Mental Health Problems

3. Psychiatric Epidemiology: An Overview of Methods and
    Findings
    Sarah Rosenfield   45

4. Special Problem Populations: The Chronically Mentally Ill,
    Elderly, Children, Minorities, and Substance Abusers
    Evelyn J. Bromet and Herbert C. Schulberg   67

Part 3. Mental Health Policy Development

5. From the Asylum to the Community in U.S. Mental Health
    Care: A Historical Overview
    Leland V. Bell   89

6. A National Community Mental Health Program: Policy
    Initiation and Progress
    James M. Cameron   121

7. The Alcohol, Drug Abuse, and Mental Health Block Grant:
    Origins, Design, and Impact
    David A. Rochefort and Bruce M. Logan   143

8. Mental Health Policymaking in the United States: Patterns,
    Process, and Structures
    Philip K. Armour   173

Part 4. Evaluating the Community Mental Health Movement

9. An Evaluative Overview of the Community Mental Health
    Centers Program
    David A. Dowell and James A. Ciarlo   195

10. Community Residential Care
    Steven P. Segal and Pamela Kotler   237

11. Nursing Homes as Community Mental Health Facilities
    Margaret W. Linn and Shayna Stein   267

12. Homelessness as a Public Mental Health Problem
    Irene Shifren Levine and Loretta K. Haggard   293

13. The Changing Role of the Public Mental Hospital
    Joseph P. Morrissey   311

Part 5. Financing, Legal, and Service System Issues

14. Mental Health Insurance
    M. Susan Ridgely and Howard H. Goldman   341

15. Legal Issues in Mental Health Care: Current Perspectives
    Ingo Keilitz   363

16. Administrative and Service Provision Issues
    Jeanette M. Jerrell and S. Lee Jerrell   385

17. Preventive Services in Mental Health
    Raymond P. Lorion and LaRue Allen   403

Part 6.   Planning for Mental Health Services

18. Needs Assessment Techniques
    Phillip M. Massad and Barrie E. Blunt   435

19. Mental Health System Strategic Planning
    David Goodrick   449

Part 7.   Enduring Problems and Opportunities

20. Toward the Year 2000 in U.S. Mental Health Policymaking
    and Administration
    David Mechanic   477

    A Guide to Sources   505
    Author Index   511
    Subject Index   525
    About the Editor and Contributors   541

Foreword

Senator Edward M. Kennedy

I welcome the opportunity to be part of this debate on mental health policy in the United States. My family and I have had a long standing interest in these issues, and I commend the participants for their thoughtful contributions.

Extensive involvement with mental health issues has convinced me that treatment for the mentally ill, research on emotional disorders, and prevention of avoidable behavioral and psychological problems are essential elements in a sound mental health system. Legislators need greater guidance from knowledgeable professionals in all three areas, and we welcome their role in shaping more effective policies for the future.

Treatment for the seriously mentally ill has been a central focus of policy efforts for the past four decades, and it has brought both hope and disappointment for the mentally ill and their families. Beginning in the early 1950s, the increasing availability of psychoactive drugs—along with evidence that long-term institutionalization created behavioral problems and violated civil rights—brought a new consensus in favor of replacing confinement of the mentally ill with a system of community care. In most cases, it was felt, hospitalization should be limited to acute episodes of illness. As President Kennedy declared in his 1963 State of the Union Message, "The abandonment of the mentally ill to the grim mercy of custodial institutions too often inflicts on them a needless cruelty which this Nation should not endure."

After passage of the Community Mental Health Centers Act of 1963, the federal government began appropriating funds for construction and operation of comprehensive community-based mental health centers. Despite the proliferation of these centers, the release of patients from mental hospitals was not matched by the growth of the community-based system of care. Instead, as several of the authors here detail, the deinstitutionalized mentally ill have too often faced a future of abandonment, homelessness and despair. It is a sad commentary on our society that a block from the White House, confused, hallucinating, mentally ill people can be found dressed in rags, talking to themselves, and sleeping on grates on the coldest days of the Washington winter.

The creation of a system of comprehensive community-based care is a matter of simple justice, but not a simple policy problem. The tragedy of homelessness among the seriously mentally ill is a prime illustration of the principle that success in addressing mental health needs depends on an integrated social and economic policy. Features that must be present in any effective community-based program of care for this seriously mentally ill include housing and support for families— matters outside the typical scope of the mental health system.

An adequate array of community-based services will be costly. However, the Community Support Program Demonstrations that have been funded on a modest scale by the federal government since 1977, as well as programs at the state and local level, have shown that community-based care is not only therapeutically effective but also cost-effective.

Despite the models available and the progress that has been made by some states and communities, the gap between good practice and typical practice remains shamefully wide, and there have been many local, state and federal contributions to this impasse. Barriers at the federal level include the failure to adapt Medicaid rules and regulations to the needs of the seriously mentally ill. In addition, the enactment of the Reagan Administration's Alcohol, Drug Abuse, and Mental Health Services Block Grant Program in 1981 and the repeal of the Mental Health Systems Act that same year seemed to signify abdication of federal responsibility for this population.

A significant trend toward increased federal commitment began with the enactment of the Comprehensive Mental Health Service Act in 1986. I introduced that legislation to require states to plan and implement a comprehensive, community-based program of care for seriously mentally ill individuals as a condition of receiving block grant funds.

In addition to requiring the plans, the 1986 Act also specified procedures for developing and implementing them. It mandated the participation and advice of service consumers and their families, the mental health community, and the various state agencies whose programs are relevant. Finally, the act requires the Department of Health and Human Services in the federal government to provide technical assistance to states by developing a model plan and by offering technical support throughout the planning and programming efforts. Technical assistance in planning is now being provided by the Division of Education and Service Systems Liaison of the National Institute of Mental Health. This type of field support ensures nationwide programming standards, and helps to identify areas in which research is most needed.

Mental health research is also receiving increasing priority. Last year, concerns expressed by parents of the seriously mentally ill and by mental health professionals and policy analysts led to a $40 million increase in appropriations for such research. Now that the mandated National Plan for Schizophrenia Research has been completed, part of this NIMH money will support research on that illness.

Finally, recent experience has shown the importance of prevention in dealing with mental health problems. A convincing case can be made for the effectiveness of such interventions. Most recently, the evidence has resulted in increased funding and higher status for the Office of Substance Abuse Prevention and state block grant funds have been set aside for prevention programs targeting specific at-risk populations.

The importance of prevention is also reflected in several legislative initiatives now pending in Congress, including increased attention to young children at risk of school failure, the incorporation of mental health benefits in a measure requiring that all workers be offered a basic package of employer-based health insurance, and earmarking funds for grants for a wide range of adolescent pregnancy prevention programs.

Developing and implementing comprehensive mental health programs, even with the best of intentions, remains a serious challenge for mental health specialists, federal and state governments, and concerned citizens in every community. Federal requirements and penalties can be catalysts for progress, but they are no guarantee that action will occur. This volume makes a genuine contribution to the task of providing high quality mental health services for all who need them. If we heed the insight and analysis offered here, the decade of the 1990s can mark the beginning of an era of real progress in this area.

Preface

This volume presents a collection of scholarly contributions on contemporary mental health problems, policies, programs, and services. Drawing simultaneously on the professional literature and current information and statistics—making use, in several instances, of previously unpublished data—each chapter addresses issues critical to an understanding and evaluation of that complex of organizational and financial relationships termed the American mental health system.

No book of even so many as twenty chapters can make claim to an exhaustive treatment of this vast topic. The task here was somewhat narrowed by a primary focus on *public* mental health care. Present arrangements are such, however, that the boundary between public and private mental health services is often an artificial one that is crossed continuously by the actual flow of dollars and patients. Analyzing this dynamic process and the structure within which it occurs has resulted in a work encompassing three centuries of historical development and delving into medical, legal, political, administrative, and social service spheres of activity.

Our intended audience comprises several different groups. Prominent among them are administrators, planners, and service providers in the public and non-profit sectors who seek an in-depth guide to issues of mental health resource allocation and management. Teachers and students of U.S. mental health policy—in public health, social work, public administration, political science, sociology, and related fields—may also find this a useful sourcebook for reading and research. A further aim is to help satisfy the information needs of those persons in government and the media who deal with mental health policy questions.

The list of contributors to this volume is suitably diverse. Disciplinary approaches represented include history, organization and management, public administration, psychiatry, psychology, social work, and sociology, among others. Many authors are faculty members at institutions of higher education; others work as practicing managers and analysts for federal, state, and local governments or in private organizations. Such variety offers powerful testament in itself to the breadth of the mental health field and the multiple methods of inquiry it invites.

No single philosophical or political stance underlies the chapters within. The reader will note varying perspectives on such matters as the relative value of different mental health service modalities, recent action to increase the role of state governments in managing community care programs, and future priorities for the investment of limited public dollars. Nonetheless, certain common themes do emerge, notably, the persistence of unmet population needs and government's responsibility to continue to improve its efforts to enhance the well-being and functioning of mentally ill persons.

The volume is organized in sections. The starting point is an introductory overview of the mental health policy arena and contemporary mental health system. Next are two chapters that review the methods of psychiatric epidemiology and summarize its major findings for the general population and selected high risk sub-groups. Part 3 of the *Handbook* traces the development of U.S. mental health policy from the seventeenth century to the decade of the 1980s, concluding with an analysis of formative patterns of policymaking and politics.

Part 4 assesses the impact of the modern community mental health movement and examines the consequences of patient placement in selected institutional and noninstitutional settings. Financing, legal, and service system issues are explored in greater detail in the volume's next section. Part 6 then turns to the technology of needs assessment and approaches for strategic planning. Based on a critical review of past trends, a capstone essay in the *Handbook*'s closing section outlines an agenda for U.S. mental health policymaking and administration into the coming century.

It is my pleasure to acknowledge the many persons and organizations that provided assistance with the preparation of this book. A National Institute of Mental Health postdoctoral fellowship enabled me to spend the 1987–1988 academic year in the Rutgers-Princeton Program in Mental Health Research at Rutgers' Institute for Health, Health Care Policy, and Aging Research. I am grateful to Director David Mechanic and the other Institute members and staff, who created an intellectually stimulating and supportive atmosphere for my work on this and other projects. Released time for research from Northeastern's Department of Political Science made it possible for me to keep the *Handbook* on track both before and after my fellowship year. Carol Boyer, at the time a fellow Rutgers ''postdoc'' and now with the New Jersey Department of Health, prepared Figure 2–1; Figures 10–1 and 14–1, initially provided by the authors of those chapters, were redrawn for reproduction purposes by Terry Beadle of Northeastern University's Center for Instructional Technology. Jan Tulloss, a former colleague at Northeastern, generously shared her computer expertise and her printer at a frantic point in my editorial work the week before the manuscript went to the publisher. Andriette Fields, my graduate research assistant, helped track down references. Michelle Apuzzo, another graduate research assistant, prepared the author index. With care and intelligence, Paula Woolley did the bulk of the work on the subject index, a formidable task indeed.

I am appreciative for the assistance and advice on varied matters that I received from the knowledgeable editorial and production staff at Greenwood Press. I particularly want to mention Margaret Brezicki, Loomis Mayer, William Neenan, Michelle Scott, and Mary Sive. Juanita Lewis copyedited the manuscript skillfully.

Using the media of the mails and the telephone, and by means of brief contacts at the occasional professional meeting, projects like this attempt to orchestrate a kind of symphony of scholarship. Unlike a musical performance, however, this is an odd collective enterprise in which the principals never convene as a group and only one person observes the emerging product. Invariably, these conditions make for unforeseen complications and a protracted process. To all of the contributors in this volume I offer my sincere thanks, again, for entrusting their work to my care and coordination and for their patience throughout.

Finally, I would like to thank my wife, Eileen, for her unwavering assistance and support, for her willingness to listen and to advise. The book is dedicated with affection to my parents.

Part I
Introduction

1

Mental Illness and Mental Health as Public Policy Concerns

DAVID A. ROCHEFORT

Current estimates are that as many as 20 percent of the adult U.S. population may suffer from an emotional or psychological disorder (U.S. Department of Health and Human Services, 1987: 67; Locke and Regier, 1985). Of this group, the chronically mentally ill (CMI)—those persons with the most severe, persistent, and dysfunctional illnesses—number from 1.7 million to 2.4 million (Goldman and Manderscheid, 1987). Only a minority of all mentally ill enter the treatment system. Still, the economic burden to society of providing mental health care is great, ranging as high as $24 billion in combined public and private funds in 1980, if one counts Social Security disability payments in addition to costs incurred in the health, human services, and specialty mental health sectors (Frank and Kamlet, 1985). Other social impacts, while difficult to measure precisely, include loss of productivity in the work place, instances of family dissolution and antisocial behavior, and community disorganization in the form of homelessness and other social problems. And for the individuals afflicted, the experience of mental illness can be ruinous, too often tragedies of frustrated personal development and lost potential.

Whether judged in demographic, fiscal, or simple human terms, then, mental illness is a problem of enormous magnitude in modern American society. As such, it has come to elicit a collective social response in the way of large-scale public policies, programs, and services. In order to establish a framework for understanding the nature of this response, and its accomplishments and failures, I begin by reviewing the genesis of mental illness and mental health as public policy concerns. I identify key features of the mental health policymaking environment and then summarize selected major contemporary trends in public mental health care.

EMERGENCE AS A PUBLIC POLICY ISSUE

Only a subset of all problems in society ever comes to receive the attention of government. To make the transition from "private" to "public" status, a problem must satisfy several conditions: its solution must be beyond the capacity of private action; its existence must be known to more than just the immediately involved parties; and the problem must generate consequences that are judged serious enough to deserve public response (Jones, 1984: 39–40). The sociologist C. Wright Mills (1959) has offered a useful distinction between "personal troubles" and "public issues." Only in the latter case is social intervention invoked in reaction to some perceived threat to established values.

The problem of mental illness remained largely within the private realm of personal troubles in the American colonies (Grob, 1973: chapter 1; Rochefort, 1981: 112–115; and chapter 5 in this volume). In this sparsely populated, agricultural society, mental illness, which was generally taken to be God's will, was not a major public concern. Such cases as existed were first and foremost family responsibilities. Public intervention occurred only when suitable family supervision was lacking, or when a mentally ill individual presented a public menace. In these circumstances, local authorities followed an ad hoc, case-by-case approach based on poor relief practices. Sometimes public funds were used to assist the family of a mentally ill person, or to house a mentally ill individual with a surrogate family in the community. Violent insane were kept in jails or otherwise confined. Then, toward the second half of the 1700s, the mentally ill often were placed in the public almshouses that were becoming increasingly common across the states. Very few institutions offering specialized mental health care were in existence prior to 1800, so "as a practical matter insane people were treated like dependents or criminals" (Leiby, 1978: 63).

The eventual development of a more systematic and large-scale public policy toward mental illness in American society was compelled by numerous forces (Grob, 1973: chapters 2 and 3; Rochefort, 1981: 115–119; and chapter 5 in this volume). Reflecting on the initiation of public policy issues, Peters (1986: 45–46) observes that "the nature of the problems themselves will have an influence on their being accepted as part of the agenda [of government]." One important aspect of a problem is the extensiveness of its effects, viewed in terms of such dimensions as extremity, concentration, and visibility. During the first half of the eighteenth century, general awareness of mental illness and the mentally ill in the United States expanded as population growth increased the incidence and prevalence of the problem. Heightened population density owing to the process of urbanization contributed to a greater conspicuousness as well.

Another factor capable of provoking new or expanded public attention to some social problem is the obvious insufficiency of existing means of response (Peters, 1986: 49–50). So it was that, in the early 1800s, rising numbers of mentally ill placed an insupportable burden on the limited almshouse and hospital facilities that were then being used for indigent cases. Operators of these facilities, in turn, appealed to public authorities for relief.

Other groups joined in the call for augmented public involvement in mental health care—social activists, physicians, and religious and political leaders. A contemporary spirit of humanitarian social improvement lent added momentum to the movement. Reformers like Dorothea Dix—who documented the inadequacy of existing provisions for the mentally ill, mobilized a coalition of public and elite supporters, and worked to influence elected officials—played a crucial role as latter-day "policy entrepreneurs" capable of sustaining the issue from its inception to legislative action (Cobb and Elder, 1983: 187).

Finally, a new "technology" (Peters, 1986: 50–51) for mental health care also became available in the early 1800s. Originating in France and England around the turn of the century, "moral treatment" advised a course of humane and individualized therapy in protected institutional settings. Nothing less than a redefined view of mental illness was taking place, from predominantly an economic and social problem to a medical one (Grob, 1973: 1).

To carry out the new mission of treatment and cure, specialized hospital facilities were built, many with private funds but increasingly under public auspices as time went on. By 1861, there were forty-eight mental institutions in America, of which the majority were funded and administered by the states. Dozens more followed in subsequent decades. These facilities were to remain the foundation of the U.S. mental health system for more than a hundred years. In 1955, when public mental hospitals in the United States reached their peak population, the year-end census counted more than 558,000 resident patients, with approximately 178,000 admissions occurring during this year (see chapter 13 in this volume).

Not until the latter half of the twentieth century did the focus of U.S. mental health policy undergo significant transformation and expansion. The origins of this process can be found in the Progressive Era preceding World War I (Grob, 1983). Simultaneous with other reform movements of the day concerned with juvenile justice, housing conditions, poverty, and public health, mental health activists sought to initiate a community-based system of care. The goal was twofold: improved aftercare services for discharged patients, and new efforts aimed at preventing the development of mental disorders in the population at large through education and early diagnosis and treatment. The perceived problem to which the system needed to respond was thus no longer merely the treatment of mental illness but the promotion of society's "mental hygiene" as well.

Establishment of the National Institute of Mental Health (NIMH) in 1946 signaled a momentous shift from the state to federal level as the locus of innovation in U.S. mental health policy (Brand, 1965). In this way it denoted, as well, continuing elevation in the status of the mental health issue. NIMH dispensed new funds for research, professional training, and community service programs, and its creation designated a central point of responsibility in the national government for data collection and policy formulation in public mental health. From colonial times to the decade of the 1940s, the problem of mental illness had made several transitions within the American political system: from a private matter to a social concern deserving of public attention first from local, then state, now federal authorities; from charity and regulation to combined management, treatment, and prevention.

Jones (1984: 52) explains that "many of the problems that eventually get to government are created by the implementation of policy. That is, government itself causes the event that is perceived and defined as a problem for an individual or group." This observation aptly describes one major thrust behind the community mental health movement that emerged in the United States during the 1950s and 1960s (Rochefort, 1984; chapter 6 in this volume). Reformers of this time defined a decrepit, overcrowded, public hospital system as anti-therapeutic, a problem needing to be addressed by U.S. mental health policy. Aided by the discovery of powerful anti-psychotic drugs, they succeeded in having enacted seminal national legislation, the Community Mental Health Centers Act of 1963 (CMHC Act), that sponsored an alternate system of care based on local facilities responsible to federal rather than state authorities. The federal-state Medicaid program and Supplemental Security Income (SSI), both established subsequently, helped underwrite this movement away from state institutions to the community and such settings as nursing homes.

At the same time, the community mental health movement also extended the Progressives' concern with the active promotion of mental health. The new "paradigm" in mental health was closely modeled after a classic "public health" approach:

Here there is a move from a focus on the individual patient to a focus on large populations. The purpose of intervention is to reduce the incidence of disability or disease in such a population. Therefore, a special value is placed on primary prevention rather than on cure, and prevention paradigms are presented along with treatment paradigms. Professional attention is placed not only on the casualties of damaging environment but on the damaging environments themselves. (Hersch, 1972: 750)

Influenced by this new perspective, some community mental health partisans endeavored to expand the scope of the mental health issue to include such matters as poverty, racism, and other forms of inequality. The line between mental health policy and social revisionism in general sometimes was difficult to distinguish.

Years from now historians may describe the 1980s as marking another crossroads in U.S. mental health policy. Federal block grants, federal funding cuts, and the growth of state programs, among other forces, have returned to the states much of the initiative in community mental health care that was lost under the original CMHC Act (Rich, 1986; chapter 7 of this volume). Also in evidence within the public mental health system, and related to this growth of state influence, is a narrowed service philosophy that is directing an increasing share of available community resources to the severely and chronically mentally ill. This trend reflects a more conservative sociopolitical climate, but also new developments in the problem at hand, namely, "the emergence of a critical mass of young, highly disturbed adults" who typically have never received long-term institutional care (Surles, 1987: 221; Talbott, 1988). Prevention and accessibility of services to all were the ideological watchwords of U.S. mental health policy in the 1960s and 1970s, and many in the field became disappointed over the system's limited success in attaining these goals. Today the more modest themes of rehabilitation and maintenance of persons most greatly in need are paramount.

This broad-brush outline of history neglects many countercurrents and exceptions that would deserve attention in a fuller account of events. Still, it suffices to underscore that mental health policymaking in the United States is a dynamic process in which the perception of the problem and proposed solutions have been constantly evolving. Existing objectives acquire new dimensions or are transformed; the scale and means of policy action are subject to revision as well. The forces of change in mental health policy have emanated both from within and without the mental health system—new etiological formulations, treatment innovations, epidemiological trends, past program successes and failures, and broader social, political, and economic currents (Rochefort, 1988).

Understanding the origins and significance of shifting public objectives is an important element of mental health policy analysis that will receive extensive consideration throughout the following chapters of this volume. A second focus will be strategy, that is, the design of programmatic mechanisms selected by public officials for achieving these objectives. Finally, whatever the formal conceptions that underlie policy, it will be necessary to evaluate actual impacts at the day-to-day level of service delivery and on the clientele being served. These topics encompass the "natural history" or "life cycle" of the policymaking process and, taken together, provide a basis for considering needed improvements in the future development of the system.

CHARACTERISTICS OF THE MENTAL HEALTH POLICY ARENA

The protean quality of policymaking—its historical pattern of issue definition–redefinition and transmuting objectives—is not unique to the mental health sphere. Such, in fact, is more the rule than the exception with other areas of American public policy, especially those, like public mental health care, whose lineages reach back over several generations. Yet an analysis of mental health policymaking in the United States does reveal several qualities that, in kind or in degree, help to differentiate it from other public involvements and define its special challenges. These have to do with the nature of the problem of mental illness, the benefits distributed by the public mental health system, the political interests that populate the mental health environment, intricacies of service delivery, and the cyclicality of mental health policy and program development.

Nature of the Problem

Mental illness is a problem of special complexity. Considered in terms of diagnosis, symptomatology, level of disability, duration of illness, epidemiologic frequency, or dangerousness, the phenomena grouped under this label are enormously heterogeneous (Leighton, 1982: 6–7; Rochefort, 1988: 138–139). No less complicated are the causes of mental illness, a condition that apparently results from the variable interplay between underlying social, demographic, biological, and personal risk factors and precipitating stresses. Not only is mental illness a complex problem, but it can also be one of the most severe and disabling personal dysfunctions. The chronic mental illnesses, chiefly certain cases of schizophrenia and other psychotic and organic illnesses, are resistant to easy management in either a clinical or social sense. The chronically mentally ill and other severely disordered persons also make up a "highly dependent patient population," a fact which "presents extraordinary problems for the administrator and staff in attempting to maintain a responsive, accountable, and humane program" (Feldman 1980: xix).

Reflecting the multidimensional nature of the problem and its uncertain etiology, debates about the definition of mental illness are ongoing (Mechanic, 1980: chapter 2). Specialists disagree, for example, whether mental illness and mental health reside at opposite ends of a single graded continuum, or whether different disorders should be viewed as distinct categorical entities. Disputes persist, too, about the boundary between mental illness and other forms of deviancy, and about the relative contribution of individual, family, and social influences in producing mental disorders.

These attributes of mental illness as a social problem exert important influence on public policy development (Mechanic, 1980: 34–38; Rochefort, 1988). Since policy design arises from problem definition, lack of consensus about the nature of the problem being dealt with works counter to a collective sense of purpose and direction in mental health policymaking. Although advocates for improved mental health care number many, their influence is often diffused in advancing different priorities for the investment of limited public resources. The situation is exacerbated by specialists' inability to reach agreement upon the boundaries of normal behavior or even the proportion of all cases of recognized abnormality severe enough to warrant public intervention. Lack of definitive knowledge about causes and cures also makes it problematic to conceive new programs in mental health care that will be cost-effective, just as it adds to the difficult task of political decision makers who must assign responsibilities and resources among the competing professional groups and service providers claiming "ownership" of this problem.

Nature and Distribution of Benefits

Improvements in the mental health status of the population are the ultimate objective of mental health policy, but this benefit cannot be bestowed directly. In this respect, the mental health policy arena differs from, say, income maintenance, in which government, wishing to increase the resources of a particular segment of society, can effect economic transfers from one group to another. Instead, mental health policy operates to ensure the availability and accessibility of mental health services, which may or may not, in their turn, yield the desired changes in emotional well-being. Feldman comments on the ambiguous character of this "output" of mental health policymaking:

In mental health our product is intangible and our degree of success is very difficult to determine and measure. The terrain is littered with ill-conceived and poorly executed evaluation studies, and the technology of mental health evaluation remains quite limited. It is, therefore, very difficult for the mental health administrator to evaluate the effectiveness of the organization, or even of individual staff members. These difficulties also exist for outside groups and organizations attempting to evaluate the utility of mental health programs. (Feldman, 1980: xix)

As to the distribution of service benefits in public mental health, most are highly concentrated. Even though community-based programs have modified the situation in recent decades, the bulk of resources in the public mental health system continues to be directed to the most severely disabled population, such as those in need of institutionalization or long-term psychological treatment and maintenance (Talbott, 1988: 51–52). This clientele constitutes a comparatively small subset of the minority of all troubled individuals who receive care. To be sure, publicly supported services are available to persons with milder difficulties, but this need is assigned lower priority within the public mental health system partly on the assumption that many of these individuals can be served on the private health insurance market or by use of other private resources. The public mental health system does deliver widely dispersed benefits in the form of preventive services such as community-wide education and consultation programs. By their very nature, however, these activities often are so broadly aimed that recipients may not even recognize a personal gain.

The upshot is that, whether warranted or not, mental health policy is generally perceived as primarily of value to a small group in society having aberrant emotional and behavioral conditions. At the same time, mental health services are poorly understood by many and are of unknown, or unappreciated, efficacy.

Organization of Interests

"The political 'market,' " according to Marmor, Wittman, and Heagy (1976: 73), "refers to institutional arrangements—the relationships among organized pressure groups, voters, authoritative governmental agencies, and affected citizens—which determine what governments do." Encompassed within the political market for mental health policy are numerous actors having varying species of interests. Discussion here will be confined to identifying those with mental health issues as their main concern, leaving to later chapters an analysis of the formal and informal decision-making structures through which these groups influence policy.

Recipients of public mental health services generally fall into the category of a "disorganized interest." Although they have the most direct stake in the quality and quantity of programs, these persons typically have been too demoralized or disabled by their conditions to organize into a coherent, effective political force (notwithstanding such efforts as the mental patients liberation movement, which has claimed some important victories in patients' rights litigation [Brown, 1981]). Weakened in the capacity to make claims in their own behalf, the mentally ill have come to be represented in the policymaking realm by various advocates acting on the basis of an "adopted interest." Included in this group are such organizations as the Mental Health Association, the Mental Health Law Project, and Alliance for the Mentally Ill. Consumers are active in some of these groups but do not comprise the sole or dominant membership.

A very powerful set of actors in mental health policymaking consists of those who deliver the services. The "provider interest" derives from the caregiving role and providers' own economic dependence on mental health programs (Frank and Kamlet, 1986: 216). This description applies equally to professional groups like the American Psychiatric Association, American Psychological Association, and National Association of Social Workers; a union like the the American Federation of State, County, and Municipal Employees; and service delivery organizations such as the National Council of Community Mental Health Centers.

Mental health policymaking in the United States also involves public sector actors having what can be called an "assigned interest" which arises from the multiple functions of allocative authority, advocacy, and political responsibility. The Alcohol, Drug Abuse, and Mental Health Administration, National Institute of Mental Health, and state and national legislative committees that exercise jurisdiction over mental health issues occupy this strategic position within the political market for mental health care. State mental health authorities, organized nationally as the National Association of State Mental Health Program Directors, are another example, with the added dimension that the state authorities are providers of care through the state mental hospital system. Though their role is a less political one in the traditional sense of this term, the courts have also significantly shaped the course of U.S. mental health policy in recent decades (Levine, 1981: chapter 6).

Experience has shown that these diverse interests can prove a formidable force for policy development when gathered behind a common cause. This, in large measure, was the case with the community mental health program of the 1950s and 1960s, which elicited broad-based support among the advocacy, provider, and public agency interests that were in existence at the time (Rochefort, 1984). On the other hand, this same constellation of interests, which has proliferated since the passage of the CMHC Act of 1963, can present just as considerable a barrier when divided in its demands, the situation that has often prevailed over the last decade or so. Consider, for example, the conflicts among state and local, institutional and community, advocacy and provider interests that enlivened consideration of the Mental Health Systems Act of 1980 (subsequently rescinded), and that linger today under the states' implementation of the Alcohol, Drug Abuse, and Mental Health (ADAMH) Block Grant (Foley and Sharfstein, 1983: chapter 5; Levine, 1981: chapter 7; and chapter 7 of this volume).

Within the context of this fluid, populous political environment, public opinion has a subtle impact on the mental health policymaking process. As already noted, most citizens are not recipients of public mental health services: according to one estimate, only 5 percent to 10 percent of the general population will ever make use of publicly financed mental health care (Frank and Kamlet, 1986: 221–222). Nor does the public identify directly with the plight of those afflicted with mental illness, which it considers a stigmatizing condition. For these reasons, the public's interest in mental health policy is a "diffuse" one, not "concentrated" as in the case of consumers, providers, or public officials (Marmor, Wittman, and Heagy, 1976: 73–74). Frank and Kamlet (1986: 221–223) portray the "median voter" with respect to mental health policy issues as simultaneously motivated by three primary concerns: control of public expenditures corresponding to a desire to limit the tax burden; some degree of compassion for the mentally ill; and a desire to maintain order in the social community. While not antithetical to the maintenance of public mental health programs, neither does this mind-set promise a wellspring of support for expansive, well-funded initiatives. And yet, an aroused public opinion can be an important stimulus behind the process of policy reform. For this, too, was demonstrated in the community mental health movement of the post–World War II period, which was fueled, in part, by popular demand for improved hospital conditions and support for alternative forms of care (Rochefort, 1984).

Complex Policymaking and Service Delivery Systems

Caring for severely and chronically mentally ill persons within the community setting requires the provision of psychiatric rehabilitation and maintenance services, but this alone is not enough. A host of social, medical, and economic supports must be made available that can respond in a systematic way to the demands of noncustodial living while promoting the fullest realization of human potential at varying levels (Mechanic and Aiken, 1987; Foley and Sharfstein, 1983: chapter 6). Depending on the needs and capacities of the individual, this spectrum of aid might encompass income support, housing assistance, medical services, employment training and placement, transportation, and recreational activities.

The problem is that policymaking structures for the human services are exceptionally fragmented. Different pockets of authority within government make decisions for different specialized areas, most of which do not view the mentally ill as a primary constituency. Administration and implementation of comprehensive community mental health programs are likewise confounded by the pluralism of the delivery system. Dominating the scene are large "categorical" bureaucracies that have typically been created to fulfill a narrow service mission oriented to particular population groups. Coordinating the activities of this heterogeneous cast of characters around the common aim of serving the mentally ill makes for a prodigious task, and issues of turf are prominent (Rochefort, 1987).

Mental health policymaking and administration in the United States also require the management of sometimes difficult relations between levels of government and public and private spheres (Brown and Stockdill, 1972: 678–680). These, of course, are not unique to the mental health field but enter into play there with special saliency. For example, because of its historical progression from a local to a national concern, today's public mental health system has a layered identity. Some programs operate under separate levels of authority, e.g., Veterans Administration facilities and state mental hospitals, while others function through joint local, state, and federal interaction, e.g., the CMHC system (Morgan and Connery, 1980: 245). Whatever the case may be, working out the responsibilities of these respective participants is a continuing political process, subject to periodic reexamination and adjustment.

Moreover, no clear dividing line distinguishes public from private action in mental health care. Not uncommonly, it is private foundations that fund, in whole or in part, the experimental programs which subsequently give rise to public innovations. Public officials, for their part, have considerable say over the activities of private providers and insurers through the powers of regulatory supervision, and the public health insurance programs of Medicare and Medicaid pay for much of the service delivered to elderly and poor patients by private mental health facilities. The present indeterminacy of precisely how much of total mental health spending in the United States represents public vs. private dollars (Frank and Kamlet 1986: 213–214)—the majority come from public sources—speaks to not only the inadequacy of existing data collection systems but also to the intertwining of these two sectors in mental health care. All in all, it is a picture of sprawling diversity in which available resources can be poorly utilized due to lack of central planning, organizational barriers, and duplication and gaps in service.

Cyclicality of Policy Development

Mental health policymaking in the United States exhibits a distinctive cyclical pattern (Rochefort, 1988; see, also, chapters 8 and 13 in this volume). Over the past three hundred years, crests of high policy and program activity have alternated with troughs of stagnation and decline as the mentally ill and their problems have moved into and out of the public spotlight. Examining the intellectual content of the field, one can also recognize how certain concepts and theories— for example, beliefs about environmental vs. somatic etiology—have recurrently risen and fallen in influence. Approaches for the organization and delivery of services, such as the emphasis given to institutional or community programs, have vacillated as well, displaying a tendency for the periodic rediscovery and revival of past program modalities.

"Issue attention cycles" are not uncommon in other areas of public policy-making (Downs, 1973), yet the multifaceted quality and long historical span of this developmental schema in mental health offer a special case in the annals of American public policy, even beyond that of antipoverty policy which holds similarities in this regard. With many arguing the failure of the policy of de-institutionalization and a need for greater reliance on public hospital facilities, it is easy to discern the presence of this same cyclical impulse today. While it is far from clear how the contemporary debate over community care will be worked out, continued instability in mental health policies and programs is predictable until and unless more effective methods of treatment and management can be demonstrated.

MENTAL HEALTH POLICY DIRECTIONS OF THE 1980s AND 1990s

An increased concern within contemporary community mental health programs with serving the severely and chronically mentally ill has already been noted and will be elaborated upon in other chapters. Added to this development, and often dictated by it, are several other recent trends in U.S. mental health poli-cymaking and administration that promise to extend into the next decade and beyond.

Ascendance of Management

Several factors in conjunction have brought issues of management and admin-istration to the forefront in contemporary public mental health care. Economic recession in the early 1980s coupled with federal funding reductions and eligi-bility restrictions in several programs on which mentally ill persons depend, including community mental health centers, Medicaid, SSI, and Social Security Disability Insurance (SSDI), has cut into the resource base for mental health care. As a result, budgets for many publicly supported agencies have not kept pace with inflation or have even declined in nominal dollars. Galvanized into action by these circumstances, managers of affected organizations have struggled to minimize the damage to existing programs, often streamlining operations to strengthen control over resource utilization (Larsen, 1987; Peterson, Austin, and Patti, 1985). Forced to reconsider mission and structure, many organizations have assigned new weight to strategic planning. In a keynote address before the annual meeting of the American College of Mental Health Administrators in 1981, James J. Callahan, Jr., poignantly summarized the situation (see, also, Shore, 1982):

In a time like this, management must be active, intrusive, accountable, and willing to take the heat. It's not possible to fake it any longer. Real deadlines exist, because at a particular point in time there will indeed be no more money. Real conflicts over the allocation of resources must be handled. Issues of what, how much, and to whom affect the entire organization, and, unless they are resolved, will exacerbate organizational conflict. (Callahan, 1982: 168–169)

Changes in intergovernmental relations that have redrawn existing lines of accountability and control have also induced administrative adaptations. Recipients of federal CMHC funds, previously distributed by the federal government but now under the authority of the states, have had to develop (or expand) a clientele relationship with those state officials responsible for the ADAMH block grant program and must satisfy the new performance criteria established in many places (Rich, 1986). State authorities, for their part, have acquired expanded administrative responsibilities pertaining to the ongoing operation of the block grant. These include procedures for public hearings, funds allocation, program monitoring, technical assistance, data collection, and auditing (U.S. General Accounting Office, 1984: chapter 4). In most cases adjustments have been minor due to existing state involvement with recipient agencies through the prior categorical CMHC program and state-funded activities. Nonetheless, block grants presented a fresh opportunity for administrative improvement and rationalization of which many state mental health departments, seeking greater efficiencies, have taken advantage (see chapter 7 in this volume).

Further contributing to the present stress on effective administration has been the desire to mount responsive multiservice programs for chronically and severely mentally ill persons in the community. To the extent that a professional consensus may be said to exist in the mental health field today, it is on this necessity (see, e.g., Mechanic and Aiken, 1987; Foley and Sharfstein, 1983: 153–156; American Hospital Association, 1986; National Mental Health Association, 1986). Seeking a solution for inadequacies of the existing fragmented public mental health "nonsystem," many have turned to managerial approaches. More will be said in following chapters about these efforts. It is enough here to note the variety of initiatives that are in progress, which range from the practice of case management to attack problems of service delivery at the level of the individual recipient (Dill, 1987), to new organizational entities capable of uniting previously unrelated funding streams and program resources (see, e.g., Robert Wood Johnson Foundation and the U.S. Department of Housing and Urban Development, 1986).

Ascendance of Financing

"Increasingly," economist Jeffrey Rubin (1987: 107) writes, "efforts to reform the mental health care system begin with changes in the way mental health services are financed." Psychiatrist Steven Sharfstein (1985: 202) echoes this notion in underscoring the need "to begin to rethink some of the fundamental assumptions of state funding of psychiatric care and the new incentives in medical care." Over the past ten years or so, interest in the financial dimensions of mental health care—in the impact of economic incentives and payment methods on the operation of the service system—has been pervasive, infiltrating thinking in the worlds of policymaking, administration, academia, and the foundation. Recent conditions of economic scarcity in public mental health care and a push for cost containment in the health sector generally have reinforced the trend.

A multitude of problems have been identified in mental health care financing. Notwithstanding the massive outflow of patients from public institutions since the mid–1950s, the lion's share of state mental health funds remains committed to institutional budgets; hence the common complaint that "dollars have not followed the patients" (Talbott, 1985: 47). Biases in the coverage of psychiatric services under public and private health insurance plans also exist. Talbott (1985: 47) summarizes, "Current inefficient reimbursement practices favor funding of inpatient over outpatient treatment, hospitalization over prevention of hospitalization, direct over indirect services, acute treatment over chronic care, and more restrictive alternatives over less restrictive ones." A sizeable group of persons in our society lack basic mental health coverage altogether. And the chronically mentally ill pose a special challenge to financing systems. Their reliance on multiple programs that cut across levels of government and mental health, health, social service, and income maintenance bureaucracies entangles them in a thicket of regulations and eligibility requirements that often obstructs the provision of service (Talbott, 1985 and 1988; Rubin, 1984).

Faced with such issues as these, mental health specialists increasingly have turned their attention to developing mechanisms for achieving a more efficient and productive distribution of mental health dollars. For example, one popular recommendation of late is for "capitation," the allocation of funds among geographical areas on the basis of such population characteristics as the incidence, prevalence, and estimated costs of mental health problems (Rubin, 1984, 1987; Talbott, 1985; Talbott and Sharfstein, 1986; Dickey and Goldman, 1986). Channeling capitated funds through federal, state, local, and private management entities has been suggested, including the idea of a Health Maintenance Organization for mental health services (Sharfstein, 1982). A more incremental kind of reform would be to correct deficiencies in existing programs that directly or indirectly fund mental health care, like Medicare, Medicaid, SSI, and SSDI, so as to match eligibility and coverage to the actual needs of mentally ill persons in the community. Work is also being done within the federal government to bring psychiatric care in general hospitals under the diagnosis-based prospective reimbursement scheme already implemented by Medicare for other forms of health services (see Kiesler and Morton [1988] for a summary of issues).

Federal Reorientation

Consolidation of the CMHC program and related alcohol and drug abuse programs on the federal level into a state-administered block grant represents another variation on the contemporary theme of system change through financial reform (Rubin, 1984: 276–277). Its object, from a policy point of view, is to shift the balance of state-federal authority in community mental health care. Rich (1986: 112) casts this development in terms of an ongoing ''transformation'' of the mental health system that began in the late 1970s and whose purpose is ''to define a 'balanced system' of inpatient and outpatient care under the direction and control of state government.'' For some observers—including, not surprisingly, many in state government—this federal reorientation is part and parcel of a long-overdue revision of intergovernmental policy that is larger than the mental health issue (see, e.g., Barfield, 1981). Others, however, view the substantial funding reductions that accompanied creation of the ADAMH block grant, together with concurrent cuts and eligibility changes in the federal disability and Medicaid programs, as heralding a retreat from the established federal role in public mental health care (see, e.g., Foley and Sharfstein, 1983: 159; Burt and Pittman, 1985: 181–183).

Reflection, Reassessment, and Renewal

Today hard questions are being asked in the mental health field. Has community mental health care worked, for whom, and why or why not? What should be the role of public mental institutions within the evolving American mental health system? How can community and institutional, public and private care systems be coordinated to deliver more effective service to the population at large? How can the performance of service activities *within* a single agency be maximized to reach the greatest number of clients in a continuous way? How will public mental health systems continue to move ahead at a time when federal deficits and popular disenchantment with large social programs have put the human services under siege? Contemplating the discourse of public mental health care in the 1980s—as presented in the pages of professional journals, on conference programs, and in the expressed concerns of public officials charged with evaluating current programs—it is hard not to be impressed by the depth of soul-searching, of painful collective self-examination that is underway.

It is also hard not to be impressed by the burgeoning of creative ideas that has taken place within this period of reflection and reassessment. Few times will strike their own inhabitants as devoid of such qualities as imagination, perseverance, and dedication. Still, the information compiled in this volume strongly suggests that a genuine regeneration of public mental health care may be taking place beneath the surface of contemporary angst and uncertainty. New directions in mental health management and financing have already been discussed. Other innovations that have been proposed or introduced on a limited basis include new types of mental health facilities (see, e.g., Gudeman and Shore, 1984; Moltzen et al., 1986), new service programs (see, eg., Gudeman, Shore, and Dickey, 1983; Paradis, 1987; Pomp and McGovern, 1988), new methods of producing services (see, e.g., Looney, 1986; Paulson, 1988), and new methods of planning and advocacy (see chapter 17 in this volume). The exact shape of the public mental health system in the United States ten or fifteen years from now is unknown at present. What is plain, however, is that such ferment is indispensable to the process of renewal.

CONCLUSION

Public involvement in the provision and financing of mental health care can be traced to the early days of American society, making this one of the oldest continuing commitments of the governmental system. Given the scale of resources invested and the scope of public services, mental health care is also a domestic activity in which government plays a distinctive leadership role. An appreciation of the history, character, and recent trends of U.S. mental health policymaking and administration, briefly surveyed in this chapter, provides the foundation for an in-depth examination of contemporary issues and problems.

ACKNOWLEDGMENT

The author is grateful to Ann E. P. Dill of Brown University who provided insightful comments on a draft of this chapter.

REFERENCES

American Hospital Association. 1986. *Caring for Patients with Chronic Mental Illness.* Chicago.
Barfield C. E. 1981. *Rethinking Federalism: Block Grants and Federal, State, and Local Responsibilities.* Washington, D.C.: American Enterprise Institute.
Brand, J. L. 1965. The National Mental Health Act of 1946: A Retrospect. *Bulletin of the History of Medicine* 39: 231–245.
Brown, B., and Stockdill, J. W. 1972. The Politics of Mental Health. In *Handbook of Community Mental Health*, eds. S. E. Golann and C. Eisdorfer. New York: Appleton-Century-Crofts.

Brown, P. 1981. The Mental Patients' Rights Movement, and Mental Health Institutional Change. *International Journal of Health Services* 11: 523–540.

Burt, M. R., and Pittman, K. J. 1985. *Testing the Social Safety Net: The Impact of Changes in Support Programs during the Reagan Administration.* Washington, D.C.: Urban Institute Press.

Callahan, J. J., Jr. 1982. Management and Leadership in Times of Scarcity: Keynote Address. *Administration in Mental Health* 9: 164–169.

Cobb, R. W., and Elder, C. D. 1983. *Participation in American Politics: The Dynamics of Agenda-Building.* 2nd ed. Baltimore: Johns Hopkins University Press.

Dickey, B., and Goldman, H. H. 1986. Public Health Care for the Chronically Mentally Ill: Financing Operating Costs: Issues and Options for Local Leadership. *Administration in Mental Health* 14: 63–77.

Dill, A. E. P. 1987. Issues in Case Management for the Chronically Mentally Ill. In *Improving Mental Health Services: What the Social Sciences Can Tell Us,* ed. D. Mechanic. *New Directions for Mental Health Services,* no. 36. San Francisco: Jossey-Bass.

Downs, A. 1973. Up and Down With Ecology: The Issue-Attention Cycle. *Public Interest* 32: 38–40.

Feldman, S. 1980. Mental Health Administration: An Appraisal. In *The Administration of Mental Health Services,* 2nd ed., ed. S. Feldman. Springfield, Ill.: Charles C Thomas.

Foley, H. A., and Sharfstein, S. S. 1983. *Madness and Government: Who Cares for the Mentally Ill?* Washington, D.C.: American Psychiatric Press.

Frank, R. G., and Kamlet, M. S. 1985. Direct Costs and Expenditures for Mental Health in the United States, 1980. In *Mental Health, United States, 1985,* eds. C. A. Taube and S. A. Barrett. DHHS Publication No. (ADM) 85–1378. Washington, D.C.: U.S. Government Printing Office.

Frank, R., and Kamlet, M. S. 1986. Nonmarket Resource Allocation in Mental Health Care. *American Behavioral Scientist* 30: 201–230.

Goldman, H. H., and Manderscheid, R. W. 1987. Chronic Mental Disorder in the United States. In *Mental Health, United States, 1987,* eds. R. W. Manderscheid and S. A. Barrett. DHHS Publication No. (ADM) 87–1518. Washington, D.C.: U.S. Government Printing Office.

Grob, G. N. 1973. *Mental Institutions in America: Social Policy to 1875.* New York: Free Press.

Grob, G. N. 1983. *Mental Illness and American Society, 1875–1940.* Princeton: Princeton University Press.

Gudeman, J. E., and Shore, M. F. 1984. Beyond Deinstitutionalization: A New Class of Facilities for the Mentally Ill. *New England Journal of Medicine* 311: 832–836.

Gudeman, J. E., Shore, M. F., and Dickey, B. 1983. Day Hospitalization and An Inn Instead of Inpatient Care for Psychiatric Patients. *New England Journal of Medicine* 308: 749–753.

Hersch, C. 1972. Social History, Mental Health, and Community Control. *American Psychologist* 27: 749–754.

Jones, C. O. 1984. *An Introduction to the Study of Public Policy.* 3rd ed. Monterey, Calif.: Brooks/Cole.

Kiesler, C. A., and Morton, T. L. 1988. Prospective Payment System for Inpatient Psychiatry: The Advantages of Controversy. *American Psychologist* 43: 141–150.

Larsen, J. K. 1987. Local Mental Health Agencies in Transition. *American Behavioral Scientist* 30: 174–187.

Leiby, J. 1978. *A History of Social Welfare and Social Work in the United States*. New York: Columbia University Press.

Leighton, A. H. 1982. *Caring for Mentally Ill People: Psychological and Social Barriers in Historical Context*. Cambridge University Press.

Levine, M. 1981. *The History and Politics of Community Mental Health*. New York: Oxford University Press.

Locke, B. Z., and Regier, D. A. 1985. Prevalence of Selected Mental Disorders. In *Mental Health, United States, 1985*, eds. C. A. Taube and S. A. Barrett. DHHS Publication No. (ADM) 85–1378. Washington, D.C.: U.S. Government Printing Office.

Looney, J. G. 1986. Vertical Integration of Psychiatric Services for Youth: A Theoretical Assessment. *Administration in Mental Health* 13: 202–211.

Marmor, T. R., Wittman, D. A., and Heagy, T. C. 1976. The Politics of Medical Care Inflation. *Journal of Health Politics, Policy and Law* 1: 69–84.

Mechanic, D. 1980. *Mental Health and Social Policy*. 2nd ed. Englewood Cliffs, N.J.: Prentice-Hall.

Mechanic, D., and Aiken, L. 1987. Improving the Care of Patients with Chronic Mental Illness. *New England Journal of Medicine* 317: 1634–1638.

Mills, C. W. 1959. *The Sociological Imagination*. New York: Oxford University Press.

Moltzen, S., Gurevitz, H., Rappaport, M., and Goldman, H. H. 1986. The Psychiatric Health Facility: An Alternative for Acute Inpatient Treatment in a Nonhospital Setting. *Hospital and Community Psychiatry* 37: 1131–1135.

Morgan, J. A., Jr., and Connery, R. H. 1980. The Governmental System. In *The Administration of Mental Health Services*, ed. S. Feldman. Springfield, Ill.: Charles C Thomas.

National Mental Health Association. 1986. *Blueprint for the Future of Mental Health Services: Report of the Future Mental Health Services Project*. Alexandria, Va.

Paradis, B. A. 1987. An Integrated Team Approach to Community Mental Health. *Social Work* 32: 101–104.

Paulson, R. I. 1988. People and Garbage Are Not the Same: Issues in Contracting for Public Mental Health Services. *Community Mental Health Journal* 24: 91–102.

Peters, B. G. 1986. *American Public Policy: Promise and Performance*. 2nd ed. Chatham, N.J.: Chatham House.

Peterson, R. S., Austin, M. J., and Patti, R. J. 1985. Cutback Management Activities in Community Mental Health Centers. *Administration in Mental Health* 13: 112–125.

Pomp, H. C., and McGovern, M. P. 1988. Integrating State Hospital and Community-Based Services for the Chronic Mentally Ill. *Hospital and Community Psychiatry* 39: 553–555.

Rich, R. F. 1986. Change and Stability in Mental Health Policy. *American Behavioral Scientist* 30: 111–142.

Robert Wood Johnson Foundation and the U.S. Department of Housing and Urban Development. 1986. *Program for the Chronically Mentally Ill*. Princeton, N. J.

Rochefort, D. A. 1981. Three Centuries of Care of the Mentally Disabled in Rhode Island and the Nation, 1650–1950. *Rhode Island History* 40: 111–132.

Rochefort, D. A. 1984. Origins of the "Third Psychiatric Revolution": The Community Mental Health Centers Act of 1963. *Journal of Health Politics, Policy and Law* 9: 1–30.

Rochefort, D. A. 1987. The Political Context of Mental Health Care. In *Improving Mental Health Services: What the Social Sciences Can Tell Us*, ed. D. Mechanic. *New Directions for Mental Health Services*, no. 36. San Francisco: Jossey-Bass.

Rochefort, D. A. 1988. Policymaking Cycles in Mental Health: Critical Examination of a Conceptual Model. *Journal of Health Politics, Policy and Law* 13: 129–153.

Rubin, J. 1984. Developments in the Financing and Economics of Mental Health Care. In *The Chronic Mental Patient Five Years Later*, ed. J. A. Talbott. Orlando, Fla.: Grune & Stratton.

Rubin, J. 1987. Financing Care for the Seriously Mentally Ill. In *Improving Mental Health Services: What the Social Sciences Can Tell Us*, ed. D. Mechanic. *New Directions for Mental Health Services*, no. 36. San Francisco: Jossey-Bass.

Sharfstein, S. S. 1982. Medicaid Cutbacks and Block Grants: Crisis or Opportunity for Community Mental Health? *American Journal of Psychiatry* 139: 466–470.

Sharfstein, S. S. 1985. State's Role in Funding Psychiatric Care. *Psychiatric Quarterly* 57: 199–202.

Shore, M. F. 1982. Leadership and Management in Times of Scarcity: The Internal Issues. *Administration in Mental Health* 9: 170–176.

Surles, R. C. 1987. Changing Organizational Structures and Relationships in Community Mental Health. *Administration in Mental Health* 14: 217–227.

Talbott, J. A. 1985. The Fate of the Public Psychiatric System. *Hospital and Community Psychiatry* 36: 46–50.

Talbott, J. A. 1988. The Chronically Mentally Ill: What Do We Now Know, and Why Aren't We Implementing What We Know? In *The Perspective of John Talbott*, ed. J. A. Talbott. *New Directions for Mental Health Services*, no. 37. San Francisco: Jossey-Bass.

Talbott, J. A., and Sharfstein, S. S. 1986. A Proposal for Future Funding of Chronic and Episodic Mental Illness. *Hospital and Community Psychiatry* 37: 1126–1130.

U.S. Department of Health and Human Services, Alcohol, Drug Abuse, and Mental Health Administration. 1987. *Alcohol and Drug Abuse and Mental Health Services Block Grant, October 1986*. Washington, D.C.: U.S. Government Printing Office, June.

U.S. General Accounting Office. 1984. *States Have Made Few Changes in Implementing the Alcohol, Drug Abuse, and Mental Health Services Block Grant*. Washington, D.C., June.

2

The Contemporary Mental Health System: Facilities, Services, Personnel, and Finances

FREDERIC G. REAMER

Imagine a dictionary of terms that became popular in the mid-twentieth century. Certainly *system* would be a prominent entry. We seem to encounter the word everywhere. Systems theory. The criminal justice system. The subway system. *The* system.

Not surprisingly, the term also is firmly entrenched in the vocabulary of mental health professionals. No analysis of mental health policy seems able to avoid it. We know that the phrase "mental health system" is vague and often misleading (some, in fact, prefer "mental health nonsystem"), but we have yet to find an adequate substitute. For better or worse, the phrase seems here to stay, like an aging but functioning automobile. We learn to live with it. After all, it seems to get us where we want to go, although not always with the greatest possible efficiency.

The term *mental health system* will appear in a variety of contexts in subsequent chapters. It is necessarily germane to a discussion of the design, implementation, and evaluation of mental health policy. It is thus important to be clear about the phrase—what the entity it refers to incorporates and what it does not. My purpose here is to describe what is ordinarily meant by the mental health system and to provide an overview of its current status in the United States, as well as recent trends in its development.

PRELIMINARY ASSUMPTIONS

The word *system* suggests a tightly organized, finely tuned, interdependent, and smoothly functioning collection of elements, be they people, organizations, or ants. We probably use the term because we like what it suggests and wish the world would operate accordingly. It would be nice, for example, if each state had a system of community mental health centers with these attributes: the centers are located in neighborhoods and towns where there is the greatest need for mental health services; referrals to and from the centers are handled efficiently; funding for services is comprehensive and coordinated; each center employs the optimum number of well-trained staff needed to provide quality care; local statutes and ordinances routinely facilitate the delivery of mental health services; and conflicts do not arise among mental health providers.

If only it were so. To our dismay, the mental health "system" too often resembles a last-place football team. It is clear *in principle* how the various components are supposed to behave. However, orchestrating them to achieve the desired end in an effective and efficient way is another matter. Human idiosyncrasies, politics, leadership, turf issues, finances, unintended consequences of good intentions, and underdeveloped or underused talent all combine to produce a noble but inevitably flawed performance.

Despite these constraints, there are presently an impressive assortment and amount of mental health services being delivered in the United States. These are provided in a wide range of settings and by a wide variety of people. This chapter will provide a general overview of the settings in which services are provided, the recipients of mental health services, the nature of the services themselves, the professionals who provide them, and the way mental health services are funded. The most recent data available from both published and unpublished sources are included; some of the information reported is drawn from several sources used in conjunction.

MENTAL HEALTH FACILITIES AND SERVICES

Service System Components

Mental health services typically are classified as inpatient or outpatient. Inpatient services are provided in settings such as state and county mental hospitals, private psychiatric hospitals, general hospitals with psychiatric units, Veterans Administration hospitals with psychiatric units, community mental health centers with inpatient units, residential treatment centers for emotionally disturbed children, nursing and personal care homes, and group residences.

The general public is most familiar with state and county mental hospitals and private psychiatric hospitals, which are the legacy of the mental hospitals and asylums first established in the United States in the late eighteenth and early nineteenth centuries. Less familiar are contemporary innovations such as community mental health centers, residential treatment centers for emotionally disturbed children, and psychiatric group residences. For example, the federal Community Mental Health Centers program began in 1963 under the supervision of the National Institute of Mental Health (NIMH). The purpose was to expand and strengthen community-based mental health services by providing inpatient and outpatient services, emergency care, and consultation to community agencies. These centers were designed to serve people of all ages with widely varying forms of mental illness.

In contrast, residential treatment centers for emotionally disturbed children were established to focus more narrowly on mentally ill patients under eighteen years of age. Some of these centers resemble psychiatric hospitals for children, although most have fifty or fewer beds. While these centers also treat a range of mental illnesses—including personality, behavior, and psychotic disorders— many do not admit children with serious drug problems (Koran and Sharfstein, 1986: 284).

Many mentally ill adults and children reside in psychiatric group residences. These facilities ordinarily provide room, board, and some supervision by in-house staff. Most have fewer than twenty-five beds and are used to prevent hospitalization or to ease a patient's transition from a psychiatric hospital to the community.

Outpatient services also are provided in different settings. Many psychiatric hospitals—both public and private—offer outpatient counseling and support services. However, most outpatient services are provided by community mental health centers, freestanding psychiatric clinics, multiservice psychiatric organizations, day treatment programs, and private practitioners. These providers offer a wide variety of services, including crisis intervention; individual, family, and group counseling; occupational counseling; medication; housing assistance; and case management. Outpatient settings typically employ staff from professions such as social work, psychology, psychiatry, nursing, and counseling. Patients who receive services from these agencies may be living on their own, with family members, or in a group residence. As I will discuss below more fully, in recent years there has been a dramatic increase in the use of outpatient services for mentally ill children and adults.

General Trends in Mental Health Care

It has been estimated that while roughly 20 percent of the U.S. adult population is afflicted with a mental disorder [based on criteria for thirty-two mental disorders that appear in the third edition of the American Psychiatric Association's *Diagnostic and Statistical Manual* (1980)], at any time only one in five receives any treatment from a mental health professional. Most (57 percent) are evaluated and "treated" by primary health care professionals, such as office-based physicians or staff in general hospital outpatient clinics and emergency rooms. A small proportion (3 percent) are patients in general hospitals or nursing homes.

The remaining 20 percent either receive no treatment or are seen by other human service providers, such as staff of social welfare agencies or clergy (Horgan, 1985: 565; Regier, Goldberg, and Taube, 1978: 685; Koran and Sharfstein, 1986: 271).

The relatively small percentage who are treated by mental health professionals receive most services in outpatient settings. In 1983, approximately three-fourths of all patient care episodes within specialty mental health organizations were outpatient in nature (National Institute of Mental Health, 1986a).[1]

But this has not always been the case. In fact, the delivery of mental health care in the United States has changed dramatically in recent years. The overriding change has been the shift from hospital-based to community-based care, due largely to the impetus provided by the National Mental Health Act of 1946 (Public Law 79–487); the Mental Health Study Act of 1955 (Public Law 84–182), which created the Joint Commission on Mental Illness and Health; the Mental Retardation Facilities and Community Mental Health Centers Construction Act of 1963 (Public Law 88–164); and the widespread use of psychotropic medication beginning in the 1950s. Other forces include the Medicaid and Medicare health insurance programs, and increased availability of federal income assistance for the mentally disabled in the community through Supplemental Security Income and Social Security Disability Insurance (Gronfein, 1985; Merwin and Ochberg, 1983).

In 1955, the institutionalized population in state and county mental hospitals peaked, with a census of 559,000 (Koran and Sharfstein, 1986: 276). By 1983, the average daily census of state and county mental hospitals was 116,236, a decline of 79 percent (National Institute of Mental Health, 1987: 128). Between 1970 and 1980, the median length of stay for admissions to state and county mental hospitals (excluding deaths) also decreased, from forty-one to twenty-three days (National Institute of Mental Health, 1985: 53). Moreover, many state and county mental hospitals have closed their doors. In 1950 there were 322 state and county mental hospitals in the United States; by 1984 there were 277, a decline of 14 percent (President's Commission on Mental Health, 1978: 94; National Institute of Mental Health, 1987: 28). Clearly, the pendulum has swung, and with profound consequences.

Along with this precipitous drop in the use of institutional mental health care has come an equally remarkable increase in services provided by outpatient psychiatric clinics, community mental health centers, day treatment centers, and community residences. In 1969, there were 1.2 million outpatient additions in specialty mental health organizations in the United States, a rate of 576 additions per 100,000 civilian population (outpatient additions include admissions, readmissions, and transfers from other programs within the same organization). By 1983 this figure more than doubled to 2.7 million, a rate of 1,148 additions per 100,000 population (National Institute of Mental Health, 1987: 38).

There is no question that the most noteworthy trend in recent mental health history has been the marked decline in hospital-based care and the growth of outpatient or community-based services. However, what this simple conclusion masks is considerable variation in the evolution of this trend. Psychiatric hospitals did not empty at the same rate in all states and in all types of settings (Gronfein, 1985). Nor did outpatient services develop at a uniform pace. As with most novel developments, this shift in mental health care met with varying degrees of enthusiasm, ideological commitment, financial support, and opposition.

Trends in Inpatient Care

It is widely assumed that the community mental health movement, begun in earnest in the early 1960s, launched a wholesale deinstitutionalization of the nation's psychiatric hospitals. In fact, this was not the case. True, the census in state and county mental hospitals declined, and many public institutions were closed as large numbers of existing patients were discharged and others at risk of admission were redirected to other settings of care. What is less well known, however, is that the number of *private* psychiatric hospitals has increased dramatically, due in part to their well-documented profitability (Koran and Sharfstein, 1986: 282; Gaylin, 1985: 154). In 1970 there were 150 private psychiatric hospitals in the United States; by 1984, there were 220 (National Institute of Mental Health, 1987: 28), an increase of 47 percent. The number of other inpatient facilities also increased substantially. General hospitals offering inpatient psychiatric services increased from 664 in 1970 to 1,259 in 1984, an increase of 59 percent. Over roughly this same period, the number of federally funded community mental health centers providing inpatient care increased from 196 to 691, an increase of 253 percent. The number of residential treatment programs for emotionally disturbed children grew from 261 to 368 (National Institute of Mental Health, 1987: 29).

Inpatient bed capacity. In the end, there has been a net decline in the number of inpatient psychiatric beds, a drop of 50 percent between 1970 (524,878 beds) and 1984 (262,673). However, while the number of beds has declined in some settings, it has increased in others. Not surprisingly, the largest drop is found in state and county mental hospitals, which moved from 413,066 beds in 1970 to 130,411 beds in 1984, a decline of 68 percent.

In contrast, the number of beds in private psychiatric hospitals grew from 14,295 in 1970 to 21,474 in 1984, an increase of 50 percent. The number of beds in general hospitals offering psychiatric services more than doubled during this same period, from 22,394 in 1970 to 46,045 fourteen years later. The number of beds in federally funded community mental health centers nearly doubled between 1970 (8,108) and 1980 (16,264). In addition, the number of beds in residential treatment centers for emotionally disturbed children increased 33 percent over the 1970s, going from an initial base of 15,129 to 20,197. Clearly the pattern of inpatient care has shifted. In 1970, state and county mental hospitals accounted for nearly four-fifths of all psychiatric beds; by 1984, this figure

Table 2–1
Number of Inpatient and Residential Treatment Days Per Thousand (Civilian Population) by Type of Mental Health Organization: United States, Selected Years 1969–1983

Type of Organization	1969	1975	1979	1981	1983
State and County Mental Hospitals	674.0	333.9	227.1	195.7	182.6
Private Psychiatric Hospitals	21.3	20.8	22.8	24.5	25.9
Non-Federal General Hospital Psychiatric Services	32.6	39.5	39.3	47.1	53.7
VA Psychiatric Services	86.4	55.5	49.5	33.3	32.0
Residential Treatment Centers for Emotionally Disturbed Children	22.7	27.9	29.3	26.9	24.9

Source: National Institute of Mental Health, 1987: 35, Table 2.5.

dropped to slightly less than half (National Institute of Mental Health, 1987: 32), although public mental hospitals still account for the greatest number of inpatient days (Table 2–1).

It is also important to note the extent to which states vary in their supply of inpatient beds in mental health organizations. In 1984, there were 113 beds per 100,000 people in the civilian U.S. population. A number of states exceeded this rate significantly, although no clear geographical pattern is evident. The list includes densely populated, industrial states (e.g., Pennsylvania, 148/100,000; New York, 211/100,000; Maryland, 132/100,000), southern states (e.g., Georgia, 156/100,000; Mississippi, 127/100,000; South Carolina, 123/100,000; Virginia, 137/100,000), and sparsely populated western states (e.g., North Dakota, 139/100,000; Wyoming, 110/100,000). There is similar variation among the states with very low rates, although western states tend to be overrepresented and industrialized states are underrepresented in this group. States with relatively low bed-to-population rates include Hawaii (45/100,000), Alaska (47/100,000), Nevada (45/100,000), New Mexico (35/100,000), Idaho (52/100,000), and Arkansas (53/100,000) (National Institute of Mental Health, 1987: 112–113).

Much variation also exists with respect to states' bed capacity in different inpatient psychiatric settings. Compared to the national rate in 1984 of 56 beds per 100,000, some states make extensive use of state and county mental hospitals (e.g., New York, 152 beds/100,000 civilian population; North Dakota, 111/100,000; and South Carolina, 102/100,000), while others use them much less (e.g., Nevada, 10/100,000; Arizona, 14/100,000; Arkansas, 17/100,000; and Utah, 20/100,000). In 1984 the national rate for private psychiatric hospitals was 9 beds per 100,000. Some states had much higher rates (e.g., Connecticut, 26/100,000; Virginia, 26/100,000; and Georgia, 22/100,000), while others had unusually low rates (e.g., Minnesota, 2/100,000; South Carolina, 3/100,000; Mississippi, 2/100,000; and Hawaii, 2/100,000) (National Institute of Mental Health, 1987: 112–113).

It is difficult to know, of course, exactly what factors account for this significant variation. Some possibilities include geographical differences in the public's acknowledgment of mental health needs, financial resources, bureaucratic compromise, quality of life and stress factors, demand for mental health care, and the unique evolution of state care systems.

Admission rates. While it is useful to examine changes in the number of organizations providing inpatient care and in the number of available beds, actual utilization of inpatient care is measured in terms of admission rates, census data, and length-of-stay data. Although the number of beds in state and county mental hospitals declined by 62 percent between 1970 and 1980, and the end-of-year inpatient census during this period dropped 61 percent, admissions during this period declined by only 10 percent, suggesting a "revolving door" phenomenon (Figure 2–1; see also Merwin and Ochberg, 1983: 101; National Institute of Mental Health, 1985: 52). In contrast, while the number of beds in private psychiatric hospitals increased 20 percent between 1970 and 1980, admissions during this period increased 62 percent. As already noted, the average length of stay in state and county mental hospitals dropped 44 percent between 1970 (forty-one days) and 1980 (twenty-three days), although there was virtually no change in the average length of stay in private psychiatric hospitals (twenty days in 1970 and nineteen days in 1980) (National Institute of Mental Health, 1985: 53).

Once again, however, we find striking variation in rates of admission and length of stay, particularly with respect to geography, patient diagnosis, and patient demographic characteristics. In 1983, the nation had a total inpatient addition rate of 701 per 100,000 civilian population. States with relatively low addition rates included Alaska (391/100,000), Hawaii (380/100,000), Idaho (285/100,000), and Montana (332/100,000), and those with relatively high rates included Georgia (1,113/100,000), Connecticut (868/100,000), Wisconsin (892/100,000), and Missouri (862/100,000). Arizona, Utah, Florida, West Virginia, and California had among the lowest addition rates for state and county mental hospitals, while North Dakota, Georgia, Delaware, and Connecticut had among the highest. For private psychiatric hospitals, Minnesota, Missouri, Hawaii, and Oregon had among the lowest addition rates, while Rhode Island, Virginia, New Mexico, and Georgia had among the highest (National Institute of Mental Health, 1987: 116–117).

In addition to geography, patients' demographic characteristics are correlated with admission rates. In 1980, males accounted for 65 percent of all admissions to state and county mental hospitals, compared with 48 percent of admissions to private psychiatric hospitals. In that same year, 28 percent of all admissions to state and county mental hospitals were of minority patients, compared with only 13 percent of admissions to private psychiatric hospitals. In 1980, there were 137 white patients admitted to state and county mental hospitals per 100,000 white civilian population, compared with 328 minority patient admissions per 100,000 civilian minority population. This is a rather compelling comparison, of course, especially in light of the comparable admission rates for private

Figure 2–1
Resident Patients and Admissions, State and County Mental Hospitals, United States, 1950–1984

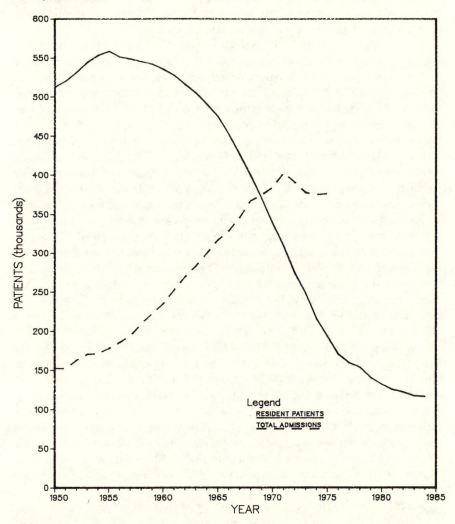

Source: National Institute of Mental Health, 1986a.

psychiatric hospitals. For these facilities, in 1980 there were 63 white patient admissions per 100,000 white population, compared with a similar rate of 58 minority patient admissions per 100,000 minority population. Nearly half of admissions to state and county mental hospitals were of patients between the ages of twenty-five and forty-four, compared with only 39 percent of patients admitted to private psychiatric hospitals (National Institute of Mental Health, 1987: 93–95).

Thus, gender, race, and age are important predictors of the setting in which inpatient care is received. Those who are young, black, or male are more likely to be admitted to a state or county mental hospital than to a private psychiatric hospital. While it is difficult to know exactly why these patterns exist, speculation is hard to avoid. Minority youths probably are less likely to have the financial resources or insurance coverage to afford private psychiatric care. Perhaps males are less likely to have diagnoses for which there tend to be higher admission rates to private psychiatric hospitals, e.g., affective disorders (National Institute of Mental Health, 1987: 79). Of course, we must also consider the possibility of institutional discrimination on the basis of age, race, and gender.

These demographic attributes also are correlated with changes in admission rates over time. The population-based admission rate for state and county mental hospitals declined 19 percent for the general population between 1970 and 1980. For males, however, this decline was only 11 percent, while for females it was 30 percent. For whites the decline was 24 percent, although for minorities it was only 9 percent. What is perhaps especially noteworthy is that between 1970 and 1980 the admission rate for state and county mental hospitals declined for every combination of gender and race (i.e., white males, white females, minority females) *except* minority males. The admission rate for this group *increased* by 9 percent.

In contrast, the overall admission rate for private psychiatric hospitals increased 45 percent between 1970 and 1980. For males, the rate increased 68 percent, while for females it increased only 28 percent. For whites the increase was 34 percent, compared with an astounding 271 percent increase in admission rates for minorities (National Institute of Mental Health, 1985: 52).

Clinical diagnosis also is related to utilization patterns, with the data suggesting that different mental health settings tend to specialize in the treatment of different psychiatric disorders. In 1980, nearly two-fifths of admissions to state and county mental hospitals were for schizophrenia, compared with only one-fifth of admissions to private psychiatric hospitals. Approximately one-fifth of admissions to state and county mental hospitals were for alcohol-related diagnoses, compared with slightly less than one-tenth of admissions to private psychiatric hospitals. In contrast, only 13 percent of admissions to state and county mental hospitals were for affective disorders, compared with over two-fifths of admissions to private psychiatric hospitals (National Institute of Mental Health, 1987: 79).

Diagnosis also is associated with different lengths of stay in various inpatient settings. State and county mental hospitals, private psychiatric hospitals, and Veterans Administration medical centers had similar median lengths of stay in 1980, when all major diagnoses are combined (twenty-three days, nineteen days, and twenty-two days, respectively). However, significant differences emerge when diagnoses are examined individually. For example, patients with schizophrenia had a median length of stay of forty-two days in state and county mental hospitals, eighteen days in private psychiatric hospitals, and twenty-four days in Veterans Administration medical centers. Patients with organic disorders had a median length of stay of seventy-one days in state and county mental hospitals, seventeen days in private psychiatric hospitals, and thirty-three days in Veterans Administration medical centers. Patients with alcohol-related diagnoses had a median length of stay of twelve days in state and county mental hospitals, twenty days in private psychiatric hospitals, and twenty-one days in Veterans Administration medical centers (National Institute of Mental Health, 1987: 80).

Some interesting changes with respect to the relationship among diagnosis, inpatient setting, and length of stay have also occurred. In state and county mental hospitals, for example, median length of stay for alcohol-related diagnoses declined sharply from thirty-three days in 1970 to twelve days in 1980, while in private psychiatric hospitals the median length of stay increased from nine days to twenty days. These trends are consistent with the decline in use of state and county mental hospitals, and the growth in private psychiatric hospitalization. For affective disorders, the median length of stay in state and county mental hospitals declined from thirty-two days in 1970 to twenty-two days in 1980, and remained constant in private psychiatric hospitals (twenty days). The median length of stay for schizophrenia declined significantly in both settings between 1970 and 1980, from fifty-eight days to forty-two days in state and county mental hospitals, and from twenty-eight days to eighteen days in private psychiatric hospitals (National Institute of Mental Health, 1985: 53).

Source of payment for the care rendered seems to contribute to differences in utilization. In 1980 patients covered by Medicare, Medicaid, their own personal resources, and those with no source of payment had significantly longer lengths of stay in state and county mental hospitals than in private psychiatric hospitals. Those covered by private insurance, by contrast, had significantly longer lengths of stay in private psychiatric hospitals than in state and county mental hospitals (National Institute of Mental Health, 1985: 49).

As to the specific treatment and services provided to inpatients, most receive some form of individual therapy, although the rates range from a low of approximately 64 percent in state and county mental hospitals and in Veterans Administration medical centers, to nearly 90 percent in private psychiatric hospitals. Family or couples therapy also is more prevalent in private psychiatric hospitals (provided to 24 percent of patients) and general hospitals with psychiatric services (15 percent of patients) than in state and county mental hospitals (7 percent) and Veterans Administration medical centers (8 percent). Group therapy is offered to the majority of inpatients, although it is somewhat more available in private psychiatric hospitals (65 percent of patients) than in Veterans Administration medical centers (57 percent), general hospitals (54 percent), and state and county mental hospitals (50 percent). Drug therapy is provided to the majority of inpatients in all settings; however, Veterans Administration medical centers offer detoxification to a much higher percentage of patients than do other settings. Veterans Administration medical centers also have the lowest rate for self-care training and social skills training (National Institute of Mental Health, 1985: 49).

Trends in Outpatient Care

Dramatic declines in the use of inpatient mental health care have been paralleled by a proliferation of outpatient services. As noted earlier, the number of federally funded community mental health centers increased two and one-half times between 1970 and 1980. Between 1970 and 1982, the number of free-standing psychiatric outpatient clinics increased by 33 percent, from 1,109 to 1,473 facilities, although recently many have closed (National Institute of Mental Health, 1987: 30). Rapid growth in outpatient facilities has been accompanied by equally impressive increases in the numbers of people served. In 1969 there were 1.2 million outpatient additions in specialty mental health organizations; by 1983 there were 2.7 million. Nearly all types of outpatient programs have participated in this dramatic increase: private psychiatric hospitals, general hospitals with psychiatric services, Veterans Administration medical centers, federally funded community mental health centers, residential treatment centers for emotionally disturbed children, and, until recently, freestanding psychiatric clinics. The one major exception has been state and county mental hospitals, whose outpatient additions declined by nearly 50 percent between 1969 and 1983, from 164,232 to 84,309 (National Institute of Mental Health, 1987: 38).

According to the most recent data available (1983), the majority of these outpatient services are provided in community-based multiservice mental health organizations (51 percent of all outpatient service additions). A large percentage of outpatient services also are provided by psychiatric outpatient clinics (20 percent) and nonfederal general hospitals with psychiatric services (18 percent). The remaining outpatient services are provided by Veterans Administration medical centers (4 percent), state and county mental hospitals (3 percent), private psychiatric hospitals (3 percent), and residential treatment centers for emotionally disturbed children (1 percent).

Recipients of outpatient services tend to be somewhat younger than recipients of inpatient care. In 1983, 20 percent of outpatients were under eighteen years of age, compared with 8 percent of inpatients. In contrast, 7 percent of outpatients were sixty-five years of age or older, compared with 21 percent of inpatients (National Institute of Mental Health, 1986b: 39).

Outpatients are also somewhat less likely to be male or black. In 1983, 52 percent of outpatients were male, compared with 63 percent of inpatients. Sixteen percent of outpatients were black, compared with 21 percent of inpatients. However, Hispanics were more likely to be outpatients (7 percent) than inpatients (4 percent) (National Institute of Mental Health, 1986b: 39).

As with inpatient services, the use of outpatient services varies considerably geographically. In 1983, there was a national rate of 1,148 outpatient additions per 100,000 civilian population. Among states with unusually high rates were

Wyoming (2,358/100,000), Vermont (2,353/100,000), Wisconsin (2,356/100,000), North Dakota (1,954/100,000), and New Mexico (1,936/100,000). States with unusually low rates included Hawaii (479/100,000), Texas (655/100,000), Louisiana (689/100,000), South Carolina (652/100,000), and Idaho (697/100,000).

It is interesting to note that some states rank above the national rate for both inpatient and outpatient additions (indicating consistently high rates of mental health care), some states rank below the national rate for both inpatient and outpatient additions (indicating consistently low rates of mental health care), and some states are above the national rate for one setting (inpatient or outpatient) and below for the other. For example, North Dakota, Wisconsin, Minnesota, and Wyoming rank above the national rate for both inpatient and outpatient additions. Idaho, Arizona, Louisiana, and Utah rank below the national rate for both inpatient and outpatient additions. Colorado, Indiana, Michigan, and Montana rank above the national rate for outpatient additions, and below for inpatient additions. And Delaware, Nebraska, Virginia, and Florida rank above the national rate for inpatient additions and below for outpatient (National Institute of Mental Health, 1987: 116–117, 136–137). Once again, these patterns may reflect differences in local philosophy about mental health care, availability of mental health services, quality of life, funding priorities, politics, and other such factors.

PERSONNEL

The Mental Health Professions

Mental health services are provided by a wide variety of staff. The four largest professional groups include psychiatrists, psychologists, social workers, and nurses. However, the majority of staff are classified as mental health workers, most of whom do not have a bachelor's degree (National Institute of Mental Health, 1986a).

Psychiatrists are medical physicians who have completed a psychiatric residency. A relatively small number—estimated to be in the vicinity of 10 percent—also obtain training in psychoanalysis (Koran and Sharfstein, 1986: 272). Psychiatrists' responsibilities in mental health settings differ considerably, depending upon their training, expertise, and interests. Some psychiatrists are actively involved in counseling, while others spend much of their time providing clinical supervision and consultation. Psychiatrists' medical background uniquely qualifies them to prescribe psychotropic medication for the treatment of mental illness.

Psychologists typically have a master's or doctoral degree in some specialization within this discipline, such as clinical, counseling, social, or experimental psychology. Their responsibilities in mental health organizations may include counseling, psychological testing, diagnosis, consultation, and other social services.

Many of these same responsibilities are shared by social workers. Trained social workers have a B.S.W., M.S.W., or doctoral degree. Many social work training programs offer students the opportunity to specialize in the field of mental health. Social workers may serve as counselors, case managers, supervisors, or administrators in mental health programs.

Nurses also perform a diversity of functions in mental health settings. Psychiatric nurses may supervise patients in residential and day treatment facilities, administer and monitor medications, and treat patients' physical health problems; some also provide individual, family, and group counseling. Some training in psychiatric nursing is included in all general nursing education programs (Koran and Sharfstein, 1986: 275).

Trends in Mental Health Staff

There have been important changes over the years in the characteristics of mental health providers. In general, the number of full-time-equivalent positions in mental health facilities has increased, from 375,984 in 1976 to 440,925 in 1984 (National Institute of Mental Health, 1987: 40). The four major mental health professions—psychiatry, psychology, social work, and nursing—make up only 30 percent of this work force. Of these, registered nurses and social workers are the most numerous. Psychologists make up 5 percent of the mental health work force, and psychiatrists only 4 percent. The remaining staff consist primarily of mental health workers, physical health professionals, and other ancillary staff (National Institute of Mental Health, 1987: 40).

According to a 1983 report published by the American Medical Association, between 1970 and 1981 the number of psychiatrists increased nationally from about 21,150 to 28,500 (Koran and Sharfstein, 1986: 272). However, the growth rate in the number of psychiatrists was lower than that for all other medical specialties. Only 20 percent of psychiatrists classify themselves as involved full-time in hospital work. Most (60 percent) have office-based practices, and most of the remainder are residents or are involved in teaching, research, or administration.

As with other physicians, psychiatrists are very unevenly distributed geographically. In 1982, for example, there were 4 psychiatrists per 100,000 population in Idaho, compared with 31 per 100,000 in New York. Psychiatrists tend to be concentrated disproportionately in urban areas (Koran and Sharfstein, 1986: 273). In 1984, psychiatrists made up 5.2 percent of the staff of mental health facilities in Washington, D.C., 5.1 percent of the staff in Delaware, and 4.5 percent in New Jersey, but only 0.8 percent of the staff in North Dakota, 1.2 percent in Wyoming, and 1.3 percent in Mississippi (National Institute of Mental Health, 1986a).

In 1982, about 28,000 psychologists were providing mental health services in facilities such as community mental health centers, psychiatric hospitals, schools, family service agencies, and in private practice (VandenBos and Stapp, 1983: 1330). Fully one-fourth were in private practice, and about one-fourth

Table 2–2
Number of Full-time-Equivalent Staff Positions in Mental Health Organizations
by Discipline: United States, Selected Years 1976–1984

Staff Discipline	1976	1978	1984
Psychiatrists	12,938	14,492	18,482
Psychologists[a]	9,443	16,501	21,052
Social Workers	17,687	28,125	36,397
Registered Nurses	31,110	42,399	54,406

Source: National Institute of Mental Health, 1987: 40, Table 2.10.

[a]For 1976–1978, this category included all psychologists with a B.A. degree and above; for 1984,
    it included only psychologists with an M.A. degree and above.

were in academic settings. About 40 percent practice primarily in mental health or social service agencies.

A 1982 survey by the National Association of Social Workers indicates that nearly two-thirds (64 percent) of the association's members are engaged in clinical mental health work. Relatively few are in private practice (approximately 12 percent list private practice as a primary setting, 8 percent as a secondary setting). A 1983 report of the National Institute of Mental Health indicates that the number of clinical social workers per 100,000 population ranged in 1982 from 9.7 in New York to 0.2 in Wyoming (Koran and Sharfstein, 1986: 274). Social workers make up over 14 percent of staff in mental health facilities in Utah, 14 percent in Vermont, and 13 percent in Michigan, but only 4 percent in Mississippi, 5 percent in Alabama, and 5 percent in Wyoming (National Institute of Mental Health, 1986a). Their role in mental health care has increased substantially in recent years, from a total of 17,687 full-time-equivalent staff positions in mental health organizations in 1976 to 36,397 in 1984 (National Institute of Mental Health, 1987: 40). As Goleman (1985) noted recently, social workers now are the largest providers of clinical mental health services in the United States. Between 1975 and 1985 the number of clinical social workers in the United States increased from 25,000 to 60,000, placing social workers first in the list of professional groups providing mental health services.

The number of registered nurses employed full-time in mental health organizations also increased in recent years, from 31,110 in 1976 to 54,406 in 1984 (National Institute of Mental Health, 1987: 40). Many are involved in psychiatric nursing. Again, states vary in the extent to which they employ registered nurses in mental health facilities. For example, they make up 13 percent of staff in mental health facilities in Rhode Island, 12 percent in Colorado, and 12 percent in Hawaii, but only 4 percent in Vermont, 5 percent in Maine, and 5 percent in Montana (National Institute of Mental Health, 1986a).

Significant changes have occurred over the years in staffing patterns in various mental health settings. Between 1972 and 1984, the total number of full-time-equivalent patient care staff in state and county mental hospitals declined 15 percent, from 138,307 to 117,630. However, much of this decline reflects cuts in the number of mental health workers without a bachelor's degree. Although the number of psychiatrists in state and county mental hospitals also declined slightly (by 6 percent), the numbers of psychologists, social workers, registered nurses, and other mental health professionals actually increased. In contrast, between 1972 and 1984 the total number of full-time-equivalent patient care staff increased for all professional groups in most other major mental health settings, including private psychiatric hospitals, freestanding day/night and multiservice organizations, residential treatment centers for emotionally disturbed children, and general hospitals offering psychiatric services (National Institute of Mental Health, 1987: 40–47).

Of special interest are changing staffing patterns in community mental health centers, given the prominence of these facilities in contemporary mental health care. Using NIMH data, Leaf (1986: 119–120) found that older community mental health centers tend to employ a greater number of psychiatrists per 1,000 additions than do more recently established centers. In contrast, more recently established centers employ significantly more psychologists per 1,000 additions than do the older centers. However, the effect of agency "age" seems to have decreased in recent years. In general, leading up to the beginning of the 1980s, there was a decline in the average number of psychiatrists in community mental health centers, and an increase in the average number of psychologists, social workers, and other mental health professionals (Cockerham, 1981: 325).

FINANCING MENTAL HEALTH

Mental Health Expenditures

Expenditures for mental health care have increased in recent years. In 1969, approximately $3.3 billion was spent to provide mental health care in state and county mental hospitals, private psychiatric hospitals, general hospitals offering psychiatric services, Veterans Administration medical centers, federally funded community mental health centers, residential treatment centers for emotionally disturbed children, freestanding psychiatric outpatient clinics, and a small group of other mental health organizations. By 1983, this figure had increased to $4.6 billion, in 1969 dollars (National Institute of Mental Health, 1987: 57).

A recent survey indicates that in 1980 total direct mental health costs (excluding governmental transfer payments) ranged as high as $19.9 billion, representing approximately 7.7 percent of total expenditures for all health care, and approximately 0.7 percent of the nation's Gross National Product (Frank and Kamlet, 1985: 165; National Institute of Mental Health, 1985: vi). Of these expenditures, approximately 54 percent were incurred in the specialty mental health sector (e.g., community mental health centers, state and county mental hospitals, private psychiatric hospitals, and office-based psychiatrists, psychologists, social workers), 31 percent in the general health sector (e.g., general hospitals without psychiatric units, nursing homes), and 16 percent in the human services and nonhealth sectors (e.g., schools, criminal justice agencies) (National Institute of Mental Health, 1985: vi).

Expenditures for state and county mental hospitals have declined in recent years, although not a great deal, while expenditures in other settings generally have increased. In 1969, $1.8 billion was spent for state and county mental hospitals; by 1983, expenditures declined to $1.7 billion (constant 1969 dollars). In contrast, expenditures for private psychiatric hospitals increased from $220 million in 1969 to $543 million in 1983. There were also significant increases in all other mental health settings, both residential and nonresidential.

In 1969, more than half (55 percent) of the expenditures for mental health organizations in the United States were devoted to state and county mental hospitals, and 7 percent to private psychiatric hospitals. By 1983, the figure for state and county mental hospitals had declined to 38 percent, and the figure for private psychiatric hospitals had grown to 12 percent (National Institute of Mental Health, 1987: 57).[2] These data suggest something of a public-to-private shift, although the matter is complicated by the fact that public programs like Medicare and Medicaid pay for some of the care delivered in private facilities.

Along with these general patterns, we again see noteworthy variation among regions and states in the United States, reflecting different degrees of financial commitment to mental health care. In 1985, state mental health agencies with unusually high expenditures per capita included New York ($90.12), Pennsylvania ($52.39), Michigan ($48.98), Massachusetts ($46.11), and Delaware ($46.05). Those with unusually low rates included Arizona ($12.06), Idaho ($14.99), Utah ($17.30), Texas ($17.33), and Kentucky ($18.82) (National Institute of Mental Health, 1987: 164–165).

In 1985, approximately two-thirds (64 percent) of state mental health agency expenditures were allocated to state mental hospitals, with approximately 32 percent going to community-based programs. Yet it has been estimated that more than three-fifths of the nation's approximately 2.4 million chronically mentally ill persons live in the community (Morganthau et al., 1986: 15). As the data reviewed thus far might lead one to predict, the proportions of state expenditures devoted to institutional and community-based care vary substantially. A number of state mental health agencies dedicate at least 50 percent of their spending to community-based programs (e.g., Wisconsin, California, Massachusetts, Hawaii, Washington), while others dedicate less than 20 percent (e.g., Iowa, Delaware, New York, Kansas, Maryland) (National Institute of Mental Health, 1987: 164–165; National Association of State Mental Health Program Directors, 1985: 90).

Mental Health Revenues

Mental health care in the United States is funded by many sources. An inventory of specialty mental health organizations conducted by the division of

Table 2–3
State Mental Health Agency Per Capita Expenditures for Major Programs, by State, Fiscal Year 1983*

State	SMHA Expenditures Per Capita	% State Hospitals	% Community Based Programs
Alabama	$27.78	79.0	18.8
Alaska	44.85	61.3	32.4
Arizona	12.06	61.2	35.9
Arkansas	23.80	57.9	33.8
California	33.51	29.4	67.3
Colorado	27.72	63.5	35.1
Connecticut	44.02	70.7	22.4
Delaware	46.05	86.3	12.4
Florida	25.52	54.4	45.6
Georgia	23.38	74.7	23.9
Hawaii	22.66	38.5	54.7
Idaho	14.99	58.5	38.0
Illinois	23.73	62.4	29.7
Indiana	27.44	59.4	39.4
Iowa	10.51	92.5	6.5
Kansas	26.85	82.4	14.4
Kentucky	18.82	65.9	31.5
Louisiana	25.62	66.8	27.9
Maine	36.15	68.9	28.4
Maryland	39.96	83.1	13.0
Massachusetts	46.11	34.1	53.4
Michigan	48.98	63.1	32.8
Minnesota	31.98	45.5	37.8
Mississippi	23.78	74.3	23.7
Missouri	27.72	53.9	42.5
Montana	29.20	69.6	29.2
Nebraska	21.29	79.5	16.7
Nevada	25.95	62.9	35.6
New Hampshire	42.02	61.8	35.0
New Jersey	35.65	67.7	20.5
New Mexico	24.60	59.6	39.5
New York	90.12	82.6	12.8
North Carolina	37.81	62.7	36.3
North Dakota	36.25	63.4	35.9
Ohio	30.41	62.1	33.8
Oklahoma	30.89	63.5	32.2
Oregon	24.89	60.7	35.4
Pennsylvania	52.39	75.7	21.6
Puerto Rico	8.38	47.5	47.0
Rhode Island	35.00	64.3	33.7
South Carolina	32.61	74.4	19.9

Table 2–3 (continued)

State	SMHA Expenditures Per Capita	% State Hospitals	% Community Based Programs
South Dakota	21.73	73.5	24.1
Tennessee	22.75	72.4	24.1
Texas	17.33	68.8	25.5
Utah	17.30	48.9	48.3
Vermont	44.35	36.6	59.6
Virginia	32.10	77.4	17.9
Washington	29.50	47.8	50.5
West Virginia	21.71	65.9	32.8
Wisconsin	27.82	30.4	68.6
Wyoming	30.52	72.9	23.3
Average	$34.62	63.9	31.8

Source: NIMH, 1987: 164–165, Table 6.2.

*Funds not allocated to state hospitals or community-based programs were allocated to other hospitals or SMHA support activities.

Biometry and Applied Sciences within the National Institute of Mental Health provides useful data on this subject, although certain types of services and organizations, most notably private office-based practitioners and non-Federal general hospitals with separate psychiatric services, are excluded. Of the $11.7 billion in revenues accounted for by this data base, the principal source is state governments, which in 1983 provided nearly half (47 percent) of all funding (excluding funds contributed by states to Medicaid). The federal government contributed 16 percent of funding, between Medicare (3 percent) and other federal subsidies (13 percent). Medicaid funds—shared by federal, state, and local governments—accounted for 12 percent of funding, and local governments contributed 7 percent. The remainder consisted of client fees and other miscellaneous sources, e.g., contracts from private agencies (National Institute of Mental Health, 1987: 58).

Of course, different kinds of mental health settings depend on different funding sources. For example, these same data show that state and county mental hospitals are very dependent on state mental health funds (62 percent) and Medicaid funds (18 percent), but receive very little revenue from clients (less than 2 percent). In contrast, private psychiatric hospitals function rather independently of state mental health agency funds (less than 3 percent), but receive over two-thirds of their funds (69 percent) from clients and their insurance companies. Multiservice mental health organizations receive substantial funding from several sources, the largest of which include state mental health agencies (45 percent), local governments (15 percent), clients and their insurance companies (10 percent), and Medicaid (9 percent) (National Institute of Mental Health, 1987: 58).

Again we find great diversity across the nation. According to data collected by the National Association of State and Mental Health Program Directors, some states rely heavily on state funds, such as Hawaii (90 percent), Montana (89 percent), Maine (93 percent), Connecticut (98 percent), and Delaware (98 percent). Others obtain a relatively small portion of their funds directly from the state, such as Iowa (35 percent), Vermont (58 percent), Virginia (60 percent). These states tend to rely more heavily than others on some combination of client fees, federal and local government funding, and Medicaid (National Institute of Mental Health, 1987: 170–71).

CONCLUSION

Contemporary descriptions of mental health in the United States necessarily are quite different from those written only a decade ago. And if we reach back to assessments of mental health in colonial America, the changes indeed are startling. The first institutional admissions in the eighteenth century to the Pennsylvania Hospital and to the first American mental asylum in Williamsburg, Virginia, inaugurated a series of profound developments in the treatment of the mentally ill. Since then, we have witnessed all manner of practices and treatments in inpatient and outpatient settings, from the use of bloodletting, purges, emetics, and psychosurgery to electroconvulsive therapy, psychotropic medication, milieu therapy, and group counseling.

We have learned many lessons along the way. We have seen some psychiatric hospitals—frequently constructed with good intentions—misused terribly, to incarcerate with minimal care and supervision a wide range of unfortunates—paupers, infirm, psychotic, retarded, and alcoholic. The developments of the 1960s eventually paved the way for the most recent chapter of "community mental health" in the nation's efforts to respond to the needs of the mentally ill.

As will be examined more thoroughly in subsequent chapters, efforts to shift from hospital-based to community-based care have had mixed results. There is no question that we have succeeded in our goal of reducing substantially the census in state and county mental hospitals. The data, as presented here, are compelling. Simultaneously, dramatic growth has occurred in the availability of outpatient services. Also, lengths of inpatient stays have dropped significantly, at least in state and county mental hospitals.

But a steep price has been paid. There is considerable evidence that institutions in many locations were emptied well before ample community-based services and resources were created to absorb the people who were discharged. Every community has its litany of horror stories, where vulnerable patients unable to negotiate life on the streets have succumbed to one or another of the world's unforgiving threats and pressures. We know now that in our haste to reduce the institutional census, thousands of patients have been discharged prematurely. To this day, large numbers of American communities are ill equipped to care adequately for the mentally ill in their midst.

Certainly there is much to applaud in contemporary efforts to care for the mentally ill. Many states and local communities have done remarkable jobs designing and administering programs and services that are at once well conceptualized, skillfully staffed, efficient, and humane. One need only examine the large number of well-planned and well-run psychiatric hospitals, group residences, day treatment centers, community mental health centers, nursing homes, and outpatient clinics to see what is possible. However, any serious and forthright student of mental health in the United States also must acknowledge the gaps and flaws.

As this review of the system makes plain, states are enormously uneven in their efforts to care for the mentally ill. There is a remarkable lack of consensus about and uniformity in mental health care. There is striking variation in the use of institutional and community-based services, admission rates, lengths of stay and service, staffing patterns, and funding. No doubt some of the variation can be explained by structural variables, such as a state's tax base, the availability of local graduate and professional schools, degree of urbanization, and population mix.

Yet it also is probable that a significant portion of the variation may be due to more idiosyncratic factors, related perhaps to politics, prejudice, and professional or civic self-interest. An understanding of these complex factors would seem essential if we are to advance the quality of mental health care in the United States. Some features of mental health policy and practice are more comprehensible than others. Our principal task here is to enhance the clarity.

NOTES

1. Patient care episodes typically are defined as the number of residents in facilities at the beginning of a year, the number of persons on the rolls of outpatient facilities at the beginning of the year, and the total number of additions to those facilities during the year. Specialty mental health organizations include state and county mental hospitals, private psychiatric hospitals, community mental health centers, freestanding psychiatric outpatient clinics, and selected other mental health facilities. The major exclusion is private psychiatric offices.

2. Due to recent changes by NIMH in the classification of some mental health organizations, expenditure trend data for other mental health settings are not available.

REFERENCES

American Psychiatric Association. 1980. *Diagnostic and Statistical Manual of Mental Disorders*. 3rd ed. Washington, D.C.

American Psychiatric Association. 1987. *Diagnostic and Statistical Manual of Mental Disorders*. 3rd ed. (Revised). Washington, D.C.

Bassuk, E. L., and Gerson, S. 1978. Deinstitutionalization and Mental Health Services. *Scientific American* 238: 46–53.

Borus, J. F. 1981. Deinstitutionalization of the Chronically Me itally Ill. *New England Journal of Medicine* 305: 339–342.

Carter, E. W. 1985. Psychiatric Nursing. In *Comprehensive Textbook of Psychiatry, Vol. 1*, eds. H. I. Kaplan and B. J. Sadock. 4th ed. Baltimore: Williams and Wilkins.

Cockerham, W. C. 1981. *Sociology of Mental Disorder*. Englewood Cliffs, N.J.: Prentice-Hall.

Fenton, W. M., Leaf, P. J., Moran, N. L., and Tischler, G. L. 1984. Trends in Psychiatric Practice, 1965–1980. *American Journal of Psychiatry* 4: 346–351.

Frank, R. G., and Kamlet, M. S. 1985. Direct Costs and Expenditures for Mental Health Care in the United States in 1980. *Hospital and Community Psychiatry* 36: 165–168.

Gaylin, W. 1985. The Coming of the Corporation and the Marketing of Psychiatry. *Hospital and Community Psychiatry* 36: 154–159.

Goleman, D. 1985. Social Workers Vault into Leading Role in Psychotherapy. *New York Times*, April 30: C–1, C–9.

Gronfein, W. 1985. Incentives and Intentions in Mental Health Policy: A Comparison of the Medicaid and Community Mental Health Programs. *Journal of Health and Social Behavior* 26: 192–206.

Horgan, C. M. 1985. Specialty and General Ambulatory Mental Health Services. *Archives of General Psychiatry* 42: 565–572.

Jonas, S., ed. 1986. *Health Care Delivery in the United States*. 3rd ed. New York: Springer.

Knesper, D. J. 1978. Psychiatric Manpower for State Mental Hospitals. *Archives of General Psychiatry* 35: 19–24.

Koran, L. M., and Sharfstein, S. S. 1986. Mental Health Services. In *Health Care Delivery in the United States*, ed. S. Jonas. 3rd ed., New York: Springer.

Lamb, H. R. 1984. Deinstitutionalization and the Homeless Mentally Ill. *Hospital and Community Psychiatry* 35: 899–907.

Leaf, P. J. 1986. Mental Health Systems Research. In *The Organization of Mental Health Services: Societal and Community Systems*, eds. W. R. Scott and B. L. Black. Beverly Hills: Sage.

Merwin, M. R., and Ochberg, F. M. 1983. The Long Voyage: Policies for Progress in Mental Health. *Health Affairs* 2:96–127.

Morganthau, T., Agrest, S., Greenberg, N. F., Doherty, S., and Raine, G. 1986. Abandoned. *Newsweek*, January 6: 14–19.

National Association of State Mental Health Program Directors. 1985. *Funding Sources and Expenditures of State Mental Health Agencies: Revenue/Expenditure Results, Fiscal Year: 1983*. Washington, D.C.

National Institute of Mental Health. 1983. *Mental Health, United States, 1983*, eds. C. A. Taube and S. A. Barrett. DHHS Publication No. (ADM) 83–1275. Rockville, Md.

National Institute of Mental Health. 1985. *Mental Health, United States, 1985*, eds. C. A. Taube and S. A. Barrett. DHHS Publication No. (ADM) 85–1378. Washington, D.C.: U.S. Government Printing Office.

National Institute of Mental Health. 1986a. Unpublished data, Division of Biometry and Applied Sciences. Washington, D.C.

National Institute of Mental Health. 1986b. Series CN No. 11, *Specialty Mental Health Organizations, United States, 1983–84*, eds. R. W. Redick, M. J. Witkin, J. E.

Atay, and R. W. Manderscheid. DHHS Publication No. (ADM) 86–1490. Washington, D.C.: U.S. Government Printing Office.

National Institute of Mental Health. 1986c. Series CN No. 10, *Trends by State in the Capacity and Volume of Inpatient Services, State and County Mental Hospitals, United States, 1976–80*, eds. J. P. Morrissey, M. J. Witkin, R. W. Manderscheid, and H. E. Bethel. DHHS Publication No. (ADM) 86–1460. Washington, D.C.: U.S. Government Printing Office.

National Institute of Mental Health. 1987. *Mental Health, United States, 1987*, eds. R. W. Manderscheid and S. A. Barrett. DHHS Publication No. (ADM) 87–1518. Washington, D.C.: U.S. Government Printing Office.

President's Commission on Mental Health. 1978. *Task Panel Reports, Vol. II: Appendix.* Washington, D.C.: U.S. Government Printing Office.

Regier, D. A., Goldberg, I. D., and Taube, C. A. 1978. The De Facto U.S. Mental Health Services System: A Public Health Perspective. *Archives of General Psychiatry* 35: 685–693.

Scott, W. R., and Black, B. L., eds. 1986. *The Organization of Mental Health Services: Societal and Community Systems.* Beverly Hills: Sage.

VandenBos, G. R., and Stapp, J. 1983. Service Providers in Psychology, Results of the 1982 APA Human Resources Survey. *American Psychologist* 38: 1330–1352.

Part 2

Epidemiologic Analysis of Mental Health Problems

3

Psychiatric Epidemiology: An Overview of Methods and Findings

SARAH ROSENFIELD

This chapter reviews selected major methodological issues and findings in psychiatric epidemiology. Psychiatric epidemiology examines the distribution of psychiatric disorders in the population as a method of determining the causes of mental illness. The degree of disorder in the population and its distribution, however, are intricately tied to the specific conceptualization and measurement of mental illness. Thus, this chapter first reviews the major categories of mental illness which have been the focus of much psychiatric epidemiologic research. Second, it reviews the specific measures that have been developed for research on mental illness, from the early studies using clinical impressions to the present diagnostic interviews using computer programs. Third, the chapter presents information on the prevalence and distribution of psychiatric disorders in the United States based on current large-scale studies using these diagnostic techniques. Finally, the chapter discusses major research issues and findings to explain the occurrence and distribution of disorders from a social psychiatric perspective, and it emphasizes major current perspectives on stressful life events and chronic conditions of stress. These findings provide suggestions for future research on the specific dynamics and mechanisms of stress that lead to mental disorder.

MAJOR CATEGORIES OF MENTAL DISORDER

The types of behaviors that psychiatry considers mental disorders are presented in the *Diagnostic and Statistical Manual* of the American Psychiatric Association (American Psychiatric Association, 1987). The most recent version of this manual, the third edition, revised (DSM-III-R), was released in 1987. The DSM-III-R describes over 250 types of mental disorders. These are organized into eighteen diagnostic categories, including disorders first evident in infancy, childhood, or adolescence, such as conduct disorders; organic mental disorders, such as senile dementia; psychoactive substance abuse disorders; schizophrenia; delusional (paranoid) disorders; and psychotic disorders not elsewhere classified, for example, brief reactive psychosis. Diagnostic categories also include mood disorders such as major depression; anxiety disorders; somatoform disorders, such as hypochondriasis; dissociative disorders, such as multiple personality; sexual disorders, such as voyeurism; sleep disorders; factitious disorders, or symptoms voluntarily produced; impulse control disorders not elsewhere classified, for example, pathological gambling; adjustment disorder; psychological factors affecting physical condition; and personality disorders.

The DSM-III-R claims to describe the symptoms of disorders without implications regarding their etiology or cause. Thus, various perspectives on etiology can use this common set of descriptions in classification and research on mental disorders. To illustrate this classification scheme in greater depth, it is useful to consider three disorders which have received major research attention: mood disorders, schizophrenia, and personality disorders.

Mood disorders include bipolar disorders and depressive disorders; major depression is an example of a depressive disorder. The primary symptoms of major depression are a mood of extreme sadness, or feeling blue, lonely, or down, or a loss of interest in usual activities. Other symptoms are difficulties with sleeping, trouble with appetite, and feelings of self-blame or self-reproach. Individuals may also experience a general loss of energy, have trouble concentrating, show psychomotor retardation or agitation, and may have suicidal thoughts or ideation. The typical course of depression suggests that although depressive episodes are debilitating, there is often no incapacitation between episodes. Individuals do not tend to deteriorate in general functioning over time, even with recurrent episodes. There is no typical age of onset for major depression, and episodes can appear at any age (Spitzer, Endicott, and Robins, 1975; American Psychiatric Association, 1987).

Schizophrenia is characterized by delusions, hallucinations, and formal thought disorder. Thought disorder is inferred from the way a person speaks, including, for example, a loosening of associations, in which the form of thought is not determined by logical and relevant associations but shifts from one apparently unconnected subject to another, or is based on sound or alliteration. Thus, the association between one idea and the next is not obvious. Other forms of thought disorder involve poverty of content of speech, in which a person talks but gives little information because of vagueness, talking past the point, or repetition. Illogical thinking is another form of thought disorder in which the facts are obscured, distorted, or omitted. The result of severe thought disorder is incoherence.

Delusions are another defining characteristic of schizophrenia. The most common types of delusions in schizophrenia include thought broadcasting, or the belief that one's thoughts are broadcast to the outside world so that other people can hear them. Thought insertion is the idea that thoughts which are not one's own are inserted into one's mind. Thought withdrawal is the belief that thoughts have been removed from one's head. The idea that one's behavior or feelings are not one's own but are imposed by an external force is referred to as delusions of being controlled.

Hallucinations involve major disturbances in perception. In contrast to delusions, which are distortions of actual stimuli, hallucinations exist in the absence of external stimulation. The most common are auditory hallucinations in which voices are heard from outside one's head. This can be one voice or many, familiar or unknown. Commonly the voices make insulting statements. They may speak directly to the person, or two voices may speak to each other. The voices often keep a running commentary on the person's behavior or thoughts.

Other symptoms of schizophrenia involve problems in affect. One example is flat affect, in which a person expresses little emotion regardless of the situation. Another is inappropriate affect, in which, for example, a person laughs or smiles when relating a tragic incident. In addition, schizophrenic disorders often involve social withdrawal or social isolation as the person becomes preoccupied with private thoughts and fantasies and suffers a distorted perception of the world. Individuals' sense of self and individuality can also be disturbed, with a loss of a sense of ego boundaries and confusion about identity. A sense of volition or self-directed activity can also be inhibited. Finally, motor behavior may be disturbed, as in catatonic forms. Individuals may stay in a rigid posture for indefinite periods of time, or may be flexible to the extent that they remain in any position in which they are moved.

The typical age of onset of schizophrenia is during adolescence or early adulthood. A particular concern in the age of deinstitutionalization is the current generation of young chronic schizophrenics, who are pervasive users of the psychiatric service system but are at the same time more hostile and rejecting of mental health treatment than earlier generations. Partly as a cause of the hostility and partly as a result, community service systems seem less prepared to treat these patients than older chronics, and young schizophrenics often fail to receive effective psychiatric care (Bachrach, 1984). The general course of schizophrenic disorders is somewhat variable, but a complete return to the level of premorbid functioning is relatively rare. Usually, there is a progressive deterioration that impairs schizophrenics' ability to care for themselves. Life expectancy is shorter than that of the general population, due to suicide and death from a variety of other causes. These causes are thought to be connected to both institutional life and the poor economic conditions under which schizophrenics often live.

The third diagnostic category encompasses the personality disorders. As opposed to the disorders presented above, which are episodic in nature, personality disorders are stable ways of thinking or behaving which are relatively consistent over time. Personality disorders signify personality traits which are maladaptive, causing psychological distress or impairment in social or occupational functioning. The personality disorders consist of the following types: paranoid, schizoid, schizotypal, antisocial, borderline, histrionic, narcissistic, avoidant, dependent, obsessive compulsive, and passive-aggressive. These are characterized by different personality traits and associated behaviors, but all have in common an onset by adolescence and continuation throughout adult life. As an example of these disorders, antisocial personality disorder involves continuous antisocial behavior in several areas. Typical behaviors before age fifteen are truancy, running away from home, persistent lying, cruelty to animals or people, destruction of others' property, and stealing. Also typical are physical fights, using weapons in fights, and forcing someone into sexual activity. According to the DSM-III-R, three or more of the above behaviors are required for a diagnosis of antisocial personality disorder. In addition, the following behaviors are typical after age fifteen: trouble sustaining work, abuse or neglect of children, illegal behavior, an inability to sustain enduring attachments to other people, and a lack of remorse. Other typical behaviors after this age are aggressiveness, financial irresponsibility, impulsiveness, lying or conning others, and recklessness with regard to driving. Four of these behaviors after age fifteen must be present in order to diagnose antisocial personality disorder by DSM-III-R criteria.

MEASURES OF MENTAL DISORDER

The disorders described above represent those diagnoses frequently investigated in psychiatric epidemiologic research and found to vary most strongly among different groups in the population, e.g., by social class and sex. However, it is important to note that the estimation of rates of mental disorders in the population depends in part on the way mental illness is measured in research. First, it should be pointed out that most studies of mental illness enumerate the prevalence rather than the incidence of mental disorders. *Incidence* refers to new cases of disorder which occur in a specified period of time. *Prevalence* refers to all cases, new or preexisting, which exist at one point in time.

Early Prevalence Studies

The wide variation in estimates of prevalence is revealed in several studies of "true" prevalence done after 1950 that are reviewed by Dohrenwend et al. (1980a). "True" prevalence studies are of community populations, which include people who are not in treatment as well as those receiving psychiatric treatment. In eight true prevalence studies done in the United States, the rates of mental disorders of all types ranged from .55 percent to 69 percent. This variation could be partly due to the samples selected for research. Some focused on urban populations, some on rural populations. Also, some included all people in institutions in the area and some did not, the latter underestimating cases of schizophrenia, which have a relatively high rate of receiving treatment, and cases of antisocial personality disorder found in prisons. But this variation in rates of mental disorders is also partly due to the way disorder has been measured in different studies. These issues of measurement involve several dimensions, including the source of information, the areas covered by the measure, the types of items included in terms of, for example, the severity of the symptomatology, and the characteristics of the interviewer.

Early studies of mental illness often used key informants as sources of information. A person who was familiar with most people in the community was asked to report on who in the community was mentally ill. But key informants most often reported more visible kinds of behavior as cases, such as antisocial behavior, omitting less obvious and less disruptive forms of disorder like depression (Dohrenwend and Dohrenwend, 1976). Consequently, in research using key informants, the rate of mental disorder is relatively low. Other early studies were done by one or a small number of clinicians who reported rates from their individual clinical interviews. Because these measures of disorder are not standardized, it is difficult to reproduce such studies and thus to evaluate the estimates of disorder on which they are based.

Use of Treated Rates

More recent measures of disorder used after World War II are structured rather than based on clinical impression, and are more often focused on self-reports of feelings and behavior rather than reports of informants. Before discussing these, however, it is necessary to review briefly one additional approach to measuring mental disorder, the use of treated rates. This method is represented in two classic studies in psychiatric epidemiology. One is Faris and Dunham's (1939) ecological research on areas of Chicago, which found the inner-city areas to have the highest concentration of institutionalized mental illness, with rates gradually declining to the outer edges of the city and into the suburbs. Also, Hollingshead and Redlich's (1958) study in New Haven used treated rates of disorder, finding a direct association between social class and schizophrenia. In this research, a one-day psychiatric census was taken from records of clinics, private psychiatrists, and institutions in Connecticut and nearby states.

There are certain advantages in using treated rates to measure mental disorder. Primarily, this is a relatively easy and efficient way of identifying cases of disorder: they are defined by the treatment staff. However, the main problem with this measure is that treated rates cannot be generalized to all cases of mental disorder, as factors other than the presence of symptomatology determine entry into treatment. It has been estimated that only approximately one-fourth of people with a significant psychiatric disorder have ever been in treatment (Dohrenwend et al., 1980a). Whether individuals get into treatment depends, for example, on their social characteristics and on factors such as the availability of services and the operating hours of those services (Rosenfield, 1983, 1984; Robins, 1978). Thus, for several reasons, treated rates have severe limitations in generalizability to rates of disorder in the general population. Partly in reaction to this limitation, instruments were developed for investigating mental disorder in the community.

Community Surveys

The first systematic measures to be used in the community were heavily influenced by the experiences of psychiatry in World War II. Psychiatrists were given the task of determining who should enter the military on the basis of mental health status. Based on the failures in this screening, a focus emerged on screening instruments and measures which would give an overall assessment of an individual's mental health. This unidimensional conception of mental health and illness was reinforced by the rejection of diagnostic categories as unreliable. Two major studies grew out of this approach: the Midtown Manhattan Study (Srole et al., 1962) and the Stirling County Study (Leighton et al., 1963). Both studies interviewed random samples of individuals within communities. Both included a large number of self-report items on symptoms which were then reviewed and assessed by psychiatrists to yield an overall rating of mental health. In the Stirling County Study, this rating was the probability of a person being a psychiatric case, ranging from almost certainly a case at one end of the scale, to no evidence of symptoms and some evidence of good adjustment and health at the other. In the Midtown Manhattan Study, the rating was of impairment and ranged from "incapacitated" to "well."

In this unidimensional approach to measuring mental disorder the underlying idea is that mental health and mental disorder exist on a single quantitative continuum, which can be identified according to an overall scale. A problem with these measures, however, is their inability to distinguish specific types of problems. This is a particular difficulty in view of the possibility that different problems or disorders may have different causes or predisposing factors.

Another example of this unidimensional approach to measuring mental disorder is the Langner twenty-two item impairment scale, which came out of the Midtown Manhattan Study (Langner, 1962). This scale is a screening device for use in large populations and is derived from those items in the Midtown Study which best differentiated between a known well group and a known ill group. Some examples of items from the scale include the frequency of feeling weak all over, having low spirits, having headaches, having a sour stomach, and wondering if anything is worthwhile. The advantage of this scale is that it is economical and efficient. However, the symptom items are heavily psychophysiological and may be confounded with physical illness. That is, it is not clear from the items whether the cause of symptoms is physical or psychological (Crandell and Dohrenwend, 1967). The Langner scale also omits many psychiatric problems, including, for example, psychoses, obsessiveness, and personality disorders. A problem this measure shares with the rating scales above is that, since it intends to measure overall impairment, it cannot delineate specific areas or types of problems.

After the Midtown and Stirling County studies were reported in the early 1960s, researchers questioned the use of a unidimensional conception of mental health and disorder. Studies began to emphasize different types of problems and differential causes for these problems. The continued idea that psychiatric diagnoses and diagnostic categories were unreliable led to a focus on specific and discrete symptom scales. The Center for Epidemiologic Studies Depression Scale (CES-D) is one example (Weissman et al., 1977). This scale is composed of twenty items asking how often in the last week individuals had trouble with, for example, eating, having the blues, concentrating, feeling lonely, having crying spells, and feeling sad. Other instruments have been developed which cover a larger variety of symptoms, such as the Psychiatric Epidemiology Research Interview (PERI) (Dohrenwend et al., 1980a). This includes a wide range of items on different types of symptoms organized into a number of separate symptom scales. These scales include, for measures of nonspecific distress or demoralization, poor self-esteem, sadness, anxiety, helplessness-hopelessness, and psychophysiological symptoms. Specific symptom scales include false beliefs and perceptions, manic characteristics, guilt, problems due to drinking, distrust, and active expression of hostility.

Symptom scales provide information on specific types of problems for investigation. Instruments like the PERI and scales like the CES-D were developed on general population groups rather than only patient groups and thus may be more applicable to community research. It is not clear how these scales relate to diagnostic categories, however. The scales also cannot distinguish the severity of symptoms. Individuals can score high or low in terms of a total number of symptoms, but specific symptoms are not differentiated. Also, it is not possible to distinguish whether the symptoms are the primary, dominant problem or a secondary problem.

Because of these criticisms of symptom scales and an increasing emphasis on the use of diagnostic categories, instruments attempting to operationalize the *Diagnostic and Statistical Manual* categories of mental disorders have been developed. The Diagnostic Interview Schedule (DIS) is an example of this approach (Robins et al., 1981). The DIS was developed to yield diagnoses based on the DSM-III (American Psychiatric Association, 1980). For forty-three of the psychiatric diagnostic categories in this manual, questions represent the symptoms required for diagnosing the disorder. For example, items on depression ask about feeling sad or depressed, about weight and appetite, sleeping problems, fatigue or agitation, loss of interest in sex, feelings of worthlessness, trouble concentrating, and suicidal thoughts. A computer program then evaluates the responses for symptoms of depressive disorder, considering also duration of

symptoms, and makes a diagnosis on that basis. In addition, the program evaluates responses to items which may indicate other psychiatric disorders. Unlike
earlier diagnostic interviews, such as the Schedule of Affective Disorders and
Schizophrenia (SADS), the DIS gives a total count of symptoms as well as
diagnoses (Robins et al., 1981).

Since the DIS offers both diagnoses and symptom scores, it is useful for both
patient and community samples. However, several problems have been noted
with the DIS in particular and with diagnostic interviews in general. One study
reports that the DIS underestimates the number of depressive episodes in comparison with clinical interviews (Helzer et al., 1985). In addition, the prevalence
of disorders depends on whether lay people or clinicans are interviewing respondents. Interviews by lay people less often result in diagnoses of alcoholism
and more often result in diagnoses of mania and panic disorders (Helzer et al.,
1985). The more general issue is that there are few objective criteria against
which to determine the validity of a diagnostic instrument (Robins et al., 1981).
Clinicians have low levels of agreement among themselves on diagnosis. Thus,
there is no method of producing an accurate DSM-III diagnosis against which
the DIS or any diagnostic instrument can be calibrated.

Assessment of Alternative Approaches

A problem with these structured measures of mental disorder is the inability
to assess unconscious processes which could potentially distort the reporting of
or underestimate symptoms, such as denial or repression. However, given this
limitation and the respective strengths and weaknesses of each type of measure,
the measure chosen for research should depend on the problem under investigation. To examine the causes of mental disorders, treated rates are inadequate.
To examine the types of psychiatric problems or the degree of psychological
well-being in a community, including a range of problems from mild to severe,
symptom scales are most useful. To understand the number and causes of the
more severe and less common clinical conditions best representing those states
psychiatrists define as mental illness, diagnostic instruments such as the DIS are
most appropriate.

PREVALENCE RATES

With the limitations of these alternative approaches to the measurement of
psychiatric disorders in mind, this section describes what is known to date about
the prevalence of mental illness in the United States. This review draws on two
sources of information, one which focuses on symptom scales and one on diagnostic instruments. As described above, true prevalence studies using symptom
scales and done in the United States after World War II are summarized by
Dohrenwend et al. (1980a). The most recent information on prevalence, however,
comes from the Epidemiological Catchment Area (ECA) studies done in the

United States in the early 1980s. These studies include approximately 3,000 adults interviewed in the community and approximately 500 institutionalized adults in each of five research sites across the country: St. Louis, Baltimore, New Haven, Los Angeles, and North Carolina (Regier et al., 1984). That is, about 20,000 individuals were interviewed to determine the prevalence of specific psychiatric disorders in the U.S. population. The DIS was developed for this purpose.

In reviewing rates of disorder in the United States, the studies summarized by Dohrenwend et al. (1980a) using symptom scales show a median rate of between .6 percent and 3 percent of schizophrenia in the population, the rates varying by the inclusiveness of the definition of schizophrenia. From the three ECA study sites reporting data thus far, the estimates of schizophrenia and schizophreniform disorders are, for six-month prevalence, from .6 percent to 1.1 percent of the population and, for lifetime prevalence, from 1.1 percent to 2.0 percent of the population (Myers et al., 1984; Robins et al., 1984). For affective psychosis, which includes major depression and manic depression, the review for the President's Commission estimates the prevalence as .3 percent of the population, from both European and U.S. studies. The ECA studies report between 4.6 percent and 6.5 percent of the U.S. population to have suffered from affective disorders in the last six months, 6.1 percent to 9.5 percent in their lifetime. This includes manic episodes, major depressive episodes, and dysthymia or neurotic depression. In addition, the six-month prevalence includes bereavement, while the lifetime prevalence excludes this category. It should be noted that the President's Commission reports rates of neurosis separately. Thus, the prevalence of depressive disorders and neurotic disorders cannot be directly compared in these studies and the ECA studies. This partly explains the lower rates of depressive disorders in the studies reviewed for the President's Commission, as neurotic depression or dysthymia was excluded. The review for the President's Commission reports the prevalence of all neurotic disorders to be between 8 and 15 percent. In the most similar categories, the ECA studies report a six-month prevalence of between .6 percent and 1.0 percent for panic disorders, between 1.3 percent and 2.0 percent for obsessive compulsive disorder, and .1 percent for somatization disorder. Lifetime prevalence of anxiety/somatoform disorders, including phobias, panic disorders, obsessive compulsive disorders, and somatization, is between 11.1 percent and 25.1 percent of the population.

The rate for personality disorders from the President's Commission Report, which includes alcoholism and drug addiction, is estimated to be 7 percent of the total population. The ECA studies assessed substance abuse disorders and personality disorders separately. Six-month prevalence figures show between 4.5 percent and 5.7 percent to have alcohol abuse or dependence, between 1.8 percent and 2.2 percent to have drug abuse or dependence. Over their lifetime, between 15.0 percent and 18.1 percent of the U.S. population suffers from substance abuse disorders, including drug and alcohol disorders. Assessing antisocial personality disorder only, the ECA studies find a rate of between .7 percent and

1.3 percent in prevalence over six months, and between 2.1 percent and 3.3 percent lifetime prevalence in the population.

Taking the total of the disorders covered, the prevalence of psychiatric disorders according to the Report to the President's Commission is between 16 percent and 25 percent of the population. According to the ECA studies, the six-month or current prevalence of psychiatric disorders is between 14.8 percent and 22.5 percent of the population. Lifetime prevalence of psychiatric disorders is between 28.8 percent and 38.0 percent of the U.S. population.

These rates of disorder vary across certain population groups. One of the most consistent findings in the epidemiology of mental disorders is that the lower class has higher rates of psychiatric disorders than higher social classes. This has been found in treated rates of mental illness (Faris and Dunham, 1939; Hollingshead and Redlich, 1958), as well as in impairment rates in community studies (Srole et al., 1962; Leighton et al., 1963; Dohrenwend et al., 1980a; Kessler, 1982). In terms of specific disorders, consistent differences in the same direction have been found by social class in schizophrenia (Dohrenwend et al., 1980a). Differences have also been found in psychiatric symptomatology by race. Although earlier studies claimed that higher rates of symptoms in blacks than in whites were due to differences in socioeconomic status rather than race per se (e.g., Warheit, Holzer, and Arey, 1975; Mirowsky and Ross, 1980a; Eaton and Kessler, 1981), recent analyses find an interaction between race and class. Specifically, blacks have higher rates of psychological distress than lower-class whites (Kessler and Neighbors, 1986).

Finally, consistent differences have been found between males and females in psychiatric disorders. Women have higher rates of symptoms of psychological distress or demoralization than men. In terms of specific disorders, women have higher rates of depression and anxiety than do men. Men have higher rates of personality disorders, particularly antisocial personality disorder, and substance abuse than women (Dohrenwend and Dohrenwend, 1976; Weissman and Klerman, 1978; Rosenfield, 1980; Kessler, Price, and Wortman, 1985).

ETIOLOGY

There are a number of models or theories of causation of psychiatric disorder. These different approaches are sometimes used in conjunction to construct multifactorial explanations. More often, however, they exist in competition with each other, their respective adherents drawing on different kinds of data and assumptions regarding the nature of human behavior. This section presents several of these approaches briefly and concentrates in more depth on one current perspective in the social epidemiology of mental disorders.

Psychoanalytic Model

The classical psychoanalytic model holds that the dynamics of early childhood development underlie psychiatric symptomatology (Freud, 1959, 1966a, 1966b;

Munroe, 1955; Freedman, Kaplan, and Sadock, 1976). According to a Freudian framework, disordered relationships within the family unit produce psychological conflicts within the child. These conflicts, in turn, lead to problems in psychosexual development and to emotional repression. Early maladjustments, which become ingrained by adulthood, are causally related to various forms of psychological disturbance, including anxiety, depression, sexual deviation, and psychosis. For example, psychodynamic theories analyze phobic disorders as displaced anxiety arising from an earlier, repressed source of emotional conflict. Psychotic conditions such as depression and schizophrenia represent a regression to more primitive stages of ego development than the less severe disorders such as phobias, and entail a break with the reality-testing functions of the ego. This perspective has been criticized for the difficulty of subjecting the ideas to empirical investigation. In addition, it has received criticism based on the relative inefficacy of psychodynamic treatments for severe chronic mental illnesses such as schizophrenia.

Behavioral Model

Behaviorist orientations focus on the nature and amount of reinforcements for maladaptive behavior and on the reward and punishment histories of individuals as producing disturbed behavior (Millon, 1967; Sahakian, Sahakian, and Nunn, 1986). One behavioral theory of psychopathology is that maladaptive behavior exists because it is or has been rewarded. For example, certain behavior that was rewarded in the past may not be acceptable in an individual's present circumstances. Alternatively, individuals who were not rewarded for socially acceptable behavior may have failed to learn these forms of behavior. A specific and more sophisticated example of a behaviorist or learning theory of psychopathology is the learned helplessness model of depression, which will be discussed further below. This model holds that a critical cause of depression is the belief, learned from past experiences, that the outcomes of one's actions are uncontrollable (Miller and Seligman, 1973, 1975; Seligman, 1975; Seligman et al., 1979; Abramson and Sackheim, 1977; Alloy et al., 1984).

Biological Model

Biological theories center on physiological, biochemical, and genetic causes of psychopathology (Andreasen, 1984). The underlying assumption is that disturbances in thinking, feeling, and behavior result from bodily malfunction or abnormality just as physical illnesses do. Though the biological approach has been applied to a wide range of disorders, including nonpsychotic disturbances such as panic attacks, its primary concern lies with the severe and chronic forms of mental illness such as schizophrenia (Rosenthal and Kety, 1968; Mednick et al., 1974; Torrey, 1983). Biological theory research is medically oriented, emphasizing sophisticated diagnostic testing, genetic transmission studies, and biomedical intervention.

Stressful Life Events Model

The last etiological approach considers stressful life events as causal agents. Currently this is a dominant model in the study of pyschosocial epidemiology, and for this reason, I will focus on it in some depth. The stress model and its revisions have been used to explain psychiatric disorders in general as well as social class and sex differences. In discussing this explanatory framework, I will present the basic model first, then its application to analyzing differences among population subgroups.

Overview of the stress model. The stressful life events approach to explaining psychiatric disorders began with the formulation by Hans Selye (1956) that events in individuals' lives, because they require changes and thus adaptation, cause illness. This applies to common events such as vacations or Christmas, as well as more significant, infrequent events like marriage and loss of a spouse. According to this framework, the greater the changes required by an event, positive or negative, the more detrimental the effect on health. Research subsequently established that the more events which occurred to individuals and the greater the required change, as rated by judges in terms of life change units, the worse the individuals' physical and mental health (Holmes and Rahe, 1967; Holmes, 1979).

Based on methodological and substantive critiques of this general approach, more refined specifications of this basic model have been proposed (Dohrenwend and Dohrenwend, 1974; Rabkin and Struening, 1976; Thoits, 1983). One such critique challenged the assumption that change per se was negative for health. Studies on this issue found instead that only undesirable events, not events per se, were associated with symptomatology (Mirowsky and Ross, 1980b; Mueller, Edwards, and Yarvis, 1977). Others found that uncontrollable events such as death of a spouse were more detrimental to health compared to more controllable events such as divorce (Paykel, 1974; Thoits, 1983).

In addition, other critiques focused on the relatively low correlations between events and symptoms typically found in research. Individuals with the same number of events did not necessarily have similar symptoms. While some showed symptoms of illness, others showed little symptomatology. Consequently, it was proposed that certain factors mediated the impact of stressful events, buffering the negative effects of stress on symptomatology. These factors generally included the degree of social support individuals had and their personal or coping resources.

Social support is thought to modify the effects of stressful life events in two basic ways. First, the existence of support can positively affect the appraisal of a stressful situation, causing the interpretation of the event to be less threatening. Second, social support can affect the psychological reaction to a stressful situation by aiding in finding a practical solution, minimizing the effects on self-perceptions, or encouraging health-promoting behaviors (Cohen and Wills, 1985). Social support has been conceptualized and measured in terms of the structure of social networks as well as the functions of social contacts. Structure involves the number and types of contacts between individuals. Functions are what people receive from these social contacts, practical or material support, emotional support, and sociability. The evidence for social support as a buffer against the ill effects of stressful life events has been mixed (see Thoits, 1982; Heller and Swindle, 1983; Kessler, Price, and Wortman, 1985; Shumaker and Brownell, 1984; and Cohen and Wills, 1985 for reviews). Some researchers find no advantage of social support under stressful circumstances, while others find a significant interaction between support and life events. However, in an extensive review of the research on this issue, Cohen and Wills (1985) conclude that those studies which are most rigorous methodologically and focus on support in terms of functions show consistent evidence that social support, especially in terms of emotional and practical support, buffers the negative effects of stressful life events on psychological well-being.

A second modifier of the effects of stress is personal resources. This usually refers to some aspect of personality, either coping skills or self-perceptions. Coping is defined as "the cognitive and behavioral efforts made to master, tolerate, or reduce external and internal demands and conflicts among them" (Folkman and Lazarus, 1980: 223). Coping efforts are problem-centered, attempting to alter the situation directly, or emotion-centered, changing the view of a problem or the emotional reaction to a problem (Folkman and Lazarus, 1980; Pearlin and Schooler, 1978). Studies of the effects of coping show that the response to a problem determines the psychological effects as well as the success of the resolution of the problem (Pearlin and Schooler, 1978; Menaghan, 1982; Menaghan and Merves, 1984). For example, coping strategies which keep people committed and engaged with each other are more effective in reducing the negative effects of interpersonal problems (Pearlin and Schooler, 1978; Menaghan, 1982). On the other hand, distancing types of coping strategies are more effective in reducing stress from impersonal situations. For example, for economic problems, devaluing the importance of money, finding other sources of rewards, and selectively ignoring the problem work best to avoid distress (Pearlin and Schooler, 1978).

Personal resources involving self-perceptions concentrate on self-esteem and perceptions of mastery or control. The importance of a sense of control has been emphasized, in terms of learned helplessness, locus of control, fatalism, and mastery, as a major determinant of psychiatric symptomatology in general (Seligman, 1975; Rotter, 1966; Kohn, 1972; Wheaton, 1980, 1983; Pearlin et al., 1981). In particular, Pearlin et al. (1981) present evidence that stressful events are problematic for mental health to the extent that they compromise individuals' sense of self-esteem and mastery. Mastery involves the degree to which individuals perceive they have control over the forces that affect them. In relation to self-esteem, Pearlin et al. also argue that social support buffers the effects of stressful events because it enhances individuals' feelings of self-worth.

In sum, the current approach to life events research claims that effects of stressful life events depend on individuals' level of social support and their personal resources. When there is little emotional and practical support, when coping strategies are inadequate to the problem area, and when self-esteem and feelings of mastery are challenged, stressful events are damaging to individuals' mental health. In the face of support, appropriate coping mechanisms, and per-ceptions of positive self-worth and mastery, stressful life events have less psy-chological impact.

Chronic stress model. The above is a brief statement of the life events approach to explaining psychiatric symptomatology and disorder. Other explanatory factors which have been gaining increasing emphasis involve more chronic conditions of stress as opposed to discrete events (Kessler, Price, and Wortman, 1985; Pearlin and Schooler, 1978; Pearlin et al., 1981). Such chronic conditions of stress include interpersonal problems or conflicts (e.g., marital and parental) and financial or occupational problems. They also include chronic demands or role overload. These strains are thought to negatively affect psychological well-being in general. In addition, stressful life events may be problematic because, and to the extent that, they create such chronic conditions of stress (Pearlin et al., 1981; Pearlin and Schooler, 1978; Kessler, Price, and Wortman, 1985). Thus, it may be the chronic conditions resulting from stressful events, rather than the events themselves, that are consequential for individuals' mental health.

Social class and sex differences. Both of these models have been applied to varying rates of symptomatology in different population groups as well as to symptomatology in general. In terms of explaining social class differences, low income in itself constitutes a chronic condition of stress. In terms of life events, lower-class individuals are found to have a greater number of events in general than individuals of higher socioeconomic status (Kessler and Cleary, 1980). However, even when the number of events are controlled, lower-class individuals have higher rates of symptomatology. This difference is explained in terms of social support and personal resources. Lower-class individuals are shown to have less emotional and practical support available than those in higher social classes (Brown and Harris, 1978, 1984). In terms of resources, research has also shown that lower-class individuals more often use less effective coping strategies for problems than individuals in higher social classes. For example, Pearlin and Schooler (1978) find that lower-class people more often use coping responses that are less effective in reducing strains especially in the economic and occu-pational areas. Specifically, they are less often in a position to devalue money or to substitute intrinsic rewards for monetary rewards from work. Although this latter research can be applied to a life events model, it focuses on the effects, and thus also highlights the importance, of chronic strains as determinants of psychiatric symptoms.

Both stressful life events and chronic conditions of stress have been applied to explain sex differences in psychiatric disorders, particularly women's higher rates of anxiety and depression. Both types of explanatory frameworks focus on aspects of male and female gender roles. Women have been found to be more vulnerable to the negative effects of stressful life events than are men. One intriguing explanation for this difference concerns gender differences in terms of emotional support and empathy. It appears that women are more negatively affected than men by the stressful events that happen to those close to them. Their stronger reaction to others' events explains the excess in symptomatology that women experience as a consequence of the occurrence of life events (Kessler and McLeod, 1984; Kessler, McLeod, and Wethington, 1984).

On the other hand, another tradition of research emphasizes the chronic conditions of stress to which men and women are differentially exposed. Much of this research derives from a discussion of the effects of gender roles on mental health by Gove and Tudor (1973). Gove and Tudor argue that women in traditional female roles have higher symptomatology than men because the housewife role is intrinsically less satisfying; it brings only one source of gratification to women as opposed to two sources of rewards, work and family, for men, and it is less socially valued than the traditional male role of breadwinner. On the other hand, women who are employed also have higher symptomatology than men because their jobs are less financially rewarding and secure and place greater demands on their time as job responsibilities are added to household tasks. The two major aspects of female versus male roles seen as causal in this analysis are the power differences between men and women and the differences in the level of demands. These two explanatory factors have been subsequently emphasized in research on sex differences in symptomatology.

Research on sex differences focuses on married men and women, as differences are most pronounced within this marital status group. Tests of power differences typically concern the effects of employment on sex differences in symptoms. The argument is that employment for women, because it is associated with greater power in the family, would reduce rates of symptomatology and thus sex differences in symptoms in general (Rosenfield, 1980). There is some evidence that employed women are lower in anxious and depressive symptoms than housewives, although the results are mixed (Radloff, 1975; Kessler and McRae, 1982; Gore and Mangione, 1983; Horwitz, 1982; Gove and Geerkin, 1977; Pearlin, 1975; Cleary and Mechanic, 1983; Barnett and Baruch, 1985; Rosenfield, 1980). However, even when symptoms of employed women are lower, they are still significantly higher than those of employed men.

Differences in power in terms of income from earnings cannot fully account for these higher rates among employed women versus employed men (Rosenfield, 1984). Thus, explanations related to differential demands become salient. Studies show that women have the primary responsibility for housework and children even when they work full-time (Gove and Tudor, 1973; Ross, Mirowsky, and Huber, 1983; Ross, Mirowsky, and Ulbrich, 1983). Several others show that employed women with children or, more specifically, with the primary responsibility for child care and housework are higher in symptomatology than other groups of women (Cleary and Mechanic, 1983; Radloff, 1975; Ross, Mirowsky, and Ulbrich, 1983; Kessler and McRae, 1982; Thoits, 1986). Equal familial demands among husbands and wives produce equal rates of symptomatology between men and women (Rosenfield, 1989). Thus, it appears that the greater level of demands that employed women face explains their higher symptomatology. Both greater power and lower demands appear to be necessary to reduce married women's symptomatology, among housewives and employed women, to a level equal that of married men.

Thus, several aspects of women's roles, including caretaking, lower power, and familial demands, may be involved in producing women's higher rates of symptoms. These lead to both a greater vulnerability to life events and greater exposure to chronic conditions of stress among women. In this sense, both reactions to life events and chronic conditions of strain appear to account for women's higher rates of anxious and depressive symptoms.

Areas of needed future research. Findings on sex differences as well as class differences suggest that future research needs to consider both discrete events and chronic strains in explaining distributions of psychiatric disorders. In addition, further research is needed on the processes by which life events and strains affect mental health in general. It is possible that both stressful events and chronic strains affect health by similar psychological mechanisms. And if, in fact, life events affect symptoms by creating chronic strains, the identification of such intervening processes may explain the effects of each. A promising lead in this regard concerns individuals' sense of mastery, which Pearlin et al. (1981) suggest is a crucial intervening mechanism in the effects of life events. Further evidence from studies of sex differences show that both low power and high demands increase symptomatology because they decrease individuals' sense of mastery or control (Rosenfield, 1985, 1989). Similarly, other research finds that differences in control related to feelings of fatalism account for the existence of class differences in symptoms (Wheaton, 1980, 1983). Further analyses of the specific dynamics connecting events, strains, and intervening mechanisms such as mastery are necessary to complete our understanding of the process of stress in general, and thus to identify critical points for intervention in the prevention of psychiatric disorders.

Also generally missing from these analyses is a consideration of how social structural or contextual factors influence events and chronic conditions and, in turn, psychological well-being. Catalano, Dooley, and Jackson (1985; see also Catalano, Rook, and Dooley, 1986) provide an example of such an analysis by demonstrating the impact of changes in the economy on the occurrence and experience of stress. Analyses of chronic conditions such as low income and high demands imply, and are connected to, structural factors involving positions of power and power relations. Explicit inclusion of structural factors in relation to events and chronic strains, and as determinants of personal resources, furthers our comprehension of the forces impinging on the psychological state of individuals.

SUMMARY

I have discussed the major categories and methods in the study of the epidemiology of mental illness. Conceptualization and measurement in research have become increasingly diagnostically oriented. However, different concepts and measures may be appropriate depending on the research questions and populations of interest. I have presented the most recent information on the prevalence of psychiatric disorders in the U.S. population. In addition, I have discussed major research agendas for explaining psychiatric disorders in general and in different population groups. There is evidence for both a stressful life events perspective and for the importance of chronic conditions of stress in determining mental disorders. Evidence also exists that certain social and personal resources mediate or intervene in the effects of stress on symptomatology. I conclude by emphasizing the continued need for investigating the particular dynamics by which stressful situations, both discrete events and chronic conditions, affect individuals' mental health and illness. Further specification of intervening social and psychological factors, and the role of social structural determinants, is required for a fuller understanding of this process.

REFERENCES

Abramson, L. N., and Sackheim, H. A. 1977. A Paradox in Depression: Uncontrollability and Self-Blame. *Psychological Bulletin* 84: 838–851.

Alloy, L., Peterson, C., Abramson, L., and Seligman, M. E. P. 1984. Attributional Style and the Generality of Learned Helplessness. *Journal of Personality and Social Psychology* 46: 681–687.

American Psychiatric Association. 1980. *Diagnostic and Statistical Manual of Mental Disorders*. 3rd ed. Washington, D.C.

American Psychiatric Association. 1987. *Diagnostic and Statistical Manual of Mental Disorders*. 3rd ed. (revised). Washington, D.C.

Andreasen, N. C. 1984. *The Broken Brain: The Biological Revolution in Psychiatry*. New York: Harper and Row.

Bachrach, L. L. 1984. The Young Adult Chronic Patient in an Era of Deinstitutionalization. *American Journal of Public Health* 74: 382–384.

Barnett, R. C., and Baruch, G. L. 1985. Women's Involvement in Multiple Roles and Psychological Distress. *Journal of Personality and Social Psychology* 49: 135–145.

Brown, G. W., and Harris, T. O. 1978. *Social Origins of Depression: A Study of Psychiatric Disorder in Women*. New York: Free Press.

Brown, G. W., and Harris, T. O. 1984. *Establishing Causal Links: The Bedford College Studies of Depression*. Unpublished manuscript.

Catalano, R. A., Dooley, D., and Jackson, R. L. 1985. Economic Antecedents of Help-

Seeking: Reformulation of Time-Series Tests. *Journal of Health and Social Behavior* 26: 141–152.

Catalano, R., Rook, K., and Dooley, D. 1986. Labor Markets and Help-Seeking: A Test of the Employment Security Hypothesis. *Journal of Health and Social Behavior* 27: 277–287.

Cleary, P., and Mechanic, D. 1983. Sex Differences in Psychological Distress among Married People. *Journal of Health and Social Behavior* 24: 111–121.

Cohen, S., and Wills, T. A. 1985. Stress, Social Support, and the Buffering Hypothesis. *Psychological Bulletin* 98: 310–357.

Crandell, D. L., and Dohrenwend, B. P. 1967. Some Relations among Psychiatric Symptoms, Organic Illness and Social Class. *American Journal of Psychiatry* 123: 1527–1538.

Dohrenwend, B. P., and Dohrenwend, B. S. 1974. Social and Cultural Influences on Psychopathology. *Annual Review of Psychology* 25: 417–452.

Dohrenwend, B. P., and Dohrenwend, B. S. 1976. Sex Differences in Psychiatric Disorders. *American Journal of Sociology* 81: 1447–1454.

Dohrenwend, B. P., and Dohrenwend, B. S. 1981. Socioeconomic Factors, Stress, and Psychopathology. *American Journal of Community Psychology* 9: 128–159.

Dohrenwend, B. P., Dohrenwend, B. S., Gould, M. S., Link, B., Neugebauer, R., and Wunch-Hitzig, R. 1980a. *Mental Illness in the United States: Epidemiological Estimates*. New York: Praeger.

Dohrenwend, B. P., Shrout, P., Egri, G., and Mendelsohn, F. 1980b. Nonspecific Psychological Distress and Other Dimensions of Psychopathology. *Archives of General Psychiatry* 37: 1229–1236.

Eaton, W., and Kessler, L. 1981. Rates of Symptoms of Depression in a National Sample. *American Journal of Epidemiology* 114: 528–538.

Faris, R. E. L., and Dunham, H. W. 1939. *Mental Disorders in Urban Areas*. Chicago: University of Chicago Press.

Folkman, S., and Lazarus, R. S. 1980. An Analysis of Coping in a Middle-aged Community Sample. *Journal of Health and Social Behavior* 21: 219–239.

Freedman, A. M., Kaplan, H. I., and Sadock, B. J. 1976. *Modern Synopsis of Comprehensive Textbook of Psychiatry II*. Baltimore: William and Wilkins.

Freud, S. 1959. *Collected Papers Vol. I*. New York: Basic Books.

Freud, S. 1966a. *A General Introduction to Psychoanalysis*. New York: Washington Square Press.

Freud, S. 1966b. *The Complete Introductory Lectures on Psychoanalysis*. New York: W. W. Norton.

Gore, S., and Mangione, T. 1983. Social Roles, Sex Roles and Psychological Distress: Additive and Interactive Models of Sex Differences. *Journal of Health and Social Behavior* 24: 300–312.

Gove, W., and Geerkin, M. 1977. The Effect of Children and Employment on the Mental Health of Married Men and Women. *Social Forces* 56: 66–76.

Gove, W., and Tudor, J. 1973. Adult Sex Roles and Mental Illness. *American Journal of Sociology* 78: 812–835.

Heller, K., and Swindle, R. 1983. "Social Networks, Perceived Social Support and Coping with Stress." In *Prevention Psychology: Theory, Research and Practice in Community Intervention*, eds. R. D. Felner, L. A. Jason, J. Moritsugu, and S. S. Farber. eds. New York: Pergamon.

Helzer, J. E., Robins, L. N., McEvoy, L. T., Spitznagel, E. L., Stoltzman, R. K., Farmer, A., and Brockington, I. F. 1985. A Comparison of Clinical and Diagnostic Interview Schedule Diagnoses. *Archives of General Psychiatry* 42: 657–666.

Hollingshead, A. B., and Redlich, F. C. 1958. *Social Class and Mental Illness.* New York: Wiley.

Holmes, T. H. 1979. Development and Application of Quantitative Measure of Life Change Magnitude. In *Stress and Mental Disorder*, ed. J. E. Barrett. New York: Raven.

Holmes, T. H., and Rahe, R. H. 1967. The Social Readjustment Rating Scale. *Journal of Psychosomatic Research* 11: 213–218.

Horwitz, A. 1982. Sex Role Expectations, Power, and Psychological Distress. *Sex Roles* 8: 607–623.

Kessler, R. C., 1982. A Disaggregation of the Relationship between Socioeconomic Status and Psychological Distress. *American Sociological Review* 47: 752–764.

Kessler, R. C., and Cleary, P. D. 1980. Social Class and Psychological Distress. *American Sociological Review* 45: 63–78.

Kessler, R. C., and McLeod, J. D. 1984. Sex Differences in Vulnerability to Undesirable Life Events. *American Sociological Review* 49: 620–631.

Kessler, R. C., McLeod, J. D., and Wethington E. 1984. The Costs of Caring: A Perspective on the Relationship between Sex and Psychological Distress. In *Social Support: Theory, Research and Applications*, eds. I. G. Sarason and B. R. Sarason. The Hague: Martinus Nijhof.

Kessler, R. C., and McRae, J. A. 1982. The Effect of Wives' Employment on the Mental Health of Married Men and Women. *American Sociological Review* 47: 216–227.

Kessler, R. C., and Neighbors, H. W. 1986. A New Perspective on the Relationships among Race, Social Class, and Psychological Distress. *Journal of Health and Social Behavior* 27: 107–115.

Kessler, R. C., Price, R. H., and Wortman, C. B. 1985. Social Factors in Psychopathology: Stress, Social Support, and Coping Processes. *Annual Review of Psychology* 36: 531–572.

Kohn, M. L. 1972. Class, Family, and Schizophrenia: A Reformulation. *Social Forces* 50: 295–304.

Langner, T. 1962. A Twenty-two Item Screening Score of Psychiatric Symptoms Indicating Impairment. *Journal of Health and Human Behavior* 3: 269–276.

Leighton, D. C., Harding, J. S., Macklin, D. B., Macmillan, A. M., and Leighton, A. H. 1963. *The Character of Danger.* New York: Basic Books.

Mednick, S. A., Schusinger, F., Higgins, J., and Bell, B. 1974. *Genetics, Environment, and Psychopathology.* Amsterdam: North-Holland.

Menaghan, E. G. 1982. Measuring Coping Effectiveness: A Panel Analysis of Marital Problems and Coping Efforts. *Journal of Health and Social Behavior* 23: 220–234.

Menaghan, E. G., and Merves, E. S. 1984. Coping with Occupational Problems: The Limits of Individual Efforts. *Journal of Health and Social Behavior* 25: 406–423.

Miller, W. R., and Seligman, M. E. P. 1973. Depression and the Perception of Reinforcement. *Journal of Abnormal Psychology* 82: 62–73.

Miller, W. R., and Seligman, M. E. P. 1975. Learned Helplessness, Depression, and the Perception of Reinforcement. *Behavior Research and Therapy* 14: 7–17.

Millon, T. 1967. *Theories of Psychopathology*. Philadelphia: W. B. Saunders.

Mirowsky, J., and Ross, C. E. 1980a. Minority Status, Ethnic Culture and Distress: A Comparison of Blacks, Whites, Mexicans, and Mexican-Americans. *American Journal of Sociology* 86: 479–495.

Mirowsky, J., and Ross, C. E. 1980b. Weighting Life Events: A Second Look. *Journal of Health and Social Behavior* 21: 296–300.

Mueller, D. P., Edwards, D. W., and Yarvis, R. 1977. Stressful Life Events and Psychiatric Symptomatology: Change or Undesirability? *Journal of Health and Social Behavior* 18: 307–317.

Munroe, R. 1955. *Schools of Psychoanalytic Thought*. New York: Holt, Rinehart, and Winston.

Myers, J. K., Weissman, M. M., Tischler, G. L., Holzer, C. E. III, Leaf, P. J., Orvaschel, H., Anthony, J. C., Boyd, J. H., Burke, J. D., Kramer, M., and Stoltzmen, R. 1984. Six Month Prevalence of Psychiatric Disorders in Three Communities. *Archives of General Psychiatry* 41: 959–967.

Paykel, E. S. 1974. Life Stress and Psychiatric Disorder: Application of the Clinical Approach. In *Stressful Life Events: Their Nature and Effects*, eds. B. S. Dohrenwend and B. P. Dohrenwend. New York: Wiley and Sons.

Pearlin, L. 1975. Sex Roles and Depression. In *Life-Span Developmental Psychology*, eds. N. Datan and L. H. Ginsberg. New York: Academic Press.

Pearlin, L. I., Lieberman, M. A., Menaghan, E. G., and Mullen, J. T. 1981. The Stress Process. *Journal of Health and Social Behavior* 22: 337–356.

Pearlin, L. I., and Schooler, C. 1978. The Structure of Coping. *Journal of Health and Social Behavior* 19: 2–21.

Rabkin, J. G., and Struening, E. L. 1976. Life Events, Stress, and Illness. *Science* 194: 1013–1020.

Radloff, L. 1975. Sex Differences in Depression: The Effects of Occupation and Marital Status. *Sex Roles* 1: 249–265.

Regier, D. A., Myers, J. K., Kramer, M., Robins, L. N., Blazer, D. G., Hough, R. L., Eaton, W. W., and Locke, B. Z. 1984. The NIMH Epidemiologic Catchment Area Program: Historical Context, Major Objectives, and Study Population Characteristics. *Archives of General Psychiatry* 41: 934–941.

Robins, L. N. 1978. Psychiatric Epidemiology. *Archives of General Psychiatry* 35: 697–702.

Robins, L. N., Helzer, J. E., Croughan, J., Ratcliff, K. S. 1981. National Institute of Mental Health Diagnostic Interview Schedule: Its History, Characteristics, and Validity. *Archives of General Psychiatry* 38: 381–389.

Robins, L. N., Helzer, J. E., Weissman, M. M., Overshal, H., Gruenberg, E., Burke, J. D., and Regier, D. A. 1984. Lifetime Prevalence of Specific Psychiatric Disorders in Three Sites. *Archives of General Psychiatry* 41: 949–958.

Rosenfield, S. 1980. Sex Differences in Depression: Do Women Always Have Higher Rates? *Journal of Health and Social Behavior* 21: 33–42.

Rosenfield, S. 1983. Sex Roles and Societal Reactions to Mental Illness. *Journal of Health and Social Behavior* 23: 18–24.

Rosenfield, S. 1984. Race Differences in Involuntary Hospitalization. *Journal of Health and Social Behavior* 25: 14–23.

Rosenfield, S. 1985. Sex Differences in Mental Health: Explanations for Relative Risk.

Presented at the Annual Meeting of the American Sociological Association, San Antonio.

Rosenfield, S. 1989. The Effects of Women's Employment: Personal Control and Sex Differences in Mental Health. *Journal of Health and Social Behavior* 30: 77–91.

Rosenthal, D., and Kety, S. S., eds. 1968. *The Transmission of Schizophrenia*. London: Pergamon Press.

Ross, C. E., Mirowsky, J., and Huber, J. 1983. Dividing Work, Sharing Work, and In-Between: Marriage Patterns and Depression. *American Sociological Review* 48: 809–823.

Ross, C. E., Mirowsky, J., and Ulbrich, P. 1983. Distress and the Traditional Female Role: A Comparison of Mexicans and Anglos. *American Journal of Sociology* 89: 670–682.

Rotter, J. B. 1966. Generalized Expectancies for Internal Versus External Control of Reinforcement. *Psychological Monographs* 80: 1–28.

Sahakian, W. S., Sahakian, B. J., and Nunn, P. L. S. 1986. *Psychopathology Today: The Current Status of Abnormal Behavior*. Itasca, Ill.: F. E. Peacock.

Seligman, M. E. P. 1975. *Helplessness*. San Francisco: Freeman.

Seligman, M. E. P., Abramson, L., Semmel, A., and von Baeyer, C. 1979. Depressive Attributional Style. *Journal of Abnormal Psychology* 88: 242–247.

Selye, H. 1956. *The Stress of Life*. New York: McGraw-Hill.

Shumaker, S. A., and Brownell, A. 1984. Toward a Theory of Social Support: Closing Conceptual Gaps. *Journal of Social Issues* 40: 11–36.

Spitzer, R., Endicott, J., and Robins, E. 1975. Clinical Criteria for Psychiatric Diagnosis and DSM-III. *American Journal of Psychiatry* 132: 1187–1192.

Srole, L., Langner, T. S., Michael, S. T., Opler, M. K., and Rennie, T. A. 1962. *Mental Health in the Metropolis: The Midtown Manhattan Study*. New York: McGraw-Hill.

Thoits, P. A. 1982. Conceptual, Methodological and Theoretical Problems in Studying Social Support as a Buffer against Life Stress. *Journal of Health and Social Behavior* 23: 145–159.

Thoits, P. A. 1983. Dimensions of Life Events That Influence Psychological Distress: An Evaluation and Synthesis of the Literature. In *Psychosocial Stress: Trends in Theory and Research*, ed. H. B. Kaplan. New York: Academic Press.

Thoits, P. A. 1986. Multiple Identities: Examining Gender and Marital Status Differences in Distress. *American Sociological Review* 51: 259–272.

Torrey, E. F. 1983. *Surviving Schizophrenia*. New York: Harper and Row.

Warheit, G., Holzer, C. E., and Arey, S. S. 1975. Race and Mental Illness: An Epidemiologic Update. *Journal of Health and Social Behavior* 16: 243–256.

Weissman, M. M., and Klerman, G. L. 1978. Epidemiology of Mental Disorders: Emerging Trends in the United States. *Archives of General Psychiatry* 35: 705–712.

Weissman, M. M., Sholomskas, D., Pottenger, M., Prusoff, B. A., and Locke, B. Z. 1977. Assessing Depressive Symptoms in Five Psychiatric Populations: A Validation Study. *American Journal of Epidemiology* 106: 203–214.

Wheaton, B. 1980. The Sociogenesis of Psychological Disorder: An Attributional Theory. *Journal of Health and Social Behavior* 21: 100–124.

Wheaton, B. 1983. Stress, Personal Coping Resources, and Psychiatric Symptoms: An Investigation of Interactive Models. *Journal of Health and Social Behavior* 24: 208–229.

4

Special Problem Populations: The Chronically Mentally Ill, Elderly, Children, Minorities, and Substance Abusers

EVELYN J. BROMET
and HERBERT C. SCHULBERG

The goal of this chapter is to describe the epidemiology and treatment patterns of five special populations whose needs have gained growing attention during recent years: the chronically mentally ill, the elderly, children, minorities, and substance abusers. Each of these populations is often poorly cared for by the existing mental health system, and each has been the object of concern of advocacy groups seeking to rectify problems in the supply and organization of services. In the following sections, we first discuss the extent of psychopathology observed in these respective populations, then consider social and demographic correlates of disorder, and conclude with an analysis of service utilization patterns.

CHRONICALLY MENTALLY ILL

During the last three decades, the number of chronically mentally ill individuals residing in community settings has increased dramatically. While it is difficult to determine the size of the chronically mentally ill population on a local level (Ashbaugh and Manderscheid, 1985), Bachrach (1984) estimated that there are two million chronically mentally ill people in the United States. The vast majority (93 percent) reside outside mental hospitals. The dominant diagnosis among chronically mentally ill persons living in the community is schizophrenia. According to the American Psychiatric Association's *Diagnostic and Statistical Manual-III-Revised* (DSM-III-R) (1987), the essential feature of schizophrenia is the presence of psychotic symptoms (hallucinations, delusions, and thought disorder) during active phases of the illness.

Schizophrenic illness, which has a lifetime prevalence rate of approximately 1 percent, is chronic and sometimes is characterized by a deteriorating course. Although the diagnosis of schizophrenia can be difficult to establish initially, individuals who have been observed repeatedly over a period of years can be diagnosed more reliably.

The chronically mentally ill population is thought to be composed of two subtypes: long-term inpatient residents discharged during the period of deinstitutionalization, and younger patients (primarily under age thirty-five) with a history of several brief inpatient episodes and assigned to aftercare services. The latter group is often characterized as the "Young Adult Patient" (Pepper and Ryglewicz, 1982). A third group of individuals is the homeless mentally ill, which contains both long-term and younger chronic patients and has become a major public health concern in recent years (Bassuk, 1986). A presentation of findings from epidemiologic research coupled with analysis of current treatment patterns highlights the multiple disabilities and service needs of these three groups.

Discharged Long-Term Patients

Prior to the contemporary era of community mental health, most chronically ill psychiatric patients resided in public mental hospitals. With the advent of deinstitutionalization in the 1960s and 1970s, thousands of institutionalized patients were released into the community. Mental hospital censuses decreased from 559,000 in 1955 to 132,000 in 1980. What has become of these individuals? Have they remained psychiatrically disturbed and in need of care, or have they adjusted to community environments?

Despite the masses of discharged public mental hospital patients, there have been few systematic follow-up studies assessing their adjustment to community life. Research comparing outcomes associated with mental hospital care and care provided in community alternatives was analyzed by Braun et al. (1981) and Kiesler (1982). Both reviews concluded that in no case were the outcomes of hospitalization more positive than alternative treatment; indeed, the latter typically was more effective when measured by such variables as psychiatric status, subsequent employment, and ability to live independently. More recently, reports about the long-term adjustment of patients discharged from mental hospitals suggest the outcome of schizophrenia to be more positive than thought previously. For example, a thirty-two-year longitudinal study by Harding et al. (1987) determined that twenty to twenty-five years after their index release from Vermont State Hospital, one-half to two-thirds of the patient cohort had achieved considerable improvement or recovery while residing in the community.

On the other hand, accumulating anecdotal and journalistic evidence suggests that chronic patients in the community often live in substandard housing in impoverished neighborhoods, or in some cases become homeless. Seemingly supportive of this observation, Caton (1984) found that 50 percent of a chronic schizophrenic sample in New York City moved within a one-year period. Also, when deinstitutionalization began, many patients were transferred from state hospitals to nursing homes. Research has since documented that under present staffing patterns, nursing homes are among the least beneficial settings for care of this population (Linn et al., 1985; see also chapter 11 in this volume).

Thus, both the quality and stability of the long-term patients' living arrangements are less than adequate. Detailed studies of the effects of specific aspects of these environmental circumstances, however, remain rare (Jones, Robinson, and Golightley, 1986). An exception is a study by Goldstein and Caton (1983) which determined that inadequate social support and high levels of environmental stress are strong predictors of poor community functioning.

The Young Adult Chronic Patient

The term *young adult chronic patient* entered the professional vocabulary after growth of awareness and concern about persons aged eighteen to thirty-five already displaying persistent and severe impairment in their psychological and social functioning (Pepper and Ryglewicz, 1982). Considered by many as the first generation of severely disabled psychiatric patients "to grow up in the community," these individuals require multiple mental health and social services over extended periods of time. If and when these patients are hospitalized during a state of acute disturbance, their stays are brief, and they are frequently discharged in spite of an incomplete state of remission (Caton, 1981).

Within this cohort of young chronic patients, it has been hypothesized that three distinct subgroups can be identified, each with unique characteristics and service needs (Sheets, Prevost, and Reihman, 1982). The first is the "low energy, low demand" group composed of persons initially hospitalized as children or adolescents. They have adapted to the patient role, displaying passivity and low motivation. The second is the "high energy and high demand" group composed of persons who are prone to impulsive behavior and have a low tolerance for frustration. These patients are highly mobile and tax the energies of case managers. The third is the "high functioning, high aspiration" group composed of persons who often function at a high level but who have been seriously disabled by their psychiatric disorder. They choose not to become involved with traditional mental health programs and seek to function as autonomously as possible. While this taxonomy of the young adult chronic patient remains to be validated, it raises important questions about the differential etiology and service needs of each subgroup.

The Homeless Mentally Ill

Bachrach (1986b: 342) describes the population of homeless mentally ill as consisting of "the overlap between two source populations, homeless individuals and chronically mentally ill individuals." With the increasing numbers of homeless individuals in the United States (Robertson and Cousineau, 1986), rates of mental illness among the homeless have been estimated for several cities. These range generally from 25 to 50 percent (Arce and Vergare, 1984), although a survey in Boston yielded a rate of 90 percent (Bassuk, 1984; Roth and Bean, 1986). In a survey of residents of six shelters in Allegheny County (western Pennsylvania) in which experienced clinicians assessed the presence of mental illness, the present authors (Bromet, Schulz, and Schulberg, 1985) found that 27 percent of those interviewed were assigned a diagnosis of schizophrenia (compared to 30 percent in the Boston survey); 57 percent of those diagnosed with schizophrenia also had alcohol abuse problems. However, the rate of diagnosed mental disorder varied markedly among shelters depending upon the clientele served.

Correlates of Chronic Schizophrenia

Psychiatric epidemiologic research has documented several correlates of chronic schizophrenia. Touching on both the incidence of illness and course of treatment, these include the disorder's association with low socioeconomic status; the occurrence of peak hospital admissions during the summer months; younger age at first hospital admission for males (late teens, early twenties) compared to females (late twenties); higher risk for unmarried persons, those born in the winter season, and individuals with biologic relatives who are schizophrenic; the likely presence of concomitant psychiatric disorders; and the value of psychotropic medication for maintaining adjustment outside of the hospital (Boyd et al., 1984; Eaton, 1974; 1985; Hare 1986).

The younger chronically ill patient population has been the focus of studies investigating the effects of family environment on course of illness. Both experimental and non-experimental forms of research have found that high expressed emotion in the household (high levels of criticism of the patient and overprotection) are associated with poorer outcomes following hospital treatment (Leff and Vaughn, 1984).

Utilization Patterns

Clearly, chronically mentally ill patients have multiple psychiatric, social, and medical disabilities and service needs (Bachrach, 1986a). The Epidemiologic Catchment Area (ECA) study is a major investigation of psychiatric disorder and service utilization among the general population that has been funded by the National Institute of Mental Health (NIMH) at five sites across the country, including New Haven, Baltimore, St. Louis, Los Angeles, and Durham (North Carolina). Findings are that 39–53 percent of community residents diagnosed with schizophrenia or schizophreniform disorders reported a mental health visit in the six months preceding interview; most of these visits were to a mental health specialist as opposed to a general medical provider (Shapiro et al., 1984). In a comparative analysis of the effects of different levels of resource availability, Beiser et al. (1985) found that schizophrenic patients discharged in a city with comprehensive psychiatric services had lower readmission rates and displayed better community adjustment than similar patients discharged in a city with a less rich service network.

The homeless chronically mentally ill have little access to services. In part, agencies lack both the resources and motivation to treat this segment of the population (Bachrach, 1986b). As we noted several years ago with respect to the chronically mentally ill in general, "the psychiatric and other human services required by such persons residing in communities remain fragmented, disorganized, and even lacking" (Schulberg and Bromet, 1981: 930). This analysis is particularly relevant to the current situation confronting the homeless mentally ill.

A potential remedial strategy is to adapt the conceptual framework of community support systems to the specific requirements of the homeless mentally ill. This framework, developed in the mid–1970s to resolve program gaps and fragmentation, is based on the premise that networks of interrelated mental health and social welfare services must be established with a focal point of responsibility to insure that mentally ill persons obtain proper care (Turner and TenHoor, 1978; see, also, chapters 12 and 19 in this volume). While community support systems organized within varying interorganizational structures (Grusky et al., 1985; Reinke and Greenley, 1986) have achieved significant breakthroughs to date, scarce resources and low awareness of the unique dilemmas of homeless persons have limited their availability to this population. Levine, Lezak, and Goldman (1986) therefore offer guidelines for modifying the ten functions of a community support system so that it can better meet the needs of homeless persons. For example, casefinding must be substantially redefined to place greater emphasis on medical and human service settings (e.g., soup kitchens) if individuals highly wary of professional mental health services are to be located and assisted.

THE ELDERLY

Both the number and proportion of individuals over age sixty-five are rapidly increasing. As Cooper and Bickel (1984: 81) stated: "The psychiatric disorders of late life are now recognized as a major cause of chronic ill-health and disablement in the developed industrial nations. . . . " The most prevalent psychiatric disorder among the elderly is dementia, which DSM-III-R defines as an impairment in short- and long-term memory, accompanied by impairment in intellect and judgment. Individuals with dementia often undergo personality changes and are incapable of performing normal activities of daily living.

The course of dementia depends on the underlying etiology. Primary degenerative dementia of the Alzheimer type, which is believed to be the most common type of dementia, has a deteriorating course over a period of several years. In reviewing prevalence studies of dementia, it is important to note that the differential diagnosis of dementia and major depressive disorder is sometimes difficult in the elderly. Several key symptoms of major depressive disorder overlap with dementia, including disorientation, apathy, and complaints of difficulty concentrating or of memory loss. Because of its grave consequences, dementia is currently regarded as a significant public health problem.

Prevalence of Disorder

Based on a review of thirteen studies reporting rates of psychiatric disorder among the elderly, Neugebauer (1980) estimated that the rate of organic and functional psychoses among those over sixty years of age approximates 7–9 percent. Drawing on the published literature in the area, Mortimer, Schuman, and French (1981) attempted to estimate the rate of dementia specifically among persons over the age of sixty-five. They found the rate for severe dementia to be 1.3–6.2 percent and that for milder dementia 2.6–15.4 percent. Variations across different studies were ascribed to several factors, including differences in diagnostic criteria, case ascertainment, and age distributions of the populations studied. These authors estimated the annual incidence of dementia among people sixty-five years and over at 1 percent.

Another recent source of information on the prevalence of dementia-related difficulties in the elderly is the ECA study. Across different sites, rates of severe cognitive impairment (scores of 17 or less on the Folstein Mini Mental State Examination) in people age sixty-five and over ranged from 4 percent (St. Louis) to 5.1 percent (Baltimore) (Robins et al., 1984). In a subsequent reanalysis, the Yale ECA investigators reported a rate of 3.4 percent for severe cognitive impairment, and an overall rate of 10.8 percent for any psychiatric disorder, including severe cognitive impairment (Weissman et al., 1985).

Correlates of Disorder

No consistent sex or ethnic differences seem to be associated with dementia. Heredity appears to be important in patients developing dementia under the age of sixty-five. Furthermore, compared to the general population of comparable ages, excess mortality associated with dementia decreases substantially with increasing age of onset. On the other hand, recent research on depression and depressive symptomatology in the elderly has suggested that such problems increase with age after sixty-five and are correlated with lower income, lower education, and poorer physical health (Berkman et al., 1986). Depression in the elderly has also been found to be associated with lower levels of social support, i.e., reduction in the availability of relationships with friends, neighbors, and other acquaintances (Henderson et al., 1986).

Utilization Patterns

In the ECA research, 4.5 percent (Baltimore) to 19.4 percent (St. Louis) of people over the age of sixty-five reported one or more mental health visits in the six months prior to time of interview. Among subjects with severe cognitive impairment, 3.6 percent (St. Louis) to 7.6 percent (New Haven) reported a mental health visit to either a general medical provider or a mental health specialist. Planners and clinicians have long been concerned about the disparity between the elderly's need for services and their relatively low use of them. Lebowitz (1987) cites numerous factors contributing to this situation. Among them are substantially lower Medicare reimbursement rates for psychiatric as compared to physical disorders; the lack of mental health professionals trained to work with the elderly; unfamiliarity of clinicians with state-of-the-art pharmacologic and psychosocial treatments for elderly patients; and the stigma that elderly persons associate with mental illness.

The locus of care for the elderly is predominantly in community facilities. However, those with severe illnesses requiring institutional care tend to be treated in nursing homes rather than hospitals. Lebowitz (1987), for example, estimates that approximately two-thirds of the 1.4 million U.S. nursing home residents have significant mental health problems which are inadequately recognized and treated (see chapter 11 in this volume).

CHILDREN

Prevalence studies of mental illness in children typically avoid the issue of precise classification because of lack of agreement about diagnostic criteria. Most studies focus on the global concept of "clinical maladjustment" as a gross index of the impaired population's size. In keeping with this approach, we will analyze the epidemiology of maladjustment in children as well as the current state of knowledge about more serious forms of childhood psychopathology, such as childhood autism. It is important that current nosological studies, such as those focused on depressive disorders in childhood (Kovacs et al., 1984a, 1984b), do seek to clarify these unresolved classification issues so that descriptive epidemiologic research on a range of child and adolescent disorders can be conducted in the future.

Prevalence of Disorder

Several investigators have studied the rate of impairment in preschool children. Rates obtained from the Behavior Screening Questionnaire have ranged from 6 percent in a Canadian sample to 24 percent in an American sample (for a review, see Cornely and Bromet, 1986). Gould, Wunsch-Hitzig, and Dohrenwend (1980) analyzed twenty-five studies of school-age children conducted in the United States between 1928 and 1975 which administered questionnaires or detailed interviews to either parents or teachers. Their review also included ten British studies, four of which used multimethod, multistage procedures for data collection. The average rates across these different types of studies were surprisingly similar, namely, 11 percent when relying on teacher information, 16 percent when relying on parents, and 16.5 percent in multimethod approaches. The male: female ratios were also similar, ranging from 2:1 in the multimethod studies to 2.3:1 in the teacher-report studies. Although the rates are similar, it is important to note that the specific children considered impaired may differ according to the methodology. Thus, Rutter (1981) has found that although teachers and parents identified the same percentage of children as impaired, there was in fact little overlap in the particular children so identified.

The primary site of epidemiologic research on autism has been Europe. Autism is a severe form of pervasive developmental disorder characterized by impairment in reciprocal social interaction, communication, and imaginative activity, and a restricted repertoire of activities and interests (DSM-III-R, 1987). Onset often occurs before the age of three. Two British studies and a Danish investigation reported age-specific rates of autism of 4.3-4.8 per 10,000 (DSM-III-R, 1987; Gould, Wunsch-Hitzig, and Dohrenwend, 1980). In these samples, boys were at greater risk of developing autism than girls, with the male:female sex ratio varying from 1.4:1 to 3.4:1.

Correlates of Disorder

Gender differences in the prevalence of children's mental illnesses occur in pre- rather than post-pubescent children. Males accounted for 66 percent of all inpatient admissions under age ten in 1980; the sexes were evenly split among admissions of children aged ten to seventeen. Descriptive investigations also suggest that the rate of disorder increases during adolescence. This is particularly true for inpatient psychiatric admissions. In 1980, 5 percent of all children admitted were under age ten, 28 percent were between ages ten and fourteen, and 67 percent were between the ages of fifteen and seventeen (Milazzo-Sayre et al., 1986).

Research has consistently shown that parental mental disorder is a risk factor for the development of psychiatric disorder in children (Rutter, 1987). Weissman and colleagues (Weissman et al., 1984, 1987), for example, found the risk of psychological symptoms, treatment for emotional problems, diagnostic psychiatric disorders, school problems, and suicidal behavior to be substantially higher in children of parents with major depressive disorder compared to other children. One possible hypothesis to explain this type of finding is the presence of a genetic link. Family environment effects have also been observed. Thus, disturbed children are more frequently identified in families with high levels of marital discord, temporary or permanent family breakup, and poor quality of parenting (measured by such factors as consistency, frequency or responsivity of interactions, and level of security in mother-child attachment) as compared to families without these characteristics (Rutter, 1987).

Utilization Patterns

Children with mental illness are treated within a wide range of settings. They include those operated by psychiatric specialists as well as facilities under the direction of educators, social workers, and correctional workers. Earlier studies indicate that almost all psychotic children and adolescents are known to some psychiatric treatment facility. The likelihood of treatment increases not only in relation to increasing impairment but also in relation to the mother's poorer mental health and greater education (Rutter, 1981). Despite the growing variety of care settings, services are not equally accessible to all children. Cost remains a dominant factor limiting access in the private sector while public facilities often have lengthy waiting periods (U.S. Congress, 1986).

An area of growing attention with regard to the treatment of mentally ill children is the practices of pediatricians in dealing with this subgroup of their patient population. Costello's (1986) review of earlier studies led her to conclude that pediatricians diagnose only about one-half of the mental illness episodes in their practices. Of these identified cases, rates of referral to mental health specialists again were generally about 50 percent. Given that 60 percent of all children with a mental disorder are in the care of a pediatrician rather than a psychiatric specialist, the need for improved diagnostic and treatment practices by these physicians is striking.

MINORITIES

The prevalence, correlates, and utilization patterns of clinically disturbed minorities in the United States are of increasing interest to epidemiologic researchers. Several earlier studies examined symptomatology (e.g., Fischer, 1969; Kessler and Neighbors, 1986; Warheit, Holzer, and Arey, 1975; Warheit, Holzer, and Schwab, 1973). Information on rates of diagnosable clinical disorder is now available from the ECA research program. This section presents descriptive epidemiological data for blacks and Hispanics, two minority groups that are the focus of accumulating research. Although information on minority vs. nonminority rates of disorder is reviewed, such comparisons are often complex and difficult to interpret. Especially questionable is the implicit assumption that the two groups are similar in all respects except race. Thus, until more complex modeling is performed on the clinical data, only tentative inferences may be drawn from current findings.

Prevalence of Disorder

Prevalence studies based on treated cohorts have long suggested that "Black people tend to be disproportionately diagnosed as schizophrenic, to be hospitalized sooner and longer, and to be less likely to receive behavioral or psychotherapeutic treatment" (Dressler and Badger, 1985: 212). Epidemiologists have sought to determine whether this consistent finding reflects biases in diagnosis and treatment or true population differences in morbidity. According to initial findings from three ECA sites, namely, New Haven, Baltimore, and St. Louis, lifetime prevalence rates for most of the fifteen psychiatric disorders assessed were similar among blacks and non-blacks in St. Louis, New Haven, and Baltimore (Robins et al., 1984). Specifically, no statistically significant differences in rates of these fifteen diagnostic categories were found for New Haven; blacks had elevated rates on four diagnostic categories in Baltimore (simple phobia—27.6 percent for blacks vs. 17.4 percent for non-blacks; agoraphobia—13.4 vs. 7.2 percent; drug abuse/dependence—7.3 vs. 4.9 percent; and schizophrenia—2.4 vs. 1.2 percent); and the St. Louis site reported higher rates for blacks on three categories (simple phobia—11.1 vs. 5.9 percent; cognitive impairment 2.2 vs. 0.7 percent; and manic episode 2.5 vs. 0.7 percent). Similarly, the New Haven study site uncovered no significant difference between whites and blacks in the six-month prevalence rate of all Diagnostic Interview Schedule (DIS) disorders combined, which was 17.1 percent for whites and 17.7 percent for blacks (Leaf et al., 1984).

More recently, detailed comparisons have been conducted of major depression rates in black vs. white ECA respondents from all five sites (Somervell et al., 1987). These analyses stratified the population both by site and by gender. With respect to lifetime prevalence of depression, whites had higher rates of depression in almost all of the sex/site groups. Six-month prevalence rates for major depression were generally similar (2.8 percent for whites and 3.0 percent for blacks in the New Haven site) (Leaf et al., 1986); but variations emerged when gender was considered. Specifically, in most sites white men tended to have higher prevalence rates than black men, and black women had higher prevalence rates than white women (Somervell et al., 1987). Thus, it appears that previously reported racial differences in diagnosis and treatment, which portrayed a picture of consistently greater illness among blacks, do not reflect true variations in morbidity between these racial groups.

Differences in suicide rates would also support the hypothesis that racial differences among patient populations reflect treatment bias rather than differential morbidity. Specifically, blacks of all ages have lower suicide rates than whites, with black women having the lowest rates of all. Since certain serious mental illnesses, such as depression and schizophrenia, carry a higher risk of suicide, the fact that black men and women have lower suicide rates than whites at least indirectly supports the notion that the level of morbidity for these prevalent psychiatric disorders is not higher among blacks. However, suicide rates among certain other ethnic minorities in the United States exceed those for whites. That is, age-adjusted rates for American Indians and for Chinese are higher than those for whites, whereas rates for Japanese and for blacks are lower (Kramer et al., 1972). The rising suicide rates nationwide among persons fifteen to twenty-four years of age have also occurred among U.S. Indians and Alaska natives. In fact, data gathered in the early 1980s indicate that the rate among such youth is 2.3 times that for the U.S. population of the same age (May, 1987).

Analyses have also been published recently on the lifetime (Karno et al., 1987) and six-month (Burnam et al., 1987) prevalence rates of mental disorder among Mexican Americans and non-Hispanic whites in the Los Angeles ECA. Similar patterns in lifetime rates were found for the two groups for all DIS diagnoses combined; however, the non-Hispanic whites were more likely to be assigned diagnoses of drug abuse/dependence and major depression than the Mexican American sample. It should be noted that the rates of disorder in the Los Angeles ECA resembled those found in the Baltimore, St. Louis, and New Haven ECA sites. Findings pertaining to six-month prevalence rates also revealed few differences in the rates of disorder between Los Angeles and the other ECA sites, and few differences between Mexican Americans compared to non-Hispanic whites. Exceptions were drug abuse/dependence, for which non-Hispanic whites had a higher rate than Mexican Americans, and severe cognitive impairment, with Mexican Americans having a higher prevalence. The most parsimonious interpretation of the finding on cognitive impairment is that of an ethnic and educational bias in its measurement, a central difficulty with many cognitive measures.

Correlates of Disorder

Little is known about the specific correlates of psychiatric disorder among minorities. Dressler and Badger (1985) assessed approximately 300 southern black adults using the Hopkins Symptom Checklist depression scale. They found the most symptomatic subgroups to include younger persons, women, single, divorced and separated respondents, unemployed, and those with low income. In a separate analysis, Dressler (1985) found that higher levels of economic stressors and life events were also associated with more depressive symptoms, although social support was uncorrelated with depression. Thus, with the exception of social support, the findings are similar to those widely reported in community studies of primarily white respondents.

From an epidemiologic perspective, one of the best studies of the correlates of disorder in a minority population was that conducted by Robins on drug use in a representative population of 235 young black men in St. Louis (Robins and Murphy, 1967). The sample was selected from elementary school records established twenty-five years prior to the time of research in 1965. By combining interview and record information, Robins found that 14 percent of study subjects had an official record of selling, use, or possession of narcotics; 49 percent of those interviewed admitted to having tried drugs. The risk for drug use other than marijuana increased among those whose father was absent during early childhood, among high school dropouts, and among boys who had a police or juvenile court record before age seventeen. Similar detailed analyses are currently underway using ECA data.

Finally, data on the correlates of attempted suicide among U.S. Indians reveal patterns that are again similar to those of white populations. Specifically, suicide attempters are more often female (whereas completers are usually male), young (average age of 20.8 years), and substance abusers.

Utilization Patterns

Race is a major factor affecting use of mental health services. According to Leaf et al. (1985: 1323), "When studies have controlled for level of symptomatology, whites usually have been found to be more likely than blacks to receive treatment for mental health reasons." In their analysis of service utilization in the New Haven ECA cohort, these authors report that whites were more likely to use mental health services than non-whites once level of symptomatology was considered, although clinical factors were the variables most strongly related to utilization.

An analysis of utilization patterns in the Los Angeles ECA revealed that among all respondents, somewhat fewer Mexican Americans (4.5 percent) reported a mental health visit in the past six months than non-Hispanic whites (9.0 percent). Moreover, Mexican Americans with a recently diagnosed mental disorder were only half as likely as non-Hispanic whites to have made a mental health visit. Among those who reported mental health visits, no differences were found in type of specialist seen.

SUBSTANCE ABUSERS

Until recently, there has been little systematic research on the distribution of diagnosable substance abuse disorders. On the other hand, many epidemiologic surveys have been conducted in the United States of substance use and associated problems, particularly drinking practices, alcohol-related problems, and tranquilizer use (e.g., Cahalan, Cisin, and Crossley, 1969; Fillmore and Midanik, 1984; Mellinger et al., 1974). The literature on alcoholism is far more extensive than that for drug addiction (Nathan and Lansky, 1978).

Prevalence of Disorder

Both survey research and other methodologies (e.g., examination of mortality from cirrhosis of the liver, and alcohol consumption data) have been used to estimate the extent of alcoholism in the community. Current estimates of the prevalence of alcoholism are derived from diagnostic interviews of community respondents. One source is the community follow-up survey of a representative sample of New Haven residents conducted in the mid–1970s that used the Schedule for Affective Disorders and Schizophrenia-Lifetime interview and the Research Diagnostic Criteria (Weissman, Myers, and Harding, 1980). Current point prevalence and lifetime prevalence rates (for probable and definite alcoholism) were 2.6 percent (3.6 percent for men; 1.7 percent for women) and 6.7 percent (10.1 percent for men; 4.1 percent for women), respectively. Another source of information is the ECA studies. Based on the DIS and DSM-III criteria, six-month prevalence rates were recorded ranging from 8.2 percent (New Haven) to 10.4 percent (Baltimore) for men and 1.0 percent (St. Louis) to 1.9 percent (New Haven) for women. Lifetime prevalence rates were considerably higher, ranging from 19.1 percent (New Haven) to 28.9 percent (Baltimore) for men and from 4.2 percent (Baltimore) to 4.8 percent (New Haven) for women.

These prevalence rates derived from structured interviews are quite consistent with findings from surveys on drinking problems. A survey by Cahalan, Cisin, and Crossley (1969) classified 12 percent of the population (20 percent males; 8 percent females) as problem drinkers (defined in terms of drinking almost every day and becoming intoxicated several times a month). A survey by the National Institute on Alcohol Abuse and Alcoholism similarly found that 13 percent of American adults (21 percent of men) were heavy drinkers, defined as consuming more than sixty drinks a month (Kamerow, Pincus, and Macdonald, 1986).

The six-month prevalence rate of drug abuse/dependence reported by the ECA ranged from 2.5 percent (New Haven) to 3.0 percent (Baltimore and St. Louis) for men and from 1.8 percent (New Haven) to 2.2 percent (Baltimore) for women. Lifetime rates were somewhat higher, ranging from 6.5 percent (New Haven) to 7.4 percent (St. Louis) for men and 3.8 percent (St. Louis) to 5.1 percent (New Haven) for women.

Correlates of Disorder

As noted above, a major correlate of substance abuse is gender, with men predominating. Other correlates of heavy drinking and alcohol abuse have been found repeatedly in community studies. High risk characteristics include age, with rates of disorder tending to diminish with increasing age; lower education; history of school difficulty; divorce or separation; lower income; and a family history of alcoholism (Holzer et al., 1983; Weissman, Myers, and Harding, 1980). Although racial differences in alcoholism rates tend to be small, significant differences in rates of drug abuse/dependence have been reported. In addition, alcoholism is more common among residents of rural than urban areas, particularly among rural blacks (Blazer, Crowell, and George, 1987). Certain occupations also have higher prevalence rates of alcoholism, based on cirrhosis data. These include waiters, bartenders, longshoremen, musicians, authors, and reporters. By contrast, accountants, mail carriers, and carpenters have been shown to have lower than expected rates of alcohol abuse. Alcoholism is also higher among American Indians than among white populations living in the same region (Beigel et al., 1974).

Affective disorders and antisocial personality disorder often occur in alcoholic patients. Interestingly, a comparison of treated and untreated opiate addicts found lower rates of depressive disorders in the latter group (Rounsaville and Kleber, 1985). With respect to the interaction of gender and age, onset of alcoholism for males tends to occur in the late teens or early twenties; the illness then follows an insidious course, with first hospitalization usually occurring in the late thirties or early forties. The onset of alcoholism in females, on the other hand, is believed to occur later in life, although there are many fewer studies of treated female alcoholics.

Utilization Patterns

Individuals with substance abuse problems make extensive use of health care services. The ECA study found that 49 percent (St. Louis) to 66 percent (Baltimore) of individuals diagnosed with substance abuse had made an ambulatory health or mental health visit in the six months preceding interview. Almost one-quarter of those visits were for mental health services. Moreover, a comparison of inpatient and outpatient costs for medical services incurred by 191 alcoholics and 191 non-alcoholic controls (members of the Los Angeles Area Kaiser Permanente Medical Program) confirmed earlier reports that alcoholics are also higher users of medical services than non-alcoholics and incur greater health care costs (Forsythe, Griffiths, and Reiff, 1982).

CONCLUSION

This chapter has provided descriptive information on the rates of disorder, sociodemographic correlates, and service utilization of five distinct groups often poorly cared for by the mental health system. More research is needed to elucidate fully the epidemiologic patterns and service needs of these groups. Yet much is already understood about the somewhat unique difficulties faced by each population. Existing research suggests several practical applications for service delivery in such areas as outreach, targeting preventive measures, and removing financial and other barriers to care. We would hope for a timely implementation of needed improvements.

REFERENCES

American Psychiatric Association. 1987. *Diagnostic and Statistical Manual of Mental Disorders.* 3rd ed. (Revised). Washington, D.C.

Arce, A., and Vergare, M. 1984. Identifying and Characterizing the Mentally Ill among the Homeless. In *The Homeless Mentally Ill,* ed. H. R. Lamb. Washington, D.C.: American Psychiatric Association Press.

Ashbaugh, J. W., and Manderscheid, R. W. 1985. A Method for Estimating the Chronic Mentally Ill Population in State and Local Areas. *Hospital and Community Psychiatry* 36: 389–393.

Bachrach, L. L. 1984. Asylum and Chronically Ill Psychiatric Patients. *American Journal of Psychiatry* 141: 975–978.

Bachrach, L. L. 1986a. Dimensions of Disability in the Chronically Mentally Ill. *Hospital and Community Psychiatry* 10: 981–982.

Bachrach, L. L. 1986b. The Homeless Mentally Ill in the General Hospital: A Question of Fit. *General Hospital Psychiatry* 8: 340–349.

Bassuk, E. 1984. The Homelessness Problem. *Scientific American* 241: 40–45.

Bassuk, E., ed. 1986. *The Mental Health Needs of Homeless Persons. New Directions for Mental Health Services*, no. 30. San Francisco: Jossey-Bass.

Beigel, A., Hunter, E. J., Tamerin, J. S., Chapin, E. H., and Lowery, M. J. 1974. Planning for the Development of Comprehensive Community Alcoholism Services: I. The Prevalence Survey. *American Journal of Psychiatry* 131: 1112–1116.

Beiser, M., Shore, J. H., Peters, R., and Tatum, E. 1985. Does Community Care for the Mentally Ill Make a Difference? A Tale of Two Cities. *American Journal of Psychiatry* 142: 1047–1052.

Berkman, L. F., Berkman, C. S., Kasl, S., Freeman, D. H., Leo, L., Ostfeld, A. M., Cornoni-Huntley, J., and Brody, J. A. 1986. Depressive Symptoms in Relation to Physical Health and Functioning in the Elderly. *American Journal of Epidemiology* 124: 372–387.

Blazer, D., Crowell, B. A., Jr., and George, L. K. 1987. Alcohol Abuse and Dependence in the Rural South. *Archives of General Psychiatry* 44: 736–740.

Boyd, J. H., Burke, J. D., Gruenberg, E., Holzer, C. E., Rae, D. S., George, L. K., Karno, M., Stoltzman, R., McEvoy, L., and Nestadt, G. 1984. Exclusion Criteria of DSM-III: A Study of Co-occurrence of Hierarchy-Free Syndromes. *Archives of General Psychiatry* 41: 983–989.

Braun, P., Kochansky, G., Shapiro, R., Greenberg, S., Gudeman, J. E., Johnson, S., and Shore, M. F. 1981. Deinstitutionalization of Psychiatric Patients: A Critical Review of Outcome Studies. *American Journal of Psychiatry* 138: 736–749.

Bromet, E., Schulz, C., and Schulberg, H. 1985. *Mental Illness among the Homeless in Allegheny County*. Unpublished manuscript.

Burnam, M. A., Hough, R. L., Escobar, J. I., Karno, M., Timbers, D. M., Tells, C. A., and Locke, B. Z. 1987. Six-Month Prevalence of Specific Psychiatric Disorders among Mexican Americans and Non-Hispanic Whites in Los Angeles. *Archives of General Psychiatry* 44: 687–694.

Cahalan, D., Cisin, I., and Crossley, H. 1969. *American Drinking Practices: A National Study of Drinking Behavior and Attitudes*. Rutgers University Center for Alcohol Studies, Monograph no. 6, New Brunswick, N.J.

Caton, C. L. M. 1981. The New Chronic Patient and the System of Community Care. *Hospital and Community Psychiatry* 32: 475–478.

Caton, C. L. M. 1984. *Management of Chronic Schizophrenia*. New York: Oxford University Press.

Cooper, B., and Bickel, H. 1984. Population Screening and the Early Detection of Dementing Disorders in Old Age: A Review. *Psychological Medicine* 14: 81–95.

Cornely, P., and Bromet, E. 1986. Prevalence of Behavior Problems in Three-Year-Old

Children Living Near Three Mile Island: A Comparative Analysis. *Journal of Child Psychology and Psychiatry* 27: 489–498.

Costello, E. 1986. Primary Care Pediatrics and Child Psychopathology: A Review of Diagnostic, Treatment, and Referral Practices. *Pediatrics* 78: 1044–1051.

Dressler, W. W. 1985. Extended Family Relationships, Social Support, and Mental Health in a Southern Black Community. *Journal of Health and Social Behavior* 26: 39–48.

Dressler, W. W., and Badger, L. 1985. Epidemiology of Depressive Symptoms in Black Communities: A Comparative Analysis. *The Journal of Nervous and Mental Disease* 173: 212–220.

Eaton, W. W. 1974. Residence, Social Class, and Schizophrenia. *Journal of Health and Social Behavior* 15: 289–299.

Eaton, W. W. 1985. Epidemiology of Schizophrenia. *Epidemiologic Reviews* 7: 105–126.

Fillmore, K., and Midanik, L. 1984. Chronicity of Drinking Problems among Men: A Longitudinal Study. *Journal of Studies on Alcohol* 45: 228–236.

Fischer, J. 1969. Negroes and Whites and Rates of Mental Illness: Reconsideration of a Myth. *Psychiatry* 32: 428–446.

Forsythe, A. B., Griffiths, B., and Reiff, S. 1982. Comparison of Utilization of Medical Services by Alcoholics and Non-Alcoholics. *American Journal of Public Health* 72: 600–602.

Goldstein, J. M., and Caton, C. L. M. 1983. The Effects of the Community Environment on Chronic Psychiatric Patients. *Psychological Medicine* 13: 193–199.

Gould, M. S., Wunsch-Hitzig, R., and Dohrenwend, B. P. 1980. Formulation of Hypotheses about the Prevalence, Treatment, and Prognostic Significance of Psychiatric Disorders in Children in the United States. In *Mental Illness in the United States: Epidemiological Estimates*, eds. B. P. Dohrenwend, B. S. Dohrenwend, M. S. Gould, B. Link, R. Neugebauer, and R. Wunsch-Hitzig. New York: Praeger.

Grusky, O., Tierney, K., Manderscheid, R. W., and Grusky, D. B. 1985. Social Bonding and Community Adjustment of Chronically Mentally Ill Adults. *Journal of Health and Social Behavior* 26: 49–63.

Harding, C. M., Brooks, G. W., Ashikaga, T., Strauss, J. S., and Breier, A. 1987. The Vermont Longitudinal Study of Persons with Severe Mental Illness, I: Methodology, Study Sample, and Overall Status 32 Years Later. *American Journal of Psychiatry* 144: 718–726.

Hare, E. 1986. Aspects of the Epidemiology of Schizophrenia. *British Journal of Psychiatry* 149: 554–561.

Henderson, A. S., Grayson, D. A., Scott, R., Wilson, S. J., Rickwood, D., and Kay, D. W. K. 1986. Social Support Dementia and Depression among the Elderly Living in the Hobart Community. *Psychological Medicine* 16: 379–390.

Holzer, C. E., Robins, L. N., Myers, J. K., Weissman, M. M., Tischler, G. L., Leaf, P. J., Anthony, J., and Bednarski, P. B. 1983. Antecedents and Correlates of Alcohol Abuse and Dependence in the Elderly. Paper presented at NIAAA Workshop on the Nature and Extent of Alcohol Problems Among the Elderly, St. Louis, Mo.

Hough, R. L., Landsverk, J. A., Karno, M., Burnam, A., Timbers, D. M., Escobar, J. I., and Regier, D. A. 1987. Utilization of Health and Mental Health Services by Los Angeles Mexican Americans and Non-Hispanic Whites. *Archives of General Psychiatry* 44: 702–709.

Jones, K., Robinson, M., and Golightley, M. 1986. Long-term Psychiatric Patients in the Community. *British Journal of Psychiatry* 149: 537–540.

Kamerow, D. B., Pincus, H. A., and Macdonald, D. I. 1986. Alcohol Abuse, Other Drug Abuse, and Mental Disorders in Medical Practice. *Journal of the American Medical Association* 15: 2054–2057.

Kandel, D. B., Davies, M., Karus, D., and Yamaguchi, K. 1986. The Consequences in Young Adulthood of Adolescent Drug Involvement. *Archives of General Psychiatry* 43: 746–754.

Karno, M., Hough, R. L., Burnam, M. A., Escobar, J. I., Timbers, D. M., Santana, F., and Boyd, J. H. 1987. Lifetime Prevalence of Specific Psychiatric Disorders among Mexican Americans and Non-Hispanic Whites in Los Angeles. *Archives of General Psychiatry* 44: 695–701.

Kessler, R. C., and Neighbors, H. W. 1986. A New Perspective on the Relationships among Race, Social Class, and Psychological Distress. *Journal of Health and Social Behavior* 27: 107–115.

Kiesler, C. 1982. Mental Hospitals and Alternative Care: Noninstitutionalization as Potential Public Policy for Mental Patients. *American Psychologist* 37: 349–360.

Kovacs, M., Feinberg, T. L., Crouse-Novak, M. A., Paulauskas, S. L., and Finkelstein, R. 1984a. Depressive Disorders in Childhood, I: A Longitudinal Prospective Study of Characteristics and Recovery. *Archives of General Psychiatry* 41: 229–237.

Kovacs, M., Feinberg, T. L., Crouse-Novak, M., Paulauskas, S. L., Pollock, M., and Finkelstein, R. 1984b. Depressive Disorders in Childhood, II: A Longitudinal Study of the Risk for a Subsequent Major Depression. *Archives of General Psychiatry* 41: 643–649.

Kramer, M., Pollack, E., Redick, R., and Locke, B. 1972. *Mental Disorders/Suicide.* Cambridge, Mass.: Harvard University Press.

Leaf, P. J., Livingston, M. M., Tischler, G. L., Weissman, M. M., Holzer, C. E., and Myers, J. K. 1985. Contact with Health Professionals for the Treatment of Psychiatric and Emotional Problems. *Medical Care* 23: 1322–1337.

Leaf, P. J., Weissman, M. M., Myers, J. K., Holzer, C. E., and Tischler, G. S. 1986. Psychosocial Risks and Correlates of Major Depression in One United States Urban Community. In *Mental Disorder in the Community: Progress and Challenge*, ed. J. Barret. New York: Guilford Press.

Leaf, P. J., Weissman, M. M., Myers, J. K., Tischler, G. L., and Holzer, C. E. 1984. Social Factors Related to Psychiatric Disorder: The Yale Epidemiologic Catchment Area Study. *Social Psychiatry* 19: 53–61.

Lebowitz, B. 1987. Mental Health Services. In *Encyclopedia of Aging*, ed. G. Maddox. New York: Springer.

Leff, J., and Vaughn, C. 1984. *Expressed Emotion in Families.* New York: Guilford Press.

Levine, I. S., Lezak, A., and Goldman, H. 1986. Community Support Systems for the Homeless Mentally Ill. In *The Mental Health Needs of Homeless Persons*, ed. E. Bassuk. *New Directions for Mental Health Services*, no. 30. San Francisco: Jossey-Bass.

Linn, M. W., Gurel, L., Williford, W. O., Overall, J., Gurland, B., Laughlin, P., and Barchiesi, A. 1985. Nursing Home Care as an Alternative to Psychiatric Hospitalization: A Veterans Administration Cooperative Study. *Archives of General Psychiatry* 42: 544–551.

May, P. 1987. Suicide and Self-destruction among American Indian Youths. *American Indian and Alaska Native Mental Health Research* 1: 52–69.

Mellinger, G. D., Balter, M. B., Parry, H. J., Manheimer, D. I., and Cisin, I. H. 1974. An Overview of Psychotherapeutic Drug Use in the United States. In *Drug Use: Epidemiologic and Social Approaches*, eds. E. Josephson and E. E. Carroll. Washington, D.C.: Hemisphere.

Milazzo-Sayre, L. J., Benson, P. R., Rosenstein, M. J., and Manderscheid, R. W. 1986. Use of Inpatient Psychiatric Services by Children and Youth under Age 18, United States, 1980. *Statistical Note*, No. 175. Rockville, Md.: National Institute of Mental Health.

Mortimer, J. A., Schuman, L. M., and French, L. R. 1981. Epidemiology of Dementing Illness. In *The Epidemiology of Dementia*, eds. J. A. Mortimer and L. M. Schuman. New York: Oxford University Press.

Myers, J. K., Weissman, M. M., Tischler G. L., Holzer, C. E., Leaf, P. J., Orvaschel, H., Anthony, J. C., Boyd, J. H., Burke, J. D., Kramer, M., and Stoltzman, R. 1984. Six-Month Prevalence of Psychiatric Disorders in Three Communities. *Archives of General Psychiatry* 41: 959–967.

Nathan, P. E., and Lansky, D. 1978. Common Methodological Problems in Research on the Addictions. *Journal of Consulting and Clinical Psychology* 46: 713–726.

Neugebauer, R. 1980. Formulation of Hypotheses about the True Prevalence of Functional and Organic Psychiatric Disorders among the Elderly in the United States. In *Mental Illness In the United States: Epidemiological Estimates*, eds. B. P. Dohrenwend, B. S. Dohrenwend, M. S. Gould, B. Link, R. Neugebauer, and R. Wunsch-Hitzig, New York: Praeger.

Pepper, B., and Ryglewicz, H., eds. 1982. *The Young Adult Chronic Patient. New Directions for Mental Health Services*, no. 14. San Francisco: Jossey-Bass.

Redick, R. W., Witkin, M. J., Atay, J. E., and Manderscheid, R. W. 1983–1984. *Mental Health Service System Reports*. Rockville, Md.: National Institute of Mental Health.

Reinke, B., and Greenley, J. 1986. Organizational Analysis of Three Community Support Program Models. *Hospital and Community Psychiatry* 37: 624–629.

Robertson, M. J., and Cousineau, M. R. 1986. Health Status and Access to Health Services among the Urban Homeless. *American Journal of Public Health* 76: 561–563.

Robins, L. N., Helzer, J. E., Weissman, M. M., Orvaschel, H., Gruenberg, E., Burke, J. D., and Regier, D. A. 1984. Lifetime Prevalence of Specific Psychiatric Disorders in Three Sites. *Archives of General Psychiatry* 41: 949–958.

Robins, L. N., and Murphy, G. E., 1967. Drug Use in a Normal Population of Young Negro Men. *American Journal of Public Health* 57: 1580–1596.

Rosenstein, M. J., Milazzo-Sayre, L. J., MacAskill, R. L., and Manderscheid, R. W. 1987. *Use of Inpatient Psychiatric Services by Special Populations*. Unpublished manuscript.

Roth, D., and Bean, G. 1986. New Perspectives on Homelessness: Findings from a Statewide Epidemiological Study. *Hospital and Community Psychiatry* 37: 712–719.

Rounsaville, B. J., and Kleber, H. D. 1985. Untreated Opiate Addicts. *Archives of General Psychiatry* 42: 1072–1077.

Rutter, M. 1987. Epidemiological/Longitudinal Strategies and Causal Research in Child Psychiatry. *Journal of the American Academy of Child Psychiatry* 20: 513–544.

Rutter, M. 1987. Parental Mental Disorder as a Psychiatric Risk Factor. In *American Psychiatric Association Annual Review*, Vol. 6, eds. R. Hales and A. Frances. Washington, D.C.: American Psychiatric Press.

Schulberg, H. C., and Bromet, E. 1981. Strategies for Evaluating the Outcome of Community Services for the Chronically Mentally Ill. *American Journal of Psychiatry* 138: 930–935.

Shapiro, S., Skinner, E. A., Kessler, L. G., Von Korff, M., German, P. S., Tischler, G. L., Leaf, P. J., Benham, L., Cottler, L., and Regier, D. A. 1984. Utilization of Health and Mental Health Services: Three Epidemiologic Catchment Area Sites. *Archives of General Psychiatry* 41: 971–978.

Sheets, J., Prevost, J., and Reihman, J. 1982. The Young Adult Chronic Patient: Three Hypothesized Subgroups. In *The Young Adult Chronic Patient*, eds. B. Pepper and H. Ryglewicz. *New Directions for Mental Health Services*, no. 14. San Francisco: Jossey-Bass.

Somervell, P. D., Leaf, P. J., Weissman, M. M., Blazer, D. G., and Bruce, M. L. 1987. The Prevalence of Major Depression in Black and White Adults in Five United States Communities. Unpublished manuscript.

Taylor, J. R., Helzer, J. E., and Robins, L. N. 1986. Moderate Drinking in Ex-Alcoholics: Recent Studies. *Journal of Studies on Alcohol* 47: 115–121.

Turner, J., and Ten Hoor, W. 1978. The NIMH Community Support Program: Pilot Approach to a Needed Social Reform. *Schizophrenia Bulletin* 4: 319–348.

U.S. Congress, Office of Technology Assessment. 1986. *Children's Mental Health: Problems and Services—A Background Paper.* Washington, D.C.: U.S. Government Printing Office.

Warheit, G. J., Holzer, C. E., and Arey, S. A. 1975. Race and Mental Illness: An Epidemiologic Update. *Journal of Health and Social Behavior* 16: 243–255.

Warheit, G. J., Holzer, C. E., and Schwab, J. J. 1973. An Analysis of Social Class and Racial Differences in Depressive Symptomatology: A Community Study. *Journal of Health and Social Behavior* 14: 291–299.

Weissman, M. M., Myers, J. K., and Harding, P. S. 1980. Prevalence and Psychiatric Heterogeneity of Alcoholism in a United States Urban Community. *Journal of Studies on Alcohol* 41: 672–681.

Weissman, M. M., Myers, J. K., Tischler, G. L., Holzer, C. E., Leaf, P. J., Orvaschel, H., and Brody, J. A. 1985. Psychiatric Disorders (DSM-III) and Cognitive Impairment in the Elderly in a U.S. Urban Community. *Acta Psychiatrica Scandinavia* 71: 366–379.

Weissman, M. M., Myers, J. K., Tischler, G. L., Holzer, C. E., Leaf, P. J., Orvaschel, H., and Brody, J. A. 1985. Psychiatric Disorders (DSM-III) and Cognitive Impairment in the Elderly in a U.S. Urban Community. *Acta Psychiatrica Scandinavica* 71: 366–379.

Weissman, M. M., Wickramaratne, P., Warner, V., John, K., Prusoff, B. A., Merikangas, K. R., and Gammon, G. D. 1987. Assessing Psychiatric Disorders in Children. *Archives of General Psychiatry* 44: 747–753.

Part 3
Mental Health Policy Development

5

From the Asylum to the Community in U.S. Mental Health Care: A Historical Overview

LELAND V. BELL

A historical overview of mental health care in the United States reveals that enormous and intricate problems endure. Some of the difficulties relate to the imprecise and varied terms and concepts used in mental health work: consider the elusive and tenuous meanings behind such expressions as *lunacy, insanity, mental illness, mental health*, and *behavioral disorder*. Another difficult problem has been the ever-changing assumptions regarding the etiology of mental afflictions. Over the years, madness has been attributed to many factors including immorality, hereditarian defects, chemical or hormonal imbalances, childhood traumas, and a variety of social problems ranging from oppressive poverty to destructive family dynamics. Without an understanding of the basic causes and mechanisms of mental illness, effective treatment regimens have remained in a state of flux; and the promises of each new therapy fade when the treatment produces limited results.

One feature of American mental health care has persisted: this basic historical fact has been the institution, the asylum or mental hospital, a facility which emerged in the early decades of the nineteenth century and became a recognized part of the social order. It received no significant challenge to its legitimacy or permanency until quite recent times. Throughout its history, the mental hospital underwent fundamental changes, notably in regard to its purpose, goals, and responsibilities. It never remained solely a static place locked to a treadmill of custodialism. Societal and professional influences altered its clientele, treatment options, the nature and quality of the staff and physical plant as well as its justification for existence. Over the years, while the ideology and character of the institution changed, facilities proliferated rapidly, and the number of resident mentally ill patients increased annually, reaching over 550,000 persons in the mid–1950s. At that time, the promise of psychopharmacology, combined with the community mental health movement, opened institutional doors, encouraging and permitting patients to find a place in the community. The mental hospital, however, was not supplanted. When the deinstitutionalization drive ebbed, the mental hospital remained a major fact of the mental health care system.

ORIGINS OF THE ASYLUM

In colonial America there was no recognized need for a specific institution to house the insane. The family cared for its disturbed member and when relatives and friends were absent, or evaded this responsibility, the individual became a community ward. Indeed, mental illness was viewed as an individual matter, a local concern and not a major social problem. A variety of informal arrangements determined the care of the insane, a custom derived from the Elizabethan Poor Law of 1601 which made each town responsible for its needy. The community was identified as the legal and responsible guardian of the insane person. It accepted this obligation because the mad individual was an indigent or a threat to public order (Deutsch, 1949: 39–54; Bell, 1980: 1–5).

Colonial Americans equated madness with disruptive, bizarre behavior and believed that it resulted from either demonological possession or moral turpitude. The prominent Puritan clergyman Cotton Mather, for example, saw the mentally ill as agents of the devil, and his publications, notably *Wonders of the Invisible World* (1693), detailed the events of satanic possession. He and other ministers also believed that madness was divine punishment for an individual's immorality. This tie between sin and insanity was a powerful belief in seventeenth-century America, much more influential than the assumption that a demon could control human behavior. Religion played a dominant role in the lives of colonials; ministers urged their flocks to pursue virtuous lives, warning that God avenged the practice of immorality with ''frightful diseases'' and an early death. The insane person was viewed as a wicked being who had to be purged of sin by harsh punishments. Whippings and beatings brought retribution and saved the insane transgressor from eternal damnation as well as a life of debauchery.

The harsh treatment of the insane reflected the harsh realities of colonial life. People were preoccupied with basic issues of subsistence. They were subject to Indian attacks and faced such natural calamities as famine and epidemic disease. A stringent policy toward the indigent and the disruptive was needed to enhance cooperative group effort, the fundamental ingredient of a town's survival. Any kind of dependency was viewed with disdain and became a burden, an obstacle to community solidarity. Not only were the insane morally reprehensible, but they required controls and restrictions to prevent them from undermining the cohesive fabric of society. Jails, kennels, and almshouses provided the proper restrictive setting to house and maintain them. In these facilities, notably the almshouse, a familiar urban institution in colonial America, the insane became part of a growing clientele of undifferentiated dependents including criminals and orphans as well as the sick, the blind, the physically maimed, and the unemployed.

Dependency also qualified the mentally disturbed for acceptance to general hospitals which were established in eighteenth-century America to provide relief for the sick poor. Pennsylvania Hospital in Philadelphia offered a typical setting. Opening in the early 1750s, it admitted mental patients, placing them in basement cells. Its prime mover, Benjamin Franklin, in a petition to the Pennsylvania Colonial Assembly, noted the growing number of mentally ill persons in the community: some were violent while others wasted away and became victims of predators who took advantage of their helpless condition. He pointed to the apparent success of caring for the insane at Bethlehem Hospital in London, hoping that this achievement could be duplicated in Philadelphia (Morton, 1895; Hunter, 1955; Williams, 1976).

The establishment of an institution devoted exclusively to the mentally ill, at Williamsburg, Virginia, in 1773, was more portentous for the future of American mental health care than either the almshouse or the general hospital. Later named Eastern Lunatic Asylum, this facility was administered by a lay keeper who maintained a selective admissions policy, excluding the transient, the aged, and the alcoholic. While it remained small, unique, and local, and actually closed for a time during the tumultuous revolutionary years, it stands as the precursor of the public asylums that emerged in the decade of the 1830s, an era of optimism, reform, and experimentation (Dain, 1971).

NEW DIRECTIONS IN TREATMENT

The type of care given to the mentally disturbed in hospitals, the Williamsburg asylum, and, to a lesser degree, in jails and almshouses was largely punitive, designed to control and isolate disoriented or unruly indigents. Assuming that a quiet patient was saner than a violent one, cell keepers maintained a strict discipline and employed such restraints as chains, leg irons, and iron rings. At Pennsylvania Hospital, the "madd shirt" was applied widely; it was a canvas garment which covered and restricted a person's body from the head to below the knees. Cold showers, bloodletting, blistering, and the use of emetics, ca-thartics, and sedatives complemented the harsher techniques. Contemporary ac-counts of institutional accommodations depict patients half-naked, sleeping on dirty straw, and chained to unpainted walls in unheated basement cells. These conditions stemmed from the prevailing belief that the insane were not affected by extreme temperatures and were indifferent to their surroundings (Dain, 1975).

While this assumption lingered well into the nineteenth century, new influences were growing. The general intellectual movement, or attitude of mind, known as the Enlightenment challenged traditional values and beliefs, and by the late eighteenth century, it had become an activist philosophy which spread into and permeated all areas of society. It espoused an ideal of progress toward the perfectibility of humankind. A belief in the goodness of humanity, a faith in reason and science along with a conviction that individuals could reshape institutions into more efficient and humane patterns became dogmas to eighteenth-century philosophers. These ideals set the direction of the French and American revolutions and fueled a humanitarian movement aimed at improving the conditions of life.

A dramatic example of the impact of the new altruism upon the care of the insane came in 1793 when Philippe Pinel, physician at the Bicêtre, a Parisian asylum, ordered the chains struck from inmates, an act symbolizing the beginning of a new era in the treatment of the mentally ill. His famous book, *A Treatise on Insanity* (1806), expressed the hope of the Enlightenment. Pinel wrote that the insane were not criminals to be punished but sick people needing sympathy and humane care. Traditional methods of therapy, notably arbitrary physical punishment, he held, hindered recovery. While favoring a kind and compassionate manner in dealing with the mad, Pinel insisted on the need for restraints, including the straitjacket, and above all, advocated psychological coercion as the best means for managing mental patients (Grange, 1961; Kavka, 1949; Woods and Carlson, 1961).

Pinel's American contemporary, Benjamin Rush, a signatory of the Declaration of Independence and a physician at Pennsylvania Hospital, also called for psychological intimidation in controlling mental cases. He regarded fear and authority as essential therapeutic tools. In addition, as a somaticist, Rush attributed mental disorder to hypertension of the brain's blood vessels and believed that the strain could best be relieved by extensive bloodletting. Recognized in his time as one of America's outstanding physicians, he exerted a powerful influence upon the medical profession through his practice, lectures, and writings, particularly *Medical Inquiries and Observations Upon the Diseases of the Mind* (1812), the first important American study on mental disorder. His work helped establish the field of mental illness as a medical specialty. Like Pinel, he struck off the chains of the insane at a time when lay and professional opinion felt only dread and revulsion towards the mentally ill, and insanity itself represented a forlorn ailment, a disorder without remedy (Hawke, 1971; Wittels, 1946; Shryock, 1945).

While Benjamin Rush exerted a major impact upon the medical profession, the example of William Tuke's Retreat at York, England, provided the inspiration for the institutional care of the mentally ill in American private asylums. Founded in 1792 by the Society of Friends, the Retreat operated on a regimen termed "moral management," which signified a way of controlling patients by means of a reward-punishment system. Improper conduct was discouraged by threats and restraints; behaving well and accepting institutional discipline brought favors. The aim was to develop the patient's sense of right and wrong. By encouraging patients to recognize that self-restrained, orderly behavior was right and that erratic, disruptive conduct was wrong, the Quakers displayed kindness, understanding, and sympathy toward their wards. Close ties between English and American Friends assured that the York experiment received attention in America where it provided guidelines for the establishment of four institutions patterned after Tuke's asylum: Friends' Asylum at Frankford, Pennsylvania (1813); Bloomingdale Asylum, New York City (1821); McLean Asylum, Boston (1818); and the Hartford Retreat, Connecticut (1824) (Tuke, 1813; Eaton, 1953).

These institutions made a special contribution to the development of mental health facilities in America by implementing the moral treatment approach. Advocates of this therapy, the founders and administrators of the private asylums, were disciples of Pinel and Tuke, and exercised a commanding authority over their institutions, supervising every aspect of asylum life. They attacked the use of arbitrary force to control patients and generally avoided the application of physical restraints and such drastic medical treatments as purging and bleeding. While offering the promise of cure through persuasion and sympathetic understanding, they tried to instill in the patient a sense of morality. Other elements of moral treatment included occupational therapy, recreation, individualized care, and the removal of the patient from family and friends to an institution in a peaceful environment (Little, 1972; Page, 1913; Carlson and Chale, 1960; Dain, 1960; Eaton, 1953). In short, moral treatment placed the patient in a total therapeutic milieu which accommodated the client's psychological condition. Its greatest impact was on the next generation of asylum superintendents, who introduced moral treatment into the state institutions of the 1830s and 1840s.

Notwithstanding its positive features, the application and concept of moral treatment carried a class bias, a portentous fact for the future. A general policy of these early nineteenth-century private asylums excluded largely the insane poor who were viewed as offensive and assumed less curable than the well-to-do. Administrators generally came from the upper middle class and preferred patients from the same social stratum. An influx of insane paupers, they argued, stigmatized an institution and drove away the middle-class patients who refused association with their apparent social inferiors (Dain and Carlson, 1959). In effect, moral treatment brought optimism and hope to those who could afford its services. It also embraced middle-class values as the norms of society. In attempting to mold patient behavior, physicians emphasized order, moderation, and self-control, the hallmark of a middle-class life-style. In private asylums, where physicians and patients came from the same socially well-placed backgrounds, mutual rapport was easily established, and patients readily grasped the therapeutic techniques of their physicians. Later, when poor people sharing different values formed the majority of patient populations, moral treatment ran into difficulties.

SPREAD OF THE ASYLUM MOVEMENT

The decade of the 1830s witnessed the emergence of public asylums for the insane. Once established, these institutions proliferated throughout the remainder of the nineteenth century and well into the 1900s, demonstrating clearly that the asylum had great social significance. In 1876, fifty-eight state asylums, ten city and county asylums, nine charitable institutions, and nine private asylums held 29,558 patients. Several factors account for the appearance of the public insane asylum. The success of moral treatment in private asylums helped dispel the pessimism associated with caring for the mentally ill, giving apparent concrete evidence that insanity was curable. Especially when viewed alongside these achievements of private hospitals, the inadequate and limited public facilities for housing the insane offended middle-class reformers who felt a paternalistic responsibility for the less fortunate members of society. Their effort to better the conditions of the mentally ill formed part of a widespread reform movement which permeated American life in the 1830s and 1840s. Imbued with an optimistic sense of mission, many reformers worked to improve the lot of the blind, the deaf, the slave, the convict, the alcoholic, the mentally retarded, and the insane. Others called for the abolition of war, agitated for women's rights, demanded the extension of the system of public education, and experimented with the establishment of utopian communities. The asylum, in this context, was really a small utopia, a secure environment screened from the anxieties of the wider society. In addition to these factors, families and friends of the insane wanted a public facility that would control as well as cure the mentally ill. Also, the establishment of public insane asylums may be attributed to concern over a major social transformation associated with urbanization and immigration: the emergence of the insane poor, a sizable class of potentially disruptive unemployables. The unruly nature of this group upset the existing systems of relief and control, notably the routine and discipline of the workhouse. The asylum offered a better option; here the insane poor would be contained, treated, and, hopefully, restored to health so that they could fulfill a productive role in the economy (Grob, 1965; Rothman, 1971; Tomes, 1984; Jimenez, 1987).

In 1833, the State Lunatic Hospital at Worcester, Massachusetts, opened, marking the beginning of the first public mental institution devoted to the therapeutic treatment of the insane. Under the leadership of its medical superintendent, Samuel B. Woodward, a vigorous, optimistic, dedicated physician, the institution achieved national recognition, becoming a model for other state asylums. Woodward's success may be attributed to his utilitarian approach to the care of the mentally ill. Above all, he was an administrator attentive to the practical possibilities of therapy and to the daily tasks of running an institution. He relied on medical intervention, particularly to pacify violent patients, and remained devoted to moral treatment, stressing regular routines, individualized care, occupational therapy, and religious or moral training. He also believed that a respectful relationship between patient and physician restored the client's confidence as well as ability to develop friendships. In most respects, the Worcester superintendent sought to play the role of the kind, generous, sensitive father who, with affectionate authority, provided for the wants and needs of his "children," the patients (Grob, 1962, 1966).

Woodward's therapeutics apparently produced a significant recovery rate especially among middle-class inmates who reaped the benefits of his system. They received privileges and lived and worked with each other apart from the other groups. Woodward promoted this policy because he insisted that interactions among a homogeneous group of patients from similar social and educational backgrounds enhanced recovery. On the other hand, many poorer patients arriving from jails and almshouses often exhibited extreme behavior; they were subdued by the staff who then left them alone. In Woodward's words, they were "vulgar" and "abusive." This situation forecast future attitudes and policies which were to dominate mental institutions during the 1860s and 1870s and contribute to the transformation of the asylum into a custodial facility. Woodward did, however, help popularize the notion that insanity was curable, especially if the afflicted received early hospitalization and proper treatment. He compiled figures on the number of patients cured, showing dramatic recovery rates. Although later generations of physicians were to question the accuracy of his statistics, Woodward himself never wavered in the belief that all mentally ill could be restored to perfect health. This optimistic message was carried in his annual reports which circulated nationwide, stirring interest in mental illness and offering guidelines for other physicians concerned with improving the condition of the insane (Grob, 1966).

During the 1830s and 1840s when new facilities for the mentally ill were being built throughout the country, the study of insanity became a medical specialty. Its practitioners formed a small group of the medical profession, consisting largely of asylum administrators who had little interest in theory and remained eclectic pragmatists, borrowing notions from such varied sources as phrenology, which explained insanity in terms of underdeveloped faculties of the brain associated with physical or behavioral factors, and John Locke's sensationalist psychology (Dain, 1964; Davies, 1955). They preferred observing patients to reading about insanity and scrambled together different theories in deriving clinical applications. They found no contradiction in believing that mental illness was a somatic disease and, at the same time, that environmental factors were determinants of insanity.

In arguing that defects in the social environment contributed to the etiology of madness, asylum superintendents made a sharp critique of American society, beginning their analysis with the generalization that insanity came with civilization. This meant that all of the stresses and frivolities of living in a complex social order overtaxed the nervous system and fostered mental illness. Such a situation was aggravated by the loss of order and stability in American life. Superintendents contended that American society was too open and fluid, and it produced the driven individual who worked furiously and anxiously to reach unattainable goals, ignoring the rules of good health. This compulsive person experienced sleepless nights, lost weight, and became irritable, and, if such a life-style went unchecked, the individual drifted into insanity.

All areas of American life, particularly business, politics, and education, asylum superintendents argued, operated at a fervid pace, and even those institutions which normally provided stability, namely, religion, the school, and the family, contributed to the unsettling of society. Religious revivals startled and disoriented people; schools created tensions by instilling an overcompetitive spirit leading students to strive for goals which were beyond their means and talents; and the family had become a weak and ineffectual institution with parents simply allowing children to gratify their whims. When parental authority was restored, the asylum reports noted, mental illness would decrease (Caplan, 1969: 12–25).

This critique was not a cry of alarm or a prophecy of doom. As guardians of the nation's mental health, medical superintendents were giving warnings and guidelines for the purpose of preventing madness and improving society. And if a matrix of social tensions caused mental illness, there was a moral obligation to ameliorate the condition. Society itself could not be reconstructed; the best solution was the creation of a special environment for the insane, the asylum, a place screened from the pressures of the community and structured by a regimen of moral treatment to facilitate the recovery of its clientele.

Imbued with a powerful sense of dedication and optimism, this first generation of superintendents clearly identified the asylum as the key to curing insanity. No one accepted this mission more than Thomas S. Kirkbride, superintendent of the Pennsylvania Hospital for the Insane at West Philadelphia (Tomes, 1984). His book, *On the Construction, Organization, and General Arrangements of Hospitals for the Insane, With Some Remarks on Insanity and Its Treatment* (1854), was a basic guide to asylum building and keeping. It outlined the steps for creating an ideal mental hospital, analyzing every aspect of construction. It specified, for example, the location of water pipes and gas light fixtures as well as the size of rooms and doors. Kirkbride even commented on the correct procedure for scrubbing floors. The design of the institution followed a linear pattern with wings extending in a step pattern from each side of the central part, which housed offices, receiving rooms, and the apartment of the superintendent and his family. The facility should be located in the country, near a town, and on approximately 100 acres of land. Its maximum capacity was set at 250 patients. Kirkbride also defined the duties and responsibilities of administrators, insisting that only cheerful and trustworthy persons be employed and an attendant-patient ratio of one to ten be maintained. These principles of the West Philadelphia superintendent became known as the Kirkbride plan and served as a model for asylum building throughout the remainder of the nineteenth century.

Kirkbride, other asylum administrators, and lay reformers such as Dorothea Dix took pride in the institution and expounded on its virtues. In their view, the asylum alone provided the atmosphere and facilities in which a mentally ill person could be treated and cured. Family treatment, incarceration in a jail or almshouse, and ordinary hospital care delayed proper therapy, diminishing the patient's chances for recovery. On the other hand, the asylum offered a unique therapeutic setting. Here superintendents did remain attentive to medical treatments, but stressed the value of controlling patients by means of a calm, precise routine. Order in the institution counteracted the instability in society and, when combined with the compassion of the staff, invariably restored the health of the client. Some superintendents went further, claiming that the asylum accomplished much more than simply restoring health. It rejuvenated and morally uplifted patients, transforming them into better persons capable of assuming responsibilities and following a life-style of high ideals (Shershow, 1977; Marshall,1937).

Exaggerated claims about the success of the asylum received publicity and acceptance. Samuel Woodward of Worcester stated that over 80 percent of his patients recovered. A few superintendents asserted 100 percent rates of cure, and others boasted that their curability rates greatly increased each year. These bold statements were supported by arbitrarily compiled statistics. This happened because the definition of recovery lacked precision: a "cured" person could be one who left the asylum and then returned after suffering a relapse, and this sequence could occur many times. One patient might account for several statistical cures. Superintendents also inflated figures to impress colleagues and legislators (Deutsch, 1949: 132–157). Still, the curability pronouncements reflected an optimistic belief that the practice of moral treatment was moving the care of the insane into a new age. There now seemed concrete evidence that insanity was curable, that the asylum held the promise of a millennium for the mentally disturbed. In the history of American mental health care, the exalted confidence and hope of the 1830s and 1840s would never again appear.

The first significant American psychiatric organization, the Association of Medical Superintendents of American Institutions for the Insane, became an instrument for propagandizing the importance of the asylum. It was created in October 1844 when thirteen superintendents of mental hospitals met in Philadelphia (Overholser, 1944; McGovern, 1987). A periodical, the *American Journal of Insanity*, became its official organ. The thrust of the association focused on the management of institutions, and members were kept informed about such issues as the value of different kinds of fuels for heating hospitals, the best types of reading materials for patients, the duties of night attendants, the means of employing inmates in winter, and the need for chapels and chaplains. While concerned with these practical matters, the association also had the broader objective of educating the public about mental disorder. A stated aim of the *American Journal of Insanity* was "to popularize the study of insanity." Superintendents wanted to share their work with the community. Contacts with the lay world, they believed, would help remove prejudices about madness and improve the mental health of the nation. These early psychiatrists possessed a moral righteousness, almost a crusading zeal, emphasizing that insanity was a curable malady, that mentally disordered persons were not wild beasts, that asylums were humane establishments.

THE TURN TOWARD CUSTODIALISM

Within a few decades, by the 1870s, medical superintendents promulgated a different message. The optimism, hope, and confidence of the pre–Civil War administrators faded; the therapeutic rehabilitative goal of the asylum remained but was now largely unfulfilled. Custody rather than cure became the essential task of the public mental institution. This dramatic change was caused by a variety of factors (Bockoven, 1963; Grob, 1973; Savino and Mills, 1967).

Overcrowded facilities constituted a basic element in the story. After 1850, overcrowding was the norm in mental hospitals with the numbers of inmates in every institution ranging between 100 and 200 above capacity. Crowded wards intensified hygenic problems. The increase of clients broke down the therapeutic relationship between physician and patient. Burdened with the problems of administering several hundred patients, a superintendent could not be attentive to the needs of each inmate. And the patients' living area became more restricted. Recreational space was reduced or transformed into sleeping quarters. Inmates were no longer separated by type of illness or condition of recovery. Instead, everyone, regardless of the kind or degree of disorder, was quartered in large open wards.

New kinds of patients aggravated the difficulties stemming from congested facilities. In the early asylum years, physicians and patients shared a common middle-class background, a fact which contributed to the success of moral treatment. After mid-century, the asylum's character was altered by the influx of paupers, immigrants, the criminally insane, the mentally retarded, the aged, and the alcoholic. Many of these newcomers were chronic cases and their presence radically modified the psychological atmosphere of the institution. The attitude of superintendents toward inmates changed noticeably. Faced with increasing numbers of impoverished and foreign-born, administrators held these patients responsible for what was perceived as the prevalence of widespread chronic madness and viewed them as inferior beings without goals, incapable of controlling passions, and indifferent to habits of good health. A self-reinforcing assumption linked the poor and the immigrant to hopeless insanity. In characterizing a large segment of the new clientele in such disparaging terms, administrators lost empathy and understanding, essential qualities in treating the mentally ill. Deterioration in care followed (Jarvis, 1855, 1857; Ranney, 1850; Rosenkrantz and Vinovskis, 1978).

An indication of shifting attitudes toward the insane was the declining belief in curability. Superintendents no longer boasted about discharging large numbers of patients restored to full health. They avoided making percentage analyses of curability statistics and lamented over the increase of chronic cases in asylums. A former believer in the curability ethos, Pliny Earle, superintendent of Northampton State Hospital, Massachusetts, published the findings of his years of statistical research in *The Curability of Insanity* (1887), a book which refuted the exaggerated curability claims of the pre–Civil War generation of asylum superintendents. A profound pessimism permeated Earle's study. His observations on hospital admissions and discharges concluded with two related points: over the years recoveries constantly decreased, and with expanded hospital facilities for the mentally ill came increased numbers of chronic cases. He emphasized that a major preventive effort rather than a search for a cure offered the best way to diminish insanity in America. These pronouncements from such an influential administrator revealed the growing antipathy associated with caring for the mentally ill.

During this time of change, new etiological assumptions and psychiatric theories affected the treatment of the insane. Some interest focused on a hereditarian explanation of mental illness, a perspective which gained attention in the asylum milieu of the 1860s and 1870s. This institutional setting of crowded wards, ambivalent administrators, mixed clientele, and diminishing recoveries facilitated specious diagnoses. Heredity and incurability became synonymous. It was quick and easy to attribute madness to a person's forebears.

Though significant and widely held, this view was not universal in its appeal. Hereditarian notions were de-emphasized, for example, by John P. Gray, one of the most prominent post–Civil War asylum superintendents. Influenced by Wilhelm Griesinger, the German psychiatrist who argued that mental disorders were brain disorders, Gray held to a strict somatic view of mental illness, maintaining that insanity was a cerebral disease. Accordingly, the experience and observations of medical science would cure the insane person, an individual suffering from a diseased brain and nervous system. Insisting that such environmental factors as religious excesses, economic troubles, and political stresses could not cause madness, Gray discounted moral treatment as a philosophy "nourished in the library" completely divorced from medicine. Its chief mode of therapy, the manipulation of the patient's social milieu, had little curative impact. Insanity, he claimed, must be treated like any physical disease (Gray, 1868, 1871, 1884).

A mental hospital regimen emphasizing somatic methods of care did help patients in poor physical condition. Individuals suffering from nutritional deficiencies or alcoholism or accident injuries benefited from the administration of drugs, proper diet, rest, a comfortable room temperature and adequate ventilation. On the other hand, advocating a rigid somaticism that linked insanity to cerebral pathology without scientific verification and that repudiated moral treatment, meant offering a promise, or, in fact, presenting a mythology which placed practitioners in a therapeutic vacuum. Gray and other superintendents wanted the study of mental illness identified with medicine. They were impressed with the emerging specialties of neurology and histology as well as the refined techniques of microscopy and chemical analysis which allowed physicians to observe physiological disorders with greater sophistication. In fact, however, while believing that medical science was the panacea for understanding and treating mental illness, they produced little evidence to demonstrate any physical connection between brain lesions and mental disease. The meager scientific research conducted at mental hospitals remained on a low, superficial plane, and on its own gave no direction as to any particular kind of therapy.

The emphasis on somaticism contributed to a growing estrangement between superintendents and the lay community. These administrators, unlike asylum practitioners of the 1830s and 1840s, concentrated on technical matters which perplexed and alienated lay people; they had little interest in informing the public about insanity and mental health care; they no longer maintained strong links with reformers and prominent leaders of society. Instead, they retreated into a shell of professionalism and became skeptical and defensive about positive criticism. This professional isolation reached a crest during the 1870s and 1880s, a transitional era of readjustment for the mental institution. By this time the asylum was no longer, in word or deed, seen as a retreat, a place committed to rehabilitation and moral regeneration. The optimism and enthusiasm of the early years had faded; the institution had become a custodial facility with a major welfare role. It housed and assumed responsibility for the poor and the alien as well as many types of dependents.

Throughout this time of institutional transition and malaise, the asylum came under attack from assorted critics ranging from foreign physicians to local politicians. One focus of the criticism dealt with the use of restraining devices to control patients, a widespread practice in late nineteenth-century asylums. Many kinds of contrivances were available: steel wristlets, iron handcuffs, chair and bed straps, and the camisole or straitjacket, the most popular and widely used restraining device. Every asylum had rooms designed to isolate inmates in solitary confinement. The physical force of attendants as well as the administration of anesthetics and sedatives such as ether and chloroform constrained an individual. Superintendents claimed an absolute right to use restraints, insisting that certain kinds of patients, notably the violent or the incorrigible, could not be treated in any other way. Criticism of this policy provoked alarm; and administrators were especially indignant when a prominent English physician, John C. Bucknill, condemned the practice in his well-publicized study *Notes on Asylums for the Insane in America* (1876). The application and visibility of restraining mechanisms, he observed, accounted for the public distrust of mental institutions. This controversy remained academic, however, for the prevailing institutional realities demanded a policy of control and order; in effect, the use of mechanical restraints became a necessary option for managing patients in large overcrowded wards (Caplan, 1969; Grissom, 1884).

Another focus of criticism dealt with the institutionalization of sane persons within asylums, a circumstance popularly called false commitment. This matter received much publicity. Newspapers often printed reports of ex-patients who claimed involuntary hospitalization; a best-selling novel, *Hard Cash* (1864), by Charles Reade, an English author, dealt with the irregular admission into an asylum of a wealthy young man by business associates who wanted his fortune. The sensational Elizabeth Packard court case in the early 1860s dramatized the issues surrounding the legal procedures for admitting a person into a mental hospital (Kittrie, 1971: 64–65).

While all of this publicity regarding commitment practices aroused interest and concern, investigations of abuse and neglect in mental hospitals proved even more damaging to the image of the asylum. In 1879, for example, a special committee of the Michigan legislature conducted an inquiry into the Asylum for the Insane at Kalamazoo and uncovered examples of crude and callous maltreatment of inmates perpetrated largely by attendants. Some patients were molested, teased, and physically abused, and, unfortunately, the guilty went unpunished. These revelations at Kalamazoo pointed to a basic, long-standing problem of mental health care, the general inferior quality of institutional personnel. Throughout the nineteenth century, little formal training for asylum workers existed. McLean Asylum in Massachusetts established a school for nurses in 1882, and Buffalo State Asylum graduated its first class of psychiatric nurses in 1888. At most places, staffs consisted of transient persons without idealism or altruism who accepted low salaries, long working hours, and the difficulties of functioning in an emotionally charged and, at times, violent atmosphere. These conditions accounted for staffs remaining in a constant state of flux; an average of one-third of an institution's working force left each year. Attendants remained closest to patients, functioning largely as keepers of order and peace on the wards. Since they applied restraining devices, administered disagreeable treatments, and often engaged in such an abhorrent task as force feeding, patients viewed them with suspicion and fear. Superintendents were preoccupied with administrative duties and gave little comfort or support to institutional residents. In short, patients were isolated and caught in a web of indifference, neglect, and degradation (*Report*, 1879; Santos and Stainbrook, 1949).

A more positive development came in 1880 when the reform efforts of two new professional groups, neurologists and charity or social workers, united to create the National Association for the Protection of the Insane and the Prevention of Insanity (NAPIPI). One concern of NAPIPI was mobilizing support for asylum reform. Toward that end, it promoted critics, particularly dissident neurologists and social workers; it passed resolutions calling for state investigations of mental hospitals; it demanded a congressional inquiry of the nation's asylums; and prominent members of the organization published sharp denunciations of hospital malpractices in both popular and medical journals. Another goal of NAPIPI was to encourage the study of psychiatry in medical colleges. It also struck at the political mismanagement of asylums. In the 1870s and 1880s, corruption was rampant at all levels of government. Political jobbery extended to state mental institutions where superintendencies became political plums, awarded according to the principle of patronage. Reformers were alert to any incident of extravagance or misuse of public money and called for the elimination of politics from all appointments to mental hospitals. A new development, the noninstitutional care of the mentally ill, received the support of NAPIPI. For example, there were calls for boarding the insane with families, and neurologists, not without some self-interest, denigrated asylum care and argued that mental patients were best treated at home (National Association for the Protection of the Insane and the Prevention of Insanity, 1880; Gapin, 1879; Spitzka, 1878; Dewey, 1878; Hammond, 1879).

NAPIPI fell apart largely because of the conflict of interest between neurologists and social workers. Neurologists remained devoted to research, social workers to asylum reform. As the organization concentrated on institutions rather than promoting the scientific study of insanity, neurologists drifted away. Nevertheless, NAPIPI was significant in drawing attention to abuses and the need for reform; it contributed to the passage of new state laws which curbed excessive political influence in asylum affairs and made mental hospital administrations more efficient and subject to periodic inspections.

Although initially superintendents were intolerant and defensive about criticism, feeling slighted especially by the assaults from neurologists, they made changes. A basic institutional problem remained and taxed their energies: the fact of increased admissions and fewer recoveries. Short-term inmates returned to the community; long-term patients rarely recovered and succumbed frequently to "hospitalism" or "institutionalism," a condition characterized by apathy, loss of individualism, and total submission to asylum life. Seeking to avert this condition, to prevent patients from sinking into chronicity, asylum physicians offered some innovative therapeutics, notably massages, Turkish baths, and music therapy. A method of care known as tent treatment involved removing a small number of patients to tents on asylum grounds where they received close attention from the staff, a contrast with the idleness and monotony of stuffy crowded wards (Caplan, 1969: 263–283). Such treatments showed concern, yet they were not widespread and, in any event, failed to effect significant change in patient recovery rates.

THE PROGRESSIVE ERA AND MENTAL HEALTH CARE

Beyond the asylum setting, however, new ideas, goals, and institutions were changing the priorities of American mental health care. These developments occurred against a backdrop of social and intellectual ferment in the wider society. The years around the turn of the century marked a reform era dominated by a spirit of optimism and innovation. This idealism was complemented by concrete achievements in science and technology, particularly medicine. Diphtheria, cholera, tetanus, typhoid, hookworm, and yellow fever were conquered. To reformer and lay person alike, science appeared as the panacea for solving human and societal problems.

If the spirit of the times, the optimism, the enthusiasm, the faith in progress and science, permeated the mental health community, providing a milieu for change, specific factors within psychiatry and related professions focused attention on community care and preventive measures. Neurologists, in their private

offices, contributed to this orientation by treating a new clientele of urban professional and business persons who suffered from such nervous disorders as hy-
pochondria, insomnia, impotence, hysteria, and nervous exhaustion. These were
neurotic, often acute, illnesses and, neurologists insisted, could be cured through
intensive private care. S. Weir Mitchell, a prominent Philadelphia neurologist,
perfected a method known as the rest cure which captured international attention.
It involved strict adherence to a regimen of proper diet, seclusion, and rest in
bed. Mitchell, and other neurologists, accepted a somatic view of insanity, but
appreciated the role played by rapid social change and daily tensions in causing
erratic behavior. They also stressed the importance of psychologically manip-
ulating patients, a method which anticipated the use of psychotherapy in treating
the acutely disordered and in some ways harked back to early principles of moral
treatment (Earnest, 1950; Mitchell, 1884, 1904; Schneck, 1963; Veith, 1962;
Walter, 1970).

The value of psychology in caring for the mentally ill as well as in theorizing
about insanity, in effect, a new view of mental illness, altered the direction of
mental health care. By 1900, psychology was a well-established field with such
prominent leaders as William James and G. Stanley Hall. Rejecting Social Dar-
winism, they emphasized the malleability of human beings; an individual had
the capacity to change, and to choose options for a better life. James and Hall
also were interested in psychopathology, advocated progressive asylum care,
and worked to educate the public and the medical profession about the use of
psychology in the treatment and prevention of mental disorder (Ross, 1972;
Hale, 1971).

A strong psychotherapy movement gained momentum, a reflection of the
growing sensitivity to the psychological resolution of emotional problems. Newspapers and magazines published a flood of articles which explained and offered
cures for mental illness. Along with mind cures, religious psychotherapy struck
a wide response, spreading to many Protestant denominations. This lay popularity
of psychotherapy was accompanied by its growing professional acceptance. It
received much attention at state medical societies; psychiatric and medical journals carried numerous articles on this new treatment; some of the country's
leading psychiatrists and neurologists vigorously promoted it. By 1910, psychotherapy had achieved respectability; this was an important factor in accounting
for the positive reception of psychoanalysis in the United States (Barker, 1906;
Burnham, 1960, 1967; Cunningham, 1962; Hinkle, 1908; Prince, 1912; Gifford,
1978).

The new directions and ferment within psychiatry, neurology, and psychology
were exemplified in the life and work of Adolf Meyer, one of the leading early
twentieth-century American psychiatrists. Throughout his career, Meyer worked
to improve mental hospitals, aiming especially at upgrading staffs and integrating
research with the daily care and treatment of patients. As director of the Henry
Phipps Psychiatric Clinic, a facility associated with the Johns Hopkins University
Medical School, he was in a commanding position to influence some of the

country's best medical students, physicians, and psychiatrists. Here he developed a program of community care and prevention. Meyer also wanted an integration of psychology with biology and argued that an individual was a physical and social being, a person shaped by a unique environment and a lifetime of experiences and conflicts. The community, the individual's home and social setting, Meyer felt, contributed to the etiology of mental illness, and an understanding of its processes enhanced a practitioner's sensitivity to a client's daily troubles. Meyer aimed at relating psychiatry to the problems of everyday life. Central to this concern with community mental health was his institution, the psychiatric clinic, a facility located in the community which offered services ranging from educational and prevention programs to the care of all types of clients who were treated as outpatients (Campbell, 1937; Grob, 1963; Lief, 1948).

The Henry Phipps Clinic under Meyer represents only one example of the new types of mental health facilities emerging in early twentieth-century America. Another institutional development, the psychiatric ward in a general hospital, originated in Albany, New York, in 1902. Its director, J. Montgomery Mosher, received the title Attending Specialist in Mental Diseases, and administered a two-story building designated Pavilion F. It operated on voluntary admissions, accepting acute cases of disorder, notably persons unable to cope with the stresses and disappointments of life. Without care, their conditions might deteriorate and lapse into chronicity, and Mosher held that a general hospital could treat mental patients just as easily as it handled those suffering from physical disease. He cited statistics to buttress this point: in a six-year period, with over 1300 admissions, only 126 were committed to asylums; presumably all of the others went home either recovered or in an improved condition (Mosher, 1909, 1915).

Another new mental health facility, the first university psychopathic hospital, opened in 1906 at the University of Michigan. The director, Albert M. Barrett, a student of Adolf Meyer, specified its chief function: to care for and treat acute cases of mental disorder. Barrett had a special interest in working with juvenile delinquents and extended that activity to Detroit where a clinic was attached to the Wayne County Juvenile Court. Here a team consisting of a psychologist, a social worker, and a psychiatrist, as well as court officials, handled the cases and much of their emphasis focused on studying the family and social settings of patients before and after treatment (Barrett, 1921, 1922).

In 1912, another new institution, the first psychopathic hospital connected to a mental facility, opened as a department of Boston State Asylum. Initially it served as a refuge and an observation place for mentally distressed persons needing emergency care. Social workers were employed and, under the direction of Mary C. Jarrett, maintained close ties between hospital and community. She coined the term "psychiatric social worker" to refer to a person who investigated the home background of a patient and supervised aftercare programs to facilitate the client's return to a job and community life (Briggs, 1906; Briggs et al., 1922; Southard, 1913).

Jarrett's program coupled with the efforts of social workers at many other mental health facilities expanded outpatient activities; they also served a new and growing clientele, juvenile delinquents. In this field, they were influenced greatly by the theory and practice of William Healy, a psychiatrist at the Juvenile Psychopathic Institute in Chicago and author of *The Individual Delinquent* (1915). Healy challenged degenerate and hereditarian assumptions about criminology, concluding that delinquency should not be oversimplified by any facile theory. Cautioning social workers to scrutinize critically existing behavioral notions, he urged that each case be studied and accepted on its own merits. Healy's work also demonstrated how psychiatry could help resolve a major social problem; by exposing the root causes of crime and treating juvenile offenders, his social psychiatry offered a tool for bettering the community (Jarrett, 1919; Pumphrey, 1973).

Such a view that psychiatry might be applied to social issues was an alien concept, an unthinkable idea, in the narrow and restrictive asylum world of the 1890s. Now, in the second decade of the twentieth century, it formed part of a broad mental health perspective embracing research, an environmental etiology, and involvement in community affairs. New mental health professionals, notably psychologists and social workers, along with psychiatrists and neurologists, formed a team which operated out of such new facilities as private clinics and general hospitals as well as some traditional mental institutions. Their priorities dealt with prevention and the care of clients suffering from acute disorders, however, an approach which implicitly relegated the severely and chronically mentally ill to continued institutional oblivion (Russell, 1913; Salmon, 1917; Sicherman, 1973).

Establishment of the National Committee for Mental Hygiene in 1909 in New York City sustained the hope and optimism of this reform era and broadened the appeal, ideology, and support for mental health care. This was an opportune time for voluntary public health associations; the success of medical and lay efforts in controlling such communicable diseases as tuberculosis, hookworm, and syphilis aroused expectations and a belief that mental illness might be prevented and conquered. The key person in the mental hygiene movement was Clifford W. Beers, a businessman, ex-mental patient, and author of *A Mind That Found Itself* (1908). He was an entrepreneur of philanthropy, a skilled fundraiser and organizer who captured the support of an extraordinarily wide mix of influential persons from the worlds of education, religion, social work, business, medicine, and psychiatry. The program of Beers and other mental hygienists identified with the new trends and facilities in mental health care, notably the employment of psychologists and social workers, the development of outpatient clinics and aftercare programs, and the need for psychopathic hospitals and wards. The traditional mental hospital was downgraded as an inferior facility, a human warehouse which quartered the failures of society (Dain, 1980; Bell, 1980: 92–96). This stigmatization of the asylum strengthened the institution's custodial role.

While supporting progressive movements in the care of the insane, mental hygienists remained preoccupied with educational and informational campaigns as well as the problems associated with prevention and acute forms of mental illness. They accepted a prevailing conviction that mental problems originated in childhood. In other words, proper child rearing could prevent any behavioral disorder, an assumption that encouraged the channeling of preventive efforts toward the family and the school (Abbott, 1920; Bingham, 1925; Campbell, 1917, 1919; Gesell, 1926; Glueck, 1924; Truitt, 1927; White, 1920).

Beyond these two prime areas, other interests and activities extended to national and even international issues. For example, the designation of dangerous occupations, labor management disputes, and the affairs of the League of Nations all fell within the ambit of mental hygiene. For many, mental hygiene became a cure-all, a panacea for resolving any issue. This promotion of broad goals and programs, and its compatibility with the general reform ethic of the period, accounts for the wide support professional and lay people gave to the movement (Barker, 1917, 1918; Brown, 1933; Fisher, 1921; Lord, 1934; Southard, 1920; Pratt, 1922).

A significant result of the mental hygiene movement was the prestige it conferred on psychiatry, a development which evolved out of the work of the National Committee for Mental Hygiene during World War I. The committee helped screen the mentally ill and deficient from the armed forces and establish facilities for treating mentally disturbed soldiers. Its first president, Thomas W. Salmon, went to Europe as a psychiatric consultant to the American military units. He studied shell shock, a phenomenon of popular interest, educating people to the anguish mental illness could bring. After the war, the committee developed programs for the rehabilitation and hospitalization of mentally ill veterans (Bailey, 1918; Bond, 1950; Brown, 1920; Kindred, 1927; Rivers, 1918; Schwab, 1920). It also made an impact on professional education, promoting the teaching of psychiatry and mental hygiene in schools of medicine, nursing, and social work. Another change may be attributed to the efforts of Beers's organization, the acceptance by lay persons and professionals of the term *mental illness*, replacing the old label of *insanity* (Pratt, 1930). In sum, all of the varied programs and activities of the mental hygiene movement revealed the new directions of American mental health care. Above all, the focus was on the future, anticipating that preventive work opened new vistas for the mentally troubled. This perspective left little concern for a root problem of care, the condition and treatment of the chronic insane. In their drive to reach a greater and better future, the mental hygienists virtually wrote off this large group of patients.

CONTINUITY AND CHANGE AT MID-TWENTIETH CENTURY

Throughout the 1920s and 1930s, while the mental hygiene movement expanded and adopted diverse programs, the state mental hospital remained the primary site of care. Many of the new types of facilities, notably the psychopathic hospitals, became adjuncts of the traditional state institution. No one called for its dissolution (Rothman, 1980). Most patients received some form of occupational therapy and their tasks related largely to maintaining the self-sufficiency of the institution. These included repair work, employment on the hospital farm, laundry, kitchen, and sewing jobs as well as those involving the construction of beds, chairs, and tables. Proponents of occupational therapy testified to its efficacy, asserting that it even brought relief and hope to chronic cases (Bond, 1928; Briggs, 1923; Davis, 1930; Emch, 1935; Haas, 1925; Holland, 1931; Hunt, 1931; Pollock, 1923). Hydrotherapy never elicted such dramatic claims, but it also was a persistent feature of institutional life. Some of its equipment included the needle spray shower, the steam as well as the whirlpool bath, the continuous bath, and the cold pack. Such hydrotherapeutic measures were used primarily to calm patients, making them more manageable (Kindwall and Henry, 1934; O'Malley, 1913). State hospitals engaged in some experimental medical treatments, notably fever therapy, the removal of various organs for focal infection, and vasectomy. Psychotherapy had only limited application to hospital inmates. A few places engaged in some special therapeutics. For instance, at Danville State Hospital, Pennsylvania, a regimen called "normal living" related institutional routines to the patient's former life patterns and established a program of rest, sleep, proper nutrition, recreation, and work (Hill, 1933; Kopeloff and Cheney, 1922; Shields, 1939).

Undermining these treatment efforts were the perennial problems of institutional care: overcrowded facilities; the uncertain, fragmentary state of etiological knowledge which made it difficult to determine proper treatment; and inadequate, limited personnel. This institutional milieu actually encouraged a brain drain: research-oriented psychiatrists went to the newly established psychopathic hospitals and private and university clinics. Others established lucrative private practices or found a congenial atmosphere in such developing specialties as child or industrial psychiatry. Nurses, social workers, and psychologists showed a decreasing interest in state hospital employment. These mental health workers had other options and opportunities, notably in courts, schools, penal institutions, and general hospitals (Bock, 1933; Newer, 1936).

All of these institutional dilemmas were aggravated by the economic depression of the 1930s. It devastated mental hospitals, forcing budget reductions, the curtailment of programs, and the abandonment of plans for expansion. Patient populations increased. Many unemployed older persons, the rejects of an economically depressed society, were admitted and retained, a new development which cast the mental hospital in the role of a relief agency. Through public works programs, the federal government offered some aid and relief to mental institutions, particularly to projects which improved physical facilities. It intervened directly in the lives of patients with some educational, recreational, and occupational therapy programs. Its key objective, however, was employing people rather than resolving the problems of institutional psychiatry (Baskett, 1935; Bonsteel, 1940; Dunn, 1934; Dynes, 1939; Menninger and Chidester, 1933; Pollock, 1935; Thom, 1932).

In these depression years, relief from the problems and tedium of hospital care came, not from any government source, but from within psychiatry. A new and dramatic therapy, shock treatment, was introduced in mental institutions in the mid and late 1930s. It received an enthusiastic reception from institutional psychiatrists who assumed that here at last was a means for attacking directly the psychoses. Three basic types of shock treatment evolved in chronological sequence: first came the insulin method followed by the use of metrazol which was replaced by electroconvulsive therapy or electroshock therapy. At about the same time, a surgical procedure, prefrontal lobotomy, was adopted throughout the country. Shock treatments and lobotomy remained popular until the 1950s when pharmacotherapy gained wide acceptance (Kalinowsky and Hoch, 1962; Sackler et al., 1956).

Electric convulsive therapy (ECT) proved the most durable of the shock treatments. The use of insulin and metrazol peaked in the late 1930s; each had a definite liability. The insulin treatment process took too long and tied up too many hospital personnel; once a patient experienced metrazol that person held a profound fear of it, a fact which limited its appeal. On the other hand, ECT was quick, inexpensive, and easy to administer. Any complication to practitioners seemed but a minor inconvenience. Adherents of electric shock treatment made exorbitant claims: it decreased the rate of suicides, calmed the excited, and brought life to the depressed. Indeed, it seemed the most effective therapy, far superior to any other form of treatment. This enthusiasm dampened, however, as evidence accumulated that ECT produced less promising conflicting results, and an acrimonious controversy over its use and effectiveness ensued. Yet the merits of the pros and cons of this debate remained academic to hospital administrators. A basic institutional reality dictated the application of ECT: the alternative was custodial care. In short, shock treatment brought movement and hope to mental hospital therapeutics; it aroused interest even in treating the most difficult patients. It did not, however, diminish the number of chronic cases (Bell, 1980: 135–149).

At this time, the early 1940s, another major historical event, World War II, exerted a powerful impact on mental institutions. In many ways, the war marks a watershed in the history of American mental health care. On one account, it dramatized mental disturbance as a major problem in society. A large number of persons were rejected for military service because of some mental disorder, and a sizable number were discharged for a psychiatric reason. The wartime psychiatric experience also revealed a high incidence of neurosis and other combat-related disorders among soldiers for which a new method of treatment, group psychotherapy, was developed (Appel, 1946; Menninger, 1947, 1948; McNeel, 1946; Braceland, 1947).

Another legacy of World War II was the massive movement of the federal government into mental health areas. Before the war, federal programs were limited to the Public Health Service and such activities as the medical inspection of aliens and some projects and studies on crime and the treatment of addicts. St. Elizabeths Hospital in Washington, D.C., was an excellent federal mental institution. During the war, the severe shortage of trained personnel and the rapidly increasing number of military psychiatric casualties demanded aggressive federal intervention. A large building program of psychiatric facilities was inaugurated and soon after the war, with the National Mental Health Act of 1946 (Public Law 79–487), the federal government began a program focusing on three areas: research on etiology, prevention, and treatment; training mental health personnel; and improving local and state services. The act also created the National Institute of Mental Health, which began to operate in 1949. The psychiatric profession enthusiastically endorsed the 1946 legislation, viewing it as a major effort to upgrade the country's mental hospitals (Lowry, 1949; Felix, 1948; Brand, 1965).

Throughout the war years, the state hospital system deteriorated, the result of maintaining the austerity policy of reduced budgets and programs which was initiated early in the depression. Grim and ugly conditions developed. Shortly after the war ended, a wave of books, magazine articles, and newspaper stories exposed the oppressive state of institutional care (Deutsch, 1948; Gorman, 1954; Wright, 1947). Administrators confirmed these reports, admitting that many hospitals were indeed snakepits. One superintendent confessed that the grass around his hospital received better care than the patients inside. Chronicity remained the fundamental problem. State hospitals accumulated the most severe cases, as well as rejects from other psychiatric facilities and correctional agencies, who remained on the back wards for long periods of time. In 1950, the average institutional stay ranged between seven and ten years, and around half of the patients in the nation's mental hospitals were over fifty-five years of age.

Professional concern about these dismal conditions encouraged change and experimentation with an emphasis placed on the interaction between the patient and the social milieu of the institution. This perspective had numerous precedents: nineteenth-century moral treatment, the work of Harry Stack Sullivan at Sheppard and Enoch Pratt Hospital in the late 1920s, the "total push" method of Abraham Myerson at Boston State Hospital in the 1930s, Anna Freud's observations of war orphans, and Bruno Bettelheim's experiments with institutionalized children during World War II. After the war, and well into the 1950s, research on the social environment of the mental hospital produced an enormous literature. Social scientists, especially, analyzed such areas of institutional life as the social atmosphere of the ward, staff relationships, patient friendship patterns, the values of attendants, and staff images of patients (Belknap, 1956; Caudill, 1958; Greenblatt, Levinson, and Williams, 1957; Stanton and Schwartz, 1954). Changes growing out of this kind of research were made at a few hospitals. A notable example was Boston Psychopathic Hospital under the direction of Harry C. Solomon. Here rooms were redecorated; punitive measures eliminated; patient government inaugurated. The most important focus of change dealt with improving interpersonal relationships, particularly between attendants and patients. The staff received continuous training and stimulation by means of psychodramas, seminars, and group conferences. A basic goal remained constant: the enrichment of life on the ward. This therapeutic regimen also demanded good community-hospital relations, assuming that positive contacts with outsiders aroused interest and acceptance of treatment programs, and encouraged the participation of volunteers in hospital activities. The results of these varied therapeutics at Boston Psychopathic remained controversial. Hospital reports showed increased discharges and improved patient behavior. Administrators, however, attributed the success to the employment of all kinds of therapy, including shock treatments and lobotomy. Presumably, the creation of a permissive, enriched institutional social milieu represented only one thrust of a multifarious attack on chronicity (Greenblatt et al., 1955).

In the early 1950s, other institutions, along with Boston Psychopathic, initiated intensive treatment programs which met with success in producing increased patient discharges. These hospitals were characterized by an optimistic, aggressive leadership committed to experimentation, an enriched social milieu for patients, a continual program of training and expansion of staff, and professionals skilled in varied therapeutics. Most mental hospitals lacked such qualities, however, and remained overcrowded, understaffed, and inadequately financed. In these facilities, patients received little treatment, only care and custody.

Again, as in the past, a new treatment raised expectations, promising a way out of a distressing situation. In 1953–1954, the tranquilizing agents, the ataractic or ataraxic drugs, notably chlorpromazine (CPZ), were introduced in American mental hospitals, inaugurating a major therapeutic revolution as well as the new field of psychopharmacology. CPZ was called the miracle drug and psychiatrists in professional journals and at conferences and symposiums confirmed its dramatic impact on hospital residents, testifying how it transformed abusive, loud patients into calm and cooperative ones. Quiet, pacified patients, in turn, produced a subdued institutional atmosphere: order was maintained, the need for drastic discipline measures diminished, staff morale improved, and new treatment options emerged especially with former intractables who were now amenable to psychotherapy and recreational programs (Overholser, 1956; Swazey, 1974).

A most significant effect of the widespread and rapid application of drug treatment was the reduction of the patient population. This trend began in 1956, and the years since have witnessed a major decrease in the numbers of institutionalized mentally ill. On a drug regimen, many patients could live in the community and receive care and treatment at a general hospital or some other clinical setting. The policy worked well with younger, more acute cases of mental distress. For older chronic patients, however, drug treatments did little more than increase manageability in the institutional setting; the rate of community discharges from this patient group remained largely unchanged, though in time many would be relocated to nursing home facilities (Brill and Patton, 1957, 1959; Greenblatt et al., 1965).

Critics of drug therapy warned about its long-term effects, directing attention to a neurological condition known as tardive dyskinesia. Its syndrome includes motor disorders and bizarre facial muscular activity. Psychotherapists also made charges of drug dependency, and asserted that institutional pharmaceutical therapy tranquilized only the hospital social milieu, a fact which benefited the staff more than the patients. In other words, subduing a belligerent patient by means of drugs made that individual acceptable to staff without affecting the inmate's behavioral problem. Drug therapy, then, created a false sense of security and accomplishment by equating quiet wards with therapeutic success (Cohen, 1956; Meerloo, 1955; Bonn, 1962). This criticism was viewed with disdain by psychopharmacologists who assumed an anti-historical attitude which downgraded previous psychiatric treatments. With the pharmaceuticals, drug clinicians announced, "a truly biologic psychiatry" was emerging, "unprecedented advances" were occurring; indeed, some made reference to "the chemical conquest of mental illness" (Ayd and Blackwell, 1970; Rinkel, 1966).

The debate over the pros and cons of pharmaceutical therapy was obscured by the success of the psychotropic drugs in ameliorating disturbed behavior. This fact opened a new course for mental health care. Now patients could be released into the community, demonstrating that there were concrete alternatives to hospitalization. The way was clear for the development of community psychiatry and a new hierarchy of community mental health facilities and authorities.

Scathing criticisms of the state hospital system by prominent mental health officials accompanied, and facilitated, the drift toward community care. Robert H. Felix, for example, a president of the American Psychiatric Association and director of the National Institute of Mental Health, referred to the mental hospital as an antitherapeutic facility and called for programs which would help discharged patients adjust to normal life. In fact, by the late 1950s, a network of agencies existed which eased the transition of persons moving from hospital to community living. The most notable examples included the halfway house, the sheltered workshop, and the ex-mental patient society; each reflected the new trend toward community care programs (Felix, 1964; Solomon, 1958; Blain, 1975; Freeman and Simmons, 1963).

A major factor in the growth of the community mental health movement was the decisive intervention of the federal and the state governments. New York moved first, passing a Community Mental Health Act in 1954; over the years, other states followed suit. The federal government, authorized by the Mental Health Study Act of 1955 (Public Law 84–182), created the Joint Commission on Mental Illness and Health, which spent over five years scrutinizing the nation's mental health services. Its final report, *Action for Mental Health* (1961), proclaimed revelations about the mental health system and called for measures to improve it. One of its most distressing observations was the disclosure of general lay and professional rejection of the mentally ill, a fact which has thwarted treatment programs. In its recommendations, the commission called for an end to the construction of large mental hospitals and claimed that only 20 percent of the nation's 227 state hospitals were therapeutic centers, an observation which drew the wrath of many institutional psychiatrists. Its most important recommendation dealt with the delivery of care, a demand for the creation of a new source of outpatient treatment, a community mental health clinic. This kind of facility, offering multifarious services and staffed by a team of psychiatrists, psychologists, and social workers, would form the core of a national mental health program.

Many other agencies, committees, and conferences corroborated the recommendations of the Joint Commission, demanding more community involvement in all areas of mental health care. And it was within this context of lay and professional ferment and debate that President John F. Kennedy, in a message to Congress in February 1963, pleaded for "a bold new approach," a comprehensive community care program. Some months later, in October 1963, a few weeks before he died, Kennedy signed the Mental Retardation Facilities and Community Mental Health Centers Construction Act (Public Law 88–164), best known as the Community Mental Health Centers Act of 1963. At that time, 2,000 community mental health centers were projected. Here was a promise, perhaps a dramatic breakthrough in the delivery of care, a concrete alternative to the asylum and long-term hospitalization (Kennedy, 1964; Freeman, 1967).

CONCLUSION

Many therapies and a few central themes emerge from this historical survey of American mental health care. Each new therapy may be tagged as representing something ephemeral or trendy or unscientific; yet the constant movement and groping for effective treatments stand as a major positive development in this story. They have demonstrated the vigor, the creativity, the constant experimentation involved in the search for a way to bring solace to the mentally distressed. This carries some irony; the recipients of these varied therapeutics have been viewed generally with disdain. Over the years, society has rejected and isolated the mentally ill, and maintained an ambivalent attitude toward the mental institution. This general negativism has handicapped the development of productive strategies for the delivery of care.

The institution itself was cast into self-defeating roles which made a travesty of its basic therapeutic purpose. Most damaging, it became a welfare facility, a depository for society's downtrodden and rejects, the elderly, the deviant, the poor, the loveless and lonely, and other marginal people, the social and psychological outcasts of the wider society. In consequence, a conservative mental health order evolved, a system geared toward providing control and custody, the end product of uncertain, conflicting institutional policies and societal negligence and indifference.

A challenge to this order came in the opening years of the twentieth century, during the Progressive Era, and then, later, after World War II, with the protests reaching a climax in the mid and late 1960s. In both periods, a great articulation of discontent agitated all areas of American life and penetrated the field of mental health. In both instances, the mental institution remained, though reduced in professional prestige and stature, while innovations occurred in other fields of mental health. For example, the number and kinds of mental health workers increased; psychiatry grew more influential as an arbiter of social issues; and the public became more sensitive to mental health issues and problems. The changes and challenges after World War II were more significant. At that time, the dismal institutional scene, the result of years of apathy and financial re-trenchment, coupled with an awareness that mental illness constituted a major social problem, made positive change imperative and prepared a receptive setting for the drive and fervor of the community mental health movement.

REFERENCES

Abbott, E. S. 1920. Program for Mental Hygiene in the Public Schools. *Mental Hygiene* 4: 320–330.

Appel, J. W. 1946. Incidence of Neuropsychiatric Disorders in the United States Army in World War II. *American Journal of Psychiatry* 102: 433–436.

Ayd, F. J., Jr., and Blackwell, B., eds. 1970. *Discoveries in Biological Psychiatry*. Philadelphia: J. B. Lippincott.

Bailey, P. 1918. Care and Disposition of the Military Insane. *Mental Hygiene* 2: 345–358.

Barker, L. F. 1906. Some Experiences with the Simpler Methods of Psychotherapy and Re-Education. *American Journal of Medical Science* 132: 499–522.

Barker, L. F. 1917. The Wider Field of Work of the National Committee for Mental Hygiene. *Mental Hygiene* 1: 4–6.

Barker, L. F. 1918. The First Ten Years of the National Committee for Mental Hygiene, with Some Comments on Its Future. *Mental Hygiene* 2: 557–581.

Barrett, A. 1921. The Psychopathic Hospital. *American Journal of Insanity* 77: 309–320.

Barrett, A. 1922. The Broadened Interests of Psychiatry. *American Journal of Psychiatry* 79: 1–13.

Baskett, G. T. 1935. The Depression and Mental Health. *Mental Health Bulletin* 13: 5–7.

Beers, C. W. 1908. *A Mind That Found Itself*. New York: Doubleday.

Belknap, I. 1956. *Human Problems of a State Mental Hospital*. New York: McGraw-Hill.

Bell, L. V. 1980. *Treating the Mentally Ill: From Colonial Times to the Present*. New York: Praeger.

Bingham, A. T. 1925. The Application of Psychiatry to High School Problems. *Mental Hygiene* 9: 1–27.

Blain, D. 1975. *Twenty-Five Years of Hospital and Community Psychiatry* 26: 605–609.

Bock, A. V. 1933. Psychiatry in Private Practice. *New England Journal of Medicine* 208: 1092–1094.

Bockoven, J. S. 1963. *Moral Treatment in American Psychiatry*. New York: Springer.

Bond, E. D. 1950. *Thomas W. Salmon: Psychiatrist*. New York: W. W. Norton.

Bond, M. 1928. How Occupational Therapy Is Used in the Mental Hospital. *Modern Hospital* 30: 81–82.

Bonn E. M. 1962. Use of Drugs in a Mental Hospital: Please Pass the Pills. *Mental Hospital* 13: 208–209.

Bonsteel, R. M. 1940. A Recreation-Occupational Therapy Project at a State Hospital under WPA Auspices. *Mental Hygiene* 24: 552–565.

Braceland, F. J. 1947. Psychiatric Lessons from World War II. *American Journal of Psychiatry* 103: 587–593.

Brand, J. L. 1965. The National Mental Health Act of 1946. *Bulletin of the History of Medicine* 39: 231–245.

Briggs, L. V. 1906. Observation Hospital for Mental Disease. *Boston Medical and Surgical Journal* 154: 696–702.

Briggs, L. V. 1923. *Occupation as a Substitute for Restraint in the Treatment of the Mentally Ill*. Boston: Wright & Potter.

Briggs, L. V., and collaborators. 1922. *History of the Psychopathic Hospital, Boston, Massachusetts*. Boston: Wright & Potter.

Brill, H., and Patton, R. E. 1957. Analysis of 1955–56 Population Fall in New York State Mental Hospitals in First Year of Large Scale Use of Tranquilizing Drugs. *American Journal of Psychiatry* 114: 509–514.

Brill, H., and Patton, R. E. 1959. Analysis of Population Re-education in New York State Mental Hospitals during the First Four Years of Large Scale Therapy with Psychotropic Drugs. *American Journal of Psychiatry* 116: 495–508.

Brown, S. 1920. Nervous and Mental Disorders in Soldiers. *Mental Hygiene* 2: 404–433.

Brown, S. 1933. Community Work in Mental Hygiene. *Psychiatric Quarterly* 7: 547–562.

Bucknill, J. C. 1876. *Notes on Asylums for the Insane in America*. London: J & A Churchill.

Burnham, J. C. 1960. Psychiatry, Psychology, and the Progressive Movement. *American Quarterly* 12: 457–465.

Burnham, J. C. 1967. *Psychoanalysis and Medicine: 1894–1918. Medicine, Science, and Culture*. New York: International Universities Press.

Campbell, C. M. 1917. Educational Methods and the Fundamental Causes of Dependency. *Mental Hygiene* 1: 235–240.

Campbell, C. M. 1919. Education and Mental Hygiene. *Mental Hygiene* 3: 398–408.

Campbell, C. M. 1937. Adolf Meyer. *Archives of Neurology and Psychiatry* 37: 715–724.

Caplan, R. 1969. *Psychiatry and the Community in Nineteenth Century America*. New York: Basic Books.

Carlson, E. T., and Chale, M. F. 1960. Dr. Rufus Wyman of the McLean Asylum. *American Journal of Psychiatry* 116: 1034–1037.

Caudill, W. 1958. *The Psychiatric Hospital as a Small Society*. Cambridge: Harvard University Press.

Cohen, I. M. 1956. Complications of Chlorpromazine. *American Journal of Psychiatry* 113: 115–121.

Cunningham, R. J. 1962. The Emmanuel Movement: A Variety of American Religious Experience. *American Quarterly* 14: 48–63.

Dain, N. 1960. Milieu Therapy in the Nineteenth Century: Patient Care at the Friend's Asylum, Frankford, Pennsylvania, 1817–1861. *Journal of Nervous and Mental Disease* 131: 277–290.

Dain, N. 1964. *Concepts of Insanity in the United States, 1789–1865*. New Brunswick: Rutgers University Press.

Dain, N. 1971. *Disordered Minds: The First Century of Eastern State Hospital in Williamsburg, Virginia, 1766–1866*. Williamsburg: Colonial Williamsburg Foundation.

Dain, N. 1975. American Psychiatry in the 18th Century. In *American Psychiatry: Past, Present, and Future*, eds. G. Kriegman, R. D. Gardner, and D. W. Abse. Charlottesville: University Press of Virginia.

Dain, N. 1980. *Clifford W. Beers: Advocate for the Insane*. Pittsburgh: University of Pittsburgh Press.

Dain, N., and Carlson, E. T. 1959. Social Class and Psychological Medicine in the United States, 1789–1824. *Bulletin of the History of Medicine* 33: 45–55.

Davies, J. D. 1955. *Phrenology: Fad and Science. A 19th Century American Crusade*. New Haven: Yale University Press.

Davis, J. E. 1930. The Value of Physical Education for the Mentally Ill. *Modern Hospital* 35: 79–84.

Deutsch, A. 1948. *The Shame of the States*. New York: Harcourt, Brace.

Deutsch, A. 1949. *The Mentally Ill in America*. 2nd ed. New York: Columbia University Press.

Dewey, R. S. 1878. Present and Prospective Management of the Insane. *Journal of Nervous and Mental Disease* 5: 60–94.

Dunn, M. 1934. Psychiatric Treatment of the Effects of the Depression: Its Possibilities and Limitations. *Mental Hygiene* 18: 179–186.

Dynes, J. B. 1939. Mental Disorders in the CCC Camps. *Mental Hygiene* 23: 363–370.

Earle, P. 1887. *The Curability of Insanity: A Series of Studies*. Philadelphia: J. B. Lippincott.

Earnest, E. 1950. *S. Weir Mitchell: Novelist and Physician*. Philadelphia: University of Pennsylvania Press.

Eaton, L. 1953. Eli Todd and the Hartford Retreat. *New England Quarterly* 24: 435–454.

Eaton, L. 1957. *New England Hospitals, 1790–1813*. Ann Arbor: University of Michigan Press.

Emch, M. 1935. The Role of Occupational Therapy in Modern Psychiatry. *American Journal of Psychiatry* 92: 207–214.

Felix, R. H. 1948. The National Mental Health Program. *Public Health Reports* 63: 837–847.

Felix, R. H. 1964. Community Mental Health: A Federal Perspective. *American Journal of Psychiatry* 121: 428–432.

Fisher. B. 1921. Has Mental Hygiene a Practical Use in Industry. *Mental Hygiene* 5: 479–496.

Freeman, A. M. 1967. Historical and Political Roots of the Community Mental Health Centers Act. *American Journal of Orthopsychiatry* 37: 487–494.

Freeman, H. E., and Simmons, O. G. 1963. *The Mental Patient Comes Home*. New York: John Wiley.

Gapin, C. 1879. Some Exceptions to the Present Management of Hospitals for the Insane. *Journal of Nervous and Mental Disease* 6: 441–449.

Gesell, A. 1926. The Kindergarten as a Mental Hygiene Agency. *Mental Hygiene* 10: 27–37.

Gifford, G. E., Jr., ed. 1978. *Psychoanalysis, Psychotherapy, and the New England Medical Scene, 1894–1944*. New York: Science History Publications.

Glueck, B. 1924. Constructive Possibilities of a Mental Hygiene of Childhood. *Mental Hygiene* 8: 648–667.

Gorman, M. 1954. *Every Other Bed*. New York: World.

Grange, K. M. 1961. Pinel and Eighteenth Century Psychiatry. *Bulletin of the History of Medicine* 35: 442–453.

Gray, J. P. 1868. Insanity and Its Relation to Medicine. *American Journal of Insanity* 25: 145–172.

Gray, J. P. 1871. The Dependence of Insanity on Physical Disease. *American Journal of Insanity* 27: 377–408.

Gray, J. P. 1884. Heredity. *American Journal of Insanity* 41: 1–21.

Greenblatt, M., Levinson, D. J., Williams, R. H. 1957. *The Patient and the Mental Hospital*. Glencoe, Ill.: Free Press.

Greenblatt, M., Solomon, M. H., Evans, A. S., Brooks, G. W. 1965. *Drugs and Social Therapy in Chronic Schizophrenia*. Springfield, Ill.: Charles C Thomas.

Greenblatt, M., York, R. H., Brown, E. L., and Hyde, R. W. 1955. *From Custodial to Therapeutic Patient Care in Mental Hospitals*. New York: Russell Sage Foundation.

Grissom, E. 1884. Mechanical Protection for the Violent Insane. *American Journal of Insanity* 41: 129–150.

Grob, G. N. 1962. Samuel Woodward and the Practice of Psychiatry in Early Nineteenth Century America. *Bulletin of the History of Medicine* 36: 420–443.

Grob, G. N. 1963. Adolf Meyer on American Psychiatry in 1895. *American Journal of Psychiatry* 119: 1135–1142.

Grob, G. N. 1965. Origins of the State Mental Hospital System: A Case Study. *Bulletin of the Menninger Clinic* 27: 1–18.

Grob, G. N. 1966. *The State and the Mentally Ill.: A History of Worcester State Hospital in Massachusetts, 1830–1920*. Chapel Hill: University of North Carolina Press.

Grob, G. N. 1973. *Mental Institutions in America: Social Policy to 1875*. New York: Free Press.

Haas, L. J. 1925. Occupational Therapy—A Field of Endeavor for Men. *Modern Hospital* 25: 357–359.

Hale, N. G., Jr. 1971. *Freud and the Americans: The Beginnings of Psychoanalysis in the United States, 1876–1917*. New York: Oxford University Press.

Hammond, W. A. 1879. *The Non-Asylum Treatment of the Insane*. New York: G. P. Putnam's Sons.

Hawke, D. F. 1971. *Benjamin Rush*. New York: Bobbs-Merrill.

Healy, W. 1915. *The Individual Delinquent*. Boston: Little, Brown.

Hill, L. B. 1933. Obstacles to Psychotherapy. *American Journal of Psychiatry* 90: 679–683.

Hinkle, B. 1908. Psychotherapy, with Some of Its Results. *Journal of the American Medical Association* 50: 1495–1498.

Holland, J. A. 1931. Physical Treatment of Mental Illness. *New England Journal of Medicine* 205: 371–373.

Hunt, C. W. 1931. Pennsylvania's Mental Hospital Farms. *Mental Health Bulletin* 8: 5–7.

Hunter, R. J. 1955. *The Origin of the Philadelphia General Hospital Blockley Division.* Philadelphia: Rittenhouse Press.

Jarrett, M. C. 1919. The Psychiatric Thread Running Through All Social Case Work. *Proceedings*, National Conference of Social Work. 587–593.

Jarvis, E. 1855. *Insanity and Idiocy in Massachusetts: Report of the Commission of Lunacy, 1855.* Cambridge: Harvard University Press, 1971.

Jarvis, E. 1857. Mental and Physical Characteristics of Pauperism. *American Journal of Insanity* 13: 309–320.

Jimenez, M. A. 1987. *Changing Faces of Madness: Early American Attitudes and Treatment of the Insane.* Hanover, N. H.: University Press of New England.

Joint Commission On Mental Illness and Health. 1961. *Action for Mental Health.* New York: Basic Books.

Kalinowsky, O. B., and Hoch, P. H. 1962. *Shock Treatments, Psychosurgery, and Other Somatic Treatments in Psychiatry.* New York: Grune & Stratton.

Kavka, J. 1949. Pinel's Conception of the Psychopathic State. *Bulletin of the History of Medicine* 23: 461–468.

Kennedy, J. F. 1964. Message from the President of the United States Relative to Mental Illness and Mental Retardation. *American Journal of Psychiatry* 120: 729–737.

Kindred, J. J. 1927. The Neuro-Psychiatric and Disabled Wards of the United States Government: The Present System of Their Medical Care, Hospitalization, Rehabilitation, and Compensation Disability. *American Journal of Psychiatry* 83: 711–724.

Kindwall, J. A., and Henry, G. W. 1934. Wet Packs and Prolonged Baths. *American Journal of Psychiatry* 91: 72–94.

Kirkbride, T. S. 1854. *On the Construction, Organization, and General Arrangements of Hospitals for the Insane, With Some Remarks on Insanity and Its Treatment.* Philadelphia: Lindsay & Blackiston.

Kittrie, N. N. 1971. *The Right to Be Different.* Baltimore: Johns Hopkins University Press.

Kopeloff, N., and Cheney, C. O. 1922. Studies in Focal Infection: Its Presence and Elimination in the Functional Psychoses. *American Journal of Psychiatry* 79: 139–156.

Lief, A., ed. 1948. *The Commonsense Psychiatry of Dr. Adolf Meyer.* New York: McGraw-Hill.

Little, N. F. 1972. *Early Years of the McLean Hospital.* Boston: Francis A. Countway Library of Medicine.

Lord, J. R. 1934. The Human Factor in International Relations. *Mental Hygiene* 18: 177–188.

Lowry, J. V. 1949. How the National Mental Health Act Works. *Public Health Reports* 64: 303–312.

Marshall, H. E. 1937. *Dorothea Dix: Forgotten Samaritan.* Chapel Hill: University of North Carolina Press.

Mather, C. 1693. *Wonders of the Invisible World*. London: John Russell Smith, 1862.

McGovern, C. M. 1987. *Masters of Madness: Social Origins of the American Psychiatric Profession*. Hanover, N.H.: University Press of New England.

McNeel, B. H. 1946. War Psychiatry in Retrospect. *American Journal of Psychiatry* 102: 500–506.

Meerloo, J. A. 1955. Medication into Submission: The Danger of Therapeutic Coercion. *Journal of Nervous and Mental Disease* 122: 353–360.

Menninger, W. C. 1947. Psychiatric Experience in the War, 1941–1946. *American Journal of Psychiatry* 103: 577–586.

Menninger, W. C. 1948. *Psychiatry in a Troubled World*. New York: Macmillan.

Menninger, W. C., and Chidester, L. 1933. The Role of Financial Losses in the Precipitation of Mental Illness. *Journal of the American Medical Association* 100: 1398–1400.

Mitchell, S. W. 1884. *Fat and Blood: An Essay on the Treatment of Certain Forms of Neurasthenia and Hysteria*. Philadelphia: J. B. Lippincott.

Mitchell, S. W. 1904. The Evolution of the Rest Treatment. *Journal of Nervous and Mental Disease* 31: 368–373.

Morton, T. G. 1895. *The History of Pennsylvania Hospital, 1751–1895*. Philadelphia: Times Printing House.

Mosher, J. M. 1909. A Consideration of the Need of Better Provision for the Treatment of Mental Disease in its Early Stage. *American Journal of Insanity* 45: 499–508.

Mosher, J. M. 1915. The Treatment of Mental Disease in a General Hospital. *Modern Hospital* 5: 327–332.

National Association for the Protection of the Insane and the Prevention of Insanity. 1880. Boston: Tolman & White.

Newer, B. 1936. The Need for a Personnel Program for State Institutions. *Mental Hygiene* 20: 55–61.

O'Malley, M. 1913. Hydrotherapy in the Treatment of the Insane. *Modern Hospital* 1: 143–154.

Overholser, W. 1944. The Founding and the Founders of the Association. In *One Hundred Years of American Psychiatry*, ed. American Psychiatric Association. New York: Columbia University Press.

Overholser, W. 1956. Has Chlorpromazine Inaugurated a New Era in Mental Hospitals? *Journal of Clinical and Experimental Psychiatry* 17: 197–201.

Page, C. W. 1913. Dr. Eli Todd and the Hartford Retreat. *American Journal of Insanity* 69: 761–785.

Pinel, P. 1806. *A Treatise on Insanity*. New York: Hafner, 1962.

Pollock, H. M. 1923. Organization of Occupational Therapy in a State Hospital. *Mental Hygiene* 7: 149–153.

Pollock, H. M. 1935. The Depression and Mental Disease in New York State. *American Journal of Psychiatry* 91: 763–771.

Pratt, G. K. 1922. The Problem of the Mental Misfit in Industry. *Mental Hygiene* 6: 526–578.

Pratt, G. K. 1930. Twenty Years of the National Committee for Mental Hygiene. *Mental Hygiene* 14: 417–428.

Prince, M., ed. 1912 *Psychotherapeutics*. Boston: Richard G. Badger.

Pumphrey, R. E. 1973. Social Work and Mental Illness, 1890–1919. In *Transactions*.

Conference Group for Social and Administrative History. Madison: State Historical Society of Wisconsin.

Ranney, M. H. 1850. On Insane Foreigners. *American Journal of Insanity* 7: 55–63.

Reade, Charles. 1864. *Hard Cash*. London: S. Low.

Report of the Joint Committee of the Michigan Legislature. 1879. Lansing.

Rinkel, M. 1966. *Biological Treatment of Mental Illness*. New York: Farrar, Straus, and Giroux.

Rivers, W.H.R. 1918. War Neurosis and Military Training. *Mental Hygiene* 2: 513–533.

Rosenkrantz, B. G., and Vinovskis, M. A. 1978. The Invisible Lunatics: Old Age and Insanity in Mid-Nineteenth Century Massachusetts. In *Aging and the Elderly*, eds. S. F. Spicker, K. M. Woodward, and D. D. Van Tassel. Atlantic Highlands, N.J: Humanities Press.

Ross, D. 1972. *G. Stanley Hall: The Psychologist as Prophet*. Chicago: University of Chicago Press.

Rothman, D. J. 1971. *The Discovery of the Asylum*. Boston: Little, Brown.

Rothman, D. J. 1980. *Conscience and Convenience*. Boston: Little, Brown.

Rush, B. 1812. *Medical Inquiries and Observations Upon the Diseases of the Mind*. New York: Hafner, 1962.

Russell, W. L. 1913. The Widening Field of Practical Psychiatry. *American Journal of Insanity* 70: 459–466.

Sackler, A. M., Sackler, R. R., Sackler, M.D., and Marti-Ibanez, F., eds. 1956. *The Great Physiodynamic Therapies in Psychiatry*. New York: Paul B. Hoeber.

Salmon, T. W. 1917. Some New Fields in Neurology and Psychiatry. *Journal of Nervous and Mental Disease* 46: 90–99.

Santos, E. H., and Stainbrook, E. 1949. A History of Psychiatric Nursing in the Nineteenth Century. *Journal of the History of Medicine and Allied Sciences* 4: 48–74.

Savino, M. T., and Mills, A. B. 1967. The Rise and Fall of Moral Treatment in California Psychiatry: 1852–1870. *Journal of the History of the Behavioral Sciences* 3: 359–367.

Schneck, J. M. 1963. William Osler, S. Weir Mitchell, and the Origin of the Rest Cure. *American Journal of Psychiatry* 119: 894–895.

Schwab, S. I. 1920. Influence of War upon Concepts of Mental Diseases and Neuroses. *Mental Hygiene* 4: 654–669.

Shershow, J. C., ed. 1977. *Delicate Branch. The Vision of Moral Psychiatry*. Oceanside, N.Y.: Dabor Science Publications.

Shields, E. 1939. Normal Living: An Interpretation from the Mental Hospital. *Mental Health Bulletin* 17: 6–9.

Shryock, R. 1945. The Psychiatry of Benjamin Rush. *American Journal of Psychiatry* 101: 429–432.

Sicherman, B. 1973. From Asylum to Community: Changing Psychiatric Goals, 1880–1921. In *Transactions*. Conference Group for Social and Administrative History. Madison: State Historical Society of Wisconsin.

Solomon, H. C. 1958. Some Historical Perspectives. *Mental Hospital* 9: 5–7.

Southard, E. E. 1913. The Psychopathic Hospital Idea. *Journal of the American Medical Association* 61: 1972–1975.

Southard, E. E. 1920. Trade Unionism and Temperament. *Mental Hygiene* 4: 281–300.

Spitzka, E. C. 1878. Merits and Motives of the Movement for Asylum Reform. *Journal of Nervous and Mental Disease* 5: 694–714.

Stanton, A., and Schwartz, M. 1954. *The Mental Hospital. A Study of Institutional Participation in Psychiatric Illness and Treatment*. New York: Basic Books.

Strecker, E. A. 1944. Military Psychiatry: World War I. In *One Hundred Years of American Psychiatry*, ed. American Psychiatric Association. New York: Columbia University Press.

Swazey, J. P. 1974. *Chlorpromazine in Psychiatry: A Study of Therapeutic Innovation*. Cambridge: MIT Press.

Thom, D. 1932. Mental Hygiene and the Depression. *Mental Hygiene* 16: 564–576.

Tomes, N. J. 1984. *A Generous Confidence: Thomas Story Kirkbride and the Art of Asylum Building, 1840–1883*. Cambridge: Cambridge University Press.

Truitt, R. P. 1927. Mental Hygiene and the Public Schools. *Mental Hygiene* 11: 261–271.

Tuke, S. 1813. *Description of the Retreat*. London: Dawsons of Pall Mall, 1964.

Veith, I. 1962. S. Weir Mitchell, Psychiatrist of Women. *Modern Medicine* 30: 234–250.

Walter, R. D. 1970. *S. Weir Mitchell, M.D.—Neurologist*. Springfield, Ill.: Charles C. Thomas.

White W. A. 1920. Childhood: The Golden Period for Mental Hygiene. *Mental Hygiene* 4: 257–267.

Williams, W. H. 1976. *America's First Hospital: The Pennsylvania Hospital, 1751–1841*. Wayne, Pa.: Haverford House.

Wittels, F. 1946. The Contribution of Benjamin Rush to Psychiatry. *Bulletin of the History of Medicine* 20: 157–166.

Woods, E. A., and Carlson, E. T. 1961. The Psychiatry of Philippe Pinel. *Bulletin of the History of Medicine* 35: 14–25.

Wright, F. 1947. *Out of Sight, Out of Mind*. Philadelphia: National Mental Health Foundation.

6

A National Community Mental Health Program: Policy Initiation and Progress

JAMES M. CAMERON

Prior to World War II, mental health programs were the domain of the states, and the principal locus of care was the large state mental institutions. The national government had almost no role in mental health. This was consistent with prevailing American values. American sociopolitical philosophy had always been firmly rooted in a general distrust of centralized planning and control. The limited role of the central government reflected the philosophy of a laissez-faire capitalist economy, individual liberty, and local responsibility.

As events in the 1930s and 1940s unfolded, American values regarding the role of government, and perspectives on mental health care, changed dramatically. The roots of the community mental health movement can be traced to two historical developments of the 1930s: (1) the embracing of neo-Freudian psychoanalytic theory by American psychiatry and (2) the birth of national social welfare programs. While psychoanalytic theory absorbed, and came to dominate, medical psychiatry, it was least relevant for the treatment of serious mental illness. The proliferation of the psychoanalytic approach had the effect of moving the medical profession away from the kinds of disorders characteristic of patients in mental hospitals. These patients often were institutionalized with little active psychological treatment and little expectation that their condition would improve. The practice of psychiatry remained primarily in the private sector among a less severely disordered population.

The national welfare programs initiated during the Great Depression did not extend to health care, but they did establish the new federal role as initiator and supporter of social welfare programs. Government's willingness to intervene reflected a substantial change in public expectations regarding the role of the federal government. A new social philosophy emerged providing a firm foundation for the future growth of federally sponsored social welfare programs.

The purpose of this chapter is to review the origins and subsequent evolution of the community mental health program in the period from 1945 to 1980 from the perspective of the national movement, and its key political and legislative developments.

EMERGENCE OF THE COMMUNITY MENTAL HEALTH MOVEMENT

World War II served to focus national attention on the problem of mental illness in American society by revealing a startling number of draft rejections for reasons of neuropsychiatric disability. Twelve percent of the men examined were rejected. Moreover, a large proportion of the men inducted and later prematurely separated from the armed services were discharged specifically for neuropsychiatric reasons. During the war new methods of treatment were introduced and tested. Mental health treatment near the battlefield was often successful in rapidly returning servicemen, who experienced sudden emotional breakdowns, to active duty. The wartime successes of treatment in the situation where stress was occurring were to have considerable influence in the development of community psychiatry after the war. In addition to innovations in treatment—such as short-term therapy and group therapy—the wartime need for new psychiatric personnel led to innovations in training mental health professionals (Felix, 1967). The war thus highlighted the prevalence of mental disability within society and served to focus attention on the need for expanding the stock of mental health professionals. It also augmented the perspective that mental illness is environmentally derived and best treated by helping the patient adapt to environmental circumstances (Grinker and Spiegel, 1945).

After the war, the abysmal conditions within state and county mental hospitals were trumpeted to the American public in an increasing chorus. With manpower shortages due to the draft, thousands of conscientious objectors had been assigned to take the place of state hospital personnel who had gone to war. Horrified by conditions, they began to publicize what they found behind the closed doors. Investigative reporters also exposed the conditions of these institutions in virtually every state, creating a national climate of sympathy for the plight of the mentally ill and antipathy for the traditional state mental institution.

Out of World War II emerged the Group for the Advancement of Psychiatry, young, reform-minded psychiatrists, trained in psychoanalysis, who were eager to sponsor the new ideas of community psychiatry. Its leader was the eminent psychoanalyst William Menninger, the army's chief psychiatrist during the war and director of the Menninger Foundation, a leading agency for the spread of psychoanalysis in the United States. The group also included Francis Braceland, chief psychiatrist for the marine corps and future editor of the *American Journal of Psychiatry*; Jack Ewalt, consultant to the air force during the war and later the chairman of the U.S. Congress Joint Commission on Mental Illness; and Robert Felix of the Public Health Service, who was to become the first director of the National Institute of Mental Health (NIMH). This group would not only come to dominate the American Psychiatric Association but would forge alliances with other actors concerned with developing a national mental health policy.

The wartime experience facilitated the postwar efforts to formulate a national mental health policy. As Brown (1985: 32) suggests, with war,

there is a massive state intervention into areas previously less touched by state activities, and into some areas where no state intervention has ever occurred. This intervention carried over into the immediate postwar period when the legacy of state intervention was still strong, and when the state still retained more power due to the necessities of reconstruction.

Impressed by the apparent success of military psychiatry during the war and shocked by reports of the extent of mental disabilities in the United States, Congress passed the National Mental Health Act of 1946 (Public Law 79–487), which established the National Institute of Mental Health as the locus of leadership, research, and training in the treatment of mental illness. NIMH's creation signaled the beginning of a new federal role, one in which the federal government would initiate, organize, and fund a massive contribution to the nation's mental health system.

NIMH was charged with providing the leadership and stimulus in academic spheres to foster research and education toward conquering mental illness. Through grants, technical assistance, and direct aid to the states, pilot projects and demonstration programs for direct mental health services were begun. Between 1948 and 1962, through the use of federal grants, NIMH developed programs that drew diverse disciplines into the mental health sphere. During this period, NIMH awarded approximately 3,000 grants totaling over $120 million to academic institutions in support of research (Foley, 1975: 11).

In its training mission, NIMH supported over 1,500 university and college schools of medicine, and graduate programs in psychology, social work, public health, and nursing, drawing over 80 percent of the nation's colleges and universities into the NIMH sphere of influence by developing powerful political constituencies in these groups (Connery et al., 1968; Foley, 1975). The outcome of this support was rapid growth of the mental health professions, with the numbers of mental health professionals graduating from these programs increasing at rates far in excess of other fields, including general medicine. These personnel were to design and staff the growing number of community and private institutions which arose to serve the mentally ill, including clinics, hospitals, and private practitioners in the community.

In this same period, NIMH also used grants-in-aid to stimulate the states to develop community-based services and training programs. Funds typically were made available to separate mental health "authorities" aligned with NIMH (Ozarin, 1982). These separate "mental health authorities" were fostered to provide a network of community mental health services and demonstration projects; in time they evolved to form the Council of State and Territorial Mental Health Authorities as an advisory group to the director of NIMH.

Through the power of the purse in research and training, NIMH built a powerful network of constituencies in academic psychiatry in schools of medicine across the country. This group became favorably influenced toward the community mental health movement, and this influence had a profound effect on how mental illness and mental health services were conceptualized in the academic literature. The underlying philosophical base of the movement was thus legitimized by academia—ideas such as the importance of prevention and early intervention. NIMH also stimulated research into new psychotropic drugs, already being used in Europe, persuading the psychiatric profession of the usefulness and applicability of these drugs in controlling many symptoms of psychosis.

A central figure in the early community mental health movement was Dr. Robert Felix, who in 1946 was named the first director of the National Institute of Mental Health. Trained in the psychoanalytic/humanistic tradition in psychiatry, Felix joined the U.S. Public Health Service in 1933. His career had been oriented toward community programs within the context of public health. It was, in fact, Felix who wrote the legislative framework which was to become the National Mental Health Act of 1946, creating NIMH. Based upon his earlier experience in public health, Felix molded NIMH with a clear focus on prevention, education, and community-based services. He first built a strong base of support within his agency by selecting and recruiting staff who shared his commitment to a community-oriented approach to mental health. Felix was able to align himself with several important advocates of community mental health and social reform, including James Shannon, director of the National Institutes of Health, Mary Lasker and Florence Mahoney, wealthy Washington philanthropists, and Mike Gorman, a key lobbyist and director of the National Committee Against Mental Illness. These were to become Felix's most powerful allies and together they comprised the core of an increasingly powerful mental health lobby. In spite of differing views on a number of issues, Felix and his allies presented a united front to Congress resulting in substantial new funding for a variety of NIMH programs (Connery et al., 1968; Foley, 1975; Felicetti, 1975).

NIMH funding of research and training in community mental health established powerful constituencies among academics, mental health practitioners, and others committed to an expanded federal role. Felix and his colleagues at NIMH were able to successfully mobilize these groups into a concerted force for influencing Congress and the media. The results of NIMH-funded research were effectively used in congressional testimony and in proselytizing the media. Such research suggested that a large proportion of the American public was in need of mental health services, that mental illness was causally related to environmental circumstances, and that mental illness could be prevented by early intervention for individuals and groups at risk. NIMH-funded research thus served to provide a scientific and technical rationale for the expansion of community-oriented programs. The process of building congressional and public support for a national community-based mental health program was cumulative, based on the continuing education of Congress and the public to the new ways of thinking about mental illness and the results of scientific inquiry. By 1960, NIMH and the mental health lobby were in an excellent position to promote a national mental health program. Not only did they have powerful political sponsors in Congress and multiple outside constituencies created by NIMH funding policies, but they were to gain the support of a dynamic new president, John F. Kennedy, in support of their ideas for radical reform.

THE NEW FEDERAL STRATEGY

The first step toward a national Community Mental Health Center (CMHC) program was taken by Congress in 1955 when it passed the Mental Health Study Act (Public Law 84–182). NIMH was directed to establish a Joint Commission on Mental Illness and Health to report annually on the status of the treatment of mental illness in the United States. Reflecting a wide range of interest groups, the task of this body was to formally assess existing mental health technologies as well as to educate the public regarding the need for more adequate mental health care.

When the Joint Commission published its final report in 1960, it recommended that a national mental health program be established, funded by federal as well as state and local funds, to provide a comprehensive array of mental health services. It stressed the importance of continued support for research and professional education for nonmedical personnel. Further, the commission stated that the state mental hospitals should be reformed into mental health centers as part of the overall service package, including outpatient and aftercare facilities as well as inpatient services. This goal, however, contradicted another goal of the commission, which was the eventual elimination of the state mental hospitals. This contradiction reflected factions within the commission who were either in favor of revitalizing state hospitals or abandoning them; the views of these two factions were not to be reconciled during the three years that the commission convened. The Joint Commission's findings were subsequently released to the public as a book entitled *Action for Mental Health* (Joint Commission, 1961). This widely read volume served to generate further public interest in, and support for, a national community mental health program.

Some of the commission's recommendations found expression within a plank of the Democratic party for the 1960 presidential elections (Foley, 1975: 31). Upon taking office in 1961, JFK directed that top-level discussions begin in the

Department of Health, Education, and Welfare to develop a response to the Joint Commission's report. It was important that the commission's contradictory statements regarding the state mental hospitals be reconciled—should federal support be committed to them or not? Eventually it was decided that no federal funds should go to state institutions. Direct federal support of the state mental hospitals, it was claimed, would violate the intent of Congress, which was to avoid supporting these traditional state facilities. The focus of the federal program would be the development of comprehensive services in prevention, treatment, and the rehabilitation of mentally ill patients at the community level, ignoring existing state institutions altogether.

This approach, which went beyond the recommendations of the Joint Commission, reflected a basic shift in policy. The commission had recommended that state hospitals be modernized and that community mental health clinics be established as part of regional systems linking outpatient, inpatient, and aftercare services aimed at "reducing the need of many persons with major mental illness for prolonged or repeated hospitalization" (Joint Commission, 1961: xiv). The administration's approach was the establishment of a wholly new, independent community system composed of autonomous centers offering a full range of services. Under the new policy all federal resources would be directed toward community mental health centers. The new administration proposed a radical alternative to the existing system, one which was impelled by a new political strategy.

The community mental health center strategy of the Democratic administration must be viewed within the context of the fundamental change in American welfare policy. The social welfare agenda of the New Deal had bogged down during the 1950s. Efforts to initiate federal programs in fields such as housing, education, civil rights, delinquency prevention, and health care were blocked by competing interest groups, an internally divided Congress, and the lack of strong presidential commitment. This led to a perception that democratic political institutions were deadlocked (Burns, 1963). In the early 1960s, however, the deadlock image dissipated with a new federal offensive.

The policy agenda of the new administration was influenced by a keen awareness of the political importance of the urban poor, particularly ethnic minorities. The growth of big-city ghettos during the 1950s, resulting from the migration of blacks from the rural South, led to an increasing awareness of poverty, racism, and unemployment. Kennedy had won a close presidential race in 1960 due, in part, to capturing large majorities among the urban poor. The political agenda of the new administration was directed at consolidating and expanding this important base of political support. Poverty became a central social issue insofar as it represented serious social and economic deprivations such as racial segregation, poor housing, juvenile delinquency, unemployment, lack of health care, and inadequate education. These conditions suddenly occupied the attention of the American public in the early 1960s. Solutions to poverty and racism were sought, not only because there were growing moral indignation and demands for social justice, but because these conditions carried with them potential subversive potential; they were politically dangerous (Piven and Cloward, 1972).

The strategy of the new Democratic administration appears to have been directed toward two major objectives: (1) to provide assistance to disadvantaged groups within the population, helping them to share in the fruits of economic prosperity, and (2) to exert influence over the behavior of such groups through direct federal intervention. To initiate and carry out a broad national antipoverty and urban renewal campaign, it was recognized, would require bypassing traditional state and local governmental apparatus. Inhibited by organizational and political constraints, state and municipal governments resisted expanding or adjusting their social service domains to the new and changing demands of the increasing lower-status urban population (Kirlin, 1973). The new federal strategy entailed the development of a variety of social programs aimed primarily at ameliorating poverty and urban turmoil. This included the establishment of new institutions within the areas to be controlled with the active participation of the community itself. Directing the flow of federal funds to newly created community organizations and integrating community activists into program implementation would serve to generate community support for the new federal initiatives; moreover, it would foster strong political support among the poor and disfranchised for the Democratic party. Underlying the many social welfare programs of the 1960s was thus a coherent, federally orchestrated political strategy. Although the nature of the programs varied, they were targeted toward the same population subgroups. "It made little difference whether the funds were appropriated under delinquency-prevention, mental health, antipoverty, or model cities legislation: in the streets of the ghettos, many aspects of these programs looked very much alike" (Piven and Cloward, 1972: 261).

The community mental health centers program was designed to be one component within a multifaceted federal strategy. As with the other new social welfare proposals, it was directed mainly toward depressed urban areas. The community mental health movement was viewed as a way of combating incipient social instability. In order for the new mental health policy proposal, tied inextricably to the antipoverty campaign, to be adopted, it needed to be legitimized by a coherent ideology that had gained wide acceptance.

THE IDEOLOGY OF COMMUNITY MENTAL HEALTH

Social reform movements have generally emerged in response to social structural change and have been legitimized by a set of beliefs and values that are consistent with the pattern of changing social structure (Cameron, 1978). The social reform movements of the 1960s, of which the community mental health movement was an integral part, were prefigured by changing social conditions—the enlarged role of government growing out of the malaise of the Great Depression and the exigencies of World War II; the dramatic and sustained economic expansion following the war; the massive migration of southern blacks to northern cities during the 1950s which contributed to racial discord and urban strife; and the explosive growth in communications and the media.

The community mental health movement was justified on the basis of a relatively coherent system of beliefs, or ideological precepts. At the core of the ideology emerged a conception of the etiology of mental illness which provided the scientific and theoretical basis for the movement. This was the "environmental" conception of mental illness, which evolved from both the psychoanalytic movement and the behavioral sciences.

The burgeoning of psychoanalytic theory during the 1930s and 1940s served to direct the focus of psychiatric practice toward noninstitutional settings. While it was implicitly recognized that psychoanalysis had little utility for the treatment of chronic mental illness (characteristic of patients in state mental hospitals), it fueled the growth of psychiatric practice in the community. The perspective that detailed inquiry into an individual's internal conflicts would avert the development of more serious psychiatric disturbance gave impetus to the view that mental illness could be prevented. It also augmented the belief that inappropriate social functioning and psychological distress were largely a function of environmental, rather than biological, circumstances.

Optimism among psychiatrists in the ability to prevent serious psychiatric disorder through early intervention, and a penchant for practicing in the community, laid the groundwork for initiating the community mental health movement within the traditional public health context with its emphasis on community health and prevention. It also ensured that the scientific rationale for the movement would, of necessity, be consistent with a public health approach. Eventually, the community mental health movement achieved consensus around the belief that mental illness is caused by a complex web of environmental circumstances. Based on the assumption of a behavioral continuum in which severely disturbed behavior is part of the same continuum as minor behavioral problems (differing only in degree of seriousness), it entailed a global perspective in which the basic assumptions and theoretical formulations provided the foundation for explaining all behavior (Mechanic, 1980; Regier, 1982). The etiology of mental disorder was based on a model of cumulative stress emanating from the environment (Regier, 1982: 93):

Diagnostic groups represented quantitative distinctions along a gradient rather than discrete, qualitatively separate entities with different genetic backgrounds, precipitants, or treatment responses . . . . Varying degrees of stress could be seen as accounting for different degrees of mental disorder, ranging from normal, to neurotic, to psychotic.

By conceiving all behavior as part of the same continuum, the community mental health movement centered on early intervention and prevention. Since mental illness was considered to be environmentally derived, it could be prevented by influencing the social environment. The ideology served to delegitimize a "medical model" which was based on a clinical conception of diagnosis and treatment and focused on the individual. The new emphasis was not on the individual but on his environment.

The community mental health ideology included a strong claim to moral righteousness. Traditional state mental hospitals, where patients received little more than custodial care, were considered anachronistic vestiges of an unenlightened past. This was contrasted to community-based care where patients could be treated in a normal setting, thereby facilitating adaptation to their social environment, and where far greater numbers of patients could be served. Further, the ideology highlighted government's obligation to provide crisis intervention and mental health education services in the community given the demonstrated need for such services. Since adverse environmental circumstances, such as poverty and social discord, are associated with increased incidence of mental illness, it was reasoned, the provision of public mental health services was a moral imperative. Moreover, since intervention and education by mental health professionals in the community could help to reduce social conflict, funding of these services was the proper function of government.

The community mental health ideology provided the rationale for mental health professionals to focus on social action. As expressed by Caplan (1964: 56), probably the most influential ideological advocate of the community mental health movement, "Social action includes efforts to modify general attitudes and behavior of community members by communication through the educational system, the mass media, and through interaction between the professional and lay communities." Psychiatrists, it was argued, "must play a role in controlling the environment which man has created" (Duhl, 1963: 73). Community mental health thus included an important political dimension. "The psychiatrist must truly be a political personage in the best sense of the word" (Duhl, 1963: 73). Community mental health advocates frequently stressed that mental health specialists should seek to influence community morality, "to help the legislators and welfare authorities improve the moral atmosphere in the homes where children are being brought up" (Caplan, 1964: 59).

A specific reformist ideology, then, provided the conceptual rationale for aiding underprivileged groups through social activism, including forging alliances with other community activists in an effort to overcome local opposition to social melioration. The environmental conception of mental illness was closely linked, and provided a scientific rationale for, the belief that mental health professionals should be social change agents. It therefore provided an excellent basis for legitimizing the federal effort to develop a network of community mental health centers separate from the existing state and local mental health bureaucracies. It provided a justification for employing mental health centers as one component of a broader federal effort to increase the power and well-being of people at the grass roots.

THE COMMUNITY MENTAL HEALTH CENTERS ACT OF 1963

In 1962, President Kennedy established the President's Interagency Task Force on Mental Health, with the charge of drafting legislation to propose a "bold, new program'' to Congress. The task force consisted of the leadership of NIMH and a number of other agencies including economists from the Bureau of the Budget and the Council of Economic Advisors. It was the latter group which was to devise the fiscal aspects of the package, and they eventually argued that the plan should become a permanent federal subsidy, and that the states be bypassed in favor of direct aid to communities (Connery et al., 1968). Many key figures in the new administration had a profound distrust of state governments born out of the controversies of the civil rights movement and state and local resistance to the implementation of welfare programs. On the other hand, Felix and others argued that bypassing the states would be imprudent given the history of joint responsibility among levels of government characteristic of the federal system. Nonfederal matching of federal funds, it was argued, would increase local commitment and create a federal-state partnership in which states would redirect funds from institutional to community-based care. It was this latter view that prevailed in the drafting of the legislative package.

In his February 5, 1963, address to Congress, Kennedy (1963: 2) formally stated his goal of deinstitutionalizing the mental health system and of providing community-based care with an emphasis on prevention:

Here more than in any other area, ''an ounce of prevention is worth more than a pound of cure.'' For prevention is far more desirable for all concerned. It is far more economical and it is far more likely to be successful. Prevention will require both selected specific programs directed especially at known causes, and the general strengthening of our fundamental community, social welfare, and educational programs which can do much to eliminate or correct the harsh environmental conditions which often are associated with mental retardation and mental illness.

Kennedy's proposal reflected a radical departure from the past. As with other social reform efforts of the 1960s, the federal government would use its vast power to spend in order to influence the delivery of social welfare services.

The mental health legislative package proposed by the Kennedy administration centered around the provision of federal matching funds for a period of five years for the construction of community mental health centers offering a comprehensive range of mental health services. Based upon state population and the state's financial need, the percent of matching funds would be similar to that provided in the Hill-Burton program (the federal program for assisting communities in the construction and renovation of acute care hospitals). A second part of the bill provided budgetary support to staff the centers once they were built.

The legislation drew immediate opposition from the American Medical Association (AMA) who likened it to ''socialized medicine.'' The primary objection of organized medicine centered on the staffing provisions of the bill, not the bricks and mortar component, nor the advisability of moving the locus of care from the state institutions to the communities. Rather, the AMA considered the direct employment of psychiatrists in the centers as an invasion of the federal government into their professional domain. In deference to the AMA, the bill was subsequently stripped of its staffing provisions. It was this version of the bill which prevailed, and on October 31, 1963, President Kennedy signed into law the Community Mental Health Centers (CMHC) Act (Public Law 88–164, Title II).

Although the program had been weakened by removal of the staffing provisions, Felix and his NIMH colleagues were optimistic that the program would be more than a construction program. It was unlikely in their view that the nonfederal sources would be able to provide sufficient funding for staffing the centers once they were built, and the NIMH leadership was willing to bet that Congress would not let the program fail once the funds had been committed for construction (Foley, 1975). The CMHC Act specified that each state would be required to apply for federal funding by means of submission of a comprehensive plan for the building of community mental health centers in its state. The intention was to divide all states into service or "catchment" areas of at least 75,000 and not more than 200,000 people, and establish a location and priority ranking of the order in which centers were to be built. The community mental health center was to be an "umbrella" facility, but it remained a function of NIMH to interpret and provide the regulations that were to define the program for implementation.

Although it was controversial, the NIMH staff decided to interpret the CMHC Act as more than a construction program. They wrote specifications mandating the essential mental health services to be provided at the centers, in spite of considerable criticism that only building codes should be specified. A CMHC was defined as consisting of five required mental health services and five secondary services that the centers were to provide in the future once their financial base was established in the community. The five key services were inpatient services, outpatient services, emergency services, partial hospitalization services, and community services (to provide mental health education to other public organizations in the community). In addition, CMHC regulations mandated linkages of information, personnel, and patients in order to operationalize the public health concept of a continuum of care. The regulations thus mandated a short list of required services, viewed by its NIMH creators as a system to enhance the services already available within the state mental hospitals. CMHC services, together with those already provided by the state hospitals, were intended to provide a balanced array of services within the state.

Passage of the CMHC Act represented a triumph for the community mental health movement. Reformers had proselytized Congress, the nation's mental health professionals, general practitioners, and the public to the concept of community mental health care. However, the CMHC program would have little likelihood of success without a further federal commitment to the operation of CMHCs.

AMENDMENTS TO THE CMHC ACT

By mid–1964, it had become apparent that the CMHC Act would not be sufficient to bring the CMHC programs into actuality. Few states had submitted plans—the small states had insufficient funds and the large states insufficient incentives to implement them. President Lyndon Johnson had succeeded to the Oval Office and was committed to fulfilling the social programs agenda inherited from President Kennedy. Under the leadership of its new director, Stanley Yolles, NIMH prepared new legislation aimed at providing federal funds for staffing CMHCs and placing full control of the program within NIMH. The 1965 amendments, in the face of Kennedy's assassination and the overwhelming Democratic victory in the 1964 elections, found a receptive Congress which was also eager to approve a legacy to JFK. AMA opposition to the legislation was weak; in opposing Medicare and Medicaid legislation earlier that year, the AMA had diminished itself in the eyes of many in Congress as being fundamentally reactionary and self-serving. The mental health legislation (Public Law 89–105) passed easily and was subsequently signed into law by President Johnson on August 4, 1965.

The staffing provisions of the 1965 amendments to the CMHC Act, as with the construction provisions of the original legislation, appropriated funds that were to be matched by nonfederal funds in each catchment area. The federal share for staffing was to start at 75 percent and decrease by 15 percent each year until it reached 30 percent, after which funding would be entirely from state and local sources. The concept of providing federal "seed money" for the development of community mental health services was based on the expectation that communities would have incentives to develop their own sources of funding after start-up.

The 1965 amendments provided the necessary stimulus for implementing the CMHC program. Not only would the federal government provide for staffing CMHCs, but administration of the funds was to be controlled by NIMH, thereby bypassing the states. This reflected the general political strategy of the Democratic administration. The funds for community-based social programs were not channeled through existing governments which often had little incentive for initiating programs for the poor. Funds for new social programs could be directed more rapidly to the poor under the direction and control of federal leaders committed to social change. This expansion of federal control would also serve to mobilize public support within the communities receiving federal funds, adding to the political base of the current party in power.

The first few years of implementation of the CMHC Act were heralded as highly successful and a confident Congress extended the act for three more years. Continued decline in the population of state mental hospitals—a trend which actually predated the CMHC legislation by several years—was widely attributed to the increased availability of community mental health services. The Mental Health Amendments of 1967 (Public Law 90–31) authorized extension of construction and staffing support for an additional three years.

In response to growing public concern over alcohol and drug abuse, Congress enacted the Alcoholic and Narcotic Addict Rehabilitation Amendments of 1968

(Public Law 90–574). It seemed appropriate to integrate services for the prevention and treatment of alcohol and drug addiction into the CMHC program. Congress greatly expanded these activities with the Comprehensive Drug Abuse Prevention and Control Act of 1970 (Public Law 91–513). Whereas the 1968 legislation focused on alcohol and drug addiction, Congress now broadened its interest to include the full constellation of problems associated with substance abuse and dependence. Federal funding was targeted to these problems within the context of community mental health, thereby adding to the types of social problems falling within the purview of the mental health system (Bloom, 1975).

The process of adding categorical grants for newly defined special populations was continued with the Community Mental Health Centers Amendments of 1970 (Public Law 91–211). Just as Congress had pointed to alcohol and drug abuse as requiring specialized services, the 1970 amendments identified children as needing special mental health programs. The amendments also extended the CMHC Act for three years, authorizing continued federal funding for all previously enacted programs until June 30, 1973 (Bloom, 1975). By 1970 it had become clear that communities were having trouble finding nonfederal sources of funds to replace the gradually diminishing federal support. As a result, the 1970 amendments modified the provisions for supporting CMHC operating costs. Federal subsidization was changed from four years to eight years, with the federal portion set at 75 percent for the first two years and gradually decreasing over the remaining six years. For poverty areas, the federal subsidy was considerably more generous. In addition, Congress underscored its support for ''primary prevention,'' allocating funds specifically for consultation and education services which were considered vital activities of community mental health centers (Foley and Sharfstein, 1983).

The CMHC Act and its succeeding amendments were viewed by Congress as a long-term national commitment designed to replace traditional public mental hospitals and to establish community mental health centers in catchment areas throughout the United States. By 1970, however, the nation's political complexion had changed dramatically. The Nixon administration was strongly opposed to the CMHC program and to funding research and training in mental health. This hostility to the CMHC concept led to a protracted period of confrontation with Congress over continuation of the program.

By mid–1970, 450 CMHCs had received federal support; as of mid–1973, only 43 additional CMHCs received federal funds. The slowdown in federal allocations was primarily due to resistance by the administration to spend the money that had been authorized by Congress. During the period 1970–1973, only $50.5 million were allocated out of $340 million authorized by Congress (less than 15 percent) (Bloom, 1975: 51). The Nixon administration, ideologically opposed to federal support of community mental health and a number of other Great Society programs created during the 1960s, refused to expend funds that were congressionally authorized. Presidential ''impoundment'' of congressionally approved expenditures led to a protracted court battle; the funds were eventually released, but during the interim many centers were forced to curtail services.

In spite of administration opposition, Congress passed the Health Programs Extension Act of 1973 (Public Law 93–45), authorizing funds for a one-year extension of federal support for several health programs, including CMHCs (Bloom, 1975). The following year Congress passed a new two-year extension, but it was not enacted until the end of the legislative session, allowing President Gerald Ford to exercise a "pocket veto," whereby legislation dies for lack of a presidential signature prior to the adjournment of Congress.

The following year the amendments were reintroduced and passed by Congress (formally, Title III of the Health Revenue Sharing and Health Services Act of 1975, Public Law 94–63) (Bloom, 1975). Although the president vetoed the extension act, Congress overrode the veto a few days later. A later presidential veto of an appropriations measure (allowing for the expenditure of funds for community mental health programs) was similarly overridden by Congress. The new law substantially modified the original CMHC Act. All new and existing CMHCs were required to add seven new services in addition to those already mandated. The newly mandated services included specialized services for children and the elderly, screening services in order to promote alternatives to hospitalization, follow-up services for patients discharged from inpatient status, and programs for the prevention and treatment of alcohol and drug abuse. The legislation defined specifically the substantive areas and types of recipients to receive required consultation and education services. The legislation also insisted that consumers participate in agency governance, that CMHCs establish quality assurance programs, that they integrate and coordinate their programs and records with other existing agencies, and that they generate, where possible, reimbursement from other public and private health insurance programs (Foley and Sharfstein, 1983).

The 1975 amendments also authorized funds for initial construction and staffing, for planning and evaluation, for consultation and education grants, for assisting existing mental health centers to meet the requirements of newly mandated services, and for assisting financially distressed CMHCs. In short, the extension of the CMHC Act kept the community mental health movement alive. Although the original scope and purpose of the CMHC program had undergone significant modification, the 1975 amendments reaffirmed congressional faith in the concept of community-based care and continuing public support for the community mental health movement. The CMHC Act was renewed in 1977 for one year, and again in 1978 for two years.

IMPACT OF THE COMMUNITY MENTAL HEALTH ACT AND ITS AMENDMENTS

Chapter 9 of this volume provides a detailed review of evaluation research into the impact of CMHC services. It is appropriate here, however, to summarize selected trends that help explain the fate of the CMHC program as a national policymaking initiative. In the twelve years following initial passage of the Community Mental Health Centers Act of 1963, the federal government spent over $1 billion for CMHCs (Foley and Sharfstein, 1983: 111). Although the original intent had been that 2,000 CMHCs would eventually be built, only about one-fourth of that number were operational by 1975 (Levine, 1981). The expectation that federal "seed money" would lead to full state and local financial support of CMHCs never really materialized. State and local funding, as a percentage of CMHC funds, actually fell from 45.4 percent in 1969 to 37.9 percent in 1975 (Brown, 1985: 63). The concept of initiating federal support at a high level and gradually reducing the federal share was based on the assumption that CMHCs would become so integral to local communities that they would take over the centers' support. Few CMHCs worked to generate additional local financial support or plan for future periods (U.S. General Accounting Office, 1974). Apparently, they failed to take the seed money concept seriously, viewing federal funding as a continuous source of support.

Idealists of the CMHC movement and designers of the CMHC legislation assumed that state and local resources would follow patients discharged from state institutions. As the institutional population decreased, funds would be redirected to community-based care. This proved a faulty assumption, however, as the history of state and local support for mental health services makes clear. States were never eager to support mental health programs. Although funding of mental institutions had been a state responsibility, little more than custodial care was provided. As Grob (1966: 356) describes the mission of these state facilities, "In effect their primary responsibility was not to their patients, but to society, which demanded some form of protection against the mentally ill." The expectation that state and local governments would assume the financial burden associated with the plethora of community mental health services, as federal funding diminished, was predicated on the belief that deinstitutionalization would substantially reduce state hospital expenses and that these funds would be redirected to CMHCs. Such institutional cost savings generally did not occur. And although some states did provide substantially increased funding for mental health, state and local funding in general was woefully inadequate, especially in light of the increasing number of federally mandated services required of CMHCs.

As to third-party reimbursement, declining federal funds were only partially offset by this source of support. Many private insurance plans did not include mental health services as an allowable outpatient benefit, while those that did carried restrictions on length and cost of treatment. Medicare, the federal health insurance program for the elderly, required 50 percent coinsurance for outpatient mental health care, although it covered the cost of hospitalization in general hospitals for a stay of up to sixty days. Medicaid, which provides federal matching funds to the states for indigent health care services, also restricted the use of outpatient mental health care. Medicare and Medicaid reimbursement, which together accounted for only 12.4 percent of CMHC revenues in 1975, was available mainly for CMHC inpatient services (U.S. General Accounting Office, 1977).

In spite of the financial difficulties that emerged for many CMHCs, the CMHC program expanded the availability of mental health services in the community, particularly outpatient services (Redlich and Kellert, 1978; Windle, Bass, and Grey, 1987), and greatly increased access to mental health services for low income groups (Babigian, 1977; Stern, 1977). Moreover, the community mental health movement appears to have augmented a general shift in public attitudes that had begun in the late 1940s entailing greater public understanding and tolerance of mental illness and increased public acceptance of mental health services (Veroff, Kulka, and Donovan, 1981; Rochefort, 1984). The population served comprised primarily a low-income clientele whose age, sex, and diagnostic characteristics generally reflected those receiving mental health treatment in the private sector—predominantly women and those with nonsevere psychological disorders (Mechanic, 1980; Heiman, 1980). This was in stark contrast to public hospitals, whose population was composed of mostly young male schizophrenics. Thus, although the CMHCs provided community services to a low-income clientele that would have otherwise been underserved, it was essentially a new population which overlapped little with the seriously mentally ill being discharged from state hospitals.

Partly as a result of inadequate funding and partly because of a lack of system incentives, major gaps in service were never adequately addressed—particularly in establishing rehabilitative and aftercare services for the continued treatment of chronic mental disorders. Because the CMHC program was funded directly by the federal government, the states were left out of the equation. NIMH regulations for the CMHC program were initially vague regarding relations with state and local agencies (Chu and Trotter, 1974); and not until after the 1975 amendments were CMHCs required to provide services to discharged hospital patients. State hospitals and CMHCs operated separately with little effort made by either to coordinate the transition process from hospital to community care for the chronically mentally ill (U.S. General Accounting Office, 1974, 1977; Cameron, 1978; Morrissey, 1982). CMHCs were oriented toward meeting the needs of a new, previously underserved population, which rarely included persons with severe and chronic mental disorders (Kirk, 1976; Bassuk and Gerson, 1978; Scherl and Macht, 1979). Although a central tenet of the community mental health movement was that CMHCs would supplant state hospitals, providing services to this population was actually one of the lowest priorities of CMHCs (Kirk and Therrien, 1975; Lamb, 1976; U.S. General Accounting Office, 1977). In large part, this was because the orientation of CMHC staff, preferred treatment modalities, and types of services offered were typically inconsistent with the special needs of the seriously mentally ill (Lamb, 1976; Gruenberg and Archer, 1979; Bachrach, 1982).

One of the outcomes of the community mental health movement was a diminution of the role of psychiatry. From the outset, participation of psychiatrists in the provision of community mental health services was relatively minor, compared to the role of other mental health professionals, and continued to decline during the 1970s. NIMH estimated that in 1975 psychiatrists constituted less than 6 percent of CMHC staff and that their principal function was administrative (Bassuk and Gerson, 1978: 51). By 1979, the participation of psychiatrists had decreased to less than 4 percent of the average full-time equivalent of the centers (Wagenfeld and Jacobs, 1982: 75). The apparent reluctance of psychiatrists to practice in CMHCs has been viewed by many analysts as a reflection of the "demedicalization" of community mental health (Bassuk and Gerson, 1978; Talbott, 1979; Mollica, 1983).

Supplemental Security Income (SSI) and Medicaid provided the financial means by which states were able to divest themselves of responsibility for many mentally ill by transferring patients from state facilities to private nursing homes and board-and-care facilities in the community. Once transferred, these patients could qualify for federally supported programs or direct cash assistance. Often the chronic mental patient was left homeless by this process or forced to live in substandard unregulated for-profit accommodations (Lerman, 1982; Morrissey, 1982; Beigel, 1985; Brown, 1985; Chacko, Adams, and Gomez, 1985).

The Nixon administration's attack on the Great Society programs resulted in curtailment of most community antipoverty programs in the early 1970s. The administration was unsuccessful, however, in its battle with Congress to phase out federal involvement in the community mental health program. Amendments to the CMHC Act not only extended federal support of CMHCs, they also significantly expanded the scope of service responsibility. The CMHC program was one of the few federal antipoverty programs that survived the period because it had developed a strong national constituency. The mental health alliance included NIMH bureaucrats, local and state governments dependent upon federal dollars, academics from a variety of disciplines, and a whole generation of professionals who had been trained in community mental health concepts since the early 1950s. Whereas public support for federally initiated community programs waned in the early 1970s, advocates of community mental health were successful in maintaining federal support.

The strong ideological support of the community mental health program may have inhibited recognition by system participants of the fact that CMHCs were rarely providing services to the more seriously mentally disabled. CMHCs often quietly ignored this population even as some community mental health partisans pointed to declining state hospital populations as evidence of the beneficial impact of the presence of CMHCs for these patients. For example, the Community Mental Health Centers Amendments of 1975 were prefaced with a claim of successful treatment of the mentally ill through coordination and cooperation with other agencies ensuring continuity of care (Levine, 1981: 64). Community mental health advocates seemed impelled by a procrustean determination to make the evidence fit the theory.

During the late 1970s the attention of the Carter administration, Congress, and the attentive public turned to the problems of those who were underserved, or not served at all, by the CMHC program. Several reports pointed to the fragmentation of responsibility and lack of coherent policy in the provision of services for people needing a variety of program assistance. The chronically mentally ill, for instance, were in need of direct clinical care, education, rehabilitation, employment, housing, and income support. Yet these services were provided by different, uncoordinated agencies.

Many officials became aware that CMHCs were not coordinating effectively with other agencies, particularly regarding follow-up care for discharged state hospital patients. The 1975 amendments expressed congressional intent that CMHCs coordinate with other agencies. But the legislation provided no authority to ensure coordination, so little was accomplished. The first attempt to deal with the issue came in 1977, when the NIMH, in response to congressional criticism, initiated a pilot program for adult chronic patients discharged to CMHC jurisdictions. The program was to provide planning and service funds to states and communities together to develop comprehensive community support systems for the chronically mentally ill (Turner and TenHoor, 1978; Levine, 1981). The basic intent of the Community Support Program (CSP) was to be reflected later in the Mental Health Systems Act of 1980.

When Jimmy Carter was narrowly elected to the presidency in 1976, the CMHC program was one of only a few survivors of the Great Society of the 1960s. It had been a difficult struggle—including appropriation battles, fund impoundments, and presidential vetoes. The program was in distress. A number of CMHCs were in serious financial trouble as they attempted to wean themselves from federal support. Establishment of new centers was increasingly difficult as federal funding was diverted to rescue older programs. An additional 160 new centers were constructed between 1976 and 1979, but at a cost to the federal government of $1 billion (Foley and Sharfstein, 1983: 112).

THE MENTAL HEALTH SYSTEMS ACT

With increasing costs and growing criticisms of the viability of the CMHC program, a new focus was needed. In February 1977, as one of his first official acts, President Carter established the President's Commission on Mental Health to embark on a one-year study of the mental health needs of the nation and to make recommendations on how best to meet those needs. The thirty-five member group was composed of mental health professionals and other interested citizens representing women, minorities, and a wide variety of interest groups. Rosalynn Carter was named honorary chairwomen, reflecting the president's and her own keen interest in mental health issues.

The commission held hearings in four cities in 1977. Among other issues, testimony addressed the fragmentation of services and accessibility problems of the CMHC program. In the end, the commission produced a comprehensive four-volume report, concentrating its attention on underserved populations (President's Commission, 1978). Delivered to the president in April 1978, the report spoke to a variety of problems and issues:

- lack of third-party reimbursement for CMHC services;
- the differing needs of underserved populations, including children, adolescents, elderly, minorities, women, and those with chronic mental illness;
- the inflexibility of the system in initiating new programs; and
- the continuing need for federal support for research and training.

In all, the report provided over 100 major recommendations and findings pertaining to problems raised or exacerbated by the current system, but it did little to advocate a corrective course of action. Along with recommendations for increased flexibility in planning new programs and new services for children, adolescents, the elderly, and the special needs of minorities, the commission recommended the formulation of "a national plan for the chronically mentally ill." The planning process, it argued, should consider changes in Medicare, Medicaid, and SSI, along with certain regulations of the U.S. Department of Housing and Community Development, in order to improve the shelter and life-support opportunities for people with chronic mental disorders. Taking a functional approach to the problems of the mentally ill, the commission made recommendations designed to help the whole person, rather than treating each symptom or need separately—in other words, a case management approach.

The report did not suggest narrowing the purview of community mental health. On the contrary, it reiterated the notion that public mental health care should be available to all who need it, which may include 15 percent of the population (President's Commission, 1978: 8). Rather than recommending that services be confined to those with well-defined pathologies, the report emphasized that problems of daily living—depression, demoralization, etc.—fall within the domain of community mental health. Thus, the commission tended to reaffirm the basic principles of community mental health.

It took well over a year for HEW leaders to develop legislation based upon the commission's report. Early drafts did not go far enough to reform the system in the eyes of President and Mrs. Carter. Finally, in May of 1979, the president submitted the Mental Health Systems Act to Congress. The bill proposed six major titles, including the provision of grant funds directly to communities to plan and implement services to underserved groups, to develop comprehensive mental health services in underserved communities, to link general health and mental health care, to continue currently funded CMHCs, and to provide distress relief for older CMHCs.

The bill fared poorly in Congress, in part because of fragmentation of interests between levels of government, professional groups, and consumer advocacy groups. The glue which held the process together was the president's and Mrs. Carter's continuing strong support and promotion (Foley and Sharfstein, 1983). During the eighteen months it took for the legislation to be enacted, a series of compromises were worked out between state and local interests, resulting in a complex, highly regulatory, and somewhat contradictory product. While it advocated a systems approach and greater organizational flexibility, the legislation nevertheless created a complex series of regulatory requirements. The bill would serve for the first time to move states into the dominant role in the community mental health delivery system, but was to include strong accountability mechanisms designed to protect the interests of communities and local agencies. The Mental Health Systems Act (Public Law 96–398), which President Carter signed into law on October 7, 1980, was considered landmark legislation which continued national commitment to the CMHC movement. While state and local control of CMHCs was expanded, the federal bureaucracy was to continue its strong leadership and management role through regulation.

But the Mental Health Systems Act was not to be implemented. The will to sustain a strong federal commitment to improved care for the mentally ill in the community was supplanted by the Reagan doctrine of retrenchment. On August 13, 1981, President Ronald Reagan signed the Omnibus Budget and Reconciliation Act of 1981 (Public Law 97–35), which substantially repealed the Mental Health Systems Act of the preceding year, and turned over to the states all responsibility for the provision of community mental health services through the mechanism of a block of funds for "alcohol and drug abuse and mental health services."

REFERENCES

Babigian, H. M. 1977. The Impact of Community Mental Health Centers on the Utilization of Services. *Archives of General Psychiatry* 34: 385–394.

Bachrach, L. L. 1982. Young Adult Chronic Patients: An Analytical Review of the Literature. *Hospital and Community Psychiatry* 33: 189–197.

Bassuk, E. L., and Gerson, S. 1978. Deinstitutionalization and Mental Health Services. *Scientific American* 238: 46–53.

Beigel, A. 1985. Public Policy and the Care of the Chronic Patient. In *The Chronic Mental Patient in a Community Context*, ed. R. C. Chacko. Washington, D.C.: American Psychiatric Press.

Bloom, B. L. 1975. *Community Mental Health: A General Introduction.* Belmont, Calif.: Wadsworth.

Brown, P. 1985. *The Transfer of Care: Psychiatric Deinstitutionalization and Its After-math*. Boston: Routledge & Kegan Paul.

Burns, J. M. 1963. *The Deadlock of Democracy*. Englewood Cliffs, N.J.: Prentice-Hall.

Cameron, J. M. 1978. Ideology and Policy Termination: Restructuring California's Mental Health System. *Public Policy* 26: 533–570.

Caplan, G. 1964. *Principles of Preventive Psychiatry*. New York: Basic Books.

Chacko, R. J., Adams, G. L., and Gomez, E. 1985. The Care of the Chronic Mental Patient: A Historical Perspective. In *The Chronic Mental Patient in a Community Context*, ed. R. C. Chacko. Washington, D.C.: American Psychiatric Press.

Chu, F. D., and Trotter, S. 1974. *The Madness Establishment*. New York: Grossman.

Connery, R. H., Backstrom, C. H., Deener, D. R., Friedman, J. R., Kroll, M., Marden, R. H., McClesky, C., Meekison, P., and Morgan, J. A. 1968. *The Politics of Mental Health*. New York: Columbia University Press.

Duhl, L. 1963. *The Urban Condition*. New York: Basic Books.

Felicetti, D. A. 1975. *Mental Health and Retardation Politics: The Mind Lobbies in Congress*. New York: Praeger.

Felix, R. H. 1967. *Mental Illness: Progress and Prospects*. New York: Columbia University Press.

Foley, H. A. 1975. *Community Mental Health Legislation*. Lexington, Mass.: D. C. Heath.

Foley, H. A., and Sharfstein, S. S. 1983. *Madness and Government: Who Cares for the Mentally Ill?* Washington, D.C.: American Psychiatric Press.

Grinker, R. R., and Spiegal, J. P. 1945. *Men Under Stress*. New York: Blakiston.

Grob, G. N. 1966. *The State and the Mentally Ill*. Chapel Hill: University of North Carolina.

Gruenberg, E. M., and Archer, J. 1979. Abandonment of Responsibility for the Seriously Mentally Ill. *Milbank Memorial Fund Quarterly* 57: 485–506.

Heiman, E. M. 1980. CMHC Inpatient Unit: Private Hospital for the Poor? *Hospital and Community Psychiatry* 31: 476–479.

Joint Commission on Mental Illness and Health. 1961. *Action for Mental Health*. New York: Basic Books.

Kennedy, J. F. 1963. *Message from the President of the United States Relative to Mental Illness and Mental Retardation*. 88th Congress, 1st Session, 5 February 1963, H. R. Document 58.

Kirk, S. 1976. Effectiveness of Community Services for Discharged Mental Patients. *American Journal of Orthopsychiatry* 46: 646–659.

Kirk, S. A., and Therrien, M. E. 1975. Community Mental Health Myths and the Fate of Former Hospitalized Patients. *Psychiatry* 38: 209–217.

Kirlin, J. 1973. The Impact of Increasing Lower Status Clientele upon City Government Structures: A Model from Organization Theory. *Urban Affairs Quarterly* 8: 317–343.

Lamb, H. R., ed. 1976. *Community Survival for Long Term Patients*. San Francisco: Jossey-Bass.

Lerman, P. 1982. *Deinstitutionalization and the Welfare State*. New Brunswick, N.J.: Rutgers University Press.

Levine, M. 1981. *The History and Politics of Community Mental Health*. New York: Oxford University Press.

Mechanic, D. 1980. *Mental Health and Social Policy*. 2nd ed. Englewood Cliffs, N.J.: Prentice-Hall.

Mollica, R. F. 1983. From Asylum to Community: The Threatened Disintegration of Public Psychiatry. *New England Journal of Medicine* 308: 367–373.

Morrissey, J. P. 1982. Deinstitutionalizing the Mentally Ill: Processes, Outcomes, and New Directions. In *Deviance and Mental Illness*, ed. W. Gove. Beverly Hills, Calif.: Sage.

Musto, D. F. 1975. What Ever Happened to "Community Mental Health"? *The Public Interest* 39: 53–79.

Ozarin, L. D. 1982. Mental Health in Public Health: The Federal Perspective. In *Public Mental Health: Perspectives and Prospects*, eds. M. O. Wagenfeld, P. V. Lemkau, and B. Justice. Beverly Hills, Calif.: Sage.

Piven, F. F., and Cloward, R. A. 1972. *Regulating the Poor: The Functions of Public Welfare*. New York: Random House.

President's Commission on Mental Health. 1978. *Report to the President. Vol. I*. Washington, D.C.: U.S. Government Printing Office.

Redlich, F., and Kellert, S. 1978. Trends in American Mental Health. *American Journal of Psychiatry* 135: 22–28.

Regier, D. A. 1982. Research Progress, 1955–1980. In *Public Mental Health: Perspectives and Prospects*, eds. M. O. Wagenfeld, P. V. Lemkau, and B. Justice. Beverly Hills, Calif.: Sage.

Rochefort, D. A. 1984. Origins of the "Third Psychiatric Revolution": The Community Mental Health Centers Act of 1963. *Journal of Health Politics, Policy and Law* 9: 1–30.

Scherl, D. J., and Macht, L. B. 1979. Deinstitutionalization in the Absence of Consensus. *Hospital and Community Psychiatry* 30: 599–604.

Stern, M. S. 1977. Social Class and Psychiatric Treatment of Adults in the Mental Health Center. *Journal of Health and Social Behavior* 18: 317–325.

Talbott, J. A. 1979. Why Psychiatrists Leave the Public Sector. *Hospital and Community Psychiatry* 30: 778–782.

Turner, J. C., and TenHoor, W. J. 1978. The NIMH Community Support Program: Pilot Approach to a Needed Social Reform. *Schizophrenia Bulletin* 4: 319–348.

U.S. General Accounting Office. 1974. *Need for More Effective Management of Community Mental Health Centers Program*. Washington, D.C.: U.S. Government Printing Office.

U.S. General Accounting Office. 1977. *Returning the Mentally Disabled to the Community: Government Needs to Do More*. (HD) 76–152. Washington, D.C.: U.S. Government Printing Office.

Veroff, J., Kulka, R. A., and Donovan, E. 1981. *Mental Health in America: Patterns of Help Seeking from 1957–1976*. New York: Basic Books.

Wagenfeld, M. O., and Jacobs, J. H. 1982. The Community Mental Health Movement: Its Origins and Growth. In *Public Mental Health: Perspectives and Prospects*, eds. M. O. Wagenfeld, P. Lemkau, and B. Justice. Beverly Hills, Calif.: Sage.

Windle, C., Bass, R. D., and Grey, C. 1987. The Impact of Federally Funded CMHCs on Local Mental Health Service Systems. *Hospital and Community Psychiatry* 38: 729–734.

7

The Alcohol, Drug Abuse, and Mental Health Block Grant: Origins, Design, and Impact

DAVID A. ROCHEFORT
and BRUCE M. LOGAN

Reform of the nation's intergovernmental relations was a high policy priority for Ronald Reagan as he entered the presidency in 1981. Arguing that the primary role in domestic affairs belonged to the states, the administration committed itself to transferring control over a broad range of programs that had come to fall within the federal government's orb (Barfield, 1981: chapter 3; Nathan and Doolittle, 1987: chapter 1; Palmer, 1984: 46–51). "It is time that the states were brought back into the mainstream," explained Donald W. Moran, associate director of the Office of Management and Budget. "For too long they have been excluded and bypassed. The president intends to restore to them their rightful constitutional authority and responsibilities in the federal system" (quoted in Barfield, 1981: 24).

An important intermediate mechanism selected to help bring about this long-term transformation was the block grant. This method of distributing federal dollars combines multiple categorical programs having detailed requirements and regulations into larger grant packages that allow state authorities increased administrative flexibility. As a result of compromises reached with Congress in putting together the Omnibus Budget Reconciliation Act of 1981 (OBRA, Public Law 97–35), the Reagan administration succeeded in grouping fifty-seven existing federal aid programs into nine new or revised block grants encompassing preventive health; maternal and child health services; primary care; social services; community services; low-income energy assistance; community development; education; and alcohol, drug abuse, and mental health services (Barfield, 1981: 27–34; Stanfield, 1981; U.S. General Accounting Office, 1982).

The alcohol, drug abuse, and mental health services block grant is one of the largest, embracing ten categorical programs that previously were funded on a project or state-formula basis under the management of the Alcohol, Drug Abuse, and Mental Health Administration (ADAMHA). As specified under OBRA, each state now receives one lump sum for these services, with limited restrictions on such things as the general nature of the services to be supported; the proportion of the grant that can be allocated to administration; and the balance of funds to be used among mental health and substance abuse services. Gone are many prior specifications having to do with the exact configuration of the service system, preparation of comprehensive planning documents, and other federal requirements.

The purpose of this chapter is to evaluate the changeover from categorical to block grant funding for ADAMH services, with a special emphasis on the activities of community mental health centers (CMHCs). Since the creation of such facilities under federal legislation in 1963, an extensive nationwide network of more than 700 CMHCs has developed (see chapters 6 and 9 of this volume). Offering emergency and outpatient services as well as follow-up care for discharged mental patients, CMHCs stand at the heart of the contemporary deinstitutionalization movement and, where they exist, constitute a key element in a community's mental health system. The operation of CMHCs thus provides a sensitive barometer for assessing the changing atmosphere of federal-state relations in mental health policy.

The chapter begins with a brief history of the grant-in-aid concept. Next is a description of the ADAMH block grant mechanism, including its major provisions and funding trends over the period 1982–1988. We then review research findings on the impact of the ADAMH block grant, considering both the states' new management role and the organization and delivery of mental health services on the local level (chapter 16 of this volume looks at some of these same issues from a CMHC administrative perspective).

BLOCK GRANTS AS AN INSTRUMENT OF INTERGOVERNMENTAL REFORM

Federal funds have been dispensed to states and localities in three primary ways: categorical grants, block grants, and general revenue sharing. These types of grants are distinguished by the range of funding discretion on the part of the federal government, by the influence in selecting funded activities that is allowed the state or local recipients, and by the extensiveness of requirements on the grant program. Block grants stand somewhere in the middle of a continuum from maximum federal control (categorical grants) to maximum recipient discretion (general revenue sharing) (Barfield, 1981: 1; Advisory Commission on Inter-governmental Relations, 1977: 5–9; Nathan, 1983: 52–54).

Prior to the 1930s, federal funding to states and localities was limited. After that, categorical grants grew steadily, with a sharp increase during the Great Society years of the Johnson administration. Some 240 ''categoricals'' were added in this period, making a total of over 375 by 1968 (Barfield, 1981: 15–16; Hale and Palley, 1981: 11–14). At the start of the 1980s, there were around 600 categorical grants, which accounted for nearly 80 percent of total federal grant outlays (Barfield, 1981: 17; Hale and Palley, 1981: 108).

In keeping with contemporary policy goals, a growing proportion of these dollars was targeted to the poor and disadvantaged. During the Johnson admin-istration, for example, health and human resource programs went from 13 percent to 40 percent of total federal aid (Barfield, 1981: 15). The federal government moved into policy areas traditionally reserved for state and local governments, which were judged lax in implementing national priorities. Categorical grants, especially ''project grants'' that are awarded competitively among applicants seeking to implement specific federal initiatives, increasingly bypassed the states for a broad range of recipients at the substate level: formal local governments (such as counties), special-purpose governments (such as school districts), or even private organizations. The federal government retained control over the expenditure of funds by specifying grant conditions and monitoring recipients' performance.

In this way states and localities came to depend on federal funding to provide a host of services. By 1978, federal aid to the states equaled roughly 39 percent of states' general revenue from their own sources, up from 22 percent in 1948. State and federal aid to local governments totaled 77 percent of their local general revenue from their own sources in 1978, up from 45 percent in 1948 (Barfield, 1981: 20). This situation reflected a recognized contradiction in American fed-eralism. While the public looked to the federal government to broaden its re-sponsibilities, it resisted expansion of the federal bureaucracy. Yet it is the national government that controls the major means of generating public reve-nue—the federal income tax. Transferring federally collected revenues to state and local bureaucracies to carry out national policies is a strategy that attempts to deal with this contradiction (Barfield, 1981: 13–15).

Over time inordinate reliance on narrow-purpose categorical grants contributed to a number of dysfunctions in intergovernmental relations (Chelimsky, 1981: 95–97; Agranoff and Robins, 1984: 169–173). Increasingly, the federal govern-ment was charged with intruding into state and local affairs. With the proliferation of special-purpose grants came fragmented and uncoordinated services. Dupli-cation of effort occurred. Application and reporting procedures were often com-plex. These problems contributed to a perception of waste and inefficiency. Furthermore, a vast array of politically active special interests sprang up around categorical grants, including the private, usually nonprofit, provider agencies that the federal government frequently funded to deliver services on the local level. These groups typically interacted directly with their bureaucratic sponsors in Washington, circumventing the authority of general-purpose state and local governments and elected officials. A good case in point is the federal CMHC program, which made local centers dependent on the National Institute of Mental Health (NIMH) for funding and operational guidelines while providing for little coordination with or accountability to existing state mental health systems (Foley and Sharfstein, 1983: chapter 4).

By the start of the 1970s, reformers of all political persuasions wanted to restore a balance in federal relations more supportive of state and local discretion. Categoricals, to these critics, meant top-heavy, rigid, and inefficient administration. Significantly, this growing demand for administrative efficiency through decentralization coincided with a resurgence of political conservatism in America. Many who shared a private-market orientation, which traditionally favored a limited role for big government (especially, big *federal* government), argued for decentralization because it suited their own ideological predispositions.

President Nixon's proposed solution was general revenue sharing, a distribution of federal revenues to states and localities with virtually no strings attached. While general revenue sharing was approved by Congress, and subsequently endorsed by both Ford and Carter, it failed to stimulate the major changes hoped for within the intergovernmental system before being allowed to lapse by the Reagan administration. Concern over inadequate guarantees that states and localities would actually use federal funding for national priorities moderated liberal support for this new form of grant-in-aid. Neither was it consistent with the conservative goal of reduced federal taxation and spending. Under these political conditions, revenue sharing remained a modest program, never accounting for more than a small percentage of state or local revenues.

It was the block grant mechanism that seemed to promise a better balance between federal influence and state-local administration. Not a conservative but Lyndon Johnson inaugurated the first two block grants: the Partnership for Health Act of 1966 and the Omnibus Crime Control and Safe Streets Act of 1968. The Nixon-Ford administrations added three more: the Comprehensive Employment and Training Act of 1973; the Housing and Community Development Act of 1974; and the Title XX Amendments to the Social Security Act, also passed in 1974. Based on the common elements of these five early grant consolidations, the Advisory Commission on Intergovernmental Relations (ACIR) (1977: 6) formally defined a block grant as "a program by which funds are provided chiefly to general purpose governmental units in accordance with a statutory formula for use in a broad functional area, largely at the recipient's discretion."

In other words, on the federal level it is decided whom or what purpose to serve. The determination of eligibility and the formula for allocation are essential for doing this. Then, on the state and local levels, it is decided which activities can best meet these national objectives. Implicit in producing a new balance between federal and state-local governments is increasing the capacity of state and local bureaucracies to run their own programs. And the new balance was frankly intended to favor *state* governments. Block grant advocates sought to return the states to a more active role in American federalism, substituting a state-local axis for the federal-local axis that had developed under categorical grants.

Proponents of block grants have expected them to meet seven sometimes conflicting technical objectives: economy and efficiency (especially through consolidation of overlapping categoricals and lessened paperwork); program enlargement (consolidation creates greater visibility and should attract political support); decentralization (subnational jurisdictions assume key decision-making roles); coordination (increased cooperation within the functional area and removal of conflicting subunits); targeting (the formula targets funds to those objectively in need, while recipient flexibility allows allocation to high-priority programs); innovation (recipients can use funds to start activities they would not otherwise); and generalist control (elected chief executives, legislators, and administrators who are more accountable would replace specialists and interest groups) (Advisory Commission on Intergovernmental Relations, 1977: 8–11).

Evaluation studies of the first five block grants yielded mixed findings (Advisory Commission on Intergovernmental Relations, 1977: 38; Hale and Palley, 1981: 108–111; Barfield, 1981: 36–43). Some economy and efficiency were achieved, partly through the reduction of paperwork. Savings were below expectations, however, and varied from state to state. Decentralization was a significant success, and coordination was enhanced. Yet program enlargement generally did not occur. Innovation was limited. And although the opportunity did exist, generalist control was not really achieved, partly because of competing demands on the time of these officials. Targeting was also disappointing. ACIR noted that political compromises, even in securing initial congressional approval of the allocation formulas, made targeting the objectively needy difficult.

In retrospect, a chief problem with these original block grants may have been that strong political support for the original categoricals impeded consolidation. In some instances, powerful groups succeeded in "recategorizing" the programs that benefited them. Other relevant programs were excluded from the blocks altogether for the same reason. As a result, these pre-Reagan block grants really did not represent a sufficient proportion of total outlays in their respective functional areas—the "critical mass"—to constitute full-scale implementation. Whether they could have better met their objectives if they were fully implemented was never tested (Advisory Commission on Intergovernmental Relations, 1977: 38, 42).

The nine block grants created by the Reagan administration in 1981 represent, in most respects, a continuation of earlier efforts to implement the block grant concept. Arguments for administrative efficiency and decentralization, for example, were prominent. Increasing the role of the states was also part of the Reagan approach, with the president espousing a literal interpretation of the constitutional provision that powers not expressly delegated to the national government belong to the states or the people (Nathan and Doolittle, 1987: 358–361).

In one sense, however, the Reagan approach is distinctive, and that is the use of block grants as a means of *reducing* the federal budget. Asserting that more efficient state management would offset federal funding cuts, the administration persuaded Congress to lower authorizations for the consolidated programs. These reductions averaged 12 percent for fiscal 1982, the president's first budget year (Nathan and Doolittle, 1987: 57–59). It is important to stress that retrenchment is not inherent in the basic concept of grant consolidation. In fact, in the past it has been just the opposite, with the creation of block grants typically being accompanied by expanded outlays within the functional area. In any event, the current administration's budget reductions have further politicized relationships under the new block grants by raising the stakes for all concerned.

To summarize, one sympathetic analyst, writing near the start of the new administration, predicted the following results from Reagan's block grant policy:

a greatly enhanced role for state governments; major reduction in the direct ties between local governments and the federal government; an uncertain and hazardous future for the community-action and nonprofit organizations, which have served as quasi-public entities at the local level, dispensing social services largely with federal dollars; [and] a fifty-state "free-for-all" competition for block-grant funds among interest groups currently served by the social services, education, and health categorical grants. (Barfield, 1981: 47)

DESIGN OF THE ADAMH BLOCK GRANT

The ADAMH block grant provides the states with funds to support the planning, operation, and evaluation of services to prevent, treat, and rehabilitate persons with substance abuse problems. Another objective is to maintain the provision of community mental health services, especially those delivered to chronically mentally ill persons, severely disturbed children and adolescents, mentally ill elderly, and other underserved populations in the state.

Federal requirements under the block grant, significantly relaxed from those of the preceding multiple categorical programs, address state administrative practices as well as the substance of funded activities (U.S. General Accounting Office, 1982). States must apply to the U.S. Department of Health and Human Services (DHHS) for their ADAMH block grant award annually. There is no standardized application format, although all states must describe the intended use of funds and include a statement of assurance that these funds will be used consistently with the authorizing act's purposes. Each year the states must hold public hearings on the proposed use and distribution of ADAMH block grant funds. Other annual requirements include an audit of program expenditures and a report on block grant activities, with the detail and content of this report left largely to state discretion. Using state-established criteria, states must also conduct regular evaluations of organizations receiving block grant funds.

Certain general ground rules govern the allocation of block grant funds between and within the substance abuse and mental health areas. For fiscal 1982, the ADAMH block grant's first year, each state had to apportion its total award between mental health and substance abuse areas in keeping with prior federal funding patterns. In fiscal 1983 and 1984, 95 percent and 85 percent, respectively, had to be divided this way. When Congress reauthorized the block grant at the end of the initial three-year period, this percentage was set at 75 percent, leaving 25 percent to be distributed among the consolidated areas as states chose. In any fiscal year states must use a minimum of 35 percent of total substance abuse funds for alcohol abuse programs, and at least the same amount for drug abuse programs. No more than 10 percent of the block grant may be used by a state for administrative expenses.

OBRA and the subsequent reauthorizing legislation (Public Law 98–509) mandated that states give support to all community mental health centers which received a grant under the federal CMHC program in fiscal 1981 and would have continued to qualify for funding under that Act in the allotment year. The amount of money provided to each center was not fixed, however. Recipient centers must provide services that are easily accessible and given to patients regardless of their ability to pay. To be eligible for block grant funds a center must offer outpatient services, twenty-four-hour emergency care, day treatment or partial hospitalization, screening of patients being considered for admission to state mental health facilities, and consultation and education services.

Finally, the ADAMH block grant also requires states to reserve a fixed percentage of their award for serving designated clientele groups (U.S. General Accounting Office, 1987b). OBRA directed the states to use 20 percent of the alcohol and drug abuse portion of their grant for prevention and early treatment programs. Legislative amendments to the program in 1984 (Public Law 98–509) and 1985 (Public Law 99–117) established two additional set-asides. One obligates the states to use a minimum of 5 percent of their total ADAMH award for new or expanded alcohol and drug abuse services for women. The other specifies that 10 percent of the amount used by each state for mental health services must be allocated for new or expanded community mental health services for underserved areas or populations, especially severely disturbed children and adolescents. Entailing new constraints on state expenditures and on the principle of allowing states to define their own special target populations, these set-asides may be considered a partial recategorization of the ADAMH block grant.

BLOCK GRANT FUNDING LEVELS

Table 7–1 provides data on aggregate funding under the ADAMH block grant. During its first year of operation in fiscal 1982, the block grant operated at a level of $428.1 million, or about 28 percent below what the constituent programs

Table 7–1
ADAMH Categorical and Block Grant Funding 1980–1988

Fiscal Year	Awards to States[a] (millions)	Annual % change	% Change from 1981 (nominal $)	% Change from 1981 (real $)[b]
Pre-Block Grant				
1980	$625.1	—	—	—
1981	$541.2	− 13.4	—	—
Post-Block Grant				
1982	$428.1	− 20.9	− 20.9	− 25.5
1983	$468.0[c]	+ 9.3	− 13.5	− 21.1
1984	$462.0	− 1.3	− 14.6	− 25.3
1985	$490.0	+ 6.1	− 9.5	− 23.5
1986	$468.9	− 4.3	− 13.4	− 28.1
1987	$508.9[d]	+ 5.6	− 8.4	− 24.8
1988	$487.3	− 4.2	− 10.0	—

Source: U.S. General Accounting Office, 1984a: 5; and data provided by the National Institute of
    Mental Health, Division of Grants and Contracts Management.

[a]Total amount of appropriated funds that was distributed to the states.
[b]Adjusted using the annual average consumer price index for these years.
[c]Includes $30 million supplemental funding from the Emergency Jobs Appropriation Act of 1983
  (Public Law 98–8).
[d]Includes $13.9 million supplemental funding from the Anti-Drug Abuse Act of 1986 (Public Law
  99–570).

received immediately prior to consolidation. Since that time, the funding pattern
has been inconsistent, with increases in support occurring in certain years (fiscal
1983, 1985, and 1987) and decreases in others (fiscal 1984, 1986, and 1988).
Overall, however, the summary effect of various changes has been modest, so
that the fiscal 1988 appropriation of $487.3 million approximates the initial block
grant award and is still 10 percent below the final year of categorical support.
Measured in terms of constant dollars, the reduction is even more severe, a 24.8
percent decline between fiscal 1981 and fiscal 1987 (the latest year for which a
full consumer price index calculation is available).

Appropriations for the ADAMH block grant have not been made in a policymaking vacuum. Year-to-year funding changes reflect not only congressional
willingness to sustain the programs brought within this package, but also the
impact of contemporaneous national issues and problems. In fiscal 1983, for
example, the block grant received supplemental funding of $30 million through
the Emergency Jobs Appropriation Act of 1983 (Public Law 98–8), which provided money for job opportunities and health care, including mental health and

substance abuse services, for persons and areas affected by unemployment. In fiscal 1987, the block grant was augmented by appropriations under the Anti-Drug Abuse Act of 1986 (Public Law 99–570), which authorized new spending for alcohol abuse and drug abuse treatment and rehabilitation programs. On the other hand, funding reductions in fiscal 1986 and 1988 occurred as a result of budgetary cuts required under the Balanced Budget and Emergency Deficit Control Act of 1985 (Public Law 99–177), known popularly as the Gramm-Rudman Act.

Table 7–2 presents a breakdown of ADAMH block grant awards to the states in fiscal 1988. OBRA, the initial authorizing legislation, tied the distribution of funds to each state's level of support under the preceding categorical programs, with a base year of fiscal 1980 for alcohol and drug abuse and fiscal 1981 for mental health (U.S. Department of Health and Human Services, 1987: 13–14; U.S. General Accounting Office, 1987a). This arrangement gave to each state the same proportion of total block grant funding in these combined program areas as the state had received in the relevant base year. States that were most active in the CMHC program just prior to consolidation therefore had the advantage. In an attempt to better address the criterion of need, the Alcohol Abuse, Drug Abuse, and Mental Health Amendments of 1984 (Public Law 98–509) adjusted this formula to factor in both a state's population and its per capita income. However, due to a "hold-harmless" provision that guaranteed each state its fiscal 1984 funding level whenever total block grant appropriations at least equaled those in that budget year ($462 million), only a small proportion of block grant funds awarded subsequently have been made on the basis of the new formula. Thus concerns persist about equity of distribution (U.S. General Accounting Office, 1984b, 1987a). In 1987, Congress failed to act upon a proposed new formula that would have allocated all block grant funds among the states according to need and ability to pay for services, using refined measures of these two factors. Other bills to alter the formula were again under consideration in the House and Senate in 1988 (Moore, 1988).

It is important to note that block grant funds actually account for only a small proportion of total spending for ADAMH services. According to one estimate, state expenditures for alcohol and drug abuse community services deriving from both federal and state sources approximated $950.7 million in fiscal 1985 (cited in U.S. General Accounting Office, 1987a: 6). Only 26 percent of this sum came from the ADAMH block grant. States spent about $2.6 billion for community mental health services in this year, of which block grant support accounted for 9 percent. Data on the revenue sources of state mental health agencies (SMHA) offer another perspective on this same issue (Lutterman et al., 1987). In fiscal 1985, 14.5 percent of total SMHA revenues came from the federal government, with 20.4 percent of these federal dollars attributable to the ADAMH block grant; thus, the block grant contributed 3.0 percent of total SMHA revenues. Medicaid, by contrast, represented 58.2 percent of total federal aid for state mental health agency programs, and 8.4 percent of total SMHA revenues.

Table 7–2
Fiscal 1988 ADAMH Block Grant Distribution By State (thousands of dollars)

State	Total Awarded	Mental Health		Substance Abuse	
		%	Amount	%	Amount
Alabama	$ 9,328	67.73	$ 6,318	32.27	$ 3,010
Alaska	2,093	23.71	496	76.29	1,597
Arizona[a]	8,904	47.72	4,249	52.28	4,655
Arkansas	6,385	67.42	4,305	32.58	2,080
California	48,405	34.31	16,608	65.69	31,797
Colorado	7,004	48.55	3,400	51.45	3,604
Connecticut	6,985	36.62	2,558	63.38	4,427
Delaware	1,428	20.68	295	79.32	1,133
D.C.	2,467	14.54	359	85.46	2,108
Florida	24,033	53.49	12,855	46.51	11,178
Georgia	10,927	68.18	7,450	31.82	3,477
Hawaii	2,827	56.00	1,583	44.00	1,244
Idaho	1,632	41.57	678	58.43	954
Illinois	19,221	56.85	10,927	43.15	8,294
Indiana	19,524	86.16	16,822	13.84	2,702
Iowa	2,839	8.75	248	91.25	2,591
Kansas	3,900	58.11	2,266	41.89	1,634
Kentucky	4,432	32.57	1,444	67.43	2,988
Louisiana	5,570	15.41	858	84.59	4,712
Maine	3,733	53.72	2,005	46.28	1,728
Maryland	4,754	13.16	626	86.84	4,128
Massachusetts	18,240	55.97	10,209	44.03	8,031
Michigan	15,630	29.52	4,614	70.48	11,016
Minnesota[b]	4,692	30.41	1,427	69.59	3,265
Mississippi	5,077	73.49	3,731	26.51	1,346
Missouri	9,643	58.34	5,626	41.66	4,017
Montana	2,153	57.37	1,235	42.63	918
Nebraska	2,634	46.36	1,221	53.64	1,413
Nevada	2,897	48.02	1,391	51.98	1,506
New Hampshire	3,844	73.00	2,086	27.00	1,038
New Jersey	20,647	51.74	10,683	48.26	9,964
New Mexico	4,934	49.88	2,461	50.12	2,473
New York	40,097	23.09	9,258	76.91	30,839
North Carolina	10,771	59.58	6,417	40.42	4,354
North Dakota	1,150	32.89	378	67.11	772
Ohio	23,585	67.91	16,017	32.09	7,568
Oklahoma	7,775	74.79	5,815	25.21	1,960
Oregon	5,875	43.10	2,532	56.90	3,343
Pennsylvania	25,114	52.73	13,243	47.27	11,871
Rhode Island	4,417	57.16	2,525	42.84	1,892
South Carolina	6,583	63.97	4,211	36.03	2,372

Table 7-2 (continued)

State	Total Awarded	Mental Health		Substance Abuse	
		%	Amount	%	Amount
South Dakota	3,100	66.62	2,065	33.38	1,035
Tennessee	7,643	68.57	5,241	31.43	2,402
Texas	21,183	41.51	8,793	58.49	12,390
Utah	3,779	46.98	1,775	53.02	2,004
Vermont	3,313	66.42	2,200	33.58	1,113
Virginia	8,229	43.35	3,567	56.65	4,662
Washington	8,977	52.66	4,727	47.34	4,250
West Virginia	4,227	66.64	2,817	33.36	1,410
Wisconsin	5,114	10.29	526	89.71	4,588
Wyoming	758	42.08	319	57.92	439
American Samoa	16	00.00	0	100.00	16
Guam	536	61.55	330	38.45	206
Marshall Islands	16	00.00	0	100.00	16
Micronesia	38	00.00	0	100.00	38
Northern Mariana Islands	32	00.00	0	100.00	32
Palau	6	00.00	0	100.00	6
Puerto Rico	6,875	40.70	2,798	59.30	4,077
Virgin Islands	1,113	75.55	841	24.45	272
Phoenix Indian Health Board	100	00.00	0	100.00	100
Red Lake Band of Chippewa Indians	113	00.00	0	100.00	113
Total	$487,317		$238,149		$249,168

Source: National Institute of Mental Health, Division of Education and Service Systems Liaison, State Planning and Resource Development Branch.

[a]Does not include $100,000 for Phoenix Indians.
[b]Does not include $113,000 for Red Lake Band of Chippewa Indians.

Clearly, then, the block grant plays a modest role in the states' larger effort to finance the provision of ADAMH services. This can be expected to have lessened the impact of the shift from categorical to block grant funding. However, this impact must be gauged not only in financial terms, but also with respect to the broader issues of federal-state, public-private relations to which it is relevant (U.S. Department of Health and Human Services, 1987: 69).

ANALYZING THE IMPACT OF THE ADAMH BLOCK GRANT

The intergovernmental system brings together federal, state, and local actors in a process that distributes resources, sets policy priorities, and assigns responsibilities across the levels of the polity. In changing the role played by the federal government within this joint interaction, block grants simultaneously fashion new roles for other involved parties, namely, state government officials, local authorities, interest groups, service providers and recipients, and advocates. Such a reorientation is likely to affect not only the "inputs" but also the "outputs" of the policy equation, since, as Morgan and Connery (1980: 253) have observed, "To change the level of government at which a decision is made, or to shift the forum for decision making at a particular level, is to alter the probabilities as to what precisely will be decided. This results in large part from the simple fact that the varying institutional forms reflect and favor different political alignments" (see, also, Brown and Stockdill, 1972: 678–680; Buck, 1984; Gorman, 1984; Pond, 1982).

A historical perspective highlights the nature of the change wrought by the ADAMH block grant. In transferring responsibility for the community mental health program to state governments, the block grant policy reverses one of the most fundamental principles that underlay initial development of the CMHC Act. Originators of this legislation purposefully structured the grant-in-aid process so as to bypass state authority and state mental health priorities, identified at the time with "an obsolete emphasis on institutional care" (Grob, 1987: 27). Moreover, proponents of the national community mental health effort favored a conception of mental illness as a continuum that included but did not place special emphasis on the kinds of severe mental disorders typical of the state mental hospital population. In effect, what was created in 1963 was an alternate system of mental health care in the states, with new facilities, aims, and funding source. Now major funders and advocates of community services in their own right, the states have gained primary control over this alternate system and, with it, the ability to pursue their own programmatic objectives.

With an empirical data base of several years of operational experience now behind it, the ADAMH block grant invites a critical consideration of these issues of realignment and redirection in community mental health care. The findings are of interest to students of mental health policy and intergovernmental relations alike.

Role of the States

Replacement of lost federal funds. Creation of the block grants in 1981 coupled with funding cuts in the programs under consolidation stimulated predictions that states would be unable or unwilling to make up for the lost federal dollars (see, e.g., Beigel, 1982; Callahan, 1982; Buck 1984). To the contrary, research within the ADAMH and other areas has shown a subsequent trend toward expanded state outlays, although not always at a level sufficient to offset inflation's eroding effects.

A report completed by the U.S. General Accounting Office (1984a) traced ADAMH funding trends based on fieldwork conducted in 1983 in thirteen states that together accounted for 46 percent of block grant awards in fiscal 1982 and included 48 percent of the U.S. population. Despite federal cutbacks in the shift from categorical to block grant support, total spending in the alcohol, drug abuse, and mental health program area increased in most of these states. For nine of the eleven states for which these data were available, increases ranged from 3 percent to 24 percent. The other two states experienced decreases of less than 1 percent and 8 percent. In real dollar terms, there were total funding increases in five of eleven states (ranging from 3 percent to 14 percent), reductions in another five states (ranging from 3 percent to 15 percent), and no significant change in the remaining state.

Two factors, especially, cushioned the impact of federal funding cuts under the block grant program. First, in many states an overlap of categorical and block grant funds in fiscal 1982 permitted the carrying over of a portion of the block grant award in this and the next funding cycle to subsequent years. Second, nearly all states in the General Accounting Office (GAO) sample increased their own contributions to this program area over the study period, presumably in order to counteract federal retrenchment. The size of state increases ranged from 2 percent to 66 percent. As a result, even with overlapping federal categorical and block grant funds for many recipients in fiscal 1982, between 1981 and 1983 the majority of states examined by GAO increased the share of support for the ADAMH area deriving from their own funds.

Corroborative findings emerge from an Urban Institute survey of eighteen states from fiscal 1981 to fiscal 1984 (Peterson et al., 1986). Of twelve states in this sample that lost federal support for ADAMH services during this period (taking into account carryover funds but excluding spending from the Emergency Jobs Appropriations bill), all twelve increased expenditures from state sources. Ten states had total program spending increases measured in nominal dollars. Even after correcting for inflation, seven had overall increases. Peterson et al. (1986; see, also, Nathan and Doolittle, 1987: 13–14) note that economic recovery in the states beginning in 1984 helped to encourage supplementation. They conclude: "The block grants can be interpreted in part as a test of states' political commitment in deciding whether or not to sustain human service programs, even when not obliged to do so by the federal government and when no longer subsidized to do so by categorical matching grants. The states passed this test of commitment to a greater degree than most observers anticipated" (Peterson et al., 1986: 15).

Underlying this overall stimulative effect of block grants on state ADAMH spending, however, are noteworthy variations by state and by type of service provider. In a detailed comparative analysis, Hudson and Dubey (1985) reported that the greatest mental health spending increases between 1977 and 1983 occurred in those states with a well-developed service system, a strong constituency of providers, a high level of per capita income, and decentralized administrative structures. Further, not all types of community care benefited from supplementation: in the sample studied by these authors community mental health centers were an exception to the general trend. Adjusted for inflation and for population, state support of CMHCs fell 28 percent between 1981 and 1983, contributing to a decrease of 37 percent in combined federal-state aid to CMHCs in this same period. These authors speculate that CMHCs bore the brunt of the funding cutbacks because of what they describe as CMHCs' "historically . . . adversarial relation with state mental health departments" (Hudson and Dubey, 1985: 19).

Management performance. A principal tenet of block grant theory is that improved management performance will result from the consolidation of fragmented federal categorical programs under state-level administration. Evaluation studies of the block grants created in 1981 typically confirm this expectation, with the greatest gains in coordination and efficiency taking place in program areas, like ADAMH services, where the states had extensive prior involvement with categorical or related state programs (see, for example, Logan, Rochefort, and Cook, 1985; Peterson et al., 1986; U.S. General Accounting Office, 1984a: chapter 4; 1985b). In general, the states acted quickly to integrate ADAMH block grant funds into existing planning and administrative processes. Rather than treating these monies as coming from a separate funding source, most states incorporated block grant support into their normal fiscal cycle, utilizing whatever budgetary mechanisms were currently in place. As a rule, states have also effectively carried out their other new management responsibilities under the ADAMH block grant, including establishment of program requirements, monitoring, technical assistance, data collection, and auditing—although adopted practices in these areas vary.

Administrative improvements and efficiencies have been achieved by several means. Most states report spending less time completing paperwork, such as grant applications and reports for the federal government. Other aspects of a more "rational-comprehensive" style of decision making within the ADAMH area are structural, such as fuller integration of budgeting and planning processes, and functional, such as a more thorough consideration and evaluation of programming alternatives (Hudson and Dubey, 1986). Some of this increased rationality, it has been noted, likely results from the need of state authorities to justify block grant allocation decisions to various interest groups and oversight bodies (Hudson and Dubey, 1986: 111).

Given the gains that states have made in their administrative and policymaking capabilities over the past two decades, these findings of effective management performance should perhaps not be surprising (Thompson, 1986). In this sense, "the timing of Reagan's federalism-reform program was propitious from the point of view of supporters of social programs" (Nathan and Doolittle, 1987: 9). Not coincidentally, it is those states with the strongest administrative capacity and most fully developed mental health systems that have best utilized the expanded management control allowed them under the ADAMH block grant. In the short term at least, less prepared recipients did not seem to benefit as much or even suffered from the development of a more "politicized," more "incremental" decision-making process for ADAMH services (Hudson and Dubey, 1986).

Forecasts of the administrative cost savings to be realized by states following block grant implementation were sizable, ranging as high as 25 percent (Peterson et al., 1986: 23–24). Indeed, some administration spokespersons claimed these anticipated savings would entirely offset the enacted funding cuts. While states reported savings subsequently, they did not characterize them as commensurate with the federal reductions. A more precise statement is not possible because the types of data needed to make valid quantitative comparisons across the states are lacking (U.S. General Accounting Office, 1984a: chapter 4). Recognizing the need for more uniform national data consistent with the requirements of program evaluation, the U.S. Congress voted in 1984 to add new data collection provisions to the ADAMH block grant and four others (U.S. General Accounting Office, 1985b). In this same year, the Single Audit Act (Public Law 98–502) established new uniform auditing procedures for all federal grant programs to state and local governments, including block grants. As with the creation of set-aside provisions for delivery of services to designated populations, the thrust of such measures is to lessen the administrative flexibility of states under the block grants and, in this sense, signifies a partial return to the philosophy of the predecessor categorical system.

Allocation decisions. In determining the recommended distribution of ADAMH funds within their jurisdiction, most state authorities have relied on quantitative calculation of population-based need for services (Logan, Rochefort, and Cook, 1985; U.S. General Accounting Office, 1984a: chapter 5; Hudson and Dubey, 1986). Formulas for mental health typically combine multiple factors for substate areas, such as population, poverty level, and characteristics of the existing caseload. Another common approach, especially in the initial transition to block grants, was to base allocations on prior categorical funding, assigning eligible CMHCs a fixed percentage of this level. The two methods have not always been mutually exclusive, with prior federal funding level entering as a factor into a more comprehensive formula in some states. Selected states have also employed a two-tier allocation mechanism by distributing the majority of block grant funds according to one of these two methods, but reserving a substantial sum for discretionary use by the mental health authority.

States have universally complied with the requirement to hold public hearings on the proposed use and distribution of ADAMH funds. Generally, the state mental authority holds one or more public forums to which any interested parties—providers, consumers, interest groups, the general public—are invited. Some states also convene special legislative hearings that are open to the public, or use a combination of legislative hearings and public forums. Special advisory groups and task forces have also been formed in many places. These practices signal the expanded involvement under the block grant of legislatures and governors in making ADAMH decisions (U.S. General Accounting Office, 1984a: chapter 5).

A main objective of the Reagan administration in creating the block grants was to weaken organized private interests by dispersing their influence across a decentralized policymaking environment (Peterson, 1982: 169). Existing studies suggest this has occurred within the ADAMH area, especially as state program officials have strengthened their administrative authority. Research completed after the first couple of years of block grant experience found that most state officials preferred the block grant funding mechanism, while providers tended to favor the categorical grant approach. Many interest groups were dissatisfied with how state decisions were impacting on their constituencies (U.S. General Accounting Office, 1984a: 61–62; Logan, Rochefort, and Cook, 1985).

Whether the public itself has gained appreciable influence over ADAMH decisions is another question. The answer probably depends on what definition is given to this nebulous entity and who is considered to represent the public's views. Public hearings have helped stimulate program changes in some states, although state officials more often cite statistical data and advisory groups as important sources of information to them (U.S. General Accounting Office, 1984a: 57–58). Also, at least within the early years of the block grant, service providers and advocacy groups clearly dominated at public hearings, with comparatively few private citizens or unorganized recipients of mental health services participating (Logan, Rochefort, and Cook, 1985).

Program priorities. Legislative provisions to continue funding to specified eligible providers coupled with limitations on transfers between the substance abuse and mental health areas guaranteed a stable transition under the ADAMH block grant. Comparing funding patterns within its sample of thirteen states between fiscal 1981 and fiscal 1983, the U.S. General Accounting Office (1984a: chapter 2; 1985a: 15–16; see, also, Peterson et al., 1986: 124–128) found no major shifts in program priorities—although some states were increasing their emphasis on substance abuse prevention and early intervention services to satisfy that prevention set-aside requirement. Extensive changes in the service network had not occurred by this time but could occur in the future, with the period of "grandfathered" support for CMHCs having concluded in fiscal 1987 and with states increasingly engaging in performance-based, competitive contracting for services (Logan, Rochefort, and Cook, 1985; Hudson and Dubey, 1986).

Within this overall continuity are certain emerging state priorities for community mental health care. Service to the chronically and severely mentally ill, traditionally the population of greatest interest for state mental health systems, has received the strongest emphasis—as part of state allocation formulas, in evaluation criteria, and in program development (Logan, Rochefort, and Cook, 1985; U.S. Department of Health and Human Services, 1987: 70–80; Ahr and Holcomb, 1985; Beigel and Fine, 1984). Some states have also increased their targeting of children and the elderly. Areas receiving less emphasis currently include prevention activities and short-term outpatient services for the general population.

Impact on CMHC Operations and Services

The context. Several political and economic developments, in addition to the ADAMH block grant, acted to redefine the environment of community mental health services in the early 1980s (Surber et al., 1986; Burt and Pittman, 1985: chapter 5). The same year that the block grant was created, the Reagan administration undertook a tightening up of the Social Security Disability Insurance (SSDI) and Supplemental Security Income (SSI) programs which made it more difficult to qualify and remain eligible for disability payments. Especially in the SSI program, many of the recipients removed from the rolls were chronically mentally ill individuals dependent on federal support for maintenance in the community. The Omnibus Budget Reconciliation Act of 1981 also cut federal matching for state Medicaid expenditures, providing the states with fresh incentive for cost-containment efforts in their covered health and mental health services. And economic recession combined with the passage of restrictive property tax initiatives in some states created a condition of fiscal austerity that added to the financial difficulties of social programs, including public mental health care. Disentangling the independent effect of the block grant on CMHC functioning in this period from these other concurrent influences is a daunting task, especially as multiple forces dictated a common direction of retrenchment.

Analysis of the ADAMH block grant's impact on community mental health centers is also complicated by the very pluralism of the CMHC system. Take, for example, the important matter of dependence on federal revenues. The CMHC Act of 1963 (as amended) granted to federally funded CMHCs a fiscal life cycle of eight years. Over this time the amount of federal "seed money" gradually declined to zero and was supposed to be replaced by other sources of support. At the time the block grant was initiated, CMHCs across the country were in various stages of maturation: some had already graduated from the federal CMHC program, others were currently funded but reliant to different degrees on federal dollars, and still others were pending applicants. It is useful to consider how centers in varying situations have fared under the block grant (see, e.g., Woy and Mazade, 1982); unfortunately, the literature on CMHCs in the 1980s has not always distinguished carefully among such subgroups.

A useful framework for approaching these conceptual and analytical complexities is offered by the observation that, prior to enactment of the block grant, the federal government maintained a "protectorate" relationship with the centers it funded (Surles, 1987). Even if many had come to rely heavily on state financing over the years, so long as they received some amount of categorical grant support, CMHCs functioned under service and operational guidelines set out by the federal government. The states generally acquiesced in this arrangement, however grudgingly, in order to maintain access to federal dollars. The ADAMH block grant removed most of these federal requirements and gave to states increased authority over the operation of CMHCs just at the time a host of forces of change were reverberating through the community mental health system. For this reason the block grant's programmatic impact outweighs its direct financial significance.

Revenue effects. It has already been noted that the CMHC community suffered fiscally in association with the shift to block grant funding even as many states increased support to the ADAMH area. This occurred for many reasons. High inflation partially or entirely offset state funding increases, so that centers' purchasing power fell. State pressure for centers to target services to the chronically mentally ill, an especially resource-consuming population, exacerbated this situation (Surber et al., 1986). Moreover, CMHCs did not automatically receive all mental health block grant money channeled through their state bureaucracies. Not only did states sometimes hold back a portion of the federal award for discretionary uses, some chose to distribute block grant (and related state) funds to alternative community providers perceived as better attuned to serving the chronically mentally ill (Hudson and Dubey, 1985; Logan, Rochefort, and Cook, 1985).

Several studies suggest the extent of revenue losses sustained by CMHCs under the block grant (although no single, comprehensive data base gives the magnitude of these effects over time for different types of centers, correcting for variable state practices such as the channeling of funds through county mental health agencies). In a telephone survey conducted in the spring of 1983 among thirty-six community mental health centers in eight states, 78 percent of respondents said that they were affected by block grant changes, and nearly three-quarters of this group reported reduced federal funds (Estes and Wood, 1984). Another survey in this same year of 104 members of the National Council of Community Mental Health Centers (NCCMHC) reported that 46 percent of facilities receiving block grant funds perceived their financial status to have "deteriorated" since 1981 (cited in Okin, 1984). It should be noted, however, that this sample includes then current and previous recipients of CMHC funds as well as other community mental health agencies, and the relationship between cited funding losses and the block grant is unclear. One state which did not use its own funds to compensate CMHCs for federal grant reductions between 1981 and 1983 was Massachusetts. Here the average CMHC program sustained cuts in the neighborhood of 30–34 percent (Burt and Pittman, 1985: 92).

These aggregate data, suitable for outlining the general picture of federal fiscal contraction, obscure important differences in how individual centers experienced the shift to block grants depending on the allocation practices of their state mental health authority and on their own dependence on federal revenues.

The most stable situation was one where a state passed along block grant funds to all centers then receiving categorical support and at a percentage of previous funding dictated by the federal reductions. This arrangement made the incidence and extent of losses among a state's centers predictable, with no provider gaining at the expense of any other. Much more disruptive was statewide distribution of block grant dollars according to a population-based formula that disregarded previous reliance on direct federal grants. This made graduate centers (and other non-CMHC providers) eligible for a potential windfall, while placing categorical grant recipients at financial risk. According to the U.S. General Accounting Office (1984a: 33), Mississippi's adoption of this approach for handling the ADAMH block grant resulted in one local center's loss of 36 percent of total operating funds from 1981 to 1983.

Perhaps hardest hit of all were centers with pending applications to begin the CMHC categorical grant program at the time the block grant took its place. Burt and Pittman give an example of one facility in Massachusetts which expected a favorable disposition of its 1980 request for an initial operations grant as a federally qualified community mental health center:

The request was rescinded, converted into a block-grant request, and the money was subsequently allocated through the state rather than given directly to the clinic by the federal government. The Dorchester clinic's block-grant allocation was one-fifth to one-sixth of what it originally requested. The block-grant legislation affected *anticipated* services, which had a high probability of receiving federal support before the Reagan administration created the state-administered block grant. To develop residential programs, Dorchester had applied for funds to develop half-way houses and cooperative apartments to provide transitional, independent living situations for chronically mentally ill adults in its catchment area. Without federal funds, Dorchester could not implement this program. (Burt and Pittman, 1985: 110–111)

Other plans canceled by the clinic included a major expansion in emergency services and augmented alcohol and drug abuse treatment and senior services.

By the late 1980s, the country's community mental health facilities were markedly less dependent on federal grant funds than at the start of the decade. Data compiled by the NCCMHC (1985, 1988), for example, indicate that, on average, the ADAMH block grant accounted for 6 percent of member agencies' budgets in fiscal 1987, down from 10.9 percent just three years earlier (see, also, Jerrell and Larsen, 1984, 1986). Continuing a trend away from federal support that began in the 1970s, this development was furthered though not caused by block grants. By contrast, an increasingly important revenue source over these years was Medicaid. Even as some states implemented restrictions in this federal-state health insurance program in reaction to the federal cuts (Estes and Wood, 1984; Surber et al., 1986), others expanded Medicaid coverage of community mental health services as an alternate means of leveraging federal dollars in this area (Jerrell and Larsen, 1984; Toff, 1984, 1986). Fee-for-service and third-party payers also became more significant funding sources. Total agency budget in nominal dollars for this same sample declined slightly on average.

Service patterns. Reflecting state priorities, the populations benefiting most from recent CMHC service changes have been the chronically and severely mentally ill, including individuals previously hospitalized in state facilities and the young chronically mentally ill who have never received long-term institutional care. In a survey by Cognos Associates of seventy-one CMHCs located in fifteen states, one-half to two-thirds of those facilities implementing program changes in 1982 and 1983 expanded services to these two groups (Jerrell and Larsen, 1986). The most common stimulus cited was state policy and funding guidelines. Other studies confirm these findings (Okin, 1984; Rochefort, Logan, and Cook, 1984; Surber et al., 1986).

Specific CMHC services undergoing expansion as part of this focus on the chronically and severely mentally ill include day treatment/partial hospitalization (described as moving toward "psychosocial" and "vocational rehabilitation" models); case management; and community residential programs. Some substate mental health areas have increased their use of inpatient care services during the block grant period, but this is not a consistent trend nationally among CMHC providers (Surber et al., 1986; Jerrell and Larsen, 1984, 1985).

While some types of CMHC services have grown in volume, others have shrunk, most notably, consultation and education, prevention, and alcohol and drug abuse treatment (the latter often being available through community providers other than CMHCs). These services, formerly required of centers by the federal government, do not represent current priorities for state mental health authorities, nor are they usually income-generating. Centers have found it possible, however, to reorient selected other services to meet one or both of these objectives. For example, outpatient care increasingly has been redirected to two quite different, sometimes physically separated, clientele groups: chronic patients (e.g., for medication and for crisis visits) and privately paying patients (Jerrell and Larsen, 1984, 1985, 1986).

The status of CMHC services for the elderly and for children, two populations of specific interest under the federal mental health centers program, is ambiguous at present. According to some studies, recent funding cutbacks have not generally damaged CMHC services for the aged, this despite the block grant's removal of the requirement for specialized geriatric services in these facilities (Fox, Swan, and Estes, 1986; Swan, Fox, and Estes, 1986). Other research, however, identifies the elderly as one of the groups currently receiving reduced attention from many CMHCs (Jerrell and Larsen, 1986; Okin, 1984; Rochefort, Logan, and Cook, 1984). And even though the Congress in 1985 enacted special set-aside provisions to assure continued targeting of community mental health services to children and youths, the amount earmarked is only a small share of each state's total ADAMH award—10 percent of the mental health portion—which, in turn, tends to be spread among multiple providers and among "other underserved areas and populations" in addition to children (U.S. Congress, 1986: 133–135). More than any other single factor, it appears, the priority CMHCs currently assign to these two social groups is being determined by individual state commitment, and the level of this commitment varies around the country.

Thus, as centers have responded to the fiscal incentives emanating from their public and private markets in the 1980s, comprehensiveness of services has lessened. Local innovation, a goal of many block grant theorists, has been limited due to the top-down nature of state management under the block grant. Speaking of his own state, one CMHC survey respondent put it colorfully: "Block grants are targeted by the state solely for the chronically mentally ill. To equate block grants with flexibility is to equate Ronald Reagan with John F. Kennedy" (Rochefort, Logan, and Cook, 1984: 30). Finally, though data on this important issue are incomplete, there is evidence that overall service levels of most CMHCs held stable or even fell slightly in this period as service demands continued to increase (Okin, 1984; National Council of Community Mental Health Centers, 1985–1988).

Management and administration. For many CMHCs the 1980s has been a period of cutback management. Particularly true for centers directly hit by block grant reductions, this predicament describes the situation of other CMHCs as well, and no single theme has been more prominent in the recent literature (see, e.g., Hagan, Forman, and Gorodezky, 1982; Hoare, 1983; Goplerud, Walfish, and Broskowski, 1985). In response to the challenge, centers have undertaken strategic assessments of current services to identify optimal areas of shrinkage and growth. The operative principle has been adaptation for survival. Many have also sought to contain costs through improved efficiency and have implemented such changes as increased clinician caseloads, closure of satellite clinics, mergers with other catchment areas for the provision of selected services to larger population units, internal mergers of departments, and heightened emphasis on staff productivity (Jerrell and Larsen, 1984, 1985; Estes and Wood, 1984; Peterson, Austin, and Patti, 1985).

Examining representative national samples of CMHCs in the late 1970s and early 1980s, Landsberg (1985) identified a trend toward expanded quality assurance (QA) activities. Seventy percent of his sample had QA systems in 1977–1978, 93 percent in 1983. Centers thus have endeavored to better document utilization of services and to limit excessive lengths of stay in inpatient and outpatient programs. Partly this development reflects centers' own perception of the possible administrative and cost-control benefits of QA, partly it reflects new state directives. In this and other ways, CMHCs have expanded their monitoring of services, especially in states that allocate funds via service-specific contracts (Rochefort, Logan, and Cook, 1984).

Many researchers have described the movement of CMHCs toward a "business model" in the 1980s, referring to the adoption of practices more in keeping with private enterprise than the public and private nonprofit sectors to which CMHCs belong (Jerrell and Larsen, 1984; Okin, 1984; Rochefort, Logan, and Cook, 1984). Components of this model include more efficient billing and collection procedures; tighter financial screening of patients; improved accounting and record keeping; and development of services for populations able to pay for treatment. The subsuming philosophy is one of competition for market share.

Most centers in this period have chosen to maintain voluntarily the citizen board involvement previously required by the federal government (Jerrell and Larsen, 1984; Rochefort, Logan, and Cook, 1984). Here too, however, CMHCs have made modifications to suit their altered environment. Some centers have recruited new board members who are influential with public officials and with private funding sources. Centers have also sought to attract more members with a business orientation.

New patterns of interaction and linkage between CMHCs and other public and private actors are discernible. Seeking to replace lost revenues from traditional sources, centers have developed more service contracts with courts, school districts, and private businesses (Jerrell and Larsen, 1984). For political advantage, some centers have also formed alliances with other local human service providers in order to maximize their bargaining power with state legislatures and the state mental health authority (Edwards and Mitchell, 1987; Goplerud, Walfish, and Broskowski, 1985). More interaction between CMHCs and elements of the state bureaucracy has also become necessary under the block grant, for obvious reasons. Despite this heightened contact, however, centers typically complain of having the same or decreased influence over their allocations as under the prior categorical program (Rochefort, Logan, and Cook, 1984).

These changes in administration and in organizational behavior, prominent throughout the CMHC community in the 1980s, have not been uniform. Exceptions and variations exist among individual centers for all of the noted trends, although more systematic research is needed to identify their sources. One study by Jerrell and Jerrell (1986) examined the impact of state policy and funding environment on CMHCs' chosen management strategies and performance. Using a cluster analysis procedure, these authors defined four types of states based on the size of the state mental health authority's budget, the proportion of this budget going to community mental health programs, entitlement program policies, the nature of center-state relationships, and other policy, program, and expenditure variables. Their findings describe the type of center most able to cope productively with current policy shifts and funding cutbacks:

Overall, the best positioned centers appear to be those operating in state contexts with relatively high percentages of government funding not fluctuating precipitously over time; those that enjoy rather positive working relationships with their state mental health authority; those that can access broad or expanding entitlement reimbursements; and those that can offset reductions in government funding with revenues from nongovernment sources. . . . In taking advantage of the opportunities within the state, the best positioned centers appear to be most innovative in using a larger number of management strategies that have more internal consistency and continue to be pursued from one year to the next. Furthermore, these strategies encompass a broad range of alternatives, including service programs, personnel, governing board, interagency, and business practice changes. (Jerrell and Jerrell, 1986: 222)

Staffing developments. Contemporary fiscal retrenchment has led to personnel reductions for many centers. In Estes and Wood's (1984) survey of thirty-six centers in eight states which was conducted in the spring of 1983, 42 percent reported recent decreases in full-time personnel. Of all centers with decreases in full- or part-time staff, 61 percent linked the reductions to federal cuts. Analyzing data gathered by the Cognos Associates study of seventy-one CMHCs in fifteen states, Jerrell and Larsen (1984) found a slight increase in average total staff from 1976 to 1980, followed by a personnel decline of approximately 15 percent between 1980 and 1982. Terminations, layoffs, and hiring freezes all were accountable.

To fulfill a new organizational mission in the 1980s, many centers have reorganized and redeployed staff in both the administrative and clinical areas. What few staff additions have been made have tended to be in partial care, residential, and case management services (Jerrell and Larsen, 1986). Between 1982 and 1983, social workers gained in representation among clinical providers in CMHCs, while doctoral-level psychologists decreased and psychiatrists' involvement remained about constant. According to Jerrell and Larsen (1986: 85), the state of the morale of CMHC staff members in 1984 was mixed: "For the most part, staff morale had improved over the past two years, but some centers are still experiencing stressful conditions, accompanied by staff burnout and low morale, due to higher workloads, increased productivity demands, and staff attrition."

DISCUSSION AND SUMMARY

Community mental health care during the 1980s is in transition. To make this observation is to state a truism. Cutting across different levels of government and different public programs, the forces of change have affected both the policy framework and funding of the system. While block grants represent only one of many contemporary influences, they are perhaps the archetypal development. Federal grant reductions and a movement away from the federal community mental health center model simultaneously created the need and a possibility for new concepts of organization, financing, management, and delivery of services, all under the expanded supervision of state government. In this way, block grants helped enable and confirmed other transformations of the period.

Talk of a "Reagan revolution" notwithstanding, it is important to underscore that many recent alterations in public mental health care are extensions of developments dating back to the 1970s (Rich, 1986). For example, the desirability of greater state authority over local CMHCs was commonly recognized by the late 1970s. The importance of better targeting the chronically mentally ill (CMI) in the community was also cited by many analysts, who criticized CMHCs for slighting this needy population in part due to the service difficulties involved; in the late 1970s NIMH initiated its own collaborative effort with the states, the Community Support Program, to expand assistance to the CMI (see chapters 9 and 12 in this volume). Both of these issues were addressed in provisions of the Mental Health Systems Act of 1980, subsequently rescinded. Similarly, the progressive changeover from federal to state funding of community mental health services predated by several years the ADAMH block grant. In this sense, "the 1981 transfer of administrative authority to the states recognized the shift that had gradually occurred in the primary source of government support over the years" (Okin, 1984: 1120).

Greater involvement of state officials, improved service to the CMI population, and a new concern with accountability and efficiency of operations are some estimable effects of the ADAMH block grant on community mental health care.

At the same time, however, these and other recent developments raise some significant concerns about the system's future.

One emerging issue is geographic variability in policies and services. As states increasingly blaze their own pathways, it is inevitable that mental health programs across the country will differ to a greater extent than if the same national model were followed everywhere. Already, states' handling of the block grant displays marked variation in the criteria used for distributing funds, whether contracts or grants are the chosen allocation mechanism, the emphasis placed on serving children and the elderly, and other important matters. For some, this variability, ipso facto, is positive because it represents responsiveness to local values and conditions and is a source of creativity. Others, however, see a potential diffusion of purpose in American mental health policy and fear the abandonment of previously established objectives of access and service for diverse social groups (see, e.g., Burt and Pittman, 1985; Swan, Fox, and Estes, 1986; Frank and Kamlet, 1986). The federal government's recent revision of the block grant to include funding set-asides for specified population groups and more standard data collection requirements attests to national policymakers' own continuing ambivalence on this old question of state discretion within the federal grants system. It reminds us, as well, that negotiating the balance between permissiveness and control within the intergovernmental system is ever an unfinished process (Thompson, 1986).

Ironically, another issue in contemporary community mental health care focuses not on the system's variability but what is perhaps its most uniform aspect—the reorientation to serving the chronically mentally ill. No one disputes the severe needs of this population, nor the system's past limited success in meeting them. But, according to some observers, this new policy priority dominates to the extent that it threatens to transform CMHCs into narrow-purpose providers. Okin (1984: 1122) explains how such a development could end up harming all service populations, including the CMI: "as the history of state hospitals has shown, facilities that exclusively serve a population that is both indigent and devalued by society tend to suffer in quality, resources, and manpower." Thus is outlined the continuing dilemma of community mental health care: adopting too broad a service philosophy draws available resources, which are limited, away from the most severely disordered; yet a more specialized approach neglects other clientele and potentially undermines the program's public support. The question is one not only of mission but also of identifying the most effective means to accomplish that mission.

At the time of its enactment, mental health professionals wondered whether the ADAMH block grant represented a "crisis" or an "opportunity" for them and their clients (see, e.g., Sharfstein, 1982). The sense of crisis has now passed, largely because of most states' demonstrated willingness and capacity to accept the new responsibilities they acquired under the program. How much of an opportunity was created is yet to be answered. The present analysis, centering as it does on the initial period of transition from one policy system to another, is but a snapshot in time of a dynamic situation.

The agenda in contemporary community mental health is clear. Improved service structures, methods of coordination, and funding mechanisms must be developed to meet the mental health, health, and social service needs of the chronically mentally ill and other patient groups in a continuous and comprehensive way (Mechanic and Aiken, 1987; Visotsky, 1987). There must also be expanded outreach to persons with serious mental health problems who require but are not receiving treatment. Whether it is the states, as opposed to the federal government, that will best be able to marshal the energy, expertise, and resources to rise to this challenge is the question. As Nathan and Doolittle (1987: 362) argue, the answer may just depend on the times, with states being the preferred locus of policymaking and administration for social change advocates during conservative periods, while the central government should be looked to in liberal periods.

Public policies have been likened to working hypotheses about the best method for linking resources to goals (Wildavsky, 1979: 393). As such, they require continuing evaluation in order to correct errors of design and to reexamine, if necessary, the fundamental assumptions that guide public action. The present chapter is a summary of this ongoing research into the ADAMH block grant and related mental health policy changes of the 1980s.

ACKNOWLEDGMENTS

The authors are grateful to the following persons who shared information and expertise that contributed to the development of this chapter: Dr. Alvira Brands, National Institute of Mental Health; James K. Finley, National Council of Community Mental Health Centers; Dr. Judith Larsen, Cognos Associates; Dr. David Mechanic, Institute for Health, Health Care Policy, and Aging Research, Rutgers University; Dr. Noel Mazade, Consultant to the National Association of State Mental Health Program Directors; Gary Palsgrove, Alcohol, Drug Abuse, and Mental Health Administration; Thomas Reynolds, Alcohol, Drug Abuse, and Mental Health Administration; Dr. E. Clark Ross, National Association of State Mental Health Program Directors; Gail Toff, Intergovernmental Health Policy Project, George Washington University; and Michael J. Witkin, National Institute of Mental Health. Other persons who read and provided useful comments on a draft of the chapter were Robert Davis, National Institute on Alcohol Abuse and Alcoholism; William Fitzgerald, National Institute on Drug Abuse; George Kanuck, Alcohol, Drug Abuse, and Mental Health Administration; Ellie McCoy, Alcohol, Drug Abuse, and Mental Health Administration; and Kathryn McKnight, Alcohol, Drug Abuse, and Mental Health Administration.

REFERENCES

Advisory Commission on Intergovernmental Relations. 1977. *Block Grants: A Comparative Analysis*. Washington, D.C.: U.S. Government Printing Office.

Agranoff, R., and Robins, L. S. 1984. The Politics and Administration of Intergovernmental Relations in Health. In *Health Politics and Policy*, eds. T. J. Litman and L. S. Robins. New York: John Wiley.

Ahr, P. R., and Holcomb, W. R. 1985. State Mental Health Directors' Priorities for Mental Health Care. *Hospital and Community Psychiatry* 36: 39–45.

Barfield, C. E. 1981. *Rethinking Federalism: Block Grants and Federal, State, and Local Responsibilities*. Washington, D.C.: American Enterprise Institute.

Beigel, A. 1982. Community Mental Health Centers: A Look Ahead. *Hospital and Community Psychiatry* 33: 741–745.

Beigel, A., and Fine, T. 1984. Legislation. In *The Chronic Mental Patient Five Years Later*, ed. J. A. Talbott. Orlando, Fla.: Grune and Stratton.

Brown, B., and Stockdill, J. W. 1972. The Politics of Mental Health. In *Handbook of Community Mental Health*, eds. S. E. Golann and C. Eisdorfer. New York: Appleton-Century-Crofts.

Buck, J. A. 1984. Block Grants and Federal Promotion of Community Mental Health Services, 1946–65. *Community Mental Health Journal* 20: 236–247.

Burt, M. R., and Pittman, K. J. 1985. *Testing the Social Safety Net: The Impact of Changes in Support Programs during the Reagan Administration*. Washington, D.C.: Urban Institute Press.

Callahan, J. J., Jr. 1982. Management and Leadership in Times of Scarcity. *Administration in Mental Health* 9: 164–169.

Chelimsky, E. 1981. Making Block Grants Accountable. In *Evaluation in Change: Meeting New Government Needs*, ed. L. Datta. Beverly Hills, Calif.: Sage.

Edwards, L. G., and Mitchell, C. C. 1987. Strategies for Cutback Management in Community Mental Health Centers. *Community Mental Health Journal* 23: 140–151.

Estes, C. L., and Wood, J. B. 1984. A Preliminary Assessment of the Impact of Block Grants on Community Mental Health Centers. *Hospital and Community Psychiatry* 35: 1125–1129.

Foley, H. A., and Sharfstein, S. S. 1983. *Madness and Government: Who Cares for the Mentally Ill?* Washington, D.C.: American Psychiatric Press.

Fox, P. J., Swan, J. H., and Estes, C. L. 1986. Trends in CMHC Services to Elderly Populations. *Hospital and Community Psychiatry* 37: 937–938.

Frank, R. F., and Kamlet, M. S. 1986. Nonmarket Resource Allocation in Mental Health Care: Interdependencies in a Fragmented World. *American Behavioral Scientist* 30: 201–230.

Goplerud, E. N., Walfish, S., and Broskowski, A. 1985. Weathering the Cuts: A Delphi Survey on Surviving Cutbacks in Community Mental Health. *Community Mental Health Journal* 21: 14–27.

Gorman, P. 1984. Block Grants: Theoretical and Practical Issues in Federal/State/Local Revenue Sharing. *New England Journal of Human Services* 4: 19–23.

Grob, G. N. 1987. Mental Health Policy in Post–World War II America. In *Improving Mental Health Services: What the Social Sciences Can Tell Us*, ed. D. Mechanic. *New Directions for Mental Health Services*, no. 36. San Francisco: Jossey-Bass.

Hagan, B. J., Forman, B. D., and Gorodezky, M. J. 1982. The Impact of Economic Stress on Community Mental Health Services. *Administration in Mental Health* 10: 104–109.

Hale, G. E., and Palley, M. L. 1981. *The Politics of Federal Grants*. Washington, D.C.: Congressional Quarterly Press.

Hoare, G. 1983. Retrenchment Strategies in Mental Health: Lessons from the Private Sector. *Administration in Mental Health* 10: 259–271.

Hudson, C. G., and Dubey, S. 1985. State Mental Health Spending under the ADAMHA Block Grant: An Empirical Study. *Journal of Social Service Research* 8: 1–23.

Hudson, C. G., and Dubey, S. N. 1986. Decision Making under the ADAMH Block Grant: Four Case Studies. *Administration in Mental Health* 14: 97–116.

Jerrell, J. M., and Jerrell, S. L. 1985. Perceptions and Effectiveness in State Mental Health Systems. *Administration in Mental Health* 13: 138–148.

Jerrell, J. M., and Jerrell, S. L. 1986. The Effects of State Policy and Funding on the Performance of Mental Health Centers. *Administration in Mental Health* 13: 212–223.

Jerrell, J. M., and Larsen, J. K. 1984. Policy Shifts and Organizational Adaptation: A Review of Current Developments. *Community Mental Health Journal* 20: 282–293.

Jerrell, J. M., and Larsen, J. K. 1985. How Community Mental Health Centers Deal with Cutbacks and Competition. *Hospital and Community Psychiatry* 36: 1169–1174.

Jerrell, J. M., and Larsen, J. K. 1986. Community Mental Health Services in Transition: Who Is Benefiting? *American Journal of Orthopsychiatry* 56: 78–88.

Landsberg, G. 1985. Quality Assurance Activities in Community Mental Health Centers: Changes over Time. *Community Mental Health Journal* 21: 189–197.

Logan, B. M., Rochefort, D. A., and Cook, E. W. 1985. Block Grants for Mental Health: Elements of the State Response. *Journal of Public Health Policy* 6: 476–492.

Lutterman, T., Wurster, C. R., Mazade, N. A., and Glover, R. 1987. State Mental Health Agency Revenues and Expenditures for Mental Health Services: Trends from 1981 to 1985. In *Mental Health United States, 1987*, eds. R. W. Manderscheid and S. A. Barrett. DHHS Publication No. (ADM) 87–1518. Washington, D.C.: U.S. Government Printing Office.

Mechanic, D., and Aiken, L. H. 1987. Improving the Care of Patients with Chronic Mental Illness. *New England Journal of Medicine* 317: 1634–1638.

Moore, W. J. 1988. Anything Goes in Grants Fight. *National Journal*, April 2: 900–901.

Morgan, J. A., Jr., and Connery, R. H. 1980. The Governmental System. In *The Administration of Mental Health Services*, ed. S. Feldman. 2nd ed. Springfield, Ill.: Charles C Thomas.

Nathan, R. P. 1983. State and Local Governments under Federal Grants: Toward A Predictive Theory. *Political Science Quarterly* 98: 47–57.

Nathan, R. P., Doolittle, F. C., and Associates. 1987. *Reagan and the States*. Princeton: Princeton University Press.

National Council of Community Mental Health Centers. 1985–1988. *Membership Profile Report*. Rockville, Md.

Okin, R. L. 1984. How Community Mental Health Centers Are Coping. *Hospital and Community Psychiatry* 35: 1118–1125.

Palmer, K. T. 1984. The Evolution of Grant Policies. In *The Changing Politics of Federal Grants*, by L. D. Brown, J. W. Fossett, and K. T. Palmer. Washington, D.C.: Brookings Institution.

Peterson, G. E. 1982. The State and Local Sector. In *The Reagan Experiment*, eds. J. L. Palmer and I. V. Sawhill. Washington, D.C.: Urban Institute Press.

Peterson, G. E., Bovbjerg, R. R., Davis, B. A., Davis, W. G., Durman, E. C., and

Gullo, T. A. 1986. *The Reagan Block Grants: What Have We Learned?* Washington, D.C.: Urban Institute Press.

Peterson, R. S., Austin, M. J., and Patti, R. J. 1985. Cutback Management Activities in Community Mental Health Centers. *Administration in Mental Health* 13: 112–125.

Pond, M. A. 1982. Block Grants for Health: A Brief History of Presidential Initiatives. *Health Policy Quarterly* 2: 180–198.

Rich, R. F. 1986. Change and Stability in Mental Health Policy. *American Behavioral Scientist* 30: 111–142.

Rochefort, D. A., Logan, B. M., and Cook, E. W. 1984. Evaluating Reagan's Block Grants: The Case of Community Mental Health Services. Paper presented at the Sixteenth Annual Meeting of the Northeastern Political Science Association, Boston, November 17.

Sharfstein, S. S. 1982. Medicaid Cutbacks and Block Grants: Crisis or Opportunity for Community Mental Health? *American Journal of Psychiatry* 139: 466–470.

Stanfield, R. L. 1981. For the States, It's Time to Put Up or Shut Up on Federal Block Grants. *National Journal*, October 10: 1800–1805.

Surber, R. W., Shumway, M., Shadoan, R., and Hargreaves, W. A. 1986. Effects of Fiscal Retrenchment on Public Mental Health Services for the Chronic Mentally Ill. *Community Mental Health Journal* 22: 215–227.

Surles, R. 1987. Changing Organizational Structures and Relationships in Community Mental Health. *Administration in Mental Health* 14: 217–227.

Swan, J. H., Fox, P. J., and Estes, C. L. 1986. Community Mental Health Services and the Elderly: Retrenchment or Expansion? *Community Mental Health Journal* 22: 275–285.

Thompson, F. J. 1986. New Federalism and Health Care Policy: States and the Old Questions. *Journal of Health Politics, Policy and Law* 11: 647–669.

Toff, G. E. 1984. *Mental Health Benefits under Medicaid: A Survey of the States.* Washington, D.C.: Intergovernmental Health Policy Project, George Washington University.

Toff, G. E. 1986. *Financing Mental Health Services under Medicaid: Proceedings from A Roundtable on Mental Health Policy Issues.* Washington, D.C.: Intergovernmental Health Policy Project, George Washington University.

U.S. Congress, Office of Technology Assessment. 1986. *Children's Mental Health: Problems and Services—A Background Paper.* Washington, D.C.: U.S. Government Printing Office.

U.S. Department of Health and Human Services, Alcohol, Drug Abuse, and Mental Health Administration. 1987. *Alcohol and Drug Abuse and Mental Health Services Block Grant, October 1986.* Washington, D.C.: U.S. Government Printing Office, June.

U.S. General Accounting Office. 1982. *A Summary and Comparison of the Legislative Provisions of the Block Grants Created by the 1981 Omnibus Budget Reconciliation Act.* Washington, D.C., December 30.

U.S. General Accounting Office. 1984a. *States Have Made Few Changes in Implementing the Alcohol, Drug Abuse, and Mental Health Services Block Grant.* Washington, D.C., June.

U.S. General Accounting Office. 1984b. Improvements in the Alcohol, Drug Abuse and Mental Health Block Grant Distribution Formula Can Be Made Both Now and in the Future. Letter from William J. Anderson, Director of GAO, to Senators Lloyd M. Bentsen, William Proxmire, Orrin G. Hatch, and John G. Tower. June 21.

U.S. General Accounting Office. 1985a. *Block Grants Brought Funding Changes and Adjustments to Program Priorities*. Washington, D.C., 1985.

U.S. General Accounting Office. 1985b. *State Rather Than Federal Policies Provided the Framework for Managing Block Grants*. Washington, D.C., March 15.

U.S. General Accounting Office. 1987a. *Block Grants: Proposed Formulas for Substance Abuse, Mental Health Provide More Equity*. Washington, D.C.

U.S. General Accounting Office. 1987b. *Block Grants: Federal Set-Asides for Substance Abuse and Mental Health Services*. Washington, D.C.

Visotsky, H. M. 1987. The Great American Roundup. *New England Journal of Medicine* 317: 1662–1663.

Wildavsky, A. 1979. *Speaking Truth to Power: The Art and Craft of Policy Analysis*. Boston: Little, Brown.

Woy, J. R., and Mazade, N. A. 1982. Community Mental Health Centers in Transition: Report on A National Conference. *Administration in Mental Health* 9: 211–224.

8

Mental Health Policymaking in the United States: Patterns, Process, and Structures

PHILIP K. ARMOUR

Though public policies for the mentally ill are some of the oldest of modern nation-state programs directed at a socially dependent population, mental health analysts tend not to cast national and local initiatives within the larger context of welfare-state development where they belong. This has occurred for a couple of reasons. First, most historical works are case studies of national or local programs within one country. Lacking the comparative perspective, these case studies tend to treat a nation's policies as unique, when in fact program initiation is either stimulated by other nations' innovations or parallels their development; even when policies in a given society depart from the general norm established by other polities, understanding of the one country's actions can be enhanced by exploring the causes of deviation. Second, many programmatic studies are based in social work, social medicine, public administration, or social psychiatric disciplines. In the hands of many users, these paradigmatic stances often are not inclusive enough to encompass a presentation and assessment of mental health policies within a historical-comparative framework of public policy development.

Adopting this kind of broad analytic approach, the present chapter seeks to describe key features of the patterns, process, and structures of U.S. mental health policymaking. The purpose is not to repeat the detailed description of policy and program developments presented in earlier chapters, but to provide a conceptual overview of selected aspects of political history in order to derive general insight into forces of change and stability within the mental health arena.

THE WELFARE STATE: A STRUCTURAL UNIFORMITY OF ADVANCED SOCIETIES

The welfare state—the constellation of public policy initiatives designed to insure persons against the risks of ill health, aging, unemployment, disability, and child dependency—is one of the structural uniformities of advanced societies. As Wilensky (1975) observed, regardless of the political ideology or system, capitalist and communist nations have converged in their initiation of programs which cover diverse human conditions and social needs.

Development of national and local mental health policies must be examined in the context of the panoply of programs that governments began initiating in the nineteenth century to cover different categories of persons at risk. Over the course of the last century, approaches to the poor have taken two broad forms: those which affirm the Poor Law theory of poverty's causation and management of the dependent, and those which mark a distinct break with this tradition. The modern welfare state which emerged in the late nineteenth century was predicated on the second of these approaches. Beginning in Imperial Germany in 1883, national governments began assuming responsibility for insuring persons against the risks of work injury, ill health, and old age. While manifest and latent purposes of these policies are widely debated from several theoretical orientations (Armour and Coughlin, 1985), most students conclude that social security programs have been ameliorative.

In contrast to this social insurance approach, Poor Law methods are clearly revealed in nineteenth- and twentieth-century programs for the mentally disordered. Specifically, in nineteenth-century Britain and America, mental health policies reflected an affirmation of seventeenth-century practices that limited governmental responsibility to only the deserving among the poor, including the mentally disordered. This was a categorical approach to persons in need characterized by a fundamental hostility toward most persons seeking relief and a belief that government's role in aiding indigents must be minimized lest government foster dependency and destroy work incentives and the drive for self-sufficiency (Rothman, 1971; Jones, 1972; Grob, 1973).

In the United States, the defeat of the nineteenth-century mental health reform movement's campaign to inaugurate national assistance for the pauper insane ensured the U.S. position as a laggard in instituting modern social policies. In his 1854 veto of the "12,225,000 Acre Bill" passed by Congress after strenuous lobbying by the charismatic social reformer Dorothea L. Dix, President Franklin Pierce clearly articulated the sociopolitical and philosophical justification for a limited federal government role in aiding society's needy. If the national government was to provide for the housing and income support of the indigent insane from the sale of federal lands, Pierce maintained, then the "whole field of public beneficence [would be] thrown open to the care and culture of the federal government'' (quoted in Foley and Sharfstein, 1983: 7).

Pierce's veto blocked federal policy initiatives for the poor for nearly eighty years. Only after the economic collapse of 1929 did the policymaking environment become sufficiently auspicious for the enactment of national social programs for the aged, unemployed, disabled, blind, and dependent children. Federal programs explicitly for the mentally disordered took even longer to institute, and then once passed were subject to attack and reversal by the opponents of this federal role in mental health care (Foley, 1975; cf. Armour, 1981).

THE CYCLES OF POLICYMAKING

Policymaking for mental health care is not different from policymaking for other public concerns: it proceeds episodically, in part varying with the perceived seriousness of the problem, the competition from other pressing social concerns, the degree of mobilization of reform forces, and the opportunities presented by the presence of officials favorable to the reform agenda (Armour, 1981; cf. Schlesinger, 1986).

The cyclical perspective on public policymaking is based on several key analytic concepts. At the outset one can observe that public policymaking exhibits two distinct phases or cycles. First are distinct *long-wave cycles* which last several decades or more and are characterized by the adoption of a major theoretical or value orientation about the fundamental relations between society, its problems, and the role of the state in their solutions. Major public policy initiatives are predicated on these orientations. Second, within a specific long-wave cycle are several *short-wave cycles* of policy initiation and implementation. The guiding theories of these short-wave cycles are derived from the dominant policy paradigms of the distinct long-wave cycle.

Like the dominant scientific paradigmatic theories that permit ''normal scientific research'' affirming hegemonic theory (Kuhn, 1962), so at the outset of a new long-wave cycle of public policymaking a whole set of policy initiatives are permissible which affirm new theories of society and the state The notion of turning points is critical for demarcating new long waves in public policymaking, whose initiation often requires a conceptual shift with regard to the polity's role in solving basic human problems and addressing fundamental social concerns (see, for example, Eckstein, 1958; Howard, 1963; Heclo, 1974; Hay, 1975; Armour, 1981; Schlesinger, 1986).

Long-wave cycles entail several elements. They usually are preceded by a major socioeconomic crisis, a war, or rapid demographic changes. The post–Civil War period of public policymaking to promote equality included adopting the Thirteenth and Fourteenth amendments to the U.S. Constitution. In the late nineteenth and early twentieth centuries, the excesses of rapid industrialization fostered the Progressive Era reforms which sought to limit monopolistic capitalism. In the 1930s, the institution of social insurance legislation flowed from the crisis of the Great Depression.

Often, the problems confronted during the onset of long-wave reform cycles have been previously ignored or neglected by governments or the private sector or both. During a crisis, the relative ignorance or inattention phase comes to an end and is followed by focused attention on the probable causes and possible cures for the societal condition. Concerted remedial action is then undertaken, followed by a period of relative inattention or even forgetfulness (Matza, 1966; Armour, 1981; Schlesinger, 1986). An issue does not return to public consciousness unless propelled by a new crisis of concern.

Within a policy cycle's long wave, specific programs designed to address a problem exhibit distinct life cycles. The life cycle of a public policy consists of identifying and documenting a problem, mobilizing to solve it, proposing solutions, campaigning and lobbying to enact solutions or obtain favorable court or administrative rulings, engaging in implementation activities, evaluating program successes or failings, seeking reauthorization of the policy mandate, and working to resurrect terminated programs.

Once programs have been initiated legislatively, administratively, or judicially during one of the long-wave cycles of policy creation, public and private sector actors engage in implementation activities (Pressman and Wildavsky, 1973; Bardach, 1977). And as these public policy activities accumulate, they do not necessarily reflect an overall grand design or order. Though comparative studies reveal clear constellations of social security provision, specific national forms reflect idiosyncratic policymaking processes, timing, institutions, and concepts (Flora and Heidenheimer, 1981; Coughlin and Armour, 1983; cf. Wilensky, 1975).

Program spending is driven by the diverse commitments embodied in law and regulations, and historically has grown not only because of amendments to extant laws but also because of the tendency to increase expenditures incrementally (Wildavsky, 1964; cf. Lowi, 1969). Policies once enacted are increasingly subject to critical review and evaluation (Moynihan, 1969). In some cases, policy evaluation can lend legitimacy to program dismantling, yet when combined with lobbying efforts on behalf of a program, evaluation studies may justify reauthorization.

Thus, public policymaking is characterized by cycles. Long-wave cycles are marked at their outset by socioeconomic, political, or military crises and reflect the adoption of new dominant policy paradigms. Within these ruling paradigms new legislative, administrative, and/or judicial programmatic initiatives can occur which are predicated on the overarching sociopolitical or economic theory. Specific policymaking actions thus both derive legitimacy from and themselves work to sustain the hegemonic notions of a long-wave policy cycle. Further, the specific policy initiatives predicated on the dominant paradigm themselves demonstrate life-cycle characteristics. These include phases of birth, growth, maturation, replication, death, and rebirth.

Cycles of Policymaking for the Mentally Disordered

Applying this cyclical perspective to the analysis of policymaking for the mentally ill, one finds that the plight of the mentally disordered has only periodically penetrated the collective social consciousness. The episodic character of public consideration of the mentally disordered seems to reflect a tendency to repress awareness of these psychologically distressed persons except for brief interludes of concern. This pattern of collective sociopolitical forgetfulness and remembrance is only one variant of what Matza (1966) has labeled the "Columbus complex" in which the forgotten and neglected in society are continually subject to discovery, which then generates consternation and calls for action.

Since colonial times, America has witnessed several long-wave cycles of mental health reform which followed the discovery of the mentally disordered. The first of these cycles originated in Europe and has been labeled the "era of confinement." The products of the period were the great hospitals like Paris's L'Hôpital Général and other specialized institutions for the insane. Working with the transplanted English Poor Law notions of corporate responsibility for the deserving poor, including persons disordered in mind, Americans similarly began founding hospitals for confining and treating the mentally disordered. The Pennsylvania Hospital in Philadelphia was established in 1751 to care for both somatic and psychiatric patients; the first American institution created exclusively for the mentally disordered was the Virginia Eastern Lunatic Asylum founded in Williamsburg in 1770 (Grob, 1973).

The second phase of mental health reform was predicated not only on the sociopolitical values of freedom and liberty that spawned the American and French revolutions (Palmer, 1959), but also on new notions regarding the causes and treatment of mental disorder. Foremost among psychiatric revolutionaries in this period was Philippe Pinel, whose liberation of the chained inmates of Bicêtre and Salpêtrière recalled the storming of the Bastille and flowed from etiological theories published later in his popular *Treaté sur Insanité* (1801). The parallel innovations in moral management of Quaker tea merchant William Tuke at the York Retreat in England and by Vincenzio Chiarugi of Florence, along with their widely read publications, marked an era of optimism in treating mental disorders.

This reform movement gathered momentum in the United States in the 1820s with the founding of ameliorative institutions. Rothman observes:

In the aftermath of the [American] Revolution . . . a spark of interest appeared, lit by Enlightenment ideology and an awareness of very dramatic events in Europe. Just as [Cesare] Beccaria had insisted humane laws could eradicate crime, so men like Tuke in England and Pinel in France insisted that kind and gentle treatment would help cure the insane. (Rothman, 1971: 109–110)

Following the lead of her policymaking mentor Horace Mann, who had helped found Massachusetts' first public asylum and then moved on to champion the cause of public schools, Dorothea Lynde Dix undertook her crusade to convince state legislatures to upgrade or establish public mental hospitals capable of implementing the treatment modalities of the era of moral management.

As Rothman (1971), Jones (1972), and others have observed, the well-intentioned innovations in psychiatric treatment which the asylum movement represented resulted in failure. Hyperbolic claims of high rates of cure by mental hospital administrators were shattered by the reality of overcrowded, underfunded institutions. The asylums' degeneration into custodial facilities providing only rudimentary care for a growing and heterogeneous population of disordered, deviant, and discarded persons marked a sad conclusion to the pre–Civil War reform era.

A third long-wave era of mental health reform was a part of the larger Progressive period of policy innovation. In addition to redefining the relationship between the federal government and monopoly-inclined capitalism, policy-makers turned their attention to the plight of children and the nation's health, e.g., the 1909 White House Conference and subsequent creation of the U.S. Children's Bureau in 1912. The founding of the U.S. Public Health Service occurred in stages, building on the Marine Hospital Service (MHS) which dated from 1798. Granted power to quarantine immigrants in 1878, and later to prevent epidemics, the MHS was granted domestic authority in 1893 to manage epidemics. By 1902, Public Health was added to the MHS name, and in 1912 the Public Health Service (PHS) was formally instituted with broadened powers to conduct research as well as prevent disease (Trattner, 1979; Leiby, 1978; Patterson, 1981).

Upon this policy mandate would eventually be erected federal programs for mental health. In the 1930s, the creation of two federal drug-treatment hospitals and a Mental Hygiene Division within the PHS provided the organizational bases for mental health reformers seeking to foster an expansive federal governmental role in treating mental disorders (Deutsch, 1949; cf. Armour, 1981).

Voluntary mental health reform initiatives were spurred by the publication of Clifford Beers' *A Mind That Found Itself* (1908). The formation of a state and later National Committee on Mental Hygiene reinvigorated a moribund reform movement and forged new cooperative links between federal and state officials, public-spirited psychiatric practitioners, and the citizen reform movement.

A fourth long wave of mental health reform began in the aftermath of World War II. The exposure of conditions in underfunded state and county mental hospitals gave impetus to calls from Mental Hygiene Bureau officials in the prewar period for the formation of a separate federal mental health agency. In 1946, Congress established the National Institute of Mental Health (NIMH), whose mandate included promoting research, training, and community treatment programs. Linkages forged among NIMH, congressional allies, and mental health advocacy groups created a network supportive of other policy innovations, and ultimately resulted in the Community Mental Health Centers Act of 1963.

INSTITUTIONAL AND IDEOLOGICAL ELEMENTS OF REFORM: EXAMPLES FROM THE CYCLES OF MENTAL HEALTH POLICYMAKING

While the cyclical perspective offers useful insights into long-standing patterns of mental health policymaking, it also raises several analytic issues. For example, does variation in the institutional environment result in variation in policy outcomes? A related concern is the impact of political ideology. While neo-Marxists and other convergence theorists agree that ideology plays only a minor, legitimating role in public policy creation (Gough, 1979; Wilensky, 1975), others argue that ideology significantly shapes both the direction and substance of new policy initiatives (Lowi, 1969).

Sociopolitical, Institutional, and Ideological Constraints on Mental Health Reform

The decentralized character of the U.S. governmental system is in part responsible for the difficulties encountered by those who have sought an expanded public mental health system during the past 100 years. Another structural obstacle facing reform advocates has been the division of powers among the branches of government (executive, legislative, and judicial), and among national, state, and substate units. Further, an ideological system that resists governmental intervention accounts for a political environment inhospitable to collective solutions to social problems. Wilensky (1975) has suggested that when a decentralized polity possesses internal cleavages based on political geography, race, ethnicity, and language, national elites are likely to encounter even greater difficulties enacting and implementing social and egalitarian policies.

This framework helps explain the failure of Dorothea Dix and her allies in their campaign to expand hospital facilities for the mentally ill through federal-level support in the nineteenth century. Not only does this episode illustrate the challenge of carrying reform activity from one level of government to another in the United States, it also shows how the checks and balances system can block policy change. After being signed by both Houses of Congress, Dix's proposal was thwarted by a presidential veto which assigned to states and localities exclusive responsibility for the socially needy, including the mentally disordered, for nearly a century to come (Deutsch, 1949; Foley, 1975; Foley and Sharfstein, 1983).

Institutional Basis for Mental Health Reform

Once instituted by states and localities, the network of mental hospitals created a bureaucratic base for incremental expansion of mental health services. Professionalization of mental hospital administration began as early as 1844 with the formation of the Association of Medical Superintendents of American Institutions for the Insane (AMSAII). This group sought to disseminate knowledge about mental disorders at professional conferences and through its journal, the *American Journal of Insanity*. The association also lobbied state and local governments for increased funding (Walters, 1978).

Despite the failure of mental hospitals to fulfill the exorbitant expectations of early reformers and hospital administrators, i.e., that hospital treatment would cure all cases of mental illness, the network of hospitals grew and they became the primary facility for treating the severely mentally disordered. Though the quality of care within these institutions was highly variable and deteriorated as the numbers of patients inexorably grew without commensurate increases in state funding, mental hospitals served as important sites for the continued development of psychiatric care. Late-nineteenth-century advances in the classification of mental disorders resulted from the observation and treatment of hospital patients. In the twentieth century, as well, the search for effective treatments was often conducted with patients of public mental hospitals. Some of these treatments, of course, ultimately proved more significant than others, such as the psychoactive drugs introduced in the 1950s (Swazey, 1974).

FORCES AUSPICIOUS FOR MENTAL HEALTH REFORM IN THE POST–WORLD WAR II ERA

In the post–World War II period, mental health reform advocates achieved a goal unattainable by their nineteenth-century predecessors: a direct role for the federal government in providing and financing of mental health services. Applying the cyclical perspective to analyze the constellation of forces that permitted this policy breakthrough gives further insight into the political process of mental health policymaking in the United States.

A Sense of Crisis

First, as with many long waves in reform cycles, national crises gave rise to or lent legitimacy to the reform proposal. Public fiscal crisis induced by the Great Depression exacerbated the financial plight of public mental hospitals. The country's involvement in World War II further starved low-priority public spending programs, including mental hospitals. Second, wartime experiences suggested much higher prevalence rates of mental disorder than were popularly believed. Rudimentary screening tests administered by the U.S. Selective Service documented a frequency of neuropsychiatric problems which shocked the public and policymakers as did the rates of discharge for psychiatric disabilities.

The Mental Health Reform Movement

A revitalized mental health reform movement in this period also helped refocus attention on the mismanagement of the mentally disordered. Lobbying efforts were directed at those elements in the federal government sympathetic to the cause of community care, and eventually the development of an alliance among legislative and executive branches of government and private reformers was central to the achievement of programmatic objectives. The use of the courts to further the rights of mental patients was another important step in this most recent reform period.

The renewal of mental health reform activity in the postwar period actually occurred along several lines. Once again, the mentally disordered began to be rediscovered after decades of relative neglect, and it was scribes of the mental health reform movement who played a critical role in bringing to public consciousness the pitiful conditions in state and local hospitals. For example, Albert Deutsch's *The Shame of the States* (1948) exposed the consequences of chronic underinvestment in mental hospitals and served as an indictment of the institutional mode of managing the mentally disordered. In a parallel exposé in the tradition of "muckrake" journalism, Oklahoma newspaper reporter Mike Gorman revealed the inhumane conditions in his state's mental hospitals and won the respect of noted public health advocates and philanthropists Mary Lasker and Florence Mahoney. With Lasker and Mahoney's sponsorship Gorman moved from the local level to the national scene as a mental health reform lobbyist. By funding Gorman's National Committee Against Mental Illness, Lasker and Mahoney helped expand the network of lobbying organizations calling for a wider federal role in basic research, personnel training, and service innovations. Gorman himself also furthered the establishment of patient advocacy groups in addition to his wide-ranging lobbying and publicity activities.

By the 1940s, a degree of consensus was also emerging from certain professional quarters for an enhanced federal role in combatting mental disorders. The Group for the Advancement of Psychiatry (GAP) assisted in the development of a proposal by the PHS Division of Mental Hygiene for a national mental health institute. The GAP proposal envisioned a federal role in supporting the training of much needed personnel and the improvement of mental health services delivery. The product of this effort was the National Mental Health Act of 1946 (Public Law 79–487), which created the National Institute of Mental Health (NIMH) and authorized formula grants for the promotion of local mental health services (Foley and Sharfstein, 1983: 17–20; cf. Clausen, 1966).

Finally, ever-rising numbers of residents in state and county mental hospitals from the 1940s through the early 1950s led still another group into the coalition in support of a wider federal involvement in mental health—the state governors. National governors' conferences had drawn attention to relentless growth in hospital populations, which represented a drain on state coffers. Gorman helped focus the national debate by convincing the governors to sponsor a study and to call a special conference centering on the innovations in delivery of mental health care as well as the fiscal and managerial plight of public hospitals (Gorman, 1956: 167ff.). Hence, mental health reform in the United States had come full circle: the legacy of Dix's nineteenth-century crusade—the state mental hospital—became a powerful negative symbol for reform activists during the 1950s and 1960s.

Institutional Bases for Reform: The U.S. Congress and the Federal Bureaucracy

With the creation of NIMH, mental health activists gained a bureaucratic base. Headed by Robert Felix, who as a protégé of Division of Mental Hygiene director Dr. Lawrence Kolb had developed a proposal for a separate mental health institute prior to World War II, NIMH was well positioned to lobby for new policies. Yet successful fulfillment of NIMH's legislative mandate required continuing congressional support, including not only funding increases but new programmatic authorizations.

Enactment of new community programs for the mentally disordered thus was made possible not only by NIMH's development of formal proposals and their backing by the mental health reform lobby, but also by a network of U.S. senators and representatives favorably disposed towards reform proposals. Important channels of information and support existed among the Subcommittee on Public Health of the House Committee on Interstate and Foreign Commerce, the Subcommittee on Health of the Senate Committee on Labor and Welfare, NIMH, and lobbyist-activist organizations like the Group for the Advancement of Psychiatry and Gorman's National Committee Against Mental Illness. This informal yet well-established network guided legislative initiatives in mental health throughout the postwar period.

Lowi (1969: 79–83) has described the Kennedy-Johnson era as a triumph of interest-group liberalism characterized by an alliance between federal agencies and private-sector interest groups (cf. Moynihan, 1969). In a similar vein, Drew (1967) has termed the coalition for an expanded federal government role in health as "Washington's noble conspirators." Whatever the label, the reality was that a powerful coalescence of public and private influentials promoted federal policy initiatives for health and mental health in the 1950s and 1960s (cf. Marmor, 1973). Though fiscally a minor program when compared with the massive Medicare-Medicaid insurance systems which were also created at this time, the community mental health initiatives sprang from the same political infrastructure and embodied a common social philosophy.

Institutional Bases for Reform: The Presidency

It was John F. Kennedy's election to the presidency that gave the mental health reform group the final key element in its coalition, a White House positively disposed toward new mental health policy initiatives. As a senator from Massachusetts, Kennedy had cosponsored the 1955 legislation that created the Joint Commission on Mental Illness and Health which undertook a comprehensive study of mental health needs and services in the United States. Further, with Kennedy's own sister a victim of mental retardation, the family had a long-standing special interest in mental disabilities. A century earlier a president unfavorably disposed to an expanded federal role in mental health care had by a single act frustrated years of legislative work to achieve this end. Now it was a chief executive committed to aiding the mentally ill who led the fight for a federally sponsored community-based innovation in mental health.

The Concept of Community Care and Its Appeal

The notion of local centers serving the mentally disordered in the community setting held widespread appeal in the 1960s. Not only had the remote asylum been discredited by scientific studies, but the political-ideological climate of the day was clearly hostile to all types of large, bureaucratically operated institutions. In contrast, the notion of community-based organizations promoting health, employment, literacy, and the like had a positive association. Conjuring up favorable images of small-scale activities and structures, which by definition were considered responsive to individuals and distinctive groups (e.g., racial and ethnic minorities), the notion of community care of the mentally ill that surfaced in the 1960s was only the latest manifestation of a well-established American tradition (Nisbet, 1953; Lipset and Wolin, 1965; Berube and Gitteil, 1969; Kanter, 1972).

DOWNSWING OF THE POLICY CYCLE

With a presidential signature affixed to the Community Mental Health Centers Act of 1963 (Public Law 88–164), the mental health coalition marked the success of its struggle for federal backing of a dramatically new approach to services and treatment. Yet major challenges still lie ahead in implementing and defending this policy mandate. This subsequent phase of community mental health policymaking clearly illustrates the difficulty of sustaining a policy cycle once the initial enthusiasm for reform has begun to wane.

Community Mental Health Politics and Policymaking, 1969–1977

Dr. Stanley Yolles, a strong advocate of community care, was appointed NIMH director in 1964, thus assuring the federal bureaucracy's continued commitment to the community-based approach. Reauthorization of the CMHC Act in 1965 (Public Law 89–105) provided funding both for construction and for salaries of personnel to staff the facilities, the latter issue being a matter of great controversy in 1963. Once funds were disbursed and centers began to open, a new element joined the mental health coalition with a vested interest in continued federal funding: the staffs of the community centers. The National Council of Community Mental Health Centers (NCCMHC) became a new lobbying organization, and along with NIMH and the activist lobby, worked to enhance and defend the 1963–1965 policy mandate.

With Richard M. Nixon's election in 1968, however, the mental health co-alition faced a challenge to its federal bureaucratic base as well as funding. Ideologically dedicated to the transfer of responsibility and administrative dis-cretion back to states and localities, the Nixon administration and the subsequent administration of Gerald R. Ford repeatedly sought to phase out federal support for community mental health centers. Only by strenuous efforts of their legislative and lobbying wings did mental health supporters manage to stave off this pres-idential attack.

So it was that the Democratically controlled Congress continued to endorse the community care concept by appropriating funds. The Nixon administration, in turn, sought to eliminate the federal government's role by phasing out CHMC support in its budget requests and then impounding funds authorized by Congress. Federal court rulings ultimately ordered the release of impounded funds, though the Ford administration continued to seek elimination of these programs in its budgetary requests.

Though critical of several aspects of CMHC programs and their operations, General Accounting Office and congressional reviews of the 1963–1965 legis-lative mandates performed an important legitimation function for the CMHC system. Congress accepted recommendations for the extension of CMHC ser-vices, overriding President Ford's veto of reauthorizing legislation in 1975. A presidential veto of CMHC appropriations was similarly overturned.

Interest Groups and the Mental Health Systems Act of 1980

In a recapitulation of the Kennedy-Johnson era, the election of former Georgia governor Jimmy Carter placed an unanticipated ally of the mental health reform movement in the White House. Carter charged a presidential commission to study and report on the U.S. mental health system, with First Lady Rosalynn Carter serving as honorary chairperson. Completed in 1978, the commission's study represented a comprehensive review and analysis of extant knowledge on the etiology and social epidemiology of mental disorders; a series of policy assessments and program reviews; and a compilation of specific studies of the mental health service needs of distinctive populations, e.g., racial and ethnic minorities, the aged, drug users, and the chronically mentally ill (President's Commission on Mental Health, 1978).

Like the Joint Commission report of 1961, the report of President Carter's commission also spawned a legislative proposal. Yet in some key ways, the policymaking environment of the late 1970s differed from that of fifteen years earlier. Senator Edward M. Kennedy (D., Mass.) and Congressman Henry Wax-man (D., Calif.), heirs to the mental health legislative leadership positions once occupied by Senator Lister Hill (D., Ala.) and Congressman John Fogarty (D., R.I.), presided over the passage of the Mental Health Systems Act of 1980 (Public Law 96–398). Enactment was tortuous for several reasons, however.

First, the political arena was populated by a variety of structural-interest groups not present in the late 1950s and early 1960s, many of which were themselves the products of liberal social activism (cf. Alford, 1975). The concerns of these distinct groups often were in conflict. For example, while the lobbyists for CMHCs sought an extension and enhanced funding for CMHC services, the National Association of State Mental Health Program Directors—an organization representing the mental hospital system—noted that by the late 1970s the majority of community mental health funds were being appropriated by states and localities. Hence, this group wanted greater discretion over state mental health services in a devolution of power and authority from the federal government.

These were not the only interest-group demands. Another special interest lobbying organization, the American Federation of State, County, and Municipal Employees (AFSCME), was critical of proposals for further reductions of state mental hospital services. Its arguments for continued funding of the traditional mental hospital mode of care were in part self-interested—some of the federation's members worked in public mental hospitals—and in part reflected growing evidence that an irreducible population of chronically mentally disordered persons continued to need long-term care. Public employees also sought worker protection provisions, and were successful in adding these to the Senate version of the bill. Waxman, however, was opposed to these proposals, making a compromise on the job-guarantee provisions necessary.

Finally, deliberations over the Mental Health Systems Act also illustrate the noted tendency in social reform cycles to rediscover categorical subpopulations. In the late 1970s, the chronically mentally ill were newly found by investigative reporters for print and television media. Wing and Hailey's (1972) analysis of an English community mental health service had earlier reported on the phenomenon of the "new long-stay" population of mainly younger schizophrenics who in all probability would require periods of hospitalization throughout the course of their lives. Now the chronically mentally ill also became the object of attention of U.S. policymakers, who considered the inadequacy of existing services for this group in both community and hospital settings. Prefiguring the mid–1980s rediscovery of the homeless and other constituents of the urban underclass, scholarly findings and newspaper reports depicted what some termed "psychiatric ghettos" in most major cities. Senator Richard Schweicker (R., Penn.), who would serve as President Reagan's first secretary of Health and Human Services, was a particular champion of persons discharged from mental hospitals into communities ill equipped to house and usefully reemploy them. He and others in Congress pushed for the inclusion of provisions for expanded availability of psychological and supportive social services for the chronically mentally ill (cf. Kramer, 1977).

MENTAL HEALTH POLICYMAKING IN THE 1980s

The postwar coalition for mental health reform was able to defend its policy advances and even build upon them during the 1970s despite efforts of the Nixon and Ford administrations to cut appropriations and transfer responsibility to state and local governments. However, with Ronald Reagan's election and the Democratic party's loss of control of the U.S. Senate, mental health advocates lost several key bases from which they had defended community care legislation. As detailed in chapter 7 of this volume, under the Omnibus Budget Reconciliation Act of 1981 (Public Law 97–35), the Mental Health Systems Act was rescinded; states were granted discretion in providing community mental health care via federal block grants for mental health, alcohol, and drug abuse treatment services. At this same time, NIMH was targeted for cuts in its research and training budget.

How can we account for the defeats suffered by mental health advocates during the 1980s? Do these setbacks suggest that a new long-wave cycle in public policymaking has begun, one that is neoconservative in nature?

An Ideological Explanation

The shift in sociopolitical climate which the Reagan election symbolized already was evident during the Carter administration. In fact, the Mental Health Systems Act was somewhat out of character for the Carter presidency, which itself advanced a stringent approach to federal spending reductions usually identified with the following Republican administration. Once a neoconservative ideology had become hegemonic in the political environment of the early 1980s, it is not surprising that a program like the Mental Health Systems Act, expensive and tailored to the demands of special interest groups, would be targeted for elimination (Stockman, 1985).

The Durability of Social Insurance vs. Categorical Spending Programs

The dismantling of the Mental Health Systems Act and the retrenchment in federal funding for community care also reflect the greater difficulty categorical spending programs encounter in an era when conservative antitaxing and antispending ideologies dominate. The widespread popularity of social insurance—for example, the old age and health insurance schemes of the Social Security Act in the United States, the National Health Service in Britain, or European universal family allowances—insulates these programs against significant cutbacks or modification. In a cross-national study, Coughlin (1980) found that social insurance programs were perceived of as equitable in benefiting retired workers who have ''earned'' pensions and health coverage. In other cases, these programs enjoy wide and deep support because they protect persons against risks they have little control over, like work injuries (cf. Wilensky, 1975, 1976). In contrast, relatively minor, nonentitlement programs like NIMH's funding of community services do not spring from a widespread popular conviction that these services must be provided only by the national government.

An Age-Cohort Explanation of Public Policymaking

Another factor also accounts for the decline of the mental health reform movement as reflected in its inability to defend the Mental Health Systems Act: the attrition through electoral defeat, retirement, and death of a generation of sympathetic public officials in key policymaking positions. For example, the founding generation of NIMH leadership, as well as the Democratic presidents they served under during the 1960s, have long since passed from the scene. The death in 1987 of former Health, Education, and Welfare Secretary Wilbur Cohen, a pioneering figure in social welfare legislation in the United States, powerfully symbolized that the cohort of leaders which came of age during the Great Depression—at the onset of a long-wave policymaking cycle marked by activism and expansion—is literally passing away. Further innovation in mental health policy will likely depend on the resurgence of a strategically placed mental health coalition within Congress, the executive branch, and the private sector. Also determinative may be the degree to which mental health issues can become reconnected to concern about other causes of dependency, including poverty, ill health, and inadequate education.

The Mentally Ill: A Weak Lobbying Force

The very nature of major chronic mental disorders such as schizophrenia severely impairs the ability of their victims to act as effective advocates on their own behalf. Simply put, to effectively defend the programs that serve them, the mentally disordered would have to be less disabled and disoriented, but the very nature of severe mental disabilities induces psychological states which impair social functioning, including political activity. In contrast, the main beneficiaries of the welfare state—retirees and indirectly their offspring—are integrated socially to a much greater extent than the average client of the mental health system. Most important from a political perspective, older people and their children are more likely to vote and to engage in other political activities, including membership in special interest groups. Only with the recent formation of groups like California's Network Against Psychiatric Assault (NAPA) and the National Alliance for the Mentally Ill (NAMI) have mentally disordered persons and their families organized for direct political action. In sum, U.S. congressmen do not confront well-funded lobbyists for the mentally disordered in the halls of the Capitol, they typically do not receive large contributions to their political action committees from the residents of state and county mental hospitals or the clients of community service centers, and they do not have to calculate the electoral risks of offending a multimillion member association of former mental patients.

REPACKAGING MENTAL HEALTH REFORM FOR THE 1990s

Will another period of activism in mental health policymaking emerge featuring new laws and innovative services for that heterogeneous population of mentally disordered individuals? What strategy and tactics are available to convince elected officials that they must fund and expand community-based services and upgrade the quality of care which still must be provided by public mental institutions? In this author's view, the ability to achieve a policymaking breakthrough in this area sufficient to reverse recent defeats and to enhance funding for basic research, training, and services depends on an ability to link the mental health reform agenda to broader social concerns. These related concerns include, first, the debate over the civil rights of the mentally ill; second, the plight of the homeless; third, overcrowding in prisons and jails; and fourth, the response to the newly recognized health problems of Alzheimer's disease and Acquired Immune Deficiency Syndrome (AIDS).

Since the late 1960s, there have been a number of judicial rulings as well as revisions of the state mental health detention codes which have increased the standards required for involuntary hospitalization of the mentally disordered. For example, California's Lanterman-Petris-Short Act of 1967 sought not only to improve the community alternatives to institutionalization but also strengthened the rights of the mentally ill against involuntary detention without due process (Bardach, 1972). In Alabama, the court held in *Wyatt v. Stickney* (1971) that patients had a right to treatment and defined minimum standards of care. If the state did not provide treatment, then release was mandatory. Further, in *O'Connor v. Donaldson* (1975), courts found that a nondangerous mental patient should not be confined in an institution if that person is capable of living in the community; dangerousness did not include, in the court's view, the mere fact that the mentally disordered person was a nuisance, though the court begged the question of what a nuisance was. And in Texas in 1985, revisions of the state mental health code substantially enhanced patients' rights and strictly defined the state's capacity to involuntarily confine and commit persons in mental hospitals.

These rulings and new laws have done much to empower the mentally disordered and to protect them against arbitrary removal to a hospital setting. Yet the evidence is that deinstitutionalized and other chronically mentally ill persons can also face severe threats when in the community that in their own way rival the problems associated with involuntary institutional care. Thus, a dilemma exists. How can we balance the rights of the mentally ill against the rights of society and at the same time ensure that mentally disordered persons receive what useful care is available?

Civil suits, whose past use often has resulted in the discharge of patients from substandard public institutions to localities with inadequate supportive services, can be a stimulus for enhancing both necessary in-hospital care and encouraging community alternatives. To select an example from the author's own state, the 70th Texas Legislature, despite its present fiscal crisis, increased funding for hospital and community services of the Texas Department of Mental Health and Mental Retardation (TDMHMR) under terms of the 1981 settlement of *R.A.J. v. Miller* (1974). As part of the settlement of that lawsuit and another, *Ruiz v. Estelle* (1980), which found the state prison system violated inmates' rights, the Texas voters approved a bond program for prison and mental hospital improvements in November 1987.

Concern for the homeless provides another opportunity to address the needs of the mentally disordered in an era of deinstitutionalization and community care. Though estimates vary and are often highly impressionistic, mentally disordered persons (including substance abusers) make up a sizable proportion of the so-called urban homeless population. In Dallas, Texas, for example, estimates prepared by the city Department of Health and Human Services suggest that at least one-fourth of the city's homeless population consists of the deinstitutionalized, including former state mental hospital residents (City of Dallas, Department of Health and Human Services, 1984). Estimates from other surveys suggest the proportions could be higher (see, for example, Hopper and Baxter's 1984 review of various city profiles of the homeless presented to the U.S. House of Representatives Subcommittee on Housing and Community Development). In crafting a solution to the homelessness problem, policymakers will have to address the special needs of this subpopulation of alcoholics, other substance abusers, and the severely and chronically mentally disordered. Besides assistance in housing and employment—the former being needed by all homeless persons and the latter by many—the homeless mentally ill require psychological services, especially psychotropic drug monitoring and treatment, and a range of supportive social services. Many local solutions to the homeless problem are and will continue to be less than optimal, but they may provide a vehicle to direct attention to the plight of the chronically mentally ill in the community.

Most state prison systems are overcrowded and officials are confronted with expensive building programs which would offer at best only the prospect of keeping pace with the projected growth in demand. In several states prison systems are under federal court direction, having been found to violate prisoners' constitutional rights to proper treatment. Increased funding required by states and localities to upgrade existing facilities and to add capacity potentially could rob state mental health programs of needed funds. Yet, given the overlap in prison and mental health populations, reflecting the propensity of the criminal justice system to confine violent mentally disordered and even retarded persons in prisons, America's prison system crisis is also a mental health service system crisis. Developing solutions to the prison problem creates an opportunity to review the use of jails and prisons for mentally disabled persons, especially those who do not present a danger to themselves or others and who could be accommodated in less restrictive community-based halfway houses and sheltered workshops. Again, this would involve a rediscovery of the mentally disordered inappropriately housed in jails and prisons, harking back over a century earlier to Dorothea Dix's discovery of lunatics and feebleminded persons ill-housed and mistreated in the jails of Cambridge, Massachusetts.

Finally, certain prominent health issues of the day are stimulating mounting public concern that could also lead to enhanced services, research, and training support within the mental health field. The aging of the population will increase that segment of society vulnerable to Alzheimer's disease, a syndrome already recognized by mental health professionals as a major cause of disability, dependence, and premature death. The increasing numbers of persons suffering from Alzheimer's disease and other senile dementias will force public officials to increase funding for research and treatment regardless of political ideology or party. In addition, rising numbers of persons infected by the family of retroviruses which produce among other disorders Acquired Immune Deficiency Syndrome already have produced and will continue to result in pressure for greater governmental spending for the array of somatic and psychiatric services required by afflicted persons.

In briefly considering these loosely clustered areas of public policy concern, I have sought to suggest how the continuing unmet and growing needs of the mentally disordered can be addressed in conjunction with selected other contemporary issues. In seeking at least partial solutions to the problems confronting the mentally disordered in the context of these issues, mental health activists may further their cause in an era of limited fiscal resources and ideological hostility to new legislative initiatives.

REFERENCES

Aaron, H. J. 1973. *Why Is Welfare So Hard to Reform?* Washington, D.C.: Brookings Institution.

Alford, R. 1975. *Health Care Politics: Ideological and Interest Group Barriers to Reform.* Chicago: University of Chicago Press.

Armour, P. K. 1981. *The Cycles of Social Reform: Mental Health Policymaking in the United States, England, and Sweden.* Washington, D.C.: University Press of America.

Armour, P. K., and Coughlin, R. M. 1985. Social Control and Social Security: Theory and Research on Capitalist and Communist Nations. *Social Science Quarterly* 6: 770–788.

Bardach, E. 1972. *The Skill Factor in Politics.* Berkeley: University of California Press.

Bardach, E. 1977. *The Implementation Game.* Cambridge, Mass.: MIT Press.

Beers, C. 1944. *A Mind That Found Itself.* New York: Doubleday, [1908].

Berube, M., and Gitteil, M., eds. 1969. *Confrontation at Ocean Hill–Brownsville: The New York School Strikes of 1968.* New York: Praeger.

Clausen, J. A. 1966. Mental Disorders. In *Contemporary Social Problems*, eds. R. K. Merton and R. Nisbet. 2nd ed. New York: Harcourt, Brace and World.

Coughlin, R. M. 1980. *Ideology, Public Opinion, and Welfare Policy*. Berkeley: University of California Institute of International Studies.

Coughlin, R. M. and Armour, P. K. 1983. Sectoral Differentiation in Social Security Spending in OECD Nations. *Comparative Social Research* 6: 175–199.

Dallas, City of. Department of Health and Human Services. 1984. Health Care for the Homeless: An Application to the Robert Wood Johnson Foundation, Pew Memorial Trust.

Deutsch, A. 1948. *The Shame of the States*. New York: Harcourt, Brace.

Deutsch, A. 1949. *The Mentally Ill in America*. 2nd ed. New York: Columbia University Press.

Drew, E. 1967. The Health Syndicate: Washington's Noble Conspirators. *Atlantic* (December), pp. 75–82.

Eckstein, H. 1958. *The English Health Service: Its Origin, Structure, and Achievements*. Cambridge: Harvard University Press.

Flora, P., and Heidenheimer, A. J. 1981. *The Development of the Welfare State in Europe and America*. New Brunswick, N. J.: Transaction Books.

Foley, H. A. 1975. *Community Mental Health Legislation: The Formative Process*. Lexington, Mass.: D.C. Heath.

Foley, H. A., and Sharfstein, S. S. 1983. *Madness and Government: Who Cares for the Mentally Ill?* Washington, D.C.: American Psychiatric Press.

Goffman, E. 1961. *Asylums*. Garden City, N.Y.: Doubleday.

Gorman, M. 1956. *Every Other Bed*. Cleveland, Ohio: World.

Gough, I. 1979. *Political Economy of the Welfare State*. New Brunswick, N.J.: Transaction Books.

Grob, G. 1973. *Mental Institutions in America: Social Policy to 1875*. New York: Free Press.

Hay, J. R. 1975. *The Origins of Liberal Welfare Reforms, 1906–1914*. London: Macmillan.

Heclo, H. 1974. *Modern Social Politics in Britain and Sweden*. New Haven.: Yale University Press.

Hopper, K., and Baxter, E. 1984. "The Experiment Continues." Testimony Submitted to the Sub-Committee on Housing and Community Development, Committee on Banking, Finance, and Urban Affairs. U.S. House of Representatives. Washington, D.C., January 25. Appendix D, Serial No. 98–64; pp. 504–526.

Howard, A. 1963. We Are the Masters Now. In *The Age of Austerity*, eds. M. Sissons and P. French. London: Hodder and Stoughton.

Joint Commission on Mental Illness and Health. 1961. *Action for Mental Health*. New York: Basic Books.

Jones, K. 1972. A *History of Mental Health Services*. London: Routledge and Kegan Paul.

Kanter, R. M. 1972. *Commitment and Community*. Cambridge, Mass.: Harvard University Press.

Kramer, M. 1977. *Psychiatric Services and the Changing Institutional Scene: 1950–1975*. Washington, D.C.: U.S. Department of Health, Education and Welfare, National Institute of Mental Health, Series B, No. 12.

Kuhn. T. 1962. *The Structure of Scientific Revolutions*. Chicago: University of Chicago Press.

Leiby, J. 1978. *A History of Social Welfare and Social Work in the United States*. New York: Columbia University Press.

Lipset, S. M., and Wolin, S. S., eds. 1965. *The Berkeley Student Revolt: Facts and Interpretations*. Garden City, N.Y.: Doubleday.

Lowi, T. 1969. *The End of Liberalism: Ideology, Policy, and the Crisis of Public Authority*. New York: W. W. Norton.

Marmor, T. 1973. *The Politics of Medicare*. Chicago: Aldine.

Matza, D. 1966. The Disreputable Poor. In *Class, Status, and Power*, eds. R. Bendix and S. M. Lipset. New York: Free Press.

Moynihan, D. P. 1969. *Maximum Feasible Misunderstanding*. New York: Free Press.

Nisbet, R. 1953. *The Quest for Community*. New York: Oxford University Press.

O'Connor v. Donaldson. 1975. 422 U.S. 563.

Palmer, R. R. 1959. *The Age of Democratic Revolutions: Vol. 1: The Challenge*. Princeton, N.J.: Princeton University Press.

Patterson, J. T. 1981. *America's Struggle against Poverty, 1900–1985*. Cambridge: Harvard University Press.

President's Commission on Mental Health. 1978. *Report to the President's Commission on Mental Health*. Washington, D.C.: The White House and U.S. Government Printing Office. 4 volumes.

Pressman, J., and Wildavsky, A. 1973. *Implementation*. Berkeley: University of California Press.

R.A.J. v. Miller. 1974. C.A. 3–74–0394H.

Rothman, D. 1971. *The Discovery of the Asylum: Social Order and Disorder in the New Republic*. Boston: Little, Brown.

Ruiz v. Estelle. 1980. 503 F. Supp. 1265.

Schlesinger, A. M., Jr. 1986. *The Cycles of American History*. New York: Houghton Mifflin.

Stockman, D. 1985. *The Triumph of Politics*. New York: Harper and Row.

Swazey, J. 1974. *Chlorpromazine in Psychiatry*. Cambridge, Mass.: MIT Press.

Thurow, L. 1980. *The Zero-Sum Society*. New York: Basic Books.

Trattner, W. I. 1979. *From Poor Law to Welfare State. A History of Social Welfare in America*. 2nd ed. New York: Free Press.

Walters, R. B. 1978. *American Reformers: 1815–1860*. New York: Hill and Wang.

Wildavsky, A. 1964. *The Politics of the Budgetary Process*. Boston: Little, Brown.

Wilensky, H. L. 1975. *The Welfare State and Equality*. Berkeley: University of California Press.

Wilensky, H. T. 1976. *The "New Corporatism," Centralization, and the Welfare State*. Beverly Hills: Sage.

Wing, J. K., and Hailey, A. M. 1972. *Evaluating a Community Psychiatric Service: The Camberwell Register, 1964–1971*. London: Oxford University Press.

Wyatt v. Stickney. 1971. 325 F. Supp. 781, 784 (M.D. Ala).

Part 4

Evaluating the Community Mental Health Movement

9

An Evaluative Overview of the Community Mental Health Centers Program

DAVID A. DOWELL
and JAMES A. CIARLO

The Community Mental Health Centers (CMHC) program, initiated with federal funding in 1963, was one of the most important social experiments of the last two decades. It involved a radical restructuring of the primary locus of public mental health care and, to a lesser extent, a restructuring of the techniques of mental health services delivery (Regier and Taube, 1981; Bloom, 1977). Even at the peak of funding, the CMHC program did not account for the largest share of public expenditures for mental health services; hospitals and nursing homes each had, in the aggregate, larger budgets (Levine and Wilner, 1976). Nevertheless, the CMHC program was the centerpiece of federal mental health policy for most of two decades.

The CMHC program was implemented during a period of many changes in the mental health arena. Psychotropic drugs were becoming widely used. The population of state and county psychiatric hospitals was dropping and many state mental health systems began to increase their own community mental health services. Third-party reimbursements became available to more consumers. The supply of mental health professionals grew rapidly, albeit never to a level commensurate with need. Public awareness of mental health issues grew. All of these factors complicate our understanding of the impact of the federal CMHC program.

With Public Law 97–35 (P.L. 97–35) in 1981, the Reagan administration persuaded Congress to alter federal mental health policy by enacting block grants to states for mental health services. This effectively marked the end of federal oversight of local community mental health center activities. Despite that decision, mental health professionals have learned a great deal from the CMHC program which should and probably will shape the future of mental health policy at many levels of government.

This chapter summarizes results of evaluative studies and statistical reports on the CMHC program. It uses nine program goals as the basis for organizing information about CMHCs:

1. Increase the range and quantity of public mental health services;

2. Make services equally available and accessible to all;

3. Provide services in relation to the existing local needs;

4. Decrease state hospital admissions and residents;

5. Maximize citizen participation in community programs;

6. Prevent development of mental disorders;

7. Coordinate mental health–related services in the catchment area;

8. Provide services as efficiently as possible;

9. Provide services which reduce suffering and increase personal functioning.

Although the conceptions and relevant data of the goals overlap, these goals provide a useful framework for organizing information about the CMHC program. We present separately the pertinent information for each goal. The first seven were derived from the enabling legislation (Public Law 88–164, Title II), associated regulations, and NIMH literature. Except for prevention, these seven have been priorities for NIMH-funded evaluation studies (Feldman and Windle, 1973; Windle, Bass, and Taube, 1974). The efficiency goal was not formally articulated in CMHC legislation but is currently pressing with Reagan-era budget cuts affecting mental health services at all governmental levels. The goal of reducing suffering and increasing functioning is based upon several "overall NIMH goals" (Feldman and Windle, 1973: 177) and although difficult to assess, remains important for CMHCs.

We have defined our task as a review of evaluative data on federally funded CMHCs obtained during the 1963–1980 period (block grants are discussed in chapter 7). In a few instances, we include data from other sources which have implications for the CMHC program. We have not sought to review information on other mental health facilities such as public hospitals, freestanding clinics, and private practice. We have sought to locate and review as much of the available information as possible pertinent to these nine goals. Of course, we likely have omitted some information unintentionally.

The data derive from a fairly wide time frame. Since our purpose is not historical, we have made no effort to organize these findings to reflect the historical development of the CMHC program. Some older findings may not reflect the more recent status of the program. In some cases, we have noted this problem of generalizing over time. In all cases, we have made an effort to include the most recent and useful information available.

The following review will discuss the goals in turn and will articulate important issues relevant to each. Importance of particular issues is, of course, a judgment, and so our assessment necessarily reflects our own perspective.

INCREASE THE RANGE AND QUANTITY OF MENTAL HEALTH SERVICES

Issues pertinent to this goal include (1) increased volume of services; (2) increased number of specialized services; (3) maintenance of a community mental health orientation; and (4) fiscal viability of the centers.

Increased Services

CMHCs have increased substantially the volume of services to catchment-area residents, particularly outpatient and partial hospitalization. By October 1980, 789 centers had received over $2 billion in federal investment (National Institute of Mental Health, 1977a, 1978; Neigher et al., 1982). Between 1955 and 1977 the total number of episodes of patient care in the United States increased from 1.7 to 6.9 million. CMHCs were responsible for 32 percent of the episodes of patient care in 1977, in contrast to none in 1955 (Witkin, 1980). However, on a more negative note, about 700 catchment areas in the United States remained without CMHCs, even after the program had been operative for many years.

Windle, Bass, and Gray (1986) used a sample of sixty-three catchment areas with CMHCs and sixty-three matched catchments without CMHCs to carefully test the hypothesis that CMHCs stimulated service development. In catchment areas with CMHCs, they found evidence for increases in available and accessible services, staff, and additions while controlling for preexisting services and national trends over time. The magnitude of the observed effects was substantial. This study succeeded in controlling for two important factors which were confounded in prior research on this subject. Although quasi-experimental, this study provides the best evidence to date about the impact of the CMHC program upon service development.

In a study of fifty nonmetropolitan catchment areas comparing 1964 and 1974 service levels, Buck (1984) found that the introduction of a CMHC was associated with a net increase in services in the catchment areas. At the same time, he noted a *decrease* in independent (non–federally funded) day/night and outpatient services. This suggests that some of the growth in services associated with

CMHCs occurred through supplanting services which might otherwise have continued or been developed through other sources.

Studies focusing on specific areas of the country show that the areas which received CMHCs developed more services more rapidly than areas which did not (Babigian, 1977; National Study Service, 1972). Of mental health facilities reporting to NIMH in 1969–1971, CMHCs had the highest utilization rates and about double the rate of the nearest alternative (outpatient psychiatric services) (Taube and Cannon, 1972). Within CMHCs, outpatient care and partial care episodes grew faster (up 78 and 101 percent, respectively, over 1969–1975) than inpatient episodes (up only 21 percent).[1] In sum, it may not be too extreme to consider the shift in the primary locus of public mental health services to outpatient care as a revolutionary change that occurred in the era of federal funding to CMHCs.

Increased Specialized Services

The CMHC Amendments Act of 1975 (Public Law 94–63) increased the number of required services from five to twelve in CMHCs. This was intended to prod CMHCs into greater flexibility in meeting the needs of special groups (such as children and the elderly) and to deal more adequately with the more disturbed client who was still served primarily by the state hospitals in a series of revolving-door admissions and discharges back to community placements. This law undoubtedly stimulated development of more specialized services, including partial care, telephone and in-person emergency services, home visit programs, and paraprofessional and nonprofessional programs (Premo and Wiseman, 1981). Federal "conversion" grants became available to support increased alcohol, drug abuse, halfway-house, and special-population programs in many CMHCs. However, a limited survey of nine CMHCs funded in 1976 indicated that these requirements for comprehensive services overwhelmed some centers (Price and Associates, 1978).

Price and Associates (1978) also asked center directors to indicate their level of satisfaction with the services offered by their centers. Directors were more satisfied with outpatient, partial hospitalization, screening, and follow-up services and less satisfied with transitional care. Half of board members and staff felt there was insufficient flexibility in the requirements of Public Law 94–63 to initiate innovative services or to tailor services to unique local needs.

Maintenance of a Community Approach

According to a report by Abt Associates (Abt Associates, 1976; Naierman, Haskins, and Robinson, 1978), during their fifth through eight years of operation CMHCs managed to implement successfully much of the philosophy and goals of community mental health. However, after the eighth year and the withdrawal of federal support, a shift away from a community orientation began. Consultation and education were de-emphasized and the number of satellite clinics diminished. Services shifted toward a greater proportion of inpatients, a trend which generated greater revenues. Partial hospitalization and emergency services were reduced. These findings were confirmed by Jerrell and Larsen (1984). In their longitudinal study (1976–1980–1982) of seventy-one CMHCs, they found a trend over time toward a less comprehensive mix of services.

Woy, Wasserman, and Weiner-Pomerantz (1981) also examined CMHCs after their period of federal funding ended and found changes in services. They found evidence that changes began before the end of federal funding and that an observed increase in inpatient services was not dramatic, due, they surmised, to administrative obstacles. The essential conclusion of these studies was that termination of federal funding is associated with centers moving away "from the comprehensive balanced mix of services intended in the CMHC program" (Woy, Wasserman, and Weiner-Pomerantz, 1981: 273). A major factor in this shift is the reimbursement criteria of public and private insurers, which have continued to favor inpatient over outpatient and partial hospitalization services. This arrangement is intended to contain costs by limiting coverage to include only the services utilized by the most severely disabled patients. In fact, this strategy escalates costs by discouraging the use of outpatient and partial hospitalization services which are cheaper and probably effective with many severely disabled patients, a point to be elaborated below (Flomenhaft, Kaplan, and Langsley, 1969; Kiesler, 1980; Washburn et al., 1976).

Fiscal Viability

An NIMH study (Weiner et al., 1979) found that some centers cannot remain fiscally viable without federal support. Those that do, however, tend to have better success in capturing client fees and third-party reimbursements. Bass et al. (1985) found major differences between centers which *provide* inpatient services and those which *affiliate* with a hospital which provides inpatient services. The key difference is which organizational entity receives the reimbursement for inpatient services. Bass et al. found that revenues from services in inpatient provider centers went up over the 1971–1980 period, while those in inpatient affiliated centers went down. In inflation-adjusted dollars, revenues in inpatient affiliated centers actually *declined* over 1976–1980. These findings suggest fiscal problems for centers which are not providers of inpatient services.

Staff and board members of at least some CMHCs share this concern with fiscal viability. Respondents in a survey of nine center boards indicated that the lack of a secure financial base would cause a reduction of services when federal support expired (Price and Associates, 1978). The same assessment was reflected in the "Report on the National Conference on Graduate CMHCs" (National Institute of Mental Health, 1980a); participants called for continued funding for "post–federally funded" CMHCs.

In sum, CMHCs succeeded in substantially increasing the range and the quantity of public mental health services in the United States, particularly outpatient care and partial hospitalization. CMHCs helped to shift the primary locus of mental health care from hospital-based, inpatient locations to community-based outpatient locations. However, this success is threatened by the lack of permanent public support for CMHC programs. In many areas of the country, the "seed-money" concept did not succeed in generating adequate state and local funding to maintain the range of services demanded by the community mental health philosophy. Severe budget cuts may well undo eighteen years of hard work in public mental health services. Those CMHCs which do survive the termination of support from federal dollars are likely to shift away from the community mental health philosophy and toward a mode of services delivery which is more successful at generating revenue.

MAKE SERVICES EQUALLY AVAILABLE AND ACCESSIBLE TO ALL

The CMHC program aimed at alleviating the two-class system of care, in which well-to-do persons with mental illness received primarily private outpatient care, and disadvantaged persons, to the extent they received any services at all, were likely to receive custodial state hospitalization. This topic is complex, but will be restricted here to issues involving poverty, ethnic minorities, older adults, children, disabled persons, and rural clients. Awareness and accessibility will also be discussed.

Poverty

Data for 1974 indicate that the majority of CMHC clients (52 percent) could be considered "poor," with incomes below the poverty level for an urban family of four (National Institute of Mental Health, 1975; Rosen, 1977). Sixty percent of CMHCs funded by 1975 were in "low-median" income areas (Stockdill, 1978). These facts are partly a result of NIMH funding more CMHCs in poverty areas than in nonpoverty areas in the earlier years of the program (Windle, Bass, and Taube, 1974).

The emphasis of NIMH on funding CMHC services for disadvantaged persons may have declined in the latter program years. Slightly more than half of centers funded under Public Law 94–63 were nonpoverty centers, while nearly all "graduate" centers which received financial distress funds were poverty centers (National Institute of Mental Health, 1977b). As of 1976, although two-thirds of all CMHCs were in "low-income areas" (below $7,500 annual income), more than half of the metropolitan CMHCs were in "high-income" areas (above $7,500). Finally, there is some evidence that the percentage of poor clients using CMHCs decreased in later years of the program (Bachrach, 1974; Taube and Cannon, 1972) at least in nonmetropolitan centers (Rosenstein, 1979).

Smith (1984) examined geographic patterns of federal funding for CMHCs and per capita income. He concluded that the program overall was moderately redistributive, with more services being provided in lower-income geographic areas.

Ethnic Minority Clients

While the large majority (about four-fifths) of CMHC additions are white (National Institute of Mental Health, 1980b), the admission *rates* for different ethnic groups are more nearly equal, with nonwhites (blacks, Asians, Native Americans) actually utilizing CMHCs at a higher rate (Redick, 1976). This pattern also holds for other public psychiatric facilities and may reflect greater need for service by nonwhites. CMHCs have tended to be funded in areas with higher black populations, but there are important regional differences in this trend (Windle, Neal, and Zinn, 1979). Reporting on an effort to stimulate centers with a history of underserving minorities to improve the equity of their services, Windle and Wu (1981) found no evidence for significant improvement.

Important work on minority utilization of mental health services has been conducted by Stanley Sue and his colleagues (Sue et al., 1974; Sue, Allen, and Conaway, 1978; Sue, 1977). They studied seventeen community mental health facilities in the vicinity of Seattle, Washington, of which only a few were federally funded CMHCs.[2] Some minorities (blacks and American Indians) were admitted to services at a rate higher than their proportion of the catchment population; however, dropout rates for several minority groups (blacks, Chicanos, American Indians) were much higher than for white clients. This is confirmed by a study of an urban CMHC by Armstrong et al. (1984) and by studies in non–federally funded CMHC settings (Baekeland and Lundwall, 1975; Lorion, 1974; and Wolkon et al., 1974). These findings suggest that the encouragingly equitable minority admission rates to CMHCs do not reflect volume of services provided to minorities, which may be less equitable.

The ethnicity of staff may influence minorities' willingness to use CMHC services and the appropriateness of treatment given. NIMH data show that in 1976 there were at least as many black, Hispanic, and "other race" staff hours per 1,000 catchment-area population as white staff hours (National Institute of Mental Health, 1977c). However, other NIMH data show that minority personnel are concentrated in the staff categories of licensed practical nurse, sub–master's degree social worker, nonprofessional mental health worker, clerical/maintenance, and (surprisingly) psychiatrist (National Institute of Mental Health, 1977d). The relative scarcity of minorities in some professional groups (psychologists, social workers, psychiatric nurses) may imply that CMHC clinical services have been less attuned to minorities than might be desirable.

Older Adults

From 1969 to 1977, the percentage of CMHC additions who were elderly (sixty-five years of age and older) ranged from 3.8 to 4.0 (National Institute of

Mental Health, 1980b). However, NIMH data show that, relative to their proportion in the population, the elderly were served at one-fourth the rate of the twenty-five to forty-four age group. A study of one regional CMHC in Connecticut found that elderly use of outpatient care had not been increased by the center and the elderly, like minorities, were one of the "special patient groups" mostly treated in categorical units staffed by paraprofessionals (Center for Health Studies, 1979). Unlike children, toward whom many consultation and education services are directed, the elderly have received few indirect services (Rosenstein, 1978, 1979; National Institute of Mental Health, 1977a).

Children

Rising from an essentially zero base in 1966, CMHCs accounted for over one-quarter of episodes of child mental health care in all types of facilities in 1971 (Redick, 1973). However, relative to population, children were served at only one-third the rate of the adult group and the percentage of CMHC additions under fifteen years of age ranged from 13.0 to 17.2 (National Institute of Mental Health, 1980b).

In a study of a Virginia law permitting minors to enter treatment without parental consent, Melton (1981) found that 40 percent of CMHCs were unaware of the law nine months after it had passed. Centers that were aware of the law were more likely to have a policy of serving minors without parental consent. Minors in treatment without parental consent were all adolescents.

Public Law 94–63 called for specialized services for children and the elderly, but the issue was still problematic in 1978 when the President's Commission on Mental Health called again for more services to children, adolescents, and the elderly (President's Commission, 1978).

Disabled Clients

Seliger (1981) assessed the preparation of CMHCs to comply with section 504 of the Rehabilitation Act of 1973, the "civil rights act for the disabled." Six months before full compliance with the act was to be required by law, Seliger mailed a survey to 80 percent of all CMHCs and 26 percent responded. Fourteen percent of respondents had completed preparation for compliance. Eighty-seven percent had no equipment for telephone access for deaf clients, but 35 percent reported clinical staff with sign language skills. Accessibility for mobility impaired clients was better than for vision or hearing impaired clients. Centers threatened with sanctions by the Department of Health, Education, and Welfare were twice as likely to have taken steps toward compliance.

Rural Clients

A comprehensive NIMH contract study (Longest, Konan, and Tweed, 1976) showed that in 1973 "adequate mental health service structures" (both available and accessible services) were found in only 17 percent of rural catchment areas, while in central city and central/metropolitan ring areas the percentage was 23 percent. In terms of manpower, rural areas had only 43 person-hours per 1,000 population while central and central/ring areas had 54. Both comparisons involved not only CMHCs, but all facilities except state hospitals. In terms of CMHCs alone, by 1975 only 181 rural CMHCs had been funded in comparison to 240 urban centers; another 94 were mixed urban/rural (Bass, 1981). Rural CMHCs averaged fewer full-time-equivalent staff (64.8 vs. 105.5 in 1974) (Rosenstein, 1979), fewer trainees (Perls, Winslow, and Pathak, 1980), and averaged only 48 percent of the annual additions reported by urban centers (Bachrach, 1974). Progress in federal funding for rural CMHCs was hampered by the extensive service pattern required for funding (initially five essential services, then twelve). The Mental Health System Act of 1980 was expected to facilitate funding of rural services, but was rescinded in the first year of the Reagan administration.

Awareness and Accessibility of Services

One factor which affects accessibility is awareness of the CMHC by community members and caregivers. Windle, Bass, and Taube (1974) cite a NIMH contract study indicating that about 17 percent of the residents of several catchment areas spontaneously named their CMHC when asked about mental health services; another 8 percent knew its location. But this same study showed that only 3 percent of residents would select the CMHC as the place to go for various mental health problems. Respondents cited such discouraging factors as waiting lists, identification as a client, need for an appointment, and limits in the hours of operation. A similar study by Scott, Balch, and Flynn (1984) found that only 5 percent could name the local CMHC, while 34 percent indicated having heard of the facility. The same questions were asked of "gatekeepers," such as school personnel and clergy, of whom 19 percent could name the center and 53 percent said they had heard of it. School counselors had the highest awareness of the CMHC; 44 percent named it and 96 percent had heard of it. Clergy reported the least awareness. Munger (1981) found that 44 percent of sixty persons called in a random dialing telephone survey had heard of a local center. In a second study by Scott, Balch, and Flynn (1983), citizens interviewed had somewhat more favorable attitudes toward CMHC services than hospital services, but there was no difference in attitudes toward CMHC clients and hospital clients.

A 1970 survey of CMHC hours of operation (Bass, 1972) showed that 71 percent of outpatient units were open in the daytime only, most just five days per week. A minority were open evenings, when many employed persons would want to use services. Partial care units were only slightly more accessible, with 68 percent open only in the daytime and nighttime. Similarly, when the National Council of Community Mental Health Centers conducted an off-hours telephone survey to emergency services for ninety-nine CMHCs, thirty-two of the centers failed to answer the phone, indicating nonaccessibility for potential clients of one-third of the sample (Wolfe, 1977). A later repeat by NIMH Regional Offices, however, found a nonresponse rate of 12 percent in one region and 0 percent in another, after a concentrated effort to locate the proper emergency telephone numbers (Windle, Albert, and Sharfstein, 1978).

Overall, the CMHC program improved availability and accessibility of public mental health care for the young and old, minorities, the poor, and possibly rural residents. Yet inequities remain in accessibility for the young and very old, and possibly also for minorities, the poor, and rural residents relative to the accessibility for the adult population, aged eighteen to sixty-four. The serious budget cuts experienced by public mental health services in recent years can only exaggerate inequities as specialized and hard-to-deliver services (e.g., outreach to the elderly) are cut back to preserve standard, reimbursable inpatient and outpatient services.

PROVIDE SERVICES IN RELATION TO EXISTING NEEDS IN THE COMMUNITY

Issues to be discussed here include services to high-need populations and severely disabled patients.

High-Need Populations

Since the association of poverty with the need for mental health services is well established, the early NIMH thrust toward funding "poverty-area" centers was well directed toward meeting citizens' needs (Rosen, 1977). A sophisticated analysis of all U.S. catchment areas in terms of needs and resources (Longest, Konan, and Tweed, 1976) showed that in 1974 catchments highest in need had the highest percentage (31 percent) of "adequate service structures" in terms of service availability and accessibility. Federally funded CMHC services undoubtedly contributed to this situation; in Colorado, for example, federal funding helped the neediest catchment (Northwest/Central Denver) to establish a very large service system capable of meeting most of the need assessed. Federal funds helped develop similar comprehensive core-city programs in many large cities across the nation.

There was a strong similarity in diagnosis between the clients seen by the CMHCs and public outpatient psychiatric clinics, with the largest groups of disorders being neurosis, schizophrenia, and personality disorders (Taube, 1971a). Udell and Hornstra (1975) compared one urban CMHC caseload with a "private practice" clientele; the CMHC caseload was far more diverse, had more alcoholics and schizophrenics, was more socially disengaged, and was less inclined to stay in treatment. Compared to state hospital clientele, however, the CMHC clientele was less impaired in terms of having fewer alcoholics, schizophrenics, and persons with organic brain syndromes (Taube, 1971b). Thus,

CMHCs typically served a population with disorders intermediate in severity between hospital and private practice clienteles.

However, NIMH was criticized for failing to ensure that services were planned and funded in relation to needs. Comptroller General reports to the Congress in 1971 and 1974 both listed this deficiency, the former with respect to not funding CMHCs in areas of greatest need and the latter with respect to programs not addressed to within-catchment area needs. In a survey of nine CMHCs, Price and Associates (1978) found that many CMHC board members felt there was no relationship between needs assessments and services. Further, in a later study by NIMH (1977b), additions to services were at a higher rate in "low need" catchment areas (1,238 per 100,000) than in "moderate need" catchment areas (1,099 per 100,000); and the "low need" figure is very nearly as great as the "high need" area figure (1,471 per 100,000). As noted previously, more "non-poverty" CMHC starts were made under Public Law 94–63 than "poverty" area starts, probably increasing services in areas where the need was not the greatest.

An Abt Associates study (1972) reported that citizens identified "drinking" and "drugs" as the two most serious mental health problems in their catchments. In 1975, Public Law 94–63 mandated CMHC services to alcoholics and drug abusers (for clients not served by other catchment area programs). In 1977, alcoholics comprised about 12 percent of CMHC additions in comparison with 9 percent in 1971; but drug abuse clients decreased from 4.4 percent to 3.7 percent in that period (National Institute of Mental Health, 1980b). In the light of community residents' concern about these problems, these rates can be seen as lower than they might have been. The National Institute of Drug Abuse and the National Institute of Alcohol and Alcohol Abuse have developed and supported programs which may have dealt with some portion of these problems.

Since substance abuse is often accompanied by serious psychological disorders, special efforts to increase services to these target groups would be appropriate. However, CMHCs often find substance abusers difficult to treat and with the elimination under block grants of the requirements for substance abuse services which existed under Public Law 94–63, reductions in these services seem inevitable.

Severely Disabled Patients

Langsley (1980: 816) alleged that CMHCs increasingly shifted their focus away from treating the seriously mentally disabled patient and toward offering "counseling and crisis intervention for predictable problems of living" (cf. Yarvis, Edwards, and Langsley, 1978; Borus, 1978; Winslow, 1982). The principal evidence cited by Langsley for this conclusion derives from data provided by Goldman et al. (1980) showing a decline in the percentage of CMHC patients diagnosed as schizophrenic; between 1970 and 1975, that percentage fell from 15.1 to 10 percent. There was a similar decline in depressive disorders (20 to

13 percent) and, correspondingly, the percentage of persons apparently without mental disorder increased from 5 to 22 percent.

Other data are relevant to interpreting these changes and suggest a different conclusion. For patients admitted over 1970–1975 with the diagnosis of schizophrenia, the rate per 100,000 population rose from 25.1 to 43.5; the number of such patients increased 82 percent (50,597 to 91,914). In the same period, the number of CMHCs increased 107 percent (255 to 528). These data suggest that CMHC service to severely disordered clients was increasing over the 1970–1975 period but not as rapidly as the growth in centers, causing the observed decline in the percentage of CMHC additions who were diagnosed as schizophrenic.

Goldman et al. (1980) suggested that more rapid growth in the number of centers than in number of schizophrenic patients may indicate that some schizophrenic patients were already under treatment in other facilities. This assumes that some individuals crossed catchment boundaries for services, reducing the number needing services for severe disorders in the newer catchments. The lesser proportion of schizophrenics is apparent largely in centers established after 1972 and is barely noticeable in the older centers. A possible explanation for this is NIMH's early emphasis on funding poverty areas, which often have high concentrations of severely disordered clients.

Windle et al. (1986) found evidence that psychiatrists in CMHCs are more likely to work with schizophrenic patients than other CMHC staff. Over the years of the CMHC program, there was a declining proportion of psychiatric staff in CMHCs (Bass, 1982; Beigel, 1984), suggesting the possibility of a reduced commitment to severely and chronically ill patients.

Siegel, Astrachan, and Levine (1984) reported a study showing that the use of patient count data underestimated services to the most chronic patients. In one CMHC, schizophrenic clients comprised 10.8 percent of the *caseload* but 19.7 percent of *client contacts*. Similar patterns were found for measures of services to clients with affective disorders (9.9 percent vs. 14.3 percent), personality disorders (5.6 percent vs. 11.6 percent), organic brain syndrome (1.1 percent vs. 2.6 percent), and anxiety disorders (2.4 percent vs. 4.8 percent). The opposite pattern of caseloads vs. client contacts was found for disorders of childhood (21.1 percent vs. 7 percent) and alcohol and drug problems (15.3 percent vs. 8.5 percent). It seems very likely that the additions data on which the Langsley assertion is based similarly underestimated services to the most chronic patients.

In the latter years of the program, and in the period of block grant funding, it appears that CMHCs increased the proportion of their effort devoted to the severely and chronically disabled patients (see chapter 7 of this volume). For example, in a longitudinal study of seventy-one CMHCs, Cognos Associates (Larsen and Jerrell, 1983; Jerrell and Larsen, 1984) found evidence of increased services to this population. They reported growth in day and partial care, residential and case management services, all services directed primarily at the chronically ill. They also found an increase in the proportion of funding from

Medicaid, which supports many chronic patients; this proportion rose from 9 percent to 15 percent over 1976 to 1982.

In sum, these studies indicate that the absolute amount of CMHC resources devoted to the seriously disabled client rose over time, but more slowly than the amount of resources devoted to other clients. Near the end of the period of federal funding this trend may have been reversing. These data, together with the 1977 report of the U.S. Comptroller General, to be discussed below, which identified deficiencies in services to this population, indicate that severely and chronically ill patients deserved a higher priority than the CMHC program provided at least over most of the 1963–1980 period (cf. Winslow, 1982).

DECREASE PUBLIC PSYCHIATRIC HOSPITAL ADMISSIONS AND RESIDENTS

Issues to be discussed under this heading include reduction in state hospital admissions and residents due to CMHCs and appropriateness of hospitalization vs. community placements.

Reduced Admissions

NIMH data (Witkin, 1980) show that in 1955, three-fourths of the 1.7 million episodes of patient care in the United States were inpatient. By 1977, 70 percent of the 6.9 million episodes were outpatient, of which CMHCs provided 32 percent.

Windle, Bass, and Taube (1974) cited unpublished NIMH data showing lower state hospital utilization from CMHC catchments than from the nation as a whole. This is quite compelling because of the likelihood that CMHC catchments would normally generate higher state hospital admission rates because of their relatively less favorable sociodemographic characteristics—greater poverty, more over-crowding, etc. (Rosen, 1977). Using a summary of several studies, Windle, Bass, and Taube (1974) concluded that CMHCs did make a positive contribution to lowering state hospital admission rates. Doidge and Rogers's (1976) study of one state, Wyoming, provided a clear picture of the positive impact of both comprehensive CMHCs and clinic services upon state hospital admissions. However, Windle and Scully (1976) more recently found less support for the impact of CMHCs on state hospital care. Examining sixteen states over five years, they concluded that there is no evidence for impact on state hospital residence rates, but that "there may be a tendency for centers to lower state hospital admission rates" (Windle and Scully, 1976: 241).

This issue is not easily resolved. The advent of Medicare and Medicaid has greatly increased the role of nursing homes in caring for the mentally disabled (Regier and Taube, 1981). Other important factors include antipsychotic drugs and community-oriented programs mounted by state hospitals themselves which may have had the effect of reducing admissions and length of stay in the hospital.

In addition, the profile of psychiatric patient populations may have shifted over time, as indicated by increases in alcohol and drug abuse clients and by the increased concern about the "young adult chronic" patients[3] (Alcohol, Drug Abuse, and Mental Health Administration, 1982; Ciarlo, 1979). At any rate, we cannot conclude that the CMHC program has had a powerful impact on the reduction of state hospital populations.

Finally, it is, in a sense, remarkable that the data reviewed above are as positive as they are, considering the unimportance attached to reducing hospital admissions by CMHC staff themselves (as contrasted with NIMH). The 1977 Comptroller General report to Congress cited an NIMH contract study to the effect that 175 CMHCs ranked decreasing state hospital utilization next to last in a list of ten CMHC program goals.

Appropriateness of Hospital Placements

A finding in a longitudinal review of studies of inappropriate hospital placements (Faden and Goldman, 1979) is disturbing. Faden and Goldman expected a decrease in inappropriate hospitalization over the period of the review (1961–1977) due to increasing recognition by mental health personnel of the existence of community alternatives to hospitalization. Instead, the percentage of patients inappropriately hospitalized seemed to increase in the ten studies conducted over seventeen years. The authors' explanations were that definitions of appropriateness had changed over the years and that methods varied in the studies. Even if these explanations are correct, the lowest percentage of inappropriate placements found was 50 percent. Their findings are consistent with the 1977 Comptroller General's report, and suggest that more could have been done to develop community alternatives to hospitalization for chronic mentally disabled individuals.

MAXIMIZE CITIZEN PARTICIPATION IN COMMUNITY PROGRAMS

From its inception, the CMHC program was viewed very much as a "community-based" effort. However, citizen input into CMHCs was slow in coming (Cibulka, 1981; Flaherty and Olsen, 1978). The Comptroller General's report of 1974 noted significant community involvement in only two of twelve centers reviewed (Comptroller General, 1974). A summary of NIMH contract work and other studies on this topic (Windle, Bass, and Taube, 1974) showed little evidence of significant movement toward the goal of increased community participation in CMHCs, as well as considerable variation between regions on extent of citizens' involvement. Another review of the history of CMHCs included two examples of community-professional conflict in CMHC operations, and indicated only a few instances of considerable citizen involvement in CMHC programs (Ozarin, 1975).

Public Law 94–63 addressed, in part, this slow response by mandating citizen involvement on "representative governing or advisory bodies" and in reviewing local CMHC evaluation efforts. This federal mandate for citizen involvement in evaluation was slowly implemented for several reasons: (1) this requirement demanded a new structure foreign to CMHCs; (2) there was a lack of effective and accepted strategies to implement it; (3) staff and board members did not understand how citizen involvement could help improve services; (4) citizen members of CMHC boards saw themselves as representatives of the community and did not perceive citizens involved in evaluation as such representatives; and (5) neither board member nor non–board member citizens felt that they had time to invest in this function. In addition, the federal requirement that CMHCs promote citizen involvement in evaluation may have contained a contradiction: Why should CMHCs cooperate in creating a mechanism to encourage local citizens to express criticism of the CMHCs (Price and Associates, 1978)?

Some progress, however, was made. In Florida, a project involved seventeen citizen groups in developing recommendations for use by nine CMHCs based upon evaluation reports. Of 310 recommendations made, 71 percent were used by the centers (Bergner, Zinober, and Dinkel, 1984).

Training programs for citizen members of CMHC boards have also appeared. Manuals outlining procedures for citizen participation in setting goals and evaluating a CMHC's progress toward achieving those goals were made available (Zinober and Dinkel, 1981; MacMurray et al., 1976), and NIMH produced training programs in evaluation for CMHC board members and staff working together. Annual evaluation reports which incorporated citizen, board member, and community input, and responses of CMHC managers to that input, were required of all CMHCs.

A special issue of the *Community Mental Health Journal* (1981, Number 1) documented the progress and problems of citizen participation in CMHCs. It showed that, while most CMHCs came into at least superficial compliance with Public Law 94–63 citizen governance requirements, the development of a full professional-and-citizen partnership in community mental health was a rarity. In sum, the CMHC program was not able to make the enormous progress hoped for in this area, but in fairness it should be noted that no other U.S. health service delivery had even attempted to develop (much less attained) the level of citizen-provider cooperation sought by the CMHC program (Simpson, 1981).

PREVENT THE DEVELOPMENT OF MENTAL DISORDERS

We cannot here review the enormous literature on prevention of mental disorder or "promotion of mental health . . . which focuses on improving the quality of life and well-being, not merely averting pathology" (Goldston, Ojemann, and Nelson, 1975: 52). Prevention and promotion activities have received uneven acceptance by mental health service providers in most settings (e.g., Schwartz, 1982; Walsh, 1982). More evidence for effectiveness of prevention activities exists now than was available during the era of direct federal funding of CMHCs. The American Psychological Association Task Force on Prevention recently selected fourteen exemplary programs which have generated evidence of effectiveness in follow-up studies done from two to nineteen years after the initial interventions (Wolfe and Swift, 1986). For example, there is now good evidence that well-designed social problem-solving skills training, directed on a fairly intensive basis to children, has beneficial adjustment outcomes several years later (see also chapter 17 in this volume).

However, such data were not available during the era of federal funding for CMHCs and prevention efforts through consultation and education (C&E) activities by CMHCs generally differed sharply from the more recently developed models of effective prevention. It is interesting that none of the exemplary programs selected by the American Psychological Association Task Force on Prevention were developed in federally funded CMHC settings. We will confine the review here mainly to data generated by the CMHC program for which it could claim at least partial responsibility, and we will review weaknesses in prevention activities as practiced by CMHCs.

Evidence for Effectiveness of Prevention

Studies document that C&E efforts aimed at prevention of mental disorders did have positive effects upon the knowledge, attitudes, and sometimes behavior of CMHC consultees, including police, other health professionals, and teachers (Carter and Cazares, 1976). Such consultation was directed primarily at teachers (Rosenstein, 1978), and this focus on children should have helped to maximize any disorder-prevention potential of the consultation process. While evidence of actual impact on children is absent from many reports, behavior changes in social interaction, learning effort, and academic performance have been noted in a few studies (Carter and Cazares, 1976).

Weaknesses in Practice

There appear to have been three major weaknesses in the CMHC prevention effort. First, resources committed to prevention activities were small in relation to direct services. Snow and Newton (1976) argued that the continuous demand associated with direct services put C&E activities at a disadvantage in claiming the energies of staff, since C&E activities required staff initiative. A 1974 sample of staff's self-reported activities over one week showed that about 6 percent of staff hours went into C&E, while direct care accounted for 78 percent (National Institute of Mental Health, 1975). In 1975, only 4 percent of CMHC budgets went into C&E activities and to public information and public education (National Institute of Mental Health, 1977e). According to a survey by Vayda and Perlmutter (1977), *primary* prevention activities, usually defined as efforts to prevent the onset of mental disorders in persons with no past or current symptoms, comprised slightly less than one-half of all C&E activities and the total effort expended for all types of C&E was low. Psychologists averaged 4.6 hours per week in community activities compared to 17 hours in clinical work and 13 hours in administration (Bloom and Parad, 1978). Data from 1975 and 1976 showed successive declines in C&E activity—1976 was down 29 percent compared to 1974 (National Institute of Mental Health, 1977e).

To make matters even less optimistic, a study (Abt Associates, 1976; Naierman, Haskins, and Robinson, 1978) of centers beyond their eighth year of operation found that C&E activities were among the first services cut in response to fiscal pressures. The same finding appeared in a longitudinal study of seventy-one CMHCs in the early 1980s by Cognos Associates (Jerrell and Larsen, 1984). The trend away from C&E is undoubtedly due in part to the lack of third-party reimbursements for C&E in an era when funds for clinical services are growing scarce (cf. Snow and Swift, 1985). There were, however, two exceptions to the declining trend reported in the Cognos study. Declines were not observed where C&E services were (1) under contract to courts, schools, and business and (2) performed by CMHCs in states which imposed guidelines for C&E services.

The second major weakness was in the C&E activities as performed. Some authors have written compellingly of the lack of knowledge and consequent ineffective practices characterizing much of C&E activity in CMHCs (Moed and Muhich, 1972; Borus, 1978); other experts visiting CMHCs noted the lack of understanding among CMHC staff about what consultation is and what it is supposed to accomplish (Glasscote et al., 1969: 27; Joint Information Service, 1978). Snow and Newton (1976) argued that C&E was never defined as a major task for CMHCs by program documents such as the National Council of Community Mental Health Centers' *Policy and Standards Manual* (see Snow and Wolfe, 1983).

Third, there was a paucity of data demonstrating the effectiveness of consultation as a primary prevention technique in mental health (Carter and Cazares, 1976; Bloom, 1968). CMHC staff cited this as their reason for lack of interest in prevention (Glasscote et al., 1969), and this appears to be at least partly responsible for the "confused status" and "mixture of optimism and pessimism" about prevention noted by other writers (Carter and Cazares, 1976).

It is frequently said that the CMHC program overstated its capacity for prevention in the early days of the program (e.g., Musto, 1975); the available data, unfortunately, do little to refute this assertion. Moreover, current funding trends make significant prevention activity by CMHCs even less likely in the future.

COORDINATE MENTAL HEALTH SERVICES IN THE CATCHMENT AREA

The issues discussed under this heading include coordination of services within the structure of CMHCs, coordination of services with other agencies, and services provided to other community agencies.

Coordination Within CMHCs

By its very structure, a CMHC integrates a range of direct services into a "comprehensive service system" facilitating the delivery of whichever type of treatment is needed by a client. An early study in one urban CMHC found that transfers of clients between different service elements resulted in continued service at the receiving end about half the time. Improvements in paper-flow and interelement communications procedures gradually increased this number to about two-thirds.[4] This was a higher percentage than is typical for non-CMHC interagency referrals (Dowell and Jones, 1980). Other studies documented increasing staff communications, broadening of focus to more target groups, and establishment of common intake points among different services unified in a CMHC (Ozarin, 1975).

One important problem in maintaining continuity of care is patients who drop out of treatment. Estimates of the proportion of clients dropping out of CMHC services can be derived from NIMH data. In an early study, CMHC therapists succeeded in continuing clients in treatment until recommended termination in 62 percent of their cases (Bass and Windle, 1972). One source of data on all CMHCs in 1974 (National Institute of Mental Health, 1977a) states that over 35 percent of discontinued clients were not referred to another resource even though they were judged to be in need of further services. For 90 percent of these cases, the reason given for nonreferral was that the client dropped out of treatment. Another 10 percent were not referred due to lack of appropriate resources. Another NIMH source (Rosenstein, 1979) stated that in 1974 about 25 percent of discontinued clients were not referred to another resource because of dropping out although they were judged to be in need of further services; 2.5 percent were not referred for lack of an appropriate facility.

Coordination with Other Agencies

One of the most significant issues for CMHCs involves coordination of the discharge of chronic patients into the community. The Comptroller General's 1977 report found that some CMHCs *did* discuss individual clients' needs with state hospital caregivers but more frequently there was insufficient communication which later resulted in an untimely or inappropriate readmission to the state hospital. Similar conclusions appear in an NIMH contract study that examined the relationship between CMHCs and state hospitals (Socio-Technical Systems Associates, 1973). Another study (Lueger and Marquette, 1981) suggested that poor coordination was not a consequence of staff failing to perceive the need to coordinate; CMHC and state hospital staff in this study rated goals of cooperative screening and aftercare as highly important. Yet the problem of lack of discharge coordination was still widespread.

The Comptroller General's report cited above noted that CMHCs and state hospitals developed independently of each other, were accountable to different authorities (state vs. federal/local/private organizations), tended to serve different populations, and had different funding (again, state vs. federal). Hence, there was little incentive to collaborate closely. As a result, too little joint planning with state hospitals was conducted, and community care for discharged persons was often inadequate.

On the other hand, instances of excellent coordination can be found in the CMHC literature. Sheridan and Teplin (1981) described a coordinated program in which the CMHC set up a "Police Reception Program" for police-apprehended mentally disabled individuals. Referred individuals were typically seriously disturbed and in crisis. They required an average of 2.2 hours of psychiatric evaluation (range: one-five hours) because of low motivation and inability to communicate due to the severity of the crisis reactions. In a comparison of police-referred cases in the two prior years with two years of program referrals, the program group had significantly fewer total hospital days (137 vs. 33 average days). The cost savings as well as treatment implications of this program are an important example of effective CMHC coordination of services in the community.

Raschko (1985) described a coordinated working relationship between a CMHC and an area agency on aging. Nonprofessional "gatekeepers" including clergy and meter-readers were organized to identify high-risk elderly individuals who were provided with a range of CMHC services including mental health services, case management, and in-home aid.

Zins and Hopkins (1981) described a cooperative relationship between a CMHC and a local school district which was designed to increase the number of referrals who kept initial appointments with the CMHC. Important factors included the school psychologist's expressed confidence in the CMHC, the identification of a specific service resource, and the psychologist's willingness to make the initial contact.

NIMH experimented with linking primary health care settings and CMHCs (Broskowski, 1980). In this program, mental health professionals worked in forty-seven sites at the time of the study providing services of triage, referral, and consultation. Results suggested that mental health services to medical clients were increased by such in-house coordination and consultation with mental health staff.

Services to Other Agencies

While community mental health ideology suggests that CMHCs would also provide services to other agencies and their clients, there are relatively few studies of this role for centers. Evidence does exist that centers often interacted with other agencies, since studies of prevention activities report frequent contacts with clergy, parents, day care centers, and especially teachers (Vayda and Perlmutter, 1977).

One study (Community Mental Health Project, 1980) focused on interactions with the judiciary and noted that CMHCs succeeded in providing consultation and education services to courts and police, including expertise in identifying community alternatives for mental health care prior to hospital commitment. However, the report also identified needs for more legal and community advocacy, more community placement alternatives for individuals processed through the judiciary system, more collaboration between courts and CMHCs, and more consultation and education with courts and police.

Developing a truly coordinated system of care is difficult; Pepper and Ryglewicz (1982) have described many of the complexities. The conception and implementation of CMHCs as interlinked arrays of services did a good deal to provide coordination among a wide variety of mental health services. In addition, there are examples in the literature of effective interagency linkages involving CMHCs. But this has not been enough. Community mental health ideology suggests that CMHCs should not be passive purveyors of services, but public health–oriented programs intended to stimulate increases and improvements in entire local systems of mental health services. All service needs cannot be met by one person, team, or agency. The need for better coordination of services and for filling gaps in local service networks seems evident, despite the progress made since implementation of the national CMHC program. Unfortunately, promising models such as NIMH's community support system program of a case manager helping to link multiple agency services have not yet received sufficient testing in the present era of federal budgetary cutbacks.

PROVIDE SERVICES AS EFFICIENTLY AS POSSIBLE

The most important issues under this goal are the cost of mental health services in CMHCs and efficiency problems.

Cost of Services

In 1974, the CMHC program spent about $600 million, most of which was nonfederal funds (National Institute of Mental Health, 1977a). As a category of direct mental health expenditure, it ranked far below state and county mental hospitals (Levine and Wilner, 1976; National Institute of Mental Health, 1977a). In terms of administrative overhead, the CMHC program compared favorably with other mental health facilities in administrative or maintenance (A/M) staff; only 26 percent were A/M staff, in comparison to an average of 32 percent for all other facilities.[5] Calculations from NIMH data on episodes of care per center and expenditures per center showed that the cost of the average episode of treatment rose 2 percent per year between 1971 and 1975, unadjusted for inflation (National Institute of Mental Health, 1977a). In constant dollars (corrected for inflation), the cost decreased from $328 to $270, about a 5 percent annual decline. This was accomplished through more rapid growth in outpatient episodes (up 78 percent) and partial care episodes (up 101 percent) than in more costly inpatient episodes (up only 21 percent). Still greater efficiency would likely be possible in the future if partial care were to continue rapid expansion and further replace inpatient stays.

A more recent NIMH-funded cost-finding study (Morrison, 1979) examined unit and episode costs in psychiatric hospitals, CMHCs, and free-standing clinics. CMHCs were the cheapest alternative in terms of episode costs; across all treatment modalities the average CMHC episode cost $635 compared to $653 in a freestanding clinic and $4,922 in a psychiatric hospital. (The CMHC figure is not necessarily comparable to the 1971–1975 figures cited above, since no attempt was made to reconcile cost-finding methodologies in the two studies.) These figures reflect the fact that CMHCs and free-standing clinics provide primarily outpatient services and hospitals provide primarily inpatient care.

In terms of median costs of each *type* of service, CMHCs did not appear to be quite so economical. Of the three organizational types, CMHCs were the cheapest providers of only two services: psychiatric evaluations and medication reviews. CMHCs were more expensive than hospitals for all three of the services studied which are provided by hospitals: inpatient, partial hospitalization, and emergency care. CMHCs were more expensive than freestanding clinics for partial hospitalization, emergency care, outpatient intake interviews, psychological evaluation, individual therapy, family therapy, and group therapy. The author of this study indicated that cost differences are almost wholly accounted for by differences in staffing patterns and staff-to-client ratios. Salaries were higher for CMHC clinical staff, who had more training and education than staff in other facilities; CMHCs had less time to provide "billable" services, partly due to the need to meet federal requirements for indirect services. In addition, the author noted that the small sample (five hospitals, six CMHCs, two freestanding clinics) makes generalization questionable.

Rubin (1982) compared inpatient costs for CMHCs with other provider settings using national samples of settings and costs from 1979 to 1982. An inpatient day in a CMHC cost $177 compared to $215 in a general hospital psychiatric ward, $110 in a veterans' hospital psychiatric ward, $56 in a public mental hospital, $96 in a private nonprofit hospital, and $74 in a private for-profit hospital. Rubin cautioned that these cost figures are derived from different sources and time frames and may not be comparable.

The Nader group's report on CMHCs (Chu and Trotter, 1974) criticized CMHCs for devoting nearly half of working hours to administration, staff meetings, consultation, teaching, and other non–patient care activities. It is widely reported informally that clinical contacts take up a minority of all CMHC staff hours; for example, the state mental health administrator of Georgia stated at a conference that his state's CMHCs averaged about one-third time in clinical care including record keeping. An analysis of direct and indirect service hours in a large western CMHC (Ciarlo, 1979) showed that only 35 percent of all staff time went into client or consultee contact.

Efficiency Problems

A survey of nine centers identified a variety of potential problems relating to efficiency (Price and Associates, 1978). Many respondents felt that their centers were losing revenues from insurance and other sources because of an inadequate system for handling and processing client accounts. An explanation offered was that center professionals did not consider fee management as part of their job. Nearly all board of directors members indicated that budget and expenditure accounts were not maintained in a manner which enabled the board to monitor how efficiently the center accomplished annual plans or objectives. Many respondents indicated that a lack of detailed cost data hampered effective allocation of resources. One-third of respondents indicated that record keeping had increased to the point that it was too burdensome. One-third indicated that lack of timely information on client status hampered effective treatment planning. An explanation offered was lack of resources to develop a management information system. One-fourth of respondents indicated that their centers were unable to use the process of program evaluation to improve program quality or redirect resources; justifications offered included staff resentment of the data collection burden and inadequate resources.

Comparing CMHCs to other service delivery approaches on a service-by-service basis leads to the conclusion that CMHCs may not be the most efficient approach. Yet it is questionable whether efficiency comparisons which do not take into account quality of service delivered should be a basis for assessing services. The goals of CMHCs are broader in scope than piecemeal service delivery and include the total impact of the range of services on the well-being of communities. An appropriate comparison of CMHCs with other service delivery approaches should examine the impact of integrated CMHC systems upon client functioning, burden and benefits to the family, services utilization, hospitalization and recidivism, and other indicators of community mental health. We could find no such comparisons of traditional isolated services with CMHCs. Such studies should have been a priority for community mental health research.

PROVIDE SERVICES WHICH REDUCE SUFFERING AND INCREASE PERSONAL FUNCTIONING

Under this heading we will discuss evidence for the effectiveness of community mental health services and development of methods for improving services.

Evidence of Effectiveness

That mental health services are probably effective to some degree is evident from scientific literature and clinical experience. For example, in a summary of more than 375 well-controlled studies of psychotherapy effectiveness (Smith and Glass, 1977; Glass, 1976), those receiving such therapies improved two-thirds of a standard deviation over untreated controls on outcome measures taken; hence, the average treated client moves from the fiftieth to about the seventy-fifth percentile of the score distribution. A reanalysis of these data (Landman and Dawes, 1982) reaffirmed those conclusions. Also quite important are studies that show increased effectiveness of partial care over inpatient treatment (Edwards and Yarvis, 1979; Hersen, 1979; Washburn et al., 1976; Weiss and Dubin, 1982), particularly since partial care is also less expensive than inpatient care. A review of literature on hospitalization itself shows that brief hospitalization appears to be at least as effective as longer hospitalization (Riessman, Rabkin, and Struening, 1977) in preventing readmissions and improving overall clinical and social functioning. CMHCs delivered outpatient services, partial care, and brief hospitalization on a large scale, and it is highly probable that they are effective to at least some degree in reducing client distress and improving clients' overall social and community functioning.

Several outcome studies on CMHC populations have been published. For example, from 1972 to 1980, Denver's city-operated CMHC routinely evaluated a sample of adult clients three to six months after their entry into treatment (most had terminated by that time). Follow-up results for all of 1975 showed that all types of clients had improved on the ''Psychological Distress'' dimension, that alcoholics and drug abusers improved on substance abuse scales, and that one of the most improved groups was the most severely disabled in terms of disorganization in thinking and behavior (Ciarlo and Reihman, 1977).

A more recent report from the Utah statewide system (Owen, 1984) used meta-analytic methods to quantify pretest-posttest results from 1,876 clients in nine centers across the state. (Meta-analysis is a family of techniques which converts differing outcome measures to a common metric, a standard score or Z-score, and permits the measures to be integrated into a single test of significance.) Effect sizes in Owen's study ranged from .57 to .91 over three years (1979–1981); this suggests that the outcome level of functioning of the treated clients was .57 to .91 of a standard deviation higher than that of the control subjects. Owen also found effect sizes ranging from .32 to 2.0 across nine centers. Significantly less favorable outcomes were associated with several factors: less than twelve years of education, never married status, less than thirty days in outpatient treatment, and fewer than five treatment contacts. Significant differences were not related to income, white vs. nonwhite status, age or court-referred status. About one-quarter of the outcome variance was attributable to initial level of distress or functioning. Despite these encouraging findings, the author noted the possibility that results were biased by regression effects, that is, the tendency for low scores on any measure to move toward the mean. This is suggested by the significant differences in the pretest means for the three groups sorted as ''improved,'' ''maintained,'' and ''declined.''

A Washington state mental health outcome study (Cox et al., 1978, 1982) examined outcomes on a broad range of variables for 500 clients. Results suggested effectiveness of community mental health services for various types of clients across a variety of outcome measures. An Oregon study shows some evidence for positive impact on the quality of life of clients (Brodsky et al., 1980; Bigelow et al., 1982). A substantial number of other CMHC effectiveness studies are also available in the published literature, particularly in summaries of CMHC evaluation activities (Fiester and Neigher, 1979; Schainblatt, 1972). Most studies show evidence of probable positive impact upon client functioning, and a few show improvement in clients approaching functional levels close to that of the community populations (Ciarlo and Davis, 1977; Ciarlo, 1977).

It is certainly possible to be critical of the scientific rigor of these studies of the effectiveness of community mental health (cf. Hargreaves, 1982). Few controls are available in such research, leaving results of any single study subject to question. The most problematic threat to the validity of outcome research is the likelihood that clients enter treatment at a point of low functioning in their lives and that, even without treatment, a sizable number of them would manifest improved functioning or partial recovery at a post-treatment or follow-up assessment. What is necessary to offset this threat to the validity of outcome studies are good estimates of the changes (if any) expectable in untreated CMHC populations; these, however, are unlikely to be readily (or ethically) obtainable. Alternative study designs such as comparing the outcomes of two equally ethical treatments, or comparing the gains of one CMHC's clients to those of other CMHC, hospital, or clinic clients, are increasingly being used to evaluate clinical outcomes. Currently, however, the weight of evidence for the effectiveness of community mental health care derives partly from evidence for the effectiveness of psychotherapy in non-CMHC settings and partly from the small number of outcome studies on community mental health reviewed above. The available evidence appears to warrant a conclusion of probable effectiveness for CMHC services at least to some degree. Unfortunately, too few studies are available for stronger conclusions.

Methods for Improving Effectiveness

The CMHC Amendments of 1975 (Public Law 94–63) required centers to spend 2 percent of their budgets on evaluation. There is disagreement about how useful this requirement was in improving services or advancing knowledge in community mental health (Neigher et al., 1982). Cook and Shadish (1982) conducted a meta-analysis of the 2 percent studies and concluded that little useful information had resulted from the policy and that the level of evaluation activity in local CMHCs was probably about the same before the 1975 requirement was added.

Some participants in a 1982 debate on this topic (Neigher et al., 1982) at the National Council of Community Mental Health Centers Annual Meeting argued that the return on investment obtained from the 2 percent policy was as great as could reasonably be expected. They noted that the state of the evaluation art was not sufficiently advanced in the 1960s to plan and conduct a national evaluation of the CMHC program. In addition, evaluation research itself has advanced in part because of the CMHC-based work. On the other side at this same forum it was argued that the 2 percent requirement resulted in poor quality evaluation research at the local level and that greater return could have been obtained from a more centrally directed evaluation policy.

At least three obstacles to the successful conduct of program evaluation in local centers can be identified. First, evaluation in CMHCs was (and is) difficult, as noted in the "evaluability assessment" for the CMHC program prepared for the Department of Health and Human Services during the Carter administration (Jewell et al., 1980). This report noted that the goals of community mental health were not well defined, posing a problem for goal-based evaluation efforts. Second, evaluation was resisted by local centers because it was perceived as an imposed requirement with no usefulness at the local level (Flaherty and Olsen, 1978, 1982; Solomon and Bernstein, 1985). Third, despite the requirement that 2 percent of a budget be spent for evaluation activities, centers had relatively few resources to conduct evaluation. Baker (1982) surveyed 537 center directors and evaluators from 323 CMHCs. The majority of centers reported only one full-time-equivalent evaluator or less. These evaluators had little formal education in evaluation and the majority had master's degrees or less training as their highest degree.

Yet, contributions to the field of evaluation have come from CMHC-related evaluation efforts. Fiester and Fort (1978) described an evaluation system broad in scope for use in CMHCs which relies on goal attainment scaling and client satisfaction data. The Western Interstate Commission for Higher Education (1980) developed an accountability package for CMHCs that is based partly on client outcomes and includes cost information. Ellis, Wilson, and Foster (1984) described the development of a statewide treatment outcome assessment system and the psychometric refinement of the instrument for Colorado that was based on CMHC and hospital research efforts. Ciarlo (1982) argued for the importance of such outcome evaluation efforts as a method for accountability along with quality assurance and performance-based evaluation. He noted that methods for outcome evaluation are improving and that policymakers clearly indicate that they want outcome information for decision making (cf. Hargreaves, 1982).

Closely related to outcome evaluation in CMHCs was a substantial effort aimed at determining clients' satisfaction with CMHC services. Windle and Paschall (1981) have argued for client participation in evaluation of services and reported that a 1972 survey found 35 percent of centers collected client satisfaction data in at least a part of the center. Contributions to the client satisfaction literature include the work of Essex and Fox (1981), who identified four factor-analysis–derived dimensions of client satisfaction: satisfaction with services, acceptability of the clinician, impact of services, and dignity of treatment. Several studies document generally favorable assessments of services received by CMHC clients (Balch et al., 1977; Kirchner, 1981).

A difficulty with client satisfaction methods is the uncertain relationship between clients' perceptions and other dimensions, especially clinical treatment outcomes (Edwards et al., 1978; Fiester and Fort, 1978; Flynn et al., 1981; Frank, Salzman, and Fergus, 1977; Simons et al., 1978). In addition, Baker (1982) found that evaluators had more commitment to the idea of consumer involvement in evaluation than center directors.

Quality assurance is another method for ensuring quality and improving services. Landsberg (1985) reported two surveys of CMHC quality assurance practices in 1977–1978 and 1983. Ninety-three percent of centers reported having had a quality assurance program in place in 1983, up from 70 percent in 1977–78; in addition, 34 percent had special quality assurance staff. Quality assurance was most common in inpatient, outpatient, emergency, and partial care units and least common in consultation and education. Quality assurance was rated of "great" or "some or moderate" importance by about 50–60 percent of respondents. On the other hand, problems in the application of quality assurance methods were reported in the Horizon Institute's (1980) test of an outcome-based model in a Colorado CMHC. Luft, Sampson, and Newman (1976) concluded that peer review was a useful method despite the finding that some staff felt treatment was negatively affected. In 1982, Drude and Nelson (1982) examined the current state of the art in applying quality assurance to CMHCs. They too concluded that many problems existed in the application of quality assurance methods to outpatient services due to the fact that quality assurance was historically developed for inpatient services and because no generally accepted standards of care existed for outpatient services.

Each of the major evaluation methods for improving services in CMHCs—outcome evaluation, quality assurance, and consumer feedback—is subject to criticism. Further development of these techniques in service settings is badly needed. However, more methodological resources for community mental health evaluation are now available than in the mid–1960s, due in part to contributions originating in CMHC-related evaluation efforts.

While perhaps unpleasant to contemplate, it must in fairness be recognized that other service systems, such as state psychiatric hospitals, private psychiatric hospitals, general medical practitioners, outpatient clinics, and private practitioners, are no better—and probably less well—informed about their services, costs, and treatment outcomes than CMHCs. Rigorous evaluation of treatment outcomes will be needed in all such settings if we are ever to understand the true value of the public mental health programs in which we, as a society, have been investing for over a century.

OVERVIEW OF THE NINE CMHC GOALS

Reviewing briefly the documented achievements for each of the CMHC program goals, it appears that the program had its greatest success with the first—*increasing the range and quantity of public mental health services* in catchment areas with CMHCs. There was also progress made by the program in *making services equally available and accessible* to all, for at least some of the poor and minorities, for whom CMHCs targeted a range of services. We also note partial success in *providing services in relation to existing community needs*, especially in urban areas, although we have indicated some substantial problems with respect to coverage of rural high-need areas and certain clinical target groups.

Unfortunately, these substantial achievements in public mental health care do not seem to be permanent. They are threatened by the elimination of federal funding, oversight, and leadership, and by increasing dependence upon third-party reimbursement mechanisms that do not share the community mental health service philosophy. There is also the risk that more custodially oriented state hospitals will compete successfully with community mental health centers for the shrinking state-administered mental health dollar. In addition, community programs remain threatened by the well-known tendency of states and local governments to reduce or eliminate funding of mental health services as the budgets for "more important" education, transportation, and safety functions overrun static or shrinking resources.

There may have been some degree of success (at least in some of the states studied) in *decreasing state hospital admissions and residents*, although it is unlikely the reductions in state hospital residents that have occurred are wholly attributable to CMHCs. The CMHC program had partial success in *coordinating mental health-related services in the catchment area*. Although most of this successful coordination may have occurred primarily with respect to a CMHC's own multiple services, we located instances of exemplary CMHC-based programs which coordinated with the police, agencies serving the elderly, and schools. With respect to coordination of chronic patient care and aftercare with state hospitals, the picture was generally bleak over most of the years of the CMHC program; it appears that services in this area began to improve in the latter program years. Nevertheless, the CMHCs' lack of accomplishment in coordinating services to chronic patients helped to generate a federal and state thrust toward "community support systems" which were most often based outside CMHCs.

It is difficult to evaluate CMHC performance in *providing services as efficiently as possible*. When compared to alternative delivery systems on a service-by-service basis, CMHCs cost more; but it can be argued that such comparisons are not appropriate because the CMHC is, by definition, a complex organization of multiple services that should be assessed by multiple measures. Yet it must be acknowledged that this very complexity and need for internal coordination and administration (not to mention consultation and education, evaluation, and other mandated functions) would inevitably drive costs up and lead to some inefficiencies. Similarly, we can draw only a mildly positive conclusion about whether CMHCs managed to *reduce suffering and increase personal functioning*, but for a different reason. While the available data are generally positive, there are too few well-designed studies to draw a solid conclusion.

With respect to the objective of *maximizing citizen participation in community programs*, we might give a positive grade for efforts made (especially by some NIMH regional offices) in a difficult area, but a negative assessment seems warranted with respect to degree of successful implementation of citizen participation in operating centers. Finally, with respect to *preventing the development of mental disorders*, we have extremely little evidence for any widespread success throughout the program, apart from success in helping non–mental health caregivers (physicians, schoolteachers) become more sensitive to psychological problems, and possibly facilitating earlier referral for direct treatment. This shortcoming could have been anticipated by a careful assessment of the available research literature on effective prevention methods in the early years of the CMHC program.

SOME SPECULATIONS AND DIRECTIONS FOR THE FUTURE

What can be learned from the pattern of successes and failures in the CMHC program that we have outlined? We present here some inferences that might be drawn from this review, with the understanding that others might drawn some very different conclusions. We also offer these as potential guidelines for future community-oriented mental health services delivery programs, both in terms of what should be done and what should probably be avoided. We regard these as more speculative than evaluative, in contrast to the conclusions of the preceding section which were derived from the data reviewed in the body of the chapter.

1. The enormous need for mental health services has been clearly demonstrated. Vast expansion of services under the CMHC program very probably tapped heretofore unmet need. The reality of these newly discovered persons is undeniable. Some may believe that not all of these users represent "legitimate" cases of need, in that their problems were not always classifiable as mental disorders using our current diagnostic systems. But we have witnessed a type of demand that is self-validating, in the sense of service utilization as a consequence of directly felt need for help. In the political phraseology of an earlier era, we could say that "people have voted for mental health services with their feet." There can now be no retreat from this reality by any governmental level, except for policymakers to maintain that they either cannot or will not tax their constituents for public mental health services which will be used if available.

2. Economically disadvantaged persons will use services that are available. "Mental health" and "therapy" are no longer just middle-class terms. The bulk of the CMHC clientele was either poor, or minorities, or both (in sharp contrast to the clientele served in the private sector). Persons from these groups who are in need stand ready to use mental health services of all modalities—emergency, outpatient, partial care, and inpatient care—if their communities will make them available and accessible.

At the same time, it is important that we do not ignore questions about the effectiveness and continuity of services for specific client groups such as children, the elderly, and minority clients. We have evidence from both within and outside the CMHC program that the rate of minority additions does not reflect accurately the degree to which services are actually meeting needs of minority groups because of differential dropout rates. There is a need for careful monitoring of the impact of services on minority clients and perhaps with other high-priority client groups.

   3. *Third-party reimbursement procedures are working against community mental health services.* It has been found that, as federal funds declined, CMHCs became significantly less community-oriented in their service patterns. In 1983, when completing an earlier review of the CMHC literature, we wrote that the then-current reimbursement system encouraged delivery of services diametrically opposite to those suggested by the community mental health philosophy of in-community care (outpatient or partial care), providing incentives instead for inpatient (institutional) care because of the presumably greater justification of the need for hospitalization. This problem has not been solved. Further, since the "seed-money" concept did not succeed in creating permanent local and state government funding for community mental health services, CMHCs will continue to be driven by these fiscal realities in a direction contrary to that specified by their original ideology.

   4. *CMHCs' role in working with chronic clients needs to be rethought.* The evidence suggests that CMHCs did not focus their efforts primarily on treatment of severely and chronically disabled clients. After about 1977 (the date of the Comptroller General's report on the needs of chronic patients), the emphasis upon this population increased in mental health systems at state and federal levels, including CMHCs. In 1983, we noted that it was at least arguable that because CMHCs have a strong focus on emergency care, crisis intervention, partial care, and brief inpatient hospitalization, they may be most appropriate for acute, short-term cases (and secondary prevention functions), rather than for chronic patients. NIMH's community support system (CSS) model recognized this fact implicitly with the provision that CMHCs were not always to have been "core service agencies" of the CSS. To be effective with chronic clients, CMHC staffing would need to reflect more closely the CSS model with its emphasis on coordinating basic health and welfare services as well as mental health services for clients, and meeting the residential and social needs of patients. Alternatively, well-organized state hospitals, supplemented by in-community aftercare, sheltered workshops, and various types of residential facilities, might meet the needs of the chronic clients as well as or better than CMHCs (cf. Winslow, 1982).

   5. *A new community-based thrust for chronic patient care may be needed.* Along the lines of the previous argument, sufficient experience with caring for chronic clients, in and outside of hospitals, nursing homes, and boarding homes, may now warrant a new thrust toward supportive in-community care for such disabled people. The NIMH community support system model, with its focus on case management and coordination of multiple agencies to obtain the varied

types of mental health and social welfare services needed for each client, is a start in this direction; however, this model lacks both (1) fiscal and organizational interconnection with this country's largest system for care of chronic clients, the state hospitals, and (2) greater state and local funding sources for mental health services other than hospitalization. It is not likely that third-party reimbursement systems, especially private insurers, will soon provide the dollars for in-community treatment and maintenance services. Only new governmental funds, perhaps closely tied to state hospital funding, but directed *away* from increased hospital beds and toward alternative community facilities, are currently a feasible source for this type of work.

6. *The role of prevention in CMHCs needs to be rethought.* The failure of most CMHCs to mount significant and credible prevention programs (leaving aside the issue of ultimate effectiveness) may be attributed to (1) a lack of agreement among mental health professionals about conceptualizing and implementing prevention activities, (2) a lack of staff expertise in this nonclinical area, and (3) the non–revenue generating nature of preventive services which makes them the underdog in competition with direct clinical care for agency resources. Prevention efforts continue to be hampered by these problems.

During the era of direct federal funding for CMHCs, prevention was in a developmental phase, and a rigorous knowledge base did not yet exist. Requiring CMHCs to mount prevention efforts meant demanding that staff translate this concept, about which professionals disagreed, into effective interventions. Such a task is more suitable for a research university than for a service organization.

The knowledge base for prevention has grown to a point that in 1976 the American Psychological Association (APA) could identify fourteen exemplary prevention programs with rigorous evaluation evidence of effectiveness. In addition, NIMH supports prevention research centers. This commitment to funding carefully conceived research and demonstration projects is well advised since, in the long run, prevention might be a very cost-effective investment for the shrinking mental health dollar.

CMHCs and other mental health service agencies should not be expected to invent prevention methods; rather, they should be encouraged to adopt prevention models from a small number of well-documented approaches. State and federal funders may provide technical assistance in choosing and implementing such models. This is, in effect, what the National Council of Community Mental Health Centers has been undertaking with a series of "Technology Transfer Conferences: Prevention Programs that Work." Held at various locations around the country and directed at mental health providers, these conferences provide training in the development of prevention programs based upon the fourteen programs selected by the American Psychological Association as exemplary. Experience with a few carefully chosen approaches may increase the acceptance of prevention among mental health professionals.

7. *Needs assessment technology must be improved for better services planning.* Early CMHC funding appeared to be directed primarily at high-need areas,

but funding in later years was heavily influenced by the differential ability of areas to put together the professional resources and expertise to generate a viable CMHC grant application. The NIMH could not put funds into areas that did not apply, and applications had to include plans for all basic services. Public Law 94–63, while it called for a "needs assessment" in conjunction with an application, did nothing to solve the problem that some of the most needy catchment areas were unable to assemble a proper application for federal support. The Mental Health Systems Act of 1980 did try to help by allowing community mental health services to be funded with just one or two of the basic services. But unless and until we are able to assess the numbers of persons in need in each catchment area, together with the amount of treatment resources available (including private and third-party reimbursable care), governmental funding will continue to misdirect at least part, if not most, of whatever services might be bought with the available dollars. Only a major thrust toward improvement of needs-assessment technologies, including reducing their large cost when based on direct survey, will alleviate the misdirection of public services (for further discussion of needs assessment issues, see chapter 18 of this volume).

8. *Lack of knowledge of outcomes of CMHC services hampers optimal investment of scarce resources.* We know of no studies that compare the clinical outcomes of highly comparable clients served by CMHCs, state hospitals, general hospitals, outpatient clinics, or private practitioners. We thus are forced to invest our public and private dollars blindly, basing the critical funding decisions on perceived need, ideology, and hope rather than demonstrated performance. And without such comparative client outcome data, we cannot make accurate cost-effectiveness comparisons that would further improve our decisions on how to invest our mental health service dollar. This is one of the top priorities for the federal government, as indicated in the report of a group of consultants reviewing NIMH's services research programs (Cole et al., 1981). States would also be well advised to try to develop such data for use in their current expanded role as funder of public mental health services.

9. *Mental health services need more visible public support.* The visibility of consumer and family groups, such as the National Alliance for the Mentally Ill, increased somewhat in 1975–1985; this is a welcome development. Unless the general public—including consumers and ex-consumers of community mental health services—can generate visible and active support for funding of services in their contacts with political representatives, community mental health services will probably continue to shrink. This shrinkage may be even more significant with the weakening of safeguards written into the original block grant legislation against diversion of the federal funds into areas other than mental health services. While Congress may continue to support development of a competent national system of community mental health services in opposition to unsympathetic administrations, citizen pressure on the local and state levels is likely to be the only key to long-term improvement in the quality and quantity of services.

ACKNOWLEDGMENTS

This chapter is a revision of an article by the authors which appeared in the *Community Mental Health Journal*, Summer 1983 (Dowell and Ciarlo, 1983). That article, in turn, was based on a report prepared by the second author for the President's Commission on Mental Health in 1977 which appeared in condensed form in the *Report of the Task Panel on Community Mental Health Centers Assessment* as a section titled "Review of Evaluative Data" (President's Commission, 1978, Vol. II, Appendix).

NOTES

1. Calculated from chart 6 of National Institute of Mental Health, 1977a.
2. Personal communication, Stanley Sue, 1981.
3. C. A. Taube, J. W. Thompson, M. J. Rosenstein, B. M. Rosen, and H. H. Goldman, *The "Chronic" State Mental Hospital Patient*, unpublished manuscript, undated.
4. J. A. Ciarlo, *Evaluation Report Series, 1972–74: Continuity of Care*, unpublished technical reports, Northwest Denver Mental Health Center, Denver, Colo., 1972–1974.
5. Memorandum dated August 29, 1977, to the President's Commission on Mental Health from the National Institute of Mental Health, Division of Mental Health Service Programs.

REFERENCES

Abt Associates. 1972. *A Study of the Accessibility of Community Mental Health Centers.* Springfield, Va.: National Technical Information Service. Accession No. PB–213–117.

Abt Associates. 1976. *An Evaluation of Community Mental Health Centers in Their 10th and 11th Years of Operation.* Unpublished report. National Institute of Mental Health, Contract No. 100–76–0205.

Alcohol, Drug Abuse, and Mental Health Administration. 1982. Young Adult Chronic Patients on the Increase. *ADAMHA News* 8: 1–2.

Armstrong, H. E., Ishiki, D., Heiman, J., Mundt, J., and Womack, W. 1984. Service Utilization by Black and White Clientele in an Urban Community Mental Health Center: Revised Assessment of an Old Problem. *Community Mental Health Journal* 20: 269–281.

Babigian, H. M. 1977. The Impact of Community Mental Health Centers on the Utilization of Services. *Archives of General Psychiatry* 34: 385–394.

Bachrach, L. L. 1974. Patients at Federally Funded Rural Community Mental Health Centers in 1971. *Statistical Note*, No. 102. Washington, D.C.: National Institute of Mental Health.

Baekeland, F., and Lundwall, L. 1975. Dropping Out of Treatment: A Critical Review. *Psychological Bulletin* 82: 738–783.

Baker, F. 1982. Program Evaluators in Community Mental Health Centers: Results of a National Survey. *Journal of Community Psychology* 10: 151–156.

Baker, F. 1983. Manager and Evaluator Views of Program Evaluation. *Journal of Community Psychology* 11: 213–223.

Balch, F., Ireland, J., McWilliams, S., and Lewis, S. B. 1977. Client Evaluation of

Community Mental Health Services: Relation to Demographic and Treatment Variables. *American Journal of Community Psychology* 5: 243–247.

Bass, R. D. 1972. Accessibility of Community Mental Health Centers. *Statistical Note*, No. 63. Washington, D.C.: National Institute of Mental Health.

Bass, R. D. 1981. Personal Communication Based on the National Institute of Mental Health. 1978. *CMHC Staffing: Who Minds the Store?* Department of Health, Education, and Welfare Publication No. ADM 78–686. Washington, D.C.: U.S. Government Printing Office.

Bass, R. D. 1982. Trends among Core Professionals in Organized Mental Health Settings: Where Have All the Psychiatrists Gone? *Statistical Note*, No. 160. Washington, D.C.: National Institute of Mental Health.

Bass, R. D., and Ozarin, L. D. 1977. The Community Mental Health Center Program: What Is Past Is Prologue. Presentation at the American Psychiatric Association Meeting, Toronto, May.

Bass, R. D., and Windle, C. 1972. Continuity of Care: An Approach to Measurement. *American Journal of Psychiatry* 129: 196–201.

Bass, R. D., Windle, C., Bethel, H. E., Henderson, P., and Rosen, B. M. 1985. The Contrasting Careers of Two Structural Types of CMHCs. *Community Mental Health Journal* 21: 74–94.

Beigel, A. 1984. The Remedicalization of Community Mental Health. *Hospital and Community Psychiatry* 35: 1114–1117.

Bergner, L. P., Zinober, J. W., and Dinkel, J. 1984. The Impact of Citizen Evaluation Review on Community Mental Health Programs. *Evaluation and Program Planning* 7: 57–64.

Bigelow, D. A., Brodsky, G., Stewart, L., and Olson, M. 1982. The Concept and Measurement of Quality of Life as a Dependent Variable in Evaluation of Mental Health Services. In *Innovative Approaches to Mental Health Evaluation*, eds. G. J. Stahler and W. R. Tash. New York: Academic Press.

Bloom, B. 1968. The Evaluation of Primary Prevention Programs. In *Comprehensive Mental Health and the Challenge of Evaluation*, eds. L. M. Roberts, N. J. Greenfield, and M. H. Miller. Madison: University of Wisconsin Press.

Bloom, B. 1977. *Community Mental Health: A General Introduction*. Monterey, Calif.: Brooks/Cole.

Bloom, B. 1979. Prevention of Mental Disorders: Recent Advances in Theory and Practice. *Community Mental Health Journal* 15: 179–191.

Bloom, B., and Parad, H. J. 1978. The Psychologist in the CMHC: An Analysis of Activities and Training Needs. *American Journal of Community Psychology* 6: 371–379.

Borus, J. F. 1978. Issues Critical to the Survival of Community Mental Health. *American Journal of Psychiatry* 135: 1029–1035.

Brodsky, G., Bigelow, D. A., Stewart, L. K., Olson, M. M., Howard, B. M., Smith, J. 1980. *The Oregon Program Impact Monitoring System: Final Report*. Unpublished report. National Institute of Mental Health, Contract No. 278–77–0029 (OP).

Broskowski, A. 1980. *Evaluation of the Primary Health Care—Community Mental Health Care Linkage Initiative*. Unpublished report. National Institute of Mental Health, Contract No. 278–79–0030 (OP).

Buck, J. A. 1984. Effects of the Community Mental Health Centers Program on the

Growth of Mental Health Facilities in Nonmetropolitan Areas. *American Journal of Community Psychology* 12: 609–622.

Carter, B. D., and Cazares, P. R. 1976. Consultation in Community Mental Health. *Community Mental Health Review* 1: 7–11.

Center for Health Studies, Institute for Social and Policy Studies, Yale University. 1979. *Trends in Mental Health.* Unpublished report. National Institute of Mental Health, Contract No. 278–77–0072 (OP).

Chu, F. B., and Trotter, S. 1974. *The Madness Establishment.* New York: Grossman.

Ciarlo, J. A. 1977. Evaluation in a Community Mental Health Center: I—Monitoring and Analysis of Mental Health Program Outcome Data. *Evaluation* 4: 109–114.

Ciarlo. J. A. 1979. Annual Evaluation Report for 1975 of the Northwest Denver Mental Health Center. In *Reporting Program Evaluations: Two Sample Community Mental Health Center Annual Evaluation Reports*, ed. C. W. Windle. U.S. Department of Health, Education, and Welfare Publication No. ADM 79–607. Washington, D.C.: U.S. Government Printing Office.

Ciarlo, J. A. 1982. Accountability Revisited: The Arrival of Client Outcome Evaluation. *Evaluation and Program Planning* 5: 31–36.

Ciarlo, J. A., and Davis, C. 1977. Outcomes for Adult Clients. In *Evaluating Community Mental Health: Principles and Practice*, eds. E. Davis, M. S. Guttentag, and J. Offutt. Washington, D.C.: U.S. Government Printing Office.

Ciarlo, J. A., and Reihman, J. 1977. The Denver Community Mental Health Questionnaire: Development of a Multi-Dimensional Program Evaluation Instrument. In *Program Evaluation for Mental Health* ed. R. Coursey. New York: Grune and Stratton,

Cibulka, J. G. 1981. Citizen Participation in the Governance of Community Mental Health Centers. *Community Mental Health Centers Journal* 17: 19–36.

Cole, J. O., Acosta, F. X., Ciarlo, J. A., Fink, R., Goodman, J. A., Lerman, P., May, P.R.A., Mercer, J., and Mowbray, C. 1981. *Final Report National Institute of Mental Health Services Research Cluster Planning Group.* Unpublished report. Rockville, Md.: National Institute of Mental Health.

Community Mental Health Journal. 1981. Special issue on citizen participation. 17: Number 1.

Community Mental Health Project. 1980. *Evaluation of Interactions between the Community Mental Health System and the Judiciary.* Unpublished report. National Institute of Mental Health, Contract No. 278–78–0066.

Comptroller General of the U.S. 1971. *The Community Mental Health Centers Program: Improvements Needed in Management.* Report No. 13–164031 (2). Washington, D.C.: U.S. Government Printing Office.

Comptroller General of the U.S. 1974. *Need for More Effective Management of the Community Mental Health Centers Program.* Report No. B–164031 (5). Washington, D.C.: Superintendent of Documents.

Comptroller General of the U.S. 1977. *Returning the Chronic Mentally Disabled to the Community: Congress Needs to Do More.* Publication No. HRD 76–152. Washington, D.C.: U.S. Government Printing Office.

Cook, T. D., and Shadish, W. R. 1982. Metaevaluation: An Assessment of the Congressionally Mandated Evaluation System for Community Mental Health Centers. In *Innovative Approaches to Mental Health Evaluation*, eds. G. J. Stahler and W. R. Tash. New York: Academic Press.

Cowan, E. L., Davidson, E. R., and Groten, E. L. 1980. Program Dissemination and the Modification of Delivery Practices in School Mental Health. *Professional Psychology* 11: 36–47.

Cox, G. B., Brown, T. R., Peterson, P. D., and Rowe, M. M. 1978. *Final Report, Two-State Collaborative Mental Health Outcome Study: State of Washington.* Unpublished report. National Institute of Mental Health, Contract No. 278–77–0030.

Cox, G. B., Brown, T. B., Peterson, P. D., and Rowe, M. M. 1982. A Report on a State-Wide Community Mental Health Center Outcome Study. *Community Mental Health Journal* 18: 135–150.

Doidge, J. R., and Rogers, C. W. 1976. Is National Institute of Mental Health's Dream Coming True?: Wyoming Centers Reduce State Hospital Admissions. *Community Mental Health Journal* 12: 399–404.

Dowell, D., and Ciarlo, J. 1983. Overview of the Community Mental Health Centers Program from an Evaluation Perspective. *Community Mental Health Journal* 19: 95–125.

Dowell, D., and Jones, T. 1980. A Study of Coordination of Services: Referrals. *Journal of Community Psychology* 8: 61–69.

Drude, K., and Nelson, R. 1982. Quality Assurance: A Challenge for Community Mental Health Centers. *Professional Psychology* 13: 85–90.

Edwards, D. W., and Yarvis, R. M. 1979. A Prospective Study of Day Treatment Outcome in Three Community Mental Health Centers. In *Evaluation in Practice: A Sourcebook of Program Evaluation Studies from Mental Health Care Systems in the United States*, eds. G. Landsberg, W. D. Neigher, R. J. Hammer, C. Windle, C. Woy, and J. R. Woy. DHEW Pub. No. ADM 78–763. Washington, D.C.: U.S. Government Printing Office.

Edwards, D. W., Yarvis, R. M., Meuller, D. P., and Langsley, D. G. 1978. Does Patient Satisfaction Correlate with Success? *Hospital and Community Psychiatry* 29: 188–190.

Eichler, A. 1978. *The Community Mental Health Centers Amendments of 1975 (Title III of P. L. 94–63): How Are the New CMHCs Doing?* Unpublished report. Program Analysis and Evaluation Branch, National Institute of Mental Health.

Ellis, R. H., Wilson, N. Z., and Foster, F. M. 1984. Statewide Treatment Outcome Assessment in Colorado: The Colorado Client Assessment Record (CCAR). *Community Mental Health Journal* 20: 72–89.

Essex, D., and Fox, J. 1981. The Development, Factor Analysis and Revision of a Client Satisfaction Form. *Community Mental Health Journal* 17: 226–235.

Faden, V. B., and Goldman, H. H. 1979. Appropriateness of Placement of Patients in State and County Mental Hospitals. *Statistical Note*, No. 152. Washington, D.C.: National Institute of Mental Health.

Feldman, S., and Windle, C. 1973. The National Institute of Mental Health Approach to Evaluating the Community Mental Health Centers Program. *Health Services Reports* 88: 174–180.

Fiester, A. R., and Fort, D. J. 1978. A Method of Evaluating the Impact of Services at a Comprehensive CMHC. *American Journal of Community Psychology* 6: 291–302.

Fiester, A. R., and Neigher, W. D. 1979. Client Outcome: Overview. In *Evaluation in Practice: A Sourcebook of Program Evaluation Studies from Mental Health Care*

Systems in the United States, eds. G. Landsberg, W. D. Neigher, R. J. Hammer, C. Windle, C. Woy, and J. R. Woy. DHEW Pub. No. ADM 78–763. Washington, D.C.: U.S. Government Printing Office.

Flaherty, E. W., and Olsen, K. 1978. *An Assessment of the Utility of Federally Required Program Evaluation in Community Mental Health Centers, Vol. 1*. Unpublished final report. National Institute of Mental Health, Contract No. 278–77–0067 (MH). Philadelphia: Philadelphia Health Management.

Flaherty, E. W., and Olsen, K. 1982. Impact of Federally Mandated Program Evaluation. *Community Mental Health Journal* 18: 56–71.

Flomenhaft, K., Kaplan, D. M., and Langsley, D. G. 1969. Avoiding Psychiatric Hospitalization. *Social Work* 14: 1438–1445.

Flynn, T. C., Balch, P., Lewis, S. B., and Katz, B. 1981. Predicting Client Improvement from and Satisfaction with Community Mental Health Center Services. *American Journal of Community Psychology* 9: 339–346.

Franco, J. N., and DeBlassie, R. R. 1979. A Model for Training Community Mental Health Researchers and Evaluators. *Evaluation Quarterly* 3: 490–496.

Frank, R., Salzman, K., and Fergus, E. 1977. Correlates of Consumer Satisfaction with Outpatient Therapy Assessed by Postcards. *Community Mental Health Journal* 13: 37–45.

Glass, G. V. 1976. Address at the Annual Meeting of the American Educational Research Association, Boulder, Colorado.

Glasscote, R. M., Sussex, J. N., Cummings, E., and Smith, L. H. 1969. *The Community Mental Health Centers: An Interim Appraisal*. Washington, D.C.: Joint Information Service.

Goldman, H. H., Regier, D. A., Taube, C. A., Redick, R. W., and Bass, R. D. 1980. Community Mental Health Centers and the Treatment of Severe Mental Disorder. *American Journal of Psychiatry* 137: 83–86.

Goldston, S. E., Ojemann, R. H., and Nelson, R. H. 1975. Primary Prevention and Health Promotion. In *Mental Health: The Public Health Challenge*, ed. E. J. Lieberman. Washington, D.C.: American Public Health Association.

Granville Corporation. 1980. *Final Report: Development of Performance Indicators for the CMHC Program*. Unpublished report. National Institute of Mental Health, Contract No. HHS–100–79–0057.

Hargreaves, W. 1982. Outcome Research or Treatment Research: A Reply to Ciarlo. *Evaluation and Program Planning* 5: 357–358.

Hersen, M. 1979. Research Considerations. In *Partial Hospitalization: A Current Perspective*, ed. R. F. Luber. New York: Plenum.

Horizon Institute. 1980. *The Horizon Institute's Test of an Outcome Based Quality Assurance Model at the Mental Health Center of Boulder County, Inc*. Unpublished final report. National Institute of Mental Health, Contract No. 278–78–0064 OP.

Jerrell, J. M., and Larsen, J. K. 1984. Policy Shifts and Organizational Adaptation: A Review of Current Developments. *Community Mental Health Journal* 20: 282–293.

Jewell, M., Beyna, L., Yates, E., and Walker, E. 1980. *Exploratory Evaluation of the Community Mental Health Centers Program*. Unpublished report. Department of Health and Human Services, Office of the Assistant Secretary for Planning and Evaluation, Washington, D.C., March.

Joint Information Service. 1978. *Evaluation of Primary Prevention Activities in CMHCs*.

Unpublished report. National Institute of Mental Health, Contract No. 278–76–0092 (OP).

Kiesler, C. A. 1980. Mental Health Policy as a Field of Inquiry for Psychology. *American Psychologist* 35: 1066–1080.

Kirchner, J. 1981. Patient Feedback on Satisfaction with Direct Services Received at a Community Mental Health Center: A Two Year Study. *Psychotherapy: Research and Practice* 18: 359–364.

Landman, J. T., and Dawes, R. M. 1982. Psychotherapy Outcome: Smith and Glass' Conclusions Stand Up under Scrutiny. *American Psychologist* 5: 504–516.

Landsberg, G. 1985. Quality Assurance in Community Mental Health Centers: Changes over Time. *Community Mental Health Journal* 21: 189–197.

Langsley, D. G. 1980. The Community Mental Health Center: Does It Treat Patients? *Hospital and Community Psychiatry* 31: 815–819.

Larsen, J. K., and Jerrell, J. M. 1983. *Mental Health Services in Transition (Technical Report, 83–84)*. Los Altos, Calif.: Cognos Associates.

Levine, D. S., and Wilner, S. G. 1976. The Cost of Mental Illness. *Statistical Note*, No. 125. Washington, D.C.: National Institute of Mental Health.

Longest, J., Konan, M., and Tweed, D. 1976. *A Study of Deficiencies and Differentials in the Distribution of Mental Health Resources in Facilities*. DHEW Publication No. ADM. 79–517. Washington, D.C.: U.S. Government Printing Office.

Lorion, R. P. 1974. Patient and Therapist Variables in the Treatment of Low Income Patients. *Psychological Bulletin* 81: 344–354.

Lueger, R. J., and Marquette, U. 1981. Mental Health Workers Ratings of the Importance of the Goals of a Cooperative CMHC-State Hospital Screening-Aftercare Program. *Journal of Community Psychology* 9: 355–360.

Luft, L. L., Sampson, L. M., and Newman, D. E. 1976. Effects of Peer Review on Outpatient Psychotherapy: Therapist and Patient Followup Survey. *American Journal of Psychiatry* 133: 891–895.

MacMurray, V. D., Cunningham, D. H., Carter, P. B., Swenson, N., and Bellin, S. S. 1976. *Citizen Evaluation of Mental Health Services: An Action Approach to Accountability*. New York: Human Sciences Press.

May, J. M. 1981. Psychotherapy Outcome Research and Multi-ethnic Mental Health Service Delivery. Paper presented at National Council of CMHCs, Dallas.

Melton, G. 1981. Effects of a State Law Permitting Minors to Consent to Psychotherapy. *Professional Psychology* 12: 647–654.

Moed, G., and Muhich, D. D. 1972. Some Problems and Parameters of Mental Health Consultation. *Community Mental Health Journal* 8: 232–239.

Morrison, L. J. 1979. *Final Report, Unit and Episode Costs of Mental Health Treatment*. Macro-Systems. Unpublished report. National Institute of Mental Health, Contract No. 278–78–0019 (MH).

Munger, R. 1981. Evaluation of Publicity Concerning a Mental Health Center. *Journal of Psychology* 109: 31–33.

Munoz, R. F. 1976. The Primary Prevention of Psychological Problems. *Community Mental Health Review* 1: 1–15.

Musto, D. F. 1975. Whatever Happened to ''Community Mental Health''? *Public Interest* 39: 53–79.

Naierman, N., Haskins, B., and Robinson, G. 1978. *Community Mental Health Centers— A Decade Later*. Cambridge, Mass.: Abt Associates.

National Institute of Mental Health. 1975. *Provisional Data on Federally Funded CMHC's 1973–1974*. Unpublished report. Division of Biometry and Epidemiology.

National Institute of Mental Health. 1977a. *CMHC's: The Federal Investment*. Unpublished manuscript.

National Institute of Mental Health. 1977b. *Selected Statistics for Federally Funded CMHCs by Need Status of Catchment Area, 1975*. Unpublished table. Division of Biometry and Epidemiology.

National Institute of Mental Health. 1977c. *Staff in CMHCs by Race/Ethnicity of Population of Catchment Area, Federally Funded CMHCs, Feb. 1975*. Unpublished table. Division of Biometry and Epidemiology.

National Institute of Mental Health. 1977d. *Percent Distribution of FTE Staff by Race/Ethnicity and Sex within Disciplines, Federally Funded CMHC's, Feb. 1975*. Unpublished table. Division of Biometry and Epidemiology.

National Institute of Mental Health. 1977e. *Provisional Data on Federally Funded CMHCs, 1975–76*. Unpublished report. Division of Biometry and Epidemiology, April.

National Institute of Mental Health. 1977f. *Requests for Proposals for Community Support Contracts*. Community Support Program.

National Institute of Mental Health. 1978. CMHC Program Overview, Status Paper No. 19. In *Briefing Book: Evaluation of CMHC Program*, eds. J. R. Woy and J. W. Stockdill. Unpublished manuscript.

National Institute of Mental Health. 1980a. *National Conference on Graduate CMHCs*. Unpublished report.

National Institute of Mental Health. 1980b. *Provisional Data on Federally Funded CMHCs 1977–78*. Survey and Reports Branch, Division of Biometry and Epidemiology.

National Institute of Mental Health. 1980c. *The Mental Health Systems Act and Its Implementation*. Memorandum from the Director.

National Institute of Mental Health Services Cluster Group. 1981. *Final Report: National Institute of Mental Health Services Research Cluster Planning Group*. Rockville, Md.; National Institute of Mental Health.

National Study Service. 1972. *Relative Impact of Various Factors in the Development of Mental Health Resources*. Unpublished report. National Institute of Mental Health, Contract HSM 42–20–108.

Neigher, W., Ciarlo, J., Hoven, C., Kirkhart, K., Landsberg, G., Light, E., Newman, F., Struening, E., Williams, L., Windle, C., and Woy, R. 1982. Evaluation in the Community Mental Health Centers Program: A Bold New Reproach? *Evaluation and Program Planning* 5: 283–311.

Owen, W. L. 1984. Analysis and Aggregation of CMHC Outcome Data in a Statewide Evaluation System: A Case Report. *Community Mental Health Journal* 20: 27–43.

Ozarin, L. 1975. Community Mental Health: Does It Work? Review of the Evaluation Literature. In *An Assessment of the Community Mental Health Movement*, eds. W. T. Barton and C. J. Sanborn. Lexington, Mass.: D. C. Heath.

Pepper, B., and Ryglewicz, H. 1982. Unified Services: Concept and Practice. *Hospital and Community Psychiatry* 33: 762–765.

Perls, S. R., Winslow, W. W., and Pathak, D. R. 1980. Staffing Patterns in Community Mental Health Centers. *Hospital and Community Psychiatry* 31: 119–121.

Premo, F. H., and Wiseman, L. G. 1981. *Community Mental Health Centers: Perspectives of the Seventies (An Annotated Bibliography)*. DHHS Publication No. ADM 81–1074. Rockville, Md.: National Institute of Mental Health.

President's Commission on Mental Health. 1978. *Report to the President from the President's Commission on Mental Health*. Washington, D.C.: U.S. Government Printing Office.

Price, W. S., and Associates. 1978. *Technical Report for Development of a Methodology to Evaluate Leadership Problems in Community Mental Health Centers*. Unpublished report. National Institute of Mental Health, Contract No. 278–77–0074 (OP).

Raschko, R. 1985. Systems Integration at the Program Level: Aging and Mental Health. *Gerontologist* 25: 460–463.

Redick, R. W. 1973. Utilization of Psychiatric Facilities by Persons under 18 Years of Age, United States, 1971. *Statistical Note*, No. 90. Washington, D.C.: National Institute of Mental Health.

Redick, R. W. 1976. Addition Rates to Federally Funded Community Mental Health Centers, United States, 1973. *Statistical Note*, No. 126. Washington, D.C.: National Institute of Mental Health.

Regier, D. A., and Taube, C. A. 1981. The Delivery of Mental Health Services. In *American Handbook of Psychiatry, Vol. 7*, eds. S. Arieti and H.K.H. Brodie. Washington D.C.: American Psychiatric Association.

Riessman, E., Rabkin, J. G., and Struening, E. L. 1977. Brief Versus Standard Psychiatric Hospitalization: A Critical Review of the Literature. *Community Mental Health Review* 2: 1–10.

Rosen, B. 1977. Mental Health of the Poor: Have the Gaps between the Poor and the "Non-Poor" Narrowed in the Last Decade? *Medical Care* 15: 647–661.

Rosenstein, M. 1978. The Indirect Services: Consultation and Education and Public Information, Federally Funded Community Mental Health Centers, 1975. *Statistical Note*, No. 147. Washington, D.C.: National Institute of Mental Health.

Rosenstein, M. 1979. *The Characteristics of Persons Served by the Federally Funded Community Mental Health Centers Program, 1974*. U.S. Department of Health, Education, and Welfare Publication No. ADM. 79–771. Washington, D.C.: U.S. Government Printing Office.

Rubin, J. 1982. Cost Measurement and Cost Data in Mental Health Settings. *Hospital and Community Psychiatry* 33: 750–754.

Schainblatt, A. 1972. *Monitoring the Outcomes of State Mental Health Treatment Programs: Some Initial Suggestions*. Washington, D.C.: Urban Institute.

Schwartz, S. 1982. Putting Primary Prevention to Work: Administrative Dilemmas. *Administration in Mental Health* 9: 272–280.

Scott, R. R., Balch, P., and Flynn, T. C. 1983. A Comparison of Community Attitudes toward CMHC Services and Clients with Those of Mental Hospitals. *American Journal of Community Psychology* 11: 741–749.

Scott, R. R., Balch, P., and Flynn, T. C. 1984. Assessing a CMHC's Impact: Resident and Gatekeeper Awareness of Center Services. *Journal of Community Psychology* 12: 61–66.

Seliger, J. 1981. Community Mental Health Center Readiness to Comply with Section 504 of the Rehabilitation Act. *Community Mental Health Journal* 17: 236–246.

Sharfstein, S. 1979. Community Mental Health Centers: Returning to Basics. *American Journal of Psychiatry* 136: 1077–1079.

Sheridan, E., and Teplin, L. 1981. Police Referred Psychiatric Emergencies: Advantages of Community Treatment. *Journal of Community Psychology* 9: 140–147.

Siegel, A. P., Astrachan, B. M., and Levine, M. S. 1984. Reevaluating the Work of a Community Mental Health Center: The Care of Chronic Patients. *Hospital and Community Psychiatry* 35: 1129–1132.

Simons, L. S., Morton, T. L., Wade, T. C., and McSharry, D. M. 1978. Treatment Outcome and Follow-up Evaluations Based upon Client Case Records in a Mental Health Center. *Journal of Consulting and Clinical Psychology* 46: 246–251.

Simpson, W. H. 1981. Reaction of a Harassed Administrator. *Community Mental Health Journal* 17: 98–104.

Smith, C. J. 1984. Geographic Patterns of Funding for Community Mental Health Centers. *Hospital and Community Psychiatry* 35: 1133–1140.

Smith, M., and Glass, G. 1977. Metaanalysis of Psychotherapy Outcomes. *American Psychologist* 32: 752–760.

Snow, D. L., and Newton, P. M. 1976. Task, Social Structure and Social Process in the Community Mental Health Center Movement. *American Psychologist* 31: 582–594.

Snow, D. L., and Swift, C. F. 1985. Consultation and Education in Community Mental Health: A Historical Analysis. *Journal of Primary Prevention* 6: 3–30.

Snow, D. L., and Wolfe, T. J. 1983. Developing Guidelines and Standards for the Delivery of Consultation and Education Services. *Consultation*, 38–46.

Socio-Technical Systems Associates. 1973. *Relationship between Community Mental Health Centers and State Mental Hospitals*. Unpublished report. National Institute of Mental Health, Contract No. HSM 42–70–107.

Solomon, G., and Bernstein, J. 1985. Program Evaluation in Rural Community Mental Health. *Journal of Rural Community Psychology* 6: 3–17.

Stockdill, J. W. 1978. The Community Mental Health Movement—Success or Failure? In *Briefing Book: Evaluation of CMHC Program*, eds. J. R. Woy and J. W. Stockdill. Unpublished report. National Institute of Mental Health.

Sue, S. 1977. Community Mental Health Services to Minority Groups: Some Optimism, Some Pessimism. *American Psychologist* 32: 616–620.

Sue, S., Allen, D. B., and Conaway, L. 1978. Responsiveness and Equality of Mental Health Care to Chicanos and Native Americans. *American Journal of Community Psychology* 6: 137–146.

Sue, S., McKinney, H., Allen, D., and Hall, J. 1974. Delivery of Community Mental Health Services to Black and White Clients. *Journal of Consulting and Clinical Psychology* 42: 794–801.

Taube, C. 1971a. Admissions to Outpatient Psychiatric Services by Age, Sex, and Diagnosis. *Statistical Note*, No. 48. Washington, D.C.: National Institute of Mental Health.

Taube, C. 1971b. Diagnostic Distribution of Inpatient Admissions to State and County Mental Hospitals—1969. *Statistical Note*, No. 49. Washington, D.C.: National Institute of Mental Health.

Taube, C., and Cannon, M. S. 1972. Whom Are Community Mental Health Centers Serving? *Statistical Note*, No. 67. Washington, D.C.: National Institute of Mental Health.

Tuckman, G., and Lipton, I. D. 1976. A Predischarge State Hospital Unit for Deinstitutionalization. *Research Communications in Psychiatry, Psychology, and Behavior* 1: 327–340.

Udell, B., and Hornstra, R. K. 1975. Good Patients and Bad: Therapeutic Assets and Liabilities. *Archives of General Psychiatry* 32: 1533–1537.

Vayda, A. M., and Perlmutter, F. D. 1977. Primary Prevention in Community Mental Health Centers: A Survey of Current Activity. *Community Mental Health Journal* 13: 343–351.

Walsh, J. 1982. Prevention in Mental Health: Organizational and Ideological Perspectives. *Social Work* 27: 298–301.

Washburn, S., Janicelli, M., Longabaugh, R., and Scheff, B. J. 1976. A Controlled Comparison of Psychiatric Day Treatment and Inpatient Hospitalization. *Journal of Consulting and Clinical Psychology* 44: 665–675.

Weiner, R. S., Woy, J. R., Sharfstein, S. S., and Bass, R. D. 1979. Community Mental Health Centers and the "Seed Money" Concept: The Effects of Terminating Federal Funds. *Community Mental Health Journal* 15: 129–138.

Weiss, K. J., and Dubin, W. R. 1982. Partial Hospitalization: State of the Art. *Hospital and Community Psychiatry* 33: 923–928.

Western Interstate Commission for Higher Education. 1980. *Mental Health Accountability: Further Development and Piloting of an Evaluation-Based Accountability Package and Process*. Unpublished report. National Institute of Mental Health, Contract No. 278–78–0035 (OP).

Windle, C., Albert, M. B., and Sharfstein, S. S. 1978. Collaborative Program Evaluations to Improve Emergency Services in Community Mental Health Centers. *Hospital and Community Psychiatry* 29: 708–710.

Windle, C., Bass, R. D., and Gray, L. 1986. Impact of Federally Funded CMHCs on Local Mental Health Service Systems. Unpublished manuscript.

Windle, C., Bass, R. D., and Taube, C. A. 1974. PR Aside: Initial Results from National Institute of Mental Health's Services Program Evaluation Studies. *American Journal of Community Psychology* 2: 311–327.

Windle, C., Neal, J., and Zinn, H. K. 1979. Stimulating Equity of Services to Nonwhites in Community Mental Health Centers. *Community Mental Health Journal* 15: 155–166.

Windle, C., and Paschall, N. 1981. Client Participation in CMHC Program Evaluation: Increasing Incidence, Adequate Involvement. *Community Mental Health Involvement* 17: 66–76.

Windle, C., Poppen, P., Thompson, M. D., Taube, C. A., and Marvelle, M. A. 1986. CMHC Outpatient Characteristics and Provider Discipline. Unpublished manuscript.

Windle, C., and Scully, D. 1976. Community Mental Health Centers and the Decreasing Use of State Hospitals. *Community Mental Health Journal* 12: 239–243.

Windle, C., and Wu, I. 1981. Stimulating Equity of CMHC Services to Non-Whites: A Follow-up Based on Expected Regression. *Community Mental Health Journal* 17: 306–309.

Winslow, W. W. 1982. Changing Trends in CMHCs: Keys to Survival in the Eighties. *Hospital and Community Psychiatry* 33: 273–277.

Witkin, M. J. 1980. Trends in Patient Care Episodes in Mental Health Facilities, 1955–

1977. *Statistical Note*, No. 154. Washington, D.C.: National Institute of Mental Health.

Wolfe, J. 1977. The Director. *National Council News*. Washington, D.C.: National Council of Community Mental Health Centers.

Wolfe, T., and Swift, C. 1986. Fourteen Exemplary Programs Selected by the American Psychological Association Task Force on Prevention. Paper presented at the Technology Transfer Conference, Prevention Programs That Work. Sponsored by the National Council of Community Mental Health Centers and the Pew Trust, San Francisco, September.

Wolkon, G. H., Moriwaki, S., Mandel, D., Archuleta, J., Bunje, P., and Zimmerman, S. 1974. Ethnicity and Social Class in Delivery of Services. *American Journal of Public Health* 64: 709–712.

Woy, J. R., Wasserman, D. B., and Weiner-Pomerantz, R. 1981. Community Mental Health Centers: Movement Away from the Model. *Community Mental Health Journal* 17: 265–276.

Yarvis, R. M., and Edwards, D. W. 1980. *Planning: The Design of Mental Health Programs*. Sacramento, Calif.: Pyramid Systems.

Yarvis, R. M., Edwards, D. W., and Langsley, D. G. 1978. Do CMHCs Underserve Psychotic Individuals? *Hospital and Community Psychiatry* 29: 387–388.

Zins, J., and Hopkins, R. 1981. Referral Out: Increasing the Number of Kept Appointments. *School Psychologist Review* 10: 107–111.

Zinober, J. W., and Dinkel, N. R. 1981. *A Trust of Evaluation: A Guide for Involving Citizens in Community Mental Health Program Evaluation*. Tampa, Fla.: Florida Consortium for Research and Evaluation.

10

Community Residential Care

STEVEN P. SEGAL
and PAMELA KOTLER

There is a greater need for supervised residential care for the mentally ill now than at any time since the early 1950s. Thirty-five years ago, the overwhelming need for mental hospital beds contributed to the development of the deinstitutionalization movement. The successes of the deinstitutionalization movement, however, went far toward eliminating the mental hospital as a source of supervised residential care. Unfortunately, several current statistical trends in combination document that a growing number of people now require a supervised living arrangement: (1) there has been no reduction in the incidence of long-term mental disorders (Regier et al., 1984; Shapiro et al., 1984; Murphy et al., 1984); (2) between 1965 and 1979 there was a steady increase in the number of inpatient episodes for mental disorders per 100,000 civilian population; (3) nationally the proportion of total hospital days attributable to mental disorder fell from 36 percent in 1969 to 25 percent in 1978 (Kiesler, 1982b); and (4) in the past ten years the number of homeless mentally ill has steadily increased (see chapter 12 in this volume).

Given these trends, it should be no surprise that we have had a major, unplanned increase in the number of private facilities purporting to provide at least some supervised twenty-four–hour care. Such facilities include family care, family foster care, board and care, residential care, and group care homes as well as halfway, quarterway, psychosocial rehabilitation facilities, and any number of satellite housing arrangements or hotel situations (excluding licensed nursing homes and licensed hospitals). At minimum, these facilities provide "a bed of last resort" for people who have no other place to go. At maximum, they provide a key service on the continuum of care and have been established as part of planned residential care systems, such as that incorporated in the Lanterman-Petris-Short Act in California (California Commission on Health and the Economy, 1985). Whichever is true, these facilities constitute one of the three major national systems of residential care for the adult mentally ill—the other two being the state and county mental hospital system and the nursing home industry. In fact, the residential care system now provides services for at least as many adult mentally ill as are provided in state and county mental hospitals.

Developed largely on an ad hoc basic, the residential care system in the United States raises a number of important issues with respect to public responsibility for the care and treatment of the mentally ill. Our review of information on this subject will make clear that community residential care is an essential, if undervalued, component of our community mental health effort.

COMMUNITY RESIDENTIAL CARE WITHIN A NATIONAL COMMUNITY MENTAL HEALTH PROGRAM

Three alternative models of community-based residential care for the adult mentally ill describe and theoretically define the functions of this system in a national context: (1) residential care as part of the *treatment continuum*, (2) residential care as a *residual system of custody*, and (3) residential care as a *developmental context* for the mentally ill.

Continuum of Care Model

In the continuum of care model, the residential care system is viewed as providing a range of residential alternatives to hospitalization (Bachrach, 1984; Lamb, 1984; Shadoan, 1985). This model conceptualizes residential care facilities as part and parcel of the treatment system. Compared to the hospital which offers the most intensive treatment experience, residential care provides a less intensive treatment setting either following hospitalization or as an alternative to hospitalization. People in residential care are expected to move along a continuum to greater independence. Theoretically, they move from facilities with more structure and greater treatment intensity to facilities with less structure and less intense therapeutics. Generally, the more intense the facility's treatment orientation the higher the ratio of staff to patients (Shadoan, 1985). High-intensity community treatment facilities include crisis housing, lodge programs, and halfway houses; moderate intensity settings are board and care homes; low-intensity facilities include cooperative apartments and satellite housing. California actually has written this type of model into its state Mental Health Law in the form of a Community Residential Treatment System '' designed to provide, at every level, alternatives to institutionalization'' (California Commission on Health and the Economy, 1985: 84), and including short-term crisis residences, transitional residences, long-term (two to three years), and semisupervised, independent, and structured living arrangements.

The Residual Model

In the residual model of residential care, these facilities simply represent a holding operation for the management of formerly hospitalized, long-term patients. They have little relevance to today's mentally ill because they are designed to house the docile elderly patients of the past. This model equates residential care facilities with the back wards of state mental hospitals; the development of the residential care system is thus viewed as a form of transinstitutionalization (Scull, 1977; Brown, 1985). This model has been presented in the popular press and in several government reports (see, for example, U.S. Congress, 1977; U.S. General Accounting Office, 1979; and California Commission on Health and the Economy, 1985), with particular focus on one segment of the residential care sector—board and care. This segment of the residential care system is the most criticized, the least funded, and provides the most service. According to Segal and Aviram (1978), the board-and-care system accounts for 72 percent of all residential care facilities serving the adult mentally ill between eighteen and sixty-five years old and houses 82 percent of this residential care population.

The purpose of the residual model is primarily to criticize the shortcomings of community residential care. It is not advanced as a conception of what this system ideally *should* be. In fact, the model's only relevance from a normative perspective lies in the ultimate dependence of the mental health system on the board-and-care system as a noninstitutional residential resource of last resort.

The Developmental Model

In the developmental model, residential care placement is viewed as a planned phase in the treatment and potential rehabilitation of individuals who are poor and chronically mentally ill (CMI). At its best, the system can offer patients a long-term decent living environment within the community and is varied enough in character to accommodate differing needs. Segal and Aviram (1978) and Betts, Stan, and Reynolds (1981) see this as a worthwhile, and even admirable, outcome.

According to this model, the CMI follow distinct careers leading to board-and-care placement. In one such career the poor CMI are pushed or thrown out of their families (Baumohl and Miller, 1974), have their first experience with major mental disorder, and join the street population in their late teenage or early adult years. They survive on the streets through their mid-thirties to early forties. At that point, some move into private residential care facilities, whereas, in the past, they would have moved into state mental hospitals. This patient population is socially marginal. Contacts with families are limited. Though some may live intermittently with their families, their primary residence from their early forties through their sixties is some supervised housing arrangement (i.e., a residential home). If, at a later point in their lives, they develop significant physical disabilities, these persons would then move to a nursing home.

In another career path, the young mentally ill individual becomes ill in his family home. He receives support—by way of income, room, and board—through his middle years, at which time family tolerance wears thin or aging parents seek a long-term arrangement for their disabled offspring. This process usually occurs at the time of one of several intermittent hospitalizations. Discharge from the hospital then involves board-and-care placement. When the board-and-care placement is made, contacts with the family decrease, though there may be intermittent returns to the family. The primary residence by the early forties through the early sixties is the residential home. Later, significant physical disability may lead to nursing home placement.

For both groups of chronically mentally ill people, the life cycle is characterized by sporadic stays in mental hospitals, general hospital psychiatric units, community mental health centers, and, occasionally, jail. Key characteristics of this population are its lack of "social margin"—most are poor and have minimal family supports (Segal, Baumohl, and Johnson, 1977)—and chronic mental illness. This model differs from the continuum of care model in that the focus is *not* on the transition from one treatment facility to another. Rather, it describes the development of a social career for the chronically mentally ill poor and downwardly mobile. This model also differs from the residual model of care in that facilities in this model are not "beds of last resort"; they are marginal housing environments serving a marginal population. Most important in the developmental model is the recognition that a majority of the facilities provide a very valued and adequate service. The career paths of these chronically mentally ill individuals, given their social marginality, are characterized by the use and abuse of systems of social support, treatment, and control.

These three models highlight different functions of residential care facilities in the ongoing support of those people with long-term mental illness. Yet, from the perspective of developing a national strategy for the care and treatment of the mentally ill, each model offers useful insights into an overall residential care effort. The transitional model directs attention to the placement dynamics of the system in terms of facility program structure and staffing requirements. The developmental model encourages us to appreciate the extensive handicaps experienced by the "disaffiliated" mentally ill population. The residual model emphasizes the existence of a residual population who will need long-term residential care no matter what type of program is employed, so long as we are without a cure for the major mental disorders.

DESCRIPTION OF THE COMMUNITY RESIDENTIAL CARE SYSTEM

Community-based residential care is provided via a varied system with a multiplicity of goals, facilities, funding sources, and service targets. In order to understand the uses of residential care, it is necessary to look at the descriptive parameters of that system.

Characteristics of Residential Care

Sherwood and Seltzer (1981) distinguish five characteristics of residential care facilities that set them apart from other types of arrangements for the care and treatment of the mentally ill.

First, *the facility must not be Medicaid-eligible and cannot provide medical care to clients through facility funds*. Residential care facilities distinguish themselves from hospitals or other facilities by the fact that they do not pay for medical care from facility funds. A distinction is made between medical care paid for by facility funds (however it is obtained) and medical care paid for by the residents' own funds (SSI, third-party payers, or private resources).

The second defining characteristic is that *residential care facilities provide room and board*. All facilities must provide a room, yet the definition of "board" varies considerably. While most residential facilities provide all meals for residents, some expect residents to purchase their own food and prepare their own meals. The rationale for this practice is that it is necessary for residents to practice independent community living skills under staff supervision. Technically, board is not provided to residents in such instances, but a facility is *not* disqualified as a residential care facility if there is reason to believe that the staff is responsible for ensuring that the residents eat even if these residents prepare their own meals.

The third defining characteristic of residential care is that *the facility provides some degree of protective oversight to residents (that is, some services beyond room, board, and basic maintenance such as laundry)*. This protective oversight is often conceptualized as the responsibility of the facility in addition to food and shelter. It includes such things as nighttime staff coverage, facilitating access to health and social services, recreational programming, and help with management of finances.

The fourth characteristic is that *the facility serves one or more designated categories of needy persons, such as children, the developmentally disabled, the mentally ill, and the elderly*. In the early 1970s, as facilities were developing, especially the group of facilities which we will discuss under board-and-care facilities, there was a tendency to serve anybody in need of a supervised living arrangement regardless of the designated needy group from which he or she came. This flexibility allowed residential care home owners to keep beds full, and, in effect, ensured their income. While this approach still remains a means of economic survival, state licensing provisions have made multiple population service in residential facilities more difficult, creating pressure on facilities to target their services to a specific population of the needy.

The fifth characteristic concerns *eligibility of residents for those Supplemental Security Income (SSI) payments available to persons in supervised living arrangements* (this applies only to adult residential care). Perhaps the single most important impetus to the development of the adult residential care industry has been the provision of SSI payments to eligible individuals to purchase supervised housing arrangements. As of January 1986, individuals living independently in California received $433 in SSI payments. Individuals in supervised living arrangements received $601, $531 of which went to the facility, and $70 of which was retained by the resident for personal needs. (The SSI rate for supervised living arrangements is determined by the state, contingent on the size of the state supplement to the basic federal contribution to the SSI payment.) The availability of SSI support made the development of fee-for-service adult residential care possible. However, it must be noted that the Keys Amendment to the Social Security Act (Section 1616[e]) excluded residents of public institutions with seventeen or more residents from eligibility for SSI supervised-living-arrangement payments.

Supply and Distribution of Different Types of Community Residences

There are no valid, current estimates of the number of residential care facilities serving the mentally ill or of the number of residents housed in these facilities in the United States. To some extent, this is a function of financial arrangements underlying the support of these facilities. Since most are privately owned and operated, they do not report to any federal agency.

Further complicating estimation of the size of the resident and facility populations is confusion over which facilities should be included among residential care homes. Figure 10–1 illustrates the various housing arrangements for the disabled which are often included in discussions related to residential care. McCoin (1983) has estimated that there are 300,000 boarding homes in the United States serving more than two million people. The large number of facilities estimated by McCoin as boarding houses do provide room and board but do not adopt the care function. Boarding houses have been providing residential service to the disabled, and especially the mentally ill, for a long time. This phenomenon was initially documented in the work of Faris and Dunham (1939). The mentally ill have tended to locate in areas of high concentration of boarding homes and, in fact, in the boarding homes themselves. Current attention to housing arrangements of the mentally ill has, however, focused on those facilities adopting a care function—particularly the rapidly growing board-and-care segment.

A 1982 report by the U.S. Inspector General estimates approximately 30,000 board-and-care homes nationwide (cited in Kusserow, 1982). Assuming that these homes represent 72 percent of all residential care facilities (Segal and

Figure 10–1
A Schema of Housing Arrangements for the Disabled

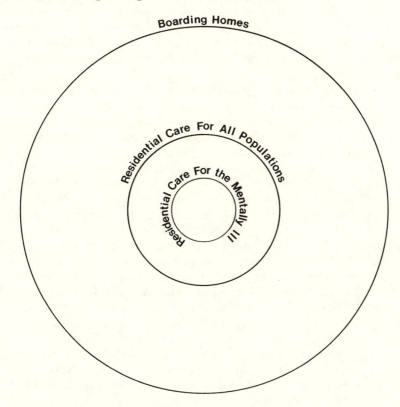

Aviram, 1978), then the number of such facilities serving all dependent groups is approximately 41,666.

Hauber et al. (1984) found approximately 13,125 residential care facilities serving the adult developmentally disabled in 1982. Segal and Aviram (1978) estimated 1,150 facilities in California serving the mentally ill between eighteen and sixty-five in 1973. Assuming 16 percent (see Hauber et al.'s [1984: 37] Table 14) of the total population of facilities were located in California, 7,187 facilities nationally would service the adult mentally ill between eighteen and sixty-five years of age. Further assuming a growth in the number of facilities equal to that found by Hauber et al. (1984) for the developmentally disabled (i.e., 8.3 percent per year), we would estimate that in 1982 there were 14,730 facilities serving the mentally ill aged eighteen to sixty-five years old. Given an estimated 41,666 facilities serving all populations in 1982—14,730 serving the eighteen- to sixty-five-year-old adult mentally ill, and 13,125 serving the developmentally disabled—the total number of residential care facilities serving the elderly and other disabled groups (i.e., non–mentally ill or developmentally disabled) would be approximately 13,811. It must be emphasized, however, that there is considerable within-facility mixing of dependent groups, particularly with regard to the aged who are frequently dually classified. These estimates of the number of facilities which would be identified with a single dependent group (with the exception of the aged) therefore represent gross overestimates of categorically defined facilities.

This mixing of dependent populations makes estimating the number of persons in residential care extremely difficult. Many studies of residential care focusing on a single dependent population count all residential care facilities and all their residents as members of a single population, thus grossly overstating the number of dependent disabled in the categorical group being served in a given facility.

Given this caveat, various studies (see National Institute of Mental Health, 1976; Melody, 1979; and U.S. General Accounting Office, 1977) indicate that there were about 400,000 chronically mentally ill persons living in boarding homes in 1980. Goldman, Gattozzi, and Taube (1981), relying on data from a service delivery assessment in the Philadelphia area for Region 3 of the U.S. Department of Health and Human Services, estimated that between 300,000 to 400,000 chronic mental patients resided in board and care facilities nationally.

Segal and Aviram's (1978) census of residential care facilities and residents in the state of California, a study which strictly sampled facilities serving the mentally ill between eighteen and sixty-five years old, estimated that only 12,400 mentally ill residents lived in 1,150 facilities. If we assume that California has 11 percent of the nation's residential care population (Hauber et al., 1984), this would mean that there were only 112,727 people in 1973 in residential care nationally who were mentally ill and between the ages of eighteen and sixty-five. Assuming that this number has remained stable (as was the case with the developmentally disabled group), then the difference between this estimate and others in the 300,000 to 400,000 range is due to the latter's inclusion of those mentally ill residents over sixty-five years old. This difference, assuming a conservative 300,000 total population, would be 187,273 elderly mentally ill. Sherwood and Seltzer (1981) estimated, however, that there are 120,000 elderly mentally ill in the nation as a whole, thus pointing to the probability of some residual measurement error in either the low estimate or the high estimate or both.

Two other trends are relevant to this descriptive summary of community residential care in the United States. First, as the country's single largest supplier of residential care services, California seems to rely on a greater number of smaller facilities. Second, the current trend nationally is toward smaller residences, as evidenced by increases in the number of facilities while the size of the clientele population has remained relatively stable.

General Client Characteristics

Males and females are equally represented in residential care (Melick and Eysaman, 1978; Sherwood and Gruenberg, 1979; Wilder, Kessel, and Caulfield,

1968; and Ditmar et al., 1983). The majority of the population is white and reflects the ethnic representation of the general population to which residents belong. Women in residential care tend to be older than their male counterparts. Three-fourths of the men have never been married, and the average age of the total population in residential care is around 50. These findings are surprisingly consistent between Segal and Aviram (1978) and Ditmar et al. (1983), the two major surveys of the residential care system. Other studies tend to focus on the demographics of specific populations such as persons in Veterans Administration foster homes in the United States (Linn, Klett, and Caffey, 1980) and Canada (Murphy, Ingelsman, and Tcheng-Laroche, 1976). These studies naturally show a higher proportion of younger males, with an average age as low as thirty. Segal and Aviram (1978) suggest that many mentally ill individuals who in the past were chronic residents of mental hospitals are now long-term residents of board-and-care homes, perhaps accounting for the age of board-and-care residents. Ditmar et al. (1983) tend to concur with this conclusion. This pattern would seem to support a residual model of the system; however, neither of these studies examined recent residents, an area of much needed research. Both studies also fail to provide the longitudinal perspective necessary to test elements of the residual model. Overall, the demographic character of the residential care population seems to have been stable from 1973 to 1983. The two major groups in the residential care system are older women and younger men.

Employment. Ditmar et al. (1983) report that 17.6 percent of residents of residential care facilities were employed: 6 percent were in sheltered workshops; 2.6 percent were employed competitively; 2.3 percent were in work training programs; 2.4 percent reported that they did volunteer work; and 4 percent reported other types of employment, primarily odd jobs. The majority of those in Ditmar's sample who reported some form of employment worked twenty or fewer hours a week (57.9 percent) and had held their current job for one year or less (61 percent). Eighteen percent of the employed said they were looking for new employment, and 14 percent of the unemployed were looking for work. These statistics show significantly higher work activity than is reported in Segal and Aviram (1978), whose data were collected seven years prior. Segal and Aviram found that only 7 percent of the residential care population was actually employed and 4 percent were looking for work.

A Typology of Residential Care Facilities

Four primary types of facilities provide residential care for the chronically mentally ill adult population. They are family care homes, board-and-care homes, halfway houses, and satellite house programs.

Family care homes. The family care home program was one of the first attempts to find alternative sheltered care or a supervised living arrangement for the mentally ill. Family care, foster family care, or adult foster care all refer to programs that place mental patients in the community with private families, usually but not always other than their own. The resident is supervised by the caretaker, who is in turn supervised by a professional, usually a social worker (Morrissey, 1967). A foster family home is defined as a small family setting; in California this is six or fewer people.

Adult family care for the mentally ill dates back to the eleventh century in Geel, Belgium. In Geel, where homes are still limited to one or two patients, patients are perceived as an integral part of society, and especially of the family. Patients have bedrooms of their own, which facilitates privacy. They share their meals and leisure activities with the family, and participate (though less today than in the past) in the family's domestic and income-producing work, thereby supplementing the modest payments for their care made by the state (Srole, 1977). Cuvelier (1975) describes foster care in Geel as a process in which the patient arrives "groupless" and homeless and then has the experience of living with a family in a normal home. The patient participates in daily home activities, is expected to behave well, and gradually becomes a family member in the sense of developing family-affective bonds as he or she learns to adapt to the day-to-day demands of a family. In short, the patient assumes a family role. Recent critical evaluations of the Geel program have pointed to the fact that, despite the effort to integrate patients into ongoing community life, patients are generally not included in the voluntary associations which form a significant part of the social relationships among "normal" community members.

In the United States similar programs were conceived as early as 1865 (Grob, 1973) and first introduced in Massachusetts in 1885, although fifty years elapsed before other states followed. Historically, the acceptance of family care has been based upon two premises: it was less expensive than hospitalization, and it would free beds for acutely ill patients (Lee, 1963). Early advocates of family care based their arguments primarily on economic grounds. It is not surprising, then, that the major growth of the program occurred in the 1930s and the 1940s, when the depression meant a lack of funds for state hospitals and the need for money among many families in the community. These converging financial conditions resulted in growth in the family care programs. During World War II, a personnel shortage in the mental hospitals also provided impetus for the family care program to relieve overcrowded, understaffed mental hospital wards. Indeed, family care programs were viewed by many at that time as "the one hopeful answer to the perennial problem of overcrowded institutions" (Morrissey, 1967: 18).

In spite of this, overall growth of the program until the early 1950s in the United States was not impressive, and, even though there was some expansion of the program during the 1950s and 1960s, it has remained relatively small. Morrissey (1967: 14) reports that, in 1963, 13,000 mentally ill resided in family care homes in the United States, plus about 4,000 in similar programs operated by the Veterans Administration. At the same time, the resident population of mental institutions in the United States was about one-half million. In the late 1950s and early 1960s, with new knowledge concerning the impact of social environment on patient outcomes, family care came to be viewed as a means of providing an alternative setting for those in need of long-term custodial care.

The goal of family care became humane treatment in the context of a normalized family relationship.

By the early 1960s, at the outset of the community mental health movement and the push to decentralize mental hospitals, family care programs generally were associated with the aftercare arm of state mental hospitals and, as such, with state-controlled mental health care. To some extent, this arrangement conflicted with the move for local control of aftercare services and, in several states, led to the demise of the family care movement as a unique type of facility sponsored through the aftercare efforts of state hospitals. On the other hand, many of these facilities merged with small board-and-care homes into small residential care facilities serving as many as six unrelated residents in a single family home. Current licensing laws in California make no distinction between the family care home and the small residential care facility, though both are usually now associated with local mental health settings. Currently, the greatest use of family care programs is by the Veterans Administration, which has about 11,000 psychiatric patients in foster care (Linn, 1981).

Halfway houses/psychosocial rehabilitation facilities. Although the formal development of halfway houses is rather recent, many informal parallels have existed for a long time. The halfway house—literally halfway between institution and community—can serve persons who cannot live independently in the community but who do not require a complete institutional regimen. The early development of halfway houses in Britain consisted of placements by the British Mental Aftercare Association of Released Psychiatric Patients into convalescent or private homes (Apte, 1968). In the 1920s, the association began accepting residents for placement directly from the community. These individuals had emotional problems that threatened their ability to function in the community. It was hoped that placing them in "hostels" (actually halfway houses) would prevent their hospitalization.

Halfway houses in the United States assumed their present form in the 1950s. Rutland Corner House in Boston, which opened in 1954, was the first halfway house that operated according to the current concept. Most definitions of the halfway house emphasize the goal of *temporary* residence in a transitional environment immediately following hospitalization and before resumption of normal independent living (Landy and Greenblatt, 1965). Glasscote, Gudeman, and Elpers (1971: 13) contend, however, that halfway houses may also serve as permanent facilities for people who are not able to move fully into the community. They define a halfway house as a "non-medical residential facility specifically intended to enhance the capability of people who are mentally ill, or who are impaired by residual deficits from mental illness, to remain in the community, participating to the fullest possible extent in community life" (Glasscote, Gudeman, and Elpers, 1971: 11).

Halfway houses, which have generally retained the notion of transition between the institution and the community, have more recently been accompanied by the quarterway house and the three-quarterway house. The former accommodates longer stays by more disabled residents and is often located on hospital grounds. The latter is closer to full participation in community life.

As transitional residences, halfway houses provide supervision and support to newly discharged patients for a limited period while their residents adjust to more independent living and reintegration into the community. The goals are to assist former patients to develop daily living skills and to improve interpersonal relationships.

More recently, many halfway houses have developed an emphasis on meaningful employment, managed use of time, resource development, and social skills training (Anthony, Cohen, and Cohen, 1984) within the framework of a rehabilitation model such as that used by Fountain House (Beard et al., 1963). Terming themselves "psychosocial rehabilitation facilities" (PRF), they emphasize concrete training in social skills more than the traditional psychotherapeutic approach of many halfway houses. In the past ten years, many halfway house facilities have become PRFs, and those which have maintained a traditional halfway house orientation have adopted many of the programs of the PRF. Boundaries related to the therapeutic efforts of these various facilities are disappearing.

Halfway houses and PRFs tend to be well staffed, often by degreed professionals, but more recently by paraprofessional help. With a definite therapeutic orientation, they attempt to serve either a treatment or rehabilitation function in addition to housing. Unlike family care homes and board-and-care homes, they often tend to be funded by mental health agencies. For this reason, they have income that is independent of a fee-for-service arrangement.

Board and care. The present system of board-and-care homes did not develop in any planned fashion or in accordance with any single model for the provision of residential care. Instead, board-and-care facilities developed to meet a need among people who were discharged from large state hospitals and others who, under a policy of deinstitutionalization, were no longer able to obtain a long-term placement in a mental hospital. The ideology of each board-and-care facility varies as a function of the background of the owner or manager. At the outset, the primary purpose of these facilities was to provide bed, board, and care. However, the unwillingness of state governments to invest in the provision of care has led to the development of a board-and-care system which is extremely inconsistent in form. It ranges from facilities that provide a very warm, caring setting in a family context, to treatment-oriented facilities which rival some halfway houses, to a large number of facilities which provide substandard environments for their residents. Because of the lack of organized leadership, and the unwillingness of the mental health community itself to accord formal legitimacy to the functions of board and care facilities, the system moves ahead without direction.

Satellite housing. This last type of residential care shows a very high potential to facilitate the reintegration of mentally disabled individuals into the community (Goldmeier, Mannino, and Shore, 1978), yet currently is used very little in this country. Satellite housing was initially used in the United States in 1963 when Fountain House leased a small number of apartments in New York City, each of which provided a placement for two mentally ill clients who were then assigned volunteer service providers (Beard et al., 1963). Satellite housing usually offers patients a lifestyle with considerable independence and opportunity for social integration. Satellite housing can include apartments, duplexes, or small single-family dwellings. The housing is usually leased by an agency, though it may be leased by a resident or in a co-ownership arrangement. Residents live in small groups of two to five without live-in staff but with professional supervision. Shopping, cooking, and housework are shared and residents are responsible for paying their own rent (either directly to the landlord or to the agency). Staff members assigned to satellite housing programs are available as needed for guidance and counseling. Satellite programs can be organized in many different ways. For example, residents of three or four apartments may form a stable group for regular meetings, sometimes with staff and sometimes without. These group meetings can be hosted by the residents within their own housing units on a rotating basis. Satellite housing programs may also exist in a single building where all apartments are owned by an agency and occupied independently by disabled resident groups. This latter arrangement, however, comes closer to board and care than to the notion of independent and integrated community living.

Comparing facility types. Very few studies have directly compared the four major types of facilities, their populations, and the needs of these populations. Generally, the family care facility has six or fewer residents living in a family setting, ideally, only one or two. A halfway house, on the other hand, is usually larger. Glasscote, Gudeman, and Elpers (1971) reported that these facilities have an average of twenty-two beds, with 9 percent of the facilities they surveyed accommodating more than forty residents. Board-and-care homes vary in size, from one resident to 300 (Segal and Aviram, 1978; Lamb, 1981). Satellite housing programs, because of the considerable variability in their form, also differ in the number of residents in the total program, yet seem to limit themselves to one to four residents per apartment or housing unit.

Relationship to community environment. Segal and Aviram's (1978) comparative study analyzed the relationship of these facilities to their community environments. Halfway houses tended to be at least a long walk from most community resources as compared to family care homes and board-and-care homes, which showed a greater variability in their distance from such resources. This is contrary to what would be expected if it is assumed that the outward-reaching orientation of the halfway house would lead to an emphasis on proximity to community resources. Halfway houses, however, were generally professionally sponsored facilities that provided easy access to medical and social services, while as many as 17 percent of the board and care facilities found such services either difficult to obtain or unobtainable. A full third of the family care facilities had this problem.

Family care homes, in contrast to board-and-care homes and halfway houses, tended to be situated in suburban, single-family-home areas rather than downtown, multiple-dwelling districts. According to Segal and Aviram (1978), 49 percent of the family care homes in their sample were in single-family-home areas, compared to 34 percent of board-and-care facilities and none of the halfway houses. Furthermore, 30 percent of the halfway houses were situated in ghetto areas featuring a combination of businesses and residential dwellings, compared to only 3 percent of the board-and-care homes and none of the family care homes. Seventy percent of the halfway houses were located in commercial areas. The location of many halfway houses in ghetto and commercial areas may account for the finding that these facilities tended to be far from general community resources.

It is important to note that, in Segal and Aviram's study, family care homes accounted for 26 percent of the facilities in California and served 14 percent of the persons in residential care. Board-and-care homes, the most criticized segment of the residential care industry, served 82 percent of the residential care population and comprised 72 percent of the facilities. Halfway houses, which have received the greatest attention from the professional mental health community, constituted only 2 percent of the facilities and served only 3 percent of the population. Despite its relatively low use, the halfway house is singularly important because it represents a professionally initiated and community-sponsored facility. As such, it is held up as a model of care and is more likely than other types of facilities to have direct access to community funding sources. Compared to board-and-care and family care homes, halfway houses are less likely to operate solely on a fee-for-service basis.

Psychopathology of residents. Facilities also differ in the type, though not necessarily the relative degree, of psychopathology reported among their residents. Generally, studies which have examined this issue report fairly consistent results. For example, Melick and Eysaman (1978) divided their sample of community residence inhabitants into three groups: Type 1, 21 percent, those with severe behavioral or physical problems or both, 70 percent of whom were judged to be difficult or impossible to motivate; Type 2, 56 percent, those with moderate problems, only 38 percent of whom were judged to be difficult to motivate; and Type 3, 24 percent, those with problems so mild that there is little interference with normal functioning, and none of whom were judged to be difficult to motivate. It is interesting to note that only Type 2 clients were considered by the authors to be appropriate for continued placement in a board-and-care home; the others were judged to have either too severe or too mild a degree of pathology.

Wilder, Kessel, and Caulfield (1968) reported a remarkably similar distribution in the severity of symptomatology among their sample of residents in a supervised apartment program in New York. They judged 16.7 percent of their sample to have severe symptomatology, 54.8 percent to have moderate symptomatology, and 28.6 percent to have mild symptomatology. Segal and Aviram (1978) divided their sample of California residential care home residents into three levels of psychopathology according to scores on the Brief Psychiatric Rating Scale (BPRS): severely disturbed (16 percent), mildly disturbed (56 percent), and no overt psychological disturbance (28 percent). Thus, all three studies yielded highly comparable results regarding the distribution of psychopathology, with approximately one-quarter of the sample members evidencing so little psycho-pathology that the reason for their residence in the board-and-care home was not clear. Van Putten and Spar (1979) also reported the predominance of a mild level of psychiatric symptomatology in their sample of forty-six Los Angeles residential care homes.

Despite apparent consistency in these comparative analyses of psychological disturbance, different types of symptoms are reported in different types of fa-cilities. Segal and Aviram (1978) show major differences in symptom patterns among residents in family care, board-and-care, and halfway houses. Whereas 25 percent of board-and-care residents lacked overt and visibly documentable symptomatology, this was true of 42 percent of family care residents, and a full 69 percent of halfway house residents. Thus, the pattern of overt disturbance and major symptoms may be much less severe among those patients involved in halfway house programs as compared to board-and-care and family care programs. Therefore, the functions of these programs may be very different. This hypothesis is further supported by Segal and Aviram's finding that reported distress among residents (as opposed to their observable symptoms) was highest among halfway house clients: a full 79 percent reported high distress levels, as compared to 47 percent in board and care, and 30 percent in family care homes. Thus, these various facilities may be serving very different populations, a pos-sibility which necessitates cautious comparisons of relative effectiveness. There may be a selection of clientele into these facilities, with the more severely disturbed population gravitating to board-and-care settings. Conversely, halfway house settings may be better at helping their clients control their overt symptom presentations.

Costs of residential care and alternatives. A number of studies have reported data on the per diem cost of residential care homes for the mentally ill. Table 10–1 expresses the relative costs of care in various types of facilities in reference to state hospital care. The table suggests a continuum of care by type of facility, ranging from the least expensive care in a foster family setting to the most expensive care in an acute psychiatric ward of a general hospital. This ordering of facility types by cost is generally comparable to ordering the facility types by amount of staff supervision, since staff costs tend to account for the majority of the budget of residential care facilities.

Emerson, Rochford, and Shaw (1981) point out, however, that considerable variation exists in the per diem costs within each facility type. For example, economically marginal large family care homes and highly capitalized larger facilities may both be categorized as group homes. Furthermore, some halfway houses or transitional facilities for acute care patients have per diem costs greater than those of state and county mental hospitals (*Mental Disability Law Reporter*,

1979). This latter phenomenon is again a function of the staffing pattern in the facility, and makes it difficult to assess costs accurately.

In Table 10–1, it can be seen that the relative cost of residential care in family care and board-and-care facilities has declined since 1973. This is consistent with the authors' own impression, which is based upon observation of a decreasing investment in long-term care service outreach efforts by community mental health agencies, an increasing isolation of board-and-care facilities from the professional community, and a reduction in their costs attributable to service utilization. Reasons for this reduction in outreach service will be discussed below as part of our analysis of the problems of the residential care system.

A second problem in assessing the cost of community-based residential care is that most residential care facilities need to have their services supplemented by other community agencies, including police, community mental health centers, and public welfare staff. Thus, actual costs which factor in these services are likely to be more equivalent (Weisbrod, Test, and Stein, 1980; Clarke, 1979) to the state hospital, which provides for its own needs in these areas.

TREATMENT EFFICACY

Information related to the treatment efficacy of residential care facilities must be considered with respect to the goals of different facilities. For example, the family-oriented foster care home generally precludes its inclusion of sophisticated psychological services and, indeed, many would debate the utility of having such services available in these facilities. The key to understanding treatment effectiveness, therefore, is first to define the goals of the facility.

Residential Care as an Alternative to Hospitalization

In studying alternatives to hospitalization, Kiesler (1982b: 1327) has noted, based upon his own and three other reviews of the literature, that "within the limits of minimal scientific methodology there has been no single *un*successful effort to discover alternative treatment. That is, alternative care always is as good or better than hospitalization regarding outcomes and always is less expensive." Among the studies on alternatives to hospitalization reviewed by Kiesler (1982a), Braun et al. (1981), and Straw (1982) are three controlled studies which look at supervised residential care as an alternative to residence in a psychiatric hospital.

The first study, by Linn et al. (1977), describes 572 chronically hospitalized patients from five Veterans Administration (VA) hospitals. The patients were randomly assigned to foster care outside the hospital or continued hospitalization. Over a four-month period, more improvement in functioning and overall adjustment was reported for the experimental than for the hospital control group.

Mosher, Menn, and Matthews (1975; see also Mosher and Menn, 1978)

Table 10–1
Per Diem Residential Care Costs as a Percentage of the Costs of Care in State and County Mental Hospitals[a]

Year	Acute Hospital	State & County Mental Hospitals	Nursing Facility	Transitional Community Residence (Halfway House)	Supervised Group Home (Lodge)	Family Care/ Board & Care
1973[b]	—	100%	65%	34%	—	26%
1979[c]	—	100%	78%	55%	43%	22%
1987[b]	186%	100%	56%	32%	29%	9%

[a]Calculations based on figures derived from Chien and Cole (1973); Watt (1970); *Mental Disability Law Reporter* (March–April 1979); Greene (1986); and Lempinen (1987).

[b] Actual costs.

[c] Actuarially estimated costs based on programming for eight clients.

conducted a controlled trial, randomly assigning sixty-three newly admitted young schizophrenic patients to either a group home employing a nonmedical, nonprofessional staff (n-33) or a short-stay, crisis-oriented, inpatient ward where drugs were emphasized (n-30). Group home patients received significantly less psychiatric aftercare and medication, were readmitted to the hospital less often than control patients, did better occupationally, and were more likely to live independently at follow-up. They did not show any significant difference from the crisis ward cases in symptomatology over a two-year follow-up period.

A third study reported by Brook (1973) capitalized on the brief closure of the inpatient unit at the Fort Logan Mental Health Center in Colorado. All patients who would have been hospitalized in this unit were instead put in a "hostel" during the closure. Forty-nine residents underwent this hostel system's intervention treatment and were compared with the last forty-nine patients admitted to the inpatient unit. Since all patients presenting themselves for treatment were included, this comes very close to a true randomized design. Most hostel patients were acutely ill: almost half were diagnosed as moderate to high suicide risks; half were schizophrenic, and half of those were chronic; one-fourth were depressed; the remaining fourth of the patients had problems with alcohol and drug abuse, adjustment reactions, marital maladies, or obsessive compulsiveness. Of the forty-nine hostel patients, eleven had been previously hospitalized.

The hostel had no residential staffing, and neighbors helped with meals and occasional problems. The focus of treatment was generally upon the interpersonal relationships of the client, particularly with his or her family. Some treatment sessions with patients were held at the hostel, including some with the family; other sessions were held at the patient's home. Individual therapy occasionally supplemented these social systems interventions. When not in an evaluation or therapy session, patients continued their normal activities. The mean stay was 5.75 days. Patients were then transferred to outpatient status and scheduled for six to eight more sessions of family or individual therapy.

No differences distinguished the two groups on eleven outcome measures, although the hostel group continued to have more symptoms. Of the forty-nine hospitalized patients, six were subsequently readmitted within six months, whereas only one of the forty-nine patients in the hostel was admitted to hospitalization within six months after discharge.

It would thus appear that, as an alternative to use of the hospital, well-monitored residential care is an appropriate therapeutic choice. This is so regardless of the cost considerations which also argue in its favor.

Residential Care as an Alternative to Community Care

Few studies compare residential care to traditional hospital aftercare programs. One well-controlled study was the Fairweather Lodge Experiment (Fairweather et al., 1969), initiated following Fairweather's efforts to train patients on a hospital ward for release into the community (Fairweather, 1964). Fairweather found that patients could be trained very well on the ward. However, the recidivism rate was quite high. He concluded that training within the hospital had limited transferability without two crucial elements in the community: (1) a supportive living situation, and (2) an opportunity for employment. The Lodge program was established to create a community-based residential facility with those crucial components. The experiment recruited volunteer patients from the hospital treatment program and matched them on age, diagnosis, and length of hospitalization. They were then randomly assigned to either aftercare in the Lodge (i.e., the community living/work situation) (n-75), or the hospital's traditional community aftercare program (n-76). An additional component was set up to phase out professional supervision from the Lodge program in a manner that would enable it to become an independent economic entity.

Results of the study demonstrated that community tenure was greatly increased among participants in the Lodge program. Lodge residents also did better in employment efforts since they were employed in the facility's janitorial service. Once the Lodge facility closed, however, the employment involvement and general experience of former patients rapidly approached those of the group in the traditional community aftercare program. It would thus appear that the supportive residential community developed by Fairweather made a significant positive contribution to the aftercare situation of its participants, but that better outcomes could not be sustained without continued involvement in the Lodge program.

Another approach to looking at outcomes of residential care is to compare different types of facilities using alternative environmental variables. Wilder, Kessel, and Caulfield (1968) developed the notion of the high-expectation environment which reinforces normalcy by requiring the individual to be responsible for his own actions. Lamb and Goertzel (1971) investigated the differential effect of high vs. low or moderate expectations on residents of board-and-care homes and found no difference in the recidivism rates of the two groups. There was, however, a significant difference in subjects' social and vocational adjustment favoring the experimental group.

Segal and Moyles (1979) classified 234 residential care facilities into client-versus management-oriented environments. Thirty-six percent of the facilities could clearly be classified as client-oriented and 29 percent of them as management-oriented, based upon descriptions provided by observers and the managers of the facilities. A sample of 119 residents living in client-centered facilities was compared to a sample of 127 residents of management-centered facilities. Management-centered environments tended to be more productive of institutional dependency similar to that found in mental hospitals.

To date, there has been very little evaluation of the effect of different environments upon the chronically mentally ill in residential care. Rigorous evaluation is crucial, however, because the primary strength of the residential care system lies in its diversity and the potential ability to match clients to that community or facility environment which would allow for maximum social integration. Two studies, one by Segal, Baumohl, and Moyles (1980) and one by Moos and Igra (1980), directly address this concept of matching. Segal, Baumohl, and Moyles (1980) report their findings based upon a social integration criterion. They developed models to predict community-based facility residents' probable level of social integration in twenty-three different combinations of facility and community environments. Using a computer simulation, they then assigned each resident to a combination of community and facility environment which would maximize his or her predicted social integration score. The frequency distribution of total assignments across the range of alternative placements turned out to be rectangular rather than normal or peaked, making it clear that many different types of environments are required to satisfy the needs presented by a heterogeneous patient population. It would further appear that residential care holds considerable promise which is yet to undergo extensive evaluative research.

ANALYSIS OF PROBLEMS

The primary problem facing the mental health system today is a lack of affordable housing to maintain mentally disabled individuals in a community environment. The consequences of this—homelessness, inappropriate use of general hospital bed facilities, and overuse of long-term locked facilities and state mental hospital facilities—have received much discussion throughout the literature. Yet, in spite of this crisis in housing for the mentally ill, recent reports indicate that some major urban areas have experienced a decrease in the number of their residential care beds. For example, San Francisco has lost 250 beds among privately owned board-and-care facilities since 1980 (Lempinen, 1987). On paper it would appear that this loss was partially offset by the creation of new beds in lodges (that is, supervised group care facilities), transitional housing arrangements, and co-op assisted independent living arrangements, which increased their bed total by 118, from 300 to 418, over this same period. However, these facilities serve a transitional population and do not provide the long-term care characteristic of privately owned board-and-care facilities.

This situation has precipitated a crisis in general hospitals in the area. Because there are fewer spaces in residential care, many people in need of long-term care end up in general hospitals, which then produces overcrowding on general hospital wards. The consequence of this overcrowding has been a demand for more long-term beds to deal with difficult patients. There has also been an investment in locked nursing homes, with beds in these facilities increasing by 72.5 percent, from 200 beds to 345 beds, since 1980. In addition, beds in general hospital wards have also increased by 25.3 percent. So there have been more beds created in high cost, highly structured, and more restrictive environments since 1980 than total placements lost in one of the least restrictive residential care environments. The real concern that must be addressed, since this is a pattern that appears to be repeating itself in many areas of the country, is why we are losing residential board-and-care beds when they offer the least expensive arrangement for supervised housing.

The answer lies in an analysis of the problems of the board-and-care facility as a component of the residential care system. Perhaps the biggest problem faced by the board-and-care industry today is its negative image. Fifteen years of muckraking activity by the press, as well as reports on system abuses by the General Accounting Office, Social Security Administration, and the Congress, have depicted the whole board-and-care system as an aggregation of shoddy residential settings run by profit-hungry owners and managers. Stories of resident exploitation, abuse, and neglect abound. This muckraking activity has been so effective that the whole system of board and care, and virtually every residential facility in it, has been tarred with a negative steretype. The system has become a political pariah, making even minimal increases in funding extremely difficult to obtain. Only recently has some recognition been given to Van Putten and Spar's (1979) observation that the responsibility for producing the residents' passive and maladaptive behavior has been incorrectly attributed to board-and-care homes. These behaviors may be due less to the adverse effects of the facility than to the type of client usually selected for board and care. For it is "precisely these negative symptoms of schizophrenia (passivity, blunted affect, and lack of initiative), mistakenly attributed to the presumed inadequacies of the board and care environment, that have given the board and care a bad press" (Van Putten and Spar, 1979: 463).

This failure to recognize the interaction between client and facility characteristics is merely emblematic of the insufficient attention paid to residential resources within the U.S. mental health system. Unfortunately, in a time of severe competition for decreasing resources, transitional facility advocates themselves have fanned the fires of opposition to board and care, claiming themselves as the only true providers of an adequate residential environment. In doing so, they, along with services advocates (that is, individuals who see residential facilities as viable only to the extent that they provide some form of internal residential service provision), have inadvertently contributed to cuts in the system and the loss of needed long-term residential care beds.

By viewing residential board and care as a viable alternative to hospitalization with significant positive potential, despite its recognized problems, we can look beyond the stigma to examine the real problems faced by this category of facilities: questionable economic viability, ambiguity in service function, and community reaction or hostility.

Questionable Economic Viability

The residential care system largely operates as a free-market economy whereby residents carry the power to select their own facility. This results from the fact that the system is based on fee-for-service payment, with the resident providing the fee through a proxy type of voucher system, sponsored largely by the federal

SSI program. Residents have at their disposal an SSI check whose amount is geared to the going rate for independent living. However, this market is not entirely free since the price of residential care (or the amount residents can pay) is actually controlled by the state with no variance allowed from one area in the state to another. Consequently, homes in high-priced urban areas, such as San Francisco, are at a significant disadvantage compared with homes located in rural areas where housing costs are much lower. For this reason, a shift has occurred in the location of residential care homes from the cities to rural or suburban areas with lower property costs.

Rapid inflation in property values and interest rates since 1975 has also posed a significant obstacle to the entrance of new board-and-care providers. Individuals getting into the business during this time of high property values—and, until recently, high interest rates—have had an increasingly difficult time paying mortgage expenses while providing adequate care for their clientele.

To make matters worse, some states, such as California, have employed a two-tier system of funding because of the differential strength of political lobbies for different disabled groups. Until recently, California paid more money to residential facilities caring for the developmentally disabled than those caring for the mentally ill. Naturally, bed availability for the mentally ill has decreased since facility operators make more money caring for the developmentally disabled.

Blaustein and Viek (1985), based on a survey of twenty-nine residential care home facilities, indicate that operators identify the inability to make a profit, high mortgage payments, and the two-tiered system of reimbursement as the most significant threats to the long-term viability of the board-and-care system. In their national sample of board and care Ditmar et al. (1983) noted that only 6 percent of the owners-operators of such facilities reported having received federal, state, or local money to open or renovate their facilities. Thus, supplemental funding for the mentally ill is not available for residential care facilities.

Service Ambiguity

A board-and-care home, by definition, must provide meals, personal care when it is needed, and protective oversight. Ditmar et al. (1983) reported that 78.4 percent of residents rated the quality of meals as good in these facilities. Special diets were provided by 59.8 percent of facilities, snacks by 81.7 percent, and special meals when the regular meal was missed by 87.3 percent. Other personal care and support services were provided as detailed in Table 10–2.

While board-and-care facilities serving the mentally ill may not provide as much personal care and support service as other residential facilities for other disabled groups (Ditmar et al., 1983), they do provide a considerable amount given their funding arrangements. Operators of facilities also report significant effort facilitating relationships with local service agencies. Only 16 percent of the sample of operators failed to identify at least one service provider who came

Table 10–2
Percent of Board-and-Care Facilities Providing Specified Personal Care and Support Services

Personal Care Services:	%
bathing	48.7
dressing	37.8
brushing of hair	35.7
shaving	33.3
eating	17.2
toileting	18.1
Support Services:	
accompanying residents shopping	73.9
shopping for residents	62.9
helping with public transportation	61.0
providing transportation—professional	81.9
providing transportation—personal	50.8
making professional service appointments	93.3
managing spending money	65.5
doing personal laundry	72.3
planning outings	79.8
giving parties for special occasions	87.4

Source: Ditmar et al. (1983: 32).

regularly to the facility and thus was familiar with residents and their service needs. Slightly more than half (55 percent) of these operators identified at least one person from a mental health agency; 32 percent identified someone from a social service agency (Ditmar et al., 1983).

The extent of services that ideally should be provided in a residential care facility remains debatable, however. Segal and Aviram (1978) agree that residential care should represent a home environment more than a hospital environment and so should not provide a full spectrum of services. Instead, operators should make use of services already available in the community. When services are not available, as they often have not been, operators should raise questions and make complaints.

Ambiguity about the service function of the board-and-care home and the special economic problems for board and care in urban areas have led to the development of two types of homes. The first, the original family care home without internal services, operates on an economic shoestring. The second is a more highly capitalized, larger facility with a service component resembling a small institution rather than a residential group home. Both facility types are poorly staffed. The family care facility cannot afford to have supplemental or relief staff because it has so few residents. The major complaint of managers of these homes concerns their inability to take vacations or have time off. Minimal staff levels are also maintained in larger board-and-care homes for economic reasons. The larger facilities find it difficult to compete with transitional residences, which are usually supplemented in their operations by mental health staffing grants from state or county level agencies.

An additional problem in the residential care industry today is the young adult chronic population (Pepper, Kirshner, and Ryglewicz, 1981) because of their propensity for disruptive behavior and negative attitudes toward the mental health system. If this latter group is to be housed in board and care, these facilities will probably require a more extensive service structure to deal with the attendant strains on owners and managers.

Community Resistance

Communities generally remain neutral or unwilling hosts of residential care facilities. While only a small percentage of facilities experience ongoing negative community reactions (Dear and Taylor, 1979; Segal, Baumohl, and Moyles, 1980), the major problem associated with community resistance relates to the development of new facilities. No count exists of the number of failed attempts to establish new facilities, though it is clear, given the siting of facilities in politically unprotected areas, that community opposition is a significant problem which contributes to the lack of adequate residential care for the mentally ill in many locales (Segal, Baumohl, and Moyles, 1980).

Research is needed to ascertain the optimal types of neighborhoods for locating homes for the mentally ill. Glasscote, Gudeman, and Elpers (1971) have recommended siting in "anonymous neighborhoods" in which residents will not be noticed, and in which the facility is close to public transportation and shopping. The advantages of such a neighborhood, they argue, include both integration and convenience. Trute and Segal (1976) agree with the first of these advantages. Using census tract data, they found that the best predictor of social integration among sheltered care residents was location in a community neither extremely socially disorganized nor strongly socially cohesive. Most studies that discuss the siting of residential care homes for the mentally ill also assert that facilities should be similarly located (e.g., Linn et al., 1977; Sandall, Hawley, and Gordon, 1975; Mosher and Menn, 1978). It is crucial, given the goal of social integration of residents, for further investigation of this question, however. Not all anonymous neighborhoods are good places for facilities. Certainly ghettos, whose appeal in the siting process derives more from political feasibility than environmental qualities relevant to residents' well-being, have been shown by Segal and Aviram (1978) to be undesirable locations.

SUMMARY AND CONCLUSION

The most optimistic view of residential care, and particularly board and care, is that it is an inexpensive and potentially salutary solution to long-term care of the mentally ill. Operating on a shoestring, this system has already demonstrated its ability to provide adequate care for many mentally ill persons. The most pessimistic view is that this private entrepreneurial system is an exploitative one which leaves people at the mercy of unscrupulous managers who provide un-stimulating and poor quality environments. Undoubtedly, exploitation of the mentally ill does occur in some of these facilities. In general, however, the environments are better than those on the back wards of public mental hospitals. To date, the potential of this residential resource remains largely unfulfilled, and much evaluative research is needed. Yet without further investment in board-and-care homes the mental health system is likely to deteriorate, leading to the increased use of locked nursing facilities at a very high cost in human terms to the mentally ill, and in economic terms to the rest of society. Residential care is thus a necessary resource and one which should be a major focus of attention in the mental health system.

ACKNOWLEDGMENT

The research and writing of this chapter have been supported by the Robert Wood Johnson Foundation and the National Institute of Mental Health.

REFERENCES

Anthony, W. A., Cohen, M. R., and Cohen, B. F. 1984. Psychiatric Rehabilitation. In *The Chronic Mental Patient: Five Years Later*, ed. J. A. Talbott. Orlando, Fla.: Grune and Stratton.

Apte, R. Z. 1968. *Halfway Houses: A New Dilemma in Institutional Care*. Occasional Papers on Social Administration No. 27. London: G. Bell.

Bachrach, L. L. 1984. Principles of Planning for Chronic Psychiatric Patients: A Syn-thesis. In *The Chronic Mental Patient*, ed. J. A. Talbott. New York: Grune and Stratton.

Baumohl, J., and Miller, H. 1974. *Down and Out in Berkeley*. Berkeley: University of California, Berkeley.

Beard, J. H., Pitt, R. B., Fisher, S. H., and Goertzel, V. 1963. Evaluating the Effec-tiveness of a Psychiatric Rehabilitation Program. *American Journal of Ortho-psychiatry* 33: 701–712.

Betts, J., Stan, J., and Reynolds, P. 1981. A Checklist for Selecting Board and Care Homes for Chronic Mental Patients. *Hospital and Community Psychiatry* 32: 488–501.

Blaustein, M., and Viek, C. 1985. Survey of Board and Care Homeowners. San Francisco: Residential Care Task Force. Unpublished memo.

Braun, P., Kochansky, G., Shapiro, R., Greenberg, S., Gudeman, J. E., Johnson, S., and Shore, M. F. 1981. Overview: Deinstitutionalization of Psychiatric Patients, A Critical Review of Outcome Studies. *American Journal of Psychiatry* 138: 736–749.

Brook, B. D. 1973. An Alternative to Psychiatric Hospitalization for Emergency Patients. *Hospital and Community Psychiatry* 24: 621–624.

Brown, P. 1985. *The Transfer of Care*. London: Routledge and Kegan Paul.

California Commission on Health and the Economy. 1985. *California Community Mental Health Services Act*. Sacramento: California State Department of Mental Health.

Chien, C. P., and Cole, J. 1973. Landlord-supervised Cooperative Apartments: A New Modality for Community-based Treatment. *American Journal of Psychiatry* 130: 156–159.

Clarke, G. J. 1979. In Defense of Deinstitutionalization. *Health and Society* 57: 461–479.

Cuvelier, F. 1975. *Patterns of Interaction between Mental Patient and Caretaker*. Paper presented at International Symposium on Foster Family Care, Geel, Belgium.

Dear, M., and Taylor, S. M. 1979. *Community Attitudes toward Neighborhood Public Facilities*. Hamilton, Ontario: Department of Geography, McMaster University.

Ditmar, N., Smith, M. A., Bell, J. C., Jones, C., and Manzaures, M. S. 1983. *Board and Care for Elderly and Mentally Disabled Populations*. Unpublished final report to USDHHS for Contract No. HEW 100–79–0117, vols. 1–5.

Emerson, R. M., Rochford, E. B., and Shaw, L. 1981. Economics and Enterprise in Board and Care Homes for the Mentally Ill. *American Behavioral Scientist* 24: 771–785.

Fairweather, G. W., ed. 1964. *Social Psychology in Treating Mental Illness: An Experimental Approach*. New York: John Wiley.

Fairweather, G. W., Sanders, D. H., Maynard, H., Cressler, D. L., and Bleck, D. S. 1969. *Community Life for the Mentally Ill: An Alternative to Institutional Care*. Chicago: Aldine.

Faris, R.E.L., and Dunham, H. W. 1939. *Mental Disorders in Urban Areas: An Ecological Study of Schizophrenia and Other Psychoses*. Chicago: University of Chicago Press.

Glasscote, R. M., Gudeman, J. E., and Elpers, J. R. 1971. *Halfway Houses for the Mentally Ill*. Joint Information Service of the American Psychiatric Association and the National Association for Mental Health.

Goldman, H. H., Gattozzi, A. A., and Taube, C. A. 1981. Defining and Counting the Chronically Mentally Ill. *Hospital and Community Psychiatry* 32: 21–27.

Goldmeier, J., Mannino, F., and Shore, M. 1978. *New Directions in Mental Health Care: Cooperative Apartments*. Rockville, Md.: USDHEW, NIMH.

Greene, S., Witkin, M. J., Atay, J., Fell, A., and Manderscheid, R. W. 1986. State and County Mental Hospitals, United States 1982–83 and 1983–84, with Trend Analyses from 1973–74 to 1983–84. *Mental Health Statistical Note No. 176*. Rockville, Md.: USDHHS.

Grob, G. N. 1973. *Mental Institutions in America: Social Policy to 1875*. New York: Free Press.

Hauber, F. A., Bruininks, R. H., Hill, B. K., Lakin, K. C., and White, C. C. 1984. *National Census of Residential Facilities: Fiscal Year 1982*. Minneapolis: Center for Residential and Community Services, University of Minnesota, Project Report No. 19.

Kiesler, C. A. 1982a. Mental Hospitals and Alternative Care: Noninstitutionalization as Potential Public Policy for Mental Patients. *American Psychologist* 37: 349–361.

Kiesler, C. A. 1982b. Public and Professional Myths about Mental Hospitalization. *American Psychologist* 37: 1323–1339.

Kusserow, R. P. 1982. *Board and Care Homes: A Study of Federal and State Actions to Safeguard the Health and Safety of Board and Care Home Residents.* Washington, D.C.: USDHHS, Office of the Inspector General.

Lamb, H. R. 1981. Board and Care Home Wanderers. *Archives of General Psychiatry* 32: 488–501.

Lamb, H. R. 1984. Alternatives to Hospitals. In *The Chronic Mental Patient: Five Years Later*, ed. J. A. Talbott. New York: Grune and Stratton.

Lamb, H. R., and Goertzel, V. 1971. Discharged Mental Patients: Are They Really in the Community? *Archives of General Psychiatry* 24: 29–34.

Landy, D., and Greenblatt, M. 1965. *Halfway House: A Sociocultural and Clinical Study of Rutland Corner House.* Washington, D.C.: USDHEW.

Lee, D. T. 1963. Family Care: Selection and Prediction. *American Journal of Psychiatry* 120: 561–566.

Lempinen, E. W. 1987. Mental Health Funds Misspent, Critics Say. *San Francisco Chronicle*, June 2, 1987, p. 4.

Linn, M. W. 1981. Can Foster Care Survive? In *New Directions for Mental Health Services: Issues in Community Residential Care*, ed. R. D. Budson. No. 11. San Francisco: Jossey-Bass.

Linn, M. W., Caffey, E. M., Klett, C. J., and Hogarty, G. 1977. Hospital Versus Community (Foster) Care for Psychiatric Patients. *Archives of General Psychiatry* 34: 78–83.

Linn, M. W., Klett, J., and Caffey, E. M. 1980. Foster Home Characteristics and Psychiatric Patient Outcome. *Archives of General Psychiatry* 37: 129–132.

McCoin, J. M. 1983. *Adult Foster Homes: Their Managers and Residents.* New York: Human Sciences Press.

Melick, C. F., and Eysaman, C. O. 1978. A Study of Former Patients Placed in Private Proprietary Homes. *Hospital and Community Psychiatry* 29: 587–589.

Melody, J. 1979. *Service Delivery Assessment of Boarding Homes.* Technical Report Region 3, DHHS, Philadelphia.

Mental Disability Law Reporter. 1979. Community-Based Residential Services for Mental Health Clients. *Mental Disability Law Reporter* 3: 150–154.

Moos, R., and Igra, A. 1980. Determinants of the Social Environments of Sheltered Care Settings. *Journal of Health and Social Behavior* 21: 88–98.

Morrissey, J. R. 1967. *The Case for Family Care of the Mentally Ill.* Community Mental Health Journal Monograph No. 2. New York: Behavioral Publications.

Mosher, L. R., and Menn, A. 1978. Community Residential Treatment for Schizophrenia: A Two Year Follow-up. *Hospital and Community Psychiatry* 29: 715–723.

Mosher, L. R., Menn, A., and Matthews, S. M. 1975. Soteria: Evaluation of a Home-based Treatment for Schizophrenia. *American Journal of Orthopsychiatry* 45: 455–467.

Murphy, M. B., Ingelsmann, F., and Tcheng-Laroche, F. 1976. The Influence of Foster-Home Care on Psychiatric Patients. *Archives of General Psychiatry* 33: 179–183.

Murphy, J. M., Sobol, A. M., Neff, R. K., Olivier, D. C., and Leighton, A. H. 1984. Stability of Prevalence: Depression and Anxiety Disorders. *Archives of General Psychiatry* 41: 990–997.

National Institute of Mental Health. 1976. *Community Living Arrangements for the Mentally Ill and Disabled: Issues and Options for Public Policy.* Rockville, Md.

Pepper, B., Kirshner, M. D., and Ryglewicz, H. 1981. The Young Adult Chronic Patient: Overview of a Population. *Hospital and Community Psychiatry* 32: 463–469.

Regier, D., Myers, J. K., Kramer, M., Robins, L. N., Blazer, D. G., Hough, R. L., Eaton, W. W., and Locke, B. Z. 1984. The NIMH Epidemiologic Catchment Area Program. *Archives of General Psychiatry* 41: 934–941.

Sandall, H., Hawley, T. T., and Gordon, G. C. 1975. The St. Louis Community Homes Program: Graduated Support for Longterm Care. *American Journal of Psychiatry* 132: 617–622.

Scull, A. T. 1977. *Decarceration*. Englewood Cliffs, N. J.: Prentice-Hall.

Segal, S. P., and Moyles, E. W. 1979. Management Style and Institutional Dependency in Sheltered Care. *Social Psychiatry* 14: 159–165.

Segal, S. P., and Aviram, U. 1978. *The Mentally Ill in Community-Based Sheltered Care: A Study of Community Care and Social Integration*. New York: John Wiley.

Segal, S. P., and Baumohl, J. 1981. Toward Harmonious Community Care Placement. In *New Directions for Mental Health Services: Issues in Community Residential Care*, ed. R. Budson. No. 11. San Francisco: Jossey-Bass.

Segal, S. P., Baumohl, J., and Johnson, E. 1977. Falling through the Cracks. *Social Problems* 24: 387–400.

Segal, S. P., Baumohl, J., and Moyles, E. W. 1980. Neighborhood Types and Community Reaction to the Mentally Ill: A Paradox of Intensity. *Journal of Health and Social Behavior* 24: 345–359.

Shadoan, R. 1985. Levels of Care for Residential Treatment in an Urban Setting. *Psychiatric Annals* 15: 639–641.

Shapiro, S., Skinner, A., Kessler, L. G., VonKorff, M., German, P. S., Tischler, G. L., Leaf, P. S., Benham, L., Cottler, L., and Regier, D. A. 1984. Utilization of Health and Mental Health Services. *Archives of General Psychiatry* 41: 971–983.

Sherwood, C. C., and Seltzer, M. M. 1981. *Evaluation of Board and Care Homes*. Boston: Boston University School of Social Work.

Sherwood, S., and Gruenberg, L. 1979. *Domiciliary Care Management Information System*. Boston, Mass.: Department of Social Gerontological Research. Mimeographed.

Srole, L. 1977. Geel, Belgium: The Natural Therapeutic Community. In *New Trends of Psychiatry in the Community*, eds. G. Serbin and B. Astrachan. Cambridge, Mass.: Ballinger.

Straw, R. B. 1982. Meta-analysis of Deinstitutionalization in Mental Health. Unpublished doctoral dissertation, Northwestern University.

Trute, B., and Segal, S. P. 1976. Census Tract Predictors and the Social Integration of Sheltered Care Residents. *Social Psychiatry* 11: 153–161.

U.S. Congress, Congressional Budget Office. 1977. *Long-term Care for the Elderly and Disabled*. Washington, D.C.

U.S. General Accounting Office. 1977. *Summary of a Report on Returning the Mentally Disabled to the Community: Government Needs to Do More, Report to the Congress*. Washington, D.C.

U.S. General Accounting Office. 1979. *Identifying Board Homes Housing the Needy, Aged, Blind, and Disabled: A Major Step toward Resolving a National Problem*. Washington, D.C.

Van Putten, T., and Spar, J. E. 1979. The Board and Care Home: Does It Deserve a Bad Press? *Hospital and Community Psychiatry* 30: 461–463.

Watt, N. 1970. Five Year Follow-up of Geriatric Chronically Ill Mental Patients in Foster Home Care. *Journal of the American Geriatric Society* 18: 310–316.

Weisbrod, B. A., Test, M. A., and Stein, L. I. 1980. Alternative to Mental Hospital Treatment, II: Economic Benefit-cost Analysis. *Archives of General Psychiatry* 37: 400–405.

Wilder, J. F., Kessel, M., and Caulfield, S. C. 1968. Follow-up of a "High Expectations" Halfway House. *American Journal of Psychiatry* 124: 103–109.

11

Nursing Homes as Community Mental Health Facilities

MARGARET W. LINN
and SHAYNA STEIN

By the year 1976, nursing homes in the United States housed more mentally ill patients than state mental hospitals (Sirrocco and Koch, 1977). Furthermore, more recent evidence suggests that this trend is continuing, with nursing homes being the largest single setting for the care of the mentally ill (U.S. Department of Health and Human Services, 1981). By 1977, the National Nursing Home Survey confirmed that nursing homes were already the number one institutional caretaker of the severely emotionally disturbed in this country. Between 1965 and 1979, the rates of institutionalization of elderly patients (sixty-five years and over) in state mental hospitals dropped from 773 per 100,000 to 164 per 100,000, a decrease of 79 percent (Taube and Barrett, 1983). This decrease was partly a result of increased placement of older residents in nursing homes. Between 1939 and 1978, the number of nursing facilities grew from 1,200 to 18,722, including 4,749 skilled nursing homes. The number of beds in nursing homes also grew during the same period from 25,000 to 1.3 million (Fox and Clauser, 1980). It has been projected that between the years 1980 and 2005, the number of nursing home residents will increase from 1,413,331 to 2,090,253 persons, an increase of 48 percent (Schmidt et al., 1977). There is evidence to suggest that the majority of these residents will have significant emotional problems. This shift in the care for mental patients from hospitals to community nursing homes has led some to call nursing homes the "new back wards in the community" (Mechanic, 1980).

This chapter will trace the history of the development of nursing homes as a locus of care for the mentally ill, describe attempts to determine prevalence of mental disorders in nursing homes, describe studies related to the outcome of psychiatric patients in nursing homes, suggest ways of improving the quality of nursing home care, and comment on consideration of alternative placements for psychiatric patients.

HISTORICAL PERSPECTIVE

Use of the community nursing home as a mental health facility is an outgrowth of contemporary public policies and legislation affecting reimbursement for medical care. The concept of providing sheltered care for the chronically mentally ill and aged developed in this country largely in response to the crusade of Dorothea Dix (Mechanic, 1980). Prior to the 1800s, relatively few attained old age. Colonial America modelled its approach to the needy after the English, with almshouses established as residences for the dependent members of society. Almshouses, supported by local governing bodies, rarely were desirable places to live. In 1923, more than half of the 78,000 almshouse residents were over sixty-five, and another 20 percent were between fifty-five and sixty-five (Vladeck, 1980). During the early 1920s, charitable private homes for the aged, supported by immigrant self-help groups, also housed about as many elderly as did almshouses. The establishment of these homes, forerunners of today's nursing homes, was largely the result of efforts by the Charitable Organization Societies, voluntary organizations whose purpose was screening applicants for outdoor relief (Moroney and Kuntz, 1975). A belief that the stigma of pauperism could not be eradicated from the administration of public charities contributed to the perception that private homes for the elderly would be more respectable than public facilities. Nevertheless, there was no organized means for delivering medical or other services in almshouses or private homes for the aged. Although local government accepted responsibility for the aged in need and for the infirm, only custodial services were provided. Partly because of the lack of services in almshouses and private homes, by 1930 more people over sixty-five resided in mental hospitals than in almshouses and private custodial homes combined (Vladeck, 1980).

Effects of Social Security

Passage of the Social Security Act of 1935 gave many elderly the financial means to make a choice about their living arrangements. Old Age and Survivors Insurance (OASI) provided monthly payments to persons sixty-five or older with benefits covered by employment, and Old Age Assistance (OAA) made payments to the needy aged. Many elderly persons were no longer forced by poverty to live in public institutions. In fact, no OAA payments could be made to persons living in a public institution. Perhaps the greatest victory of this legislation was the philosophical change it represented, lessening the stigma of immorality with which poverty in old age had been associated. With the depression of the 1930s and the newly acquired financial resources of the elderly, boarding homes, convalescent homes, and nursing homes became more numerous. The Social Security Act, however, contained no provisions for health insurance. Although voluntary health insurance and hospitals enjoyed intensified growth during this period, the elderly in boarding homes and nursing homes had no direct linkage to medical services. Moreover, emphasis was on acute care in hospitals, not on supportive care needed for the chronically ill in nursing homes. In addition, the quality of care in convalescent settings was relatively unsupervised and unregulated in the 1930s and 1940s.

Amendments to the Social Security Act in 1950 permitted federal matching of direct payments by state and local welfare agencies to parties other than beneficiaries. In other words, suppliers of health services were now eligible to receive government support for medical care to the needy. There would no longer be a prohibition on payments to residents of public medical facilities. Also, this legislation required states making such payments to residents of public institutions or to vendors of services to establish a program for licensing nursing homes. Though no specific licensing regulations or the means for enforcing them were provided, it was a beginning.

Hill-Burton Legislation and the Ideological Transformation of the Nursing Home

Medical care and the need for hospital services became paramount after World War II. In 1946, the Hospital Survey and Construction Act (Public Law 79–725), known after its principal sponsors as the Hill-Burton Act, was passed. With this large-scale infusion of new funding, instead of places to die, hospitals became identified as places to receive treatment and recover. In 1954, the legislation was amended to provide grants to public and nonprofit entities to construct nursing homes. By including nursing homes under the auspices of nonprofit and public hospitals, it was hoped that the same quality found in hospitals might prevail in nursing homes. Subsidies required that the nursing home operate in conjunction with a hospital. Even though little was actually spent on nursing homes through Hill-Burton, nursing homes would no longer be thought of as solely part of the welfare system. They were transformed, at least by definition, into medical facilities, under the jurisdiction of the Public Health Service.

The Kerr-Mills Bill

The post-World War II focus on medical care coincided with, and contributed to, the growing numbers of elderly. From 1950 to 1965, persons over age sixty-five had grown from 12.3 million to 18.2 million (U.S. Department of Health, Education, and Welfare, 1965). Severe bed shortages in hospitals developed, in part, from the increase in the elderly chronically ill. Consequently, more referrals were made to nursing homes for patients less able to pay for long-term hospital care. Passage of Medical Assistance for the Aged in 1960 (Public Law 86–778), known as the Kerr-Mills Bill, increased federal support for medical care vendor payment programs for the aged, thereby contributing to the deinstitutionalization of older patients from state mental hospitals. As a result of the Kerr-Mills Bill, the federal government became more involved in providing the funds for the health care needs of the aged and set the stage for what was to come.

The Social Security Amendments of 1965—Medicare and Medicaid

Public Law 89–97 established an individual right to medical care and a government responsibility for ensuring that right. Medicare, under Title XVIII, provided extended care benefits (100 days) if the beneficiary had spent at least three days in the hospital. Medicaid, under Title XIX, extended medical coverage to all persons, regardless of age, who received cash welfare benefits from federal programs or met state-established criteria. Medicare was viewed as an extension of Social Security, whereas Medicaid was part of the welfare administration. It was Medicaid, or Title XIX, that contributed largely to deinstitutionalization by providing financial support for the transfer of mental patients from state hospitals to community nursing homes. By transferring psychiatric patients to nursing homes, the states were able to receive 50 percent or more from the federal government for the cost of care. Despite matching federal funds, Medicaid programs put financial pressures on state budgets. States could control their costs by the manner in which they reimbursed institutions and providers. Reduction in payments to institutions, in many cases, resulted in the provision of only perfunctory care.

Medicare recipients were eligible for only 190 lifetime days in a private or public psychiatric institution, resulting in an increased use of psychiatric units in general hospitals by the elderly. These general hospitals were not subject to the same 190-day limitation since they were not considered psychiatric institutions. Patients hospitalized in state facilities before Medicare went into effect, however, were not eligible for the 190-day lifetime maximum for inpatient psychiatric care. They were able to receive nursing home benefits through Medicaid only (Stotsky and Stotsky, 1983). Partly as a result of Public Law 89–97, state mental hospital populations were reduced by two-thirds over a 15-year period as patients were placed in nursing homes and other community care facilities (Bassuk and Gerson, 1978).

The Moss Amendments

A major incentive for Medicare and Medicaid was concern over rising hospital costs, and the nursing home was considered a less costly alternative to hospital care. The extended care facility (ECF) of the Medicare program and the skilled nursing homes (SNF) of Medicaid were used increasingly as alternatives to acute care general hospitals (Moroney and Kuntz, 1975). However, concern about quality of care in nursing homes surfaced in the mid–1960s. A Subcommittee on Long-Term Care of the Senate Special Committee on Aging, headed by Senator Frank Moss (D., Utah), pointed out severe problems in the nursing home industry: poor sanitary conditions, absent or limited patient activities, untrained and inadequate administrators, shortages in staffing, fire hazards, and absent or inadequate food or diets. As a result of these findings, Moss introduced legislation calling for stricter federal standards under Medicaid, later incorporated into the Social Security Amendments of 1967. Unfortunately, the recommendations were not adhered to as proposed. Nursing standards were the central issue, with the subcommittee recommending a registered nurse (RN) as director of nursing staff and adequate nursing services twenty-four hours each day. The final version of the law substituted licensed practical nurse (LPN) for RN and all references to the number of nurses needed for adequate patient care were dropped. A major outgrowth of Moss's proposals, however, was the development of intermediate care facilities (ICFs). Fearing loss of funding with increased demands for improved patient care, nursing home operators argued that many patients did not need skilled nursing care. With Medicaid already burdened with spiraling costs for nursing homes, almost $907 million between 1965 and 1967 (Moroney and Kuntz, 1975), it was not difficult to convince Congress to enact legislation to provide for less expensive institutional care.

Public Law 90–248—The "Miller Amendment"

ICFs were established by law in 1967. Because these facilities were not medical in orientation, they were not funded under Medicaid, but rather under cash assistance titles of the Social Security Act with the federal matching share computed using Medicaid formulas. The result was the wholesale reclassification of all substandard nursing homes as ICFs with almost no sanitary or safety standards established until 1971. In 1971, ICFs were brought under Title XIX, or Medicaid. It has been estimated that by 1977, approximately 65 percent of the ICF residents were former mental patients (Shadish and Bootzin, 1981a).

Public Law 92–603

The White House Conference on Aging of 1971, and the Nixon Administration of the early 1970s, focused further on the inadequacies of nursing home care. Congress enacted Public Law 92–603, which amended Medicare and Medicaid. Professional Standards Review Organizations (PSROs) were created to monitor the quality of medical care, and Supplemental Security Income (SSI) was established in 1972, combining into one federal program the previous forms of categorical aid to the blind, disabled, and aged. Medicare's ECFs and Medicaid's

SNFs were redefined as SNFs with a single set of standards, and both SNFs and ICFs would now be subject to independent professional review.

Medicare and Medicaid in the 1980s

In 1980, about 23 million Americans received Medicaid benefits, including approximately 30 percent of the disabled recipients of SSI (Schulz, 1985). The SSI program is important in long-term care because of its relationship to Medicaid eligibility and domiciliary care. The law provides automatic Medicaid eligibility for SSI beneficiaries unless states choose to adopt more stringent standards (Harrington et al., 1985). Medicaid provides federal funds from general revenue to states establishing qualifying medical assistance programs. Federal cost sharing varies from 50 percent to 80 percent depending on a state's per capita income. Persons who have severe long-term disabilities, including those with chronic mental illness, are eligible for SSI if they have no covered employment and can establish financial need according to state standards. In many states, all SSI recipients are eligible for Medicaid. Some states place additional income and disability requirements on SSI beneficiaries. Disabled persons who do not qualify for SSI may be eligible for Medicaid in states with a "medically needy" program (Rubin, 1981). Medicaid is the largest source of public funding for long-term care, and pays the Medicare deductible and coinsurance for eligible persons. About 13 percent of those on Medicare are covered by Medicaid (Harrington et al., 1985). In 1979, about 87 percent of the $10 billion in public funding for nursing home care was provided by the Medicaid program. By contrast, Medicare paid less than 3 percent of all nursing home expenditures (Fox and Clauser, 1980). Until 1988, Medicare payments for nursing home services covered only skilled nursing care and paid for up to 100 days of service after each spell of hospitalized illness of at least three days, excluding psychiatric care. The Medicare Catastrophic Coverage Act of 1988 (Public Law 100–36) eliminated the prior hospitalization requirement for nursing home coverage, increased the days covered to 150 in any calendar year, and increased payment to psychiatrists treating patients in nursing homes to the new outpatient annual limits as set by the Omnibus Budget Reconciliation Act of 1987 (see chapter 14 in this volume). Patients with psychiatric diagnoses requiring acute psychiatric treatment with twenty-four hour supervision are not considered appropriate for nursing homes. Persons with psychiatric diagnoses who have physical conditions requiring nursing home care could be admitted to nursing homes. Although Alzheimer's disease and other forms of dementia are still considered mental disorders, they were excluded from the category of psychiatric diagnoses.

The Medicare payment rate is predetermined and based on allowable and fixed costs as defined by the program. Allowable costs under Medicaid are based on a specific state's cost and accounting principles. Even though federal contributions account for about half of Medicaid expenditures, states still have a major role in financing Medicaid. Program growth has been about one-third to one-half higher than the growth rate of state revenues (Bovbjerg and Holahan, 1982). Moreover, recent changes in the federal government's budgetary allocations, which limit the growth of federal expenditures under Medicaid, have resulted in more stringent state eligibility policies, as well as other efforts to reduce costs (Harrington et al., 1985).

Federal financial participation in state Medicaid programs has been disallowed for services rendered in nursing homes considered institutions for mental disease (IMDs). This classification has been made in situations in which more than 50 percent of the patients have mental illnesses which require inpatient treatment according to the patients' medical records (Jazwieck and Press, 1986). In 1983, this rule was modified so that residents with organic mental disorders would not count against the 50 percent ceiling (*State Medicaid Manual*, 1983). One of the major consequences of this requirement has been the failure to appropriately diagnose mental illness in nursing home patients and a subsequent lack of treatment. Actual standards for the care of psychiatric patients in nursing homes do not exist (Goldman, Feder, and Scanlon, 1986). As of 1981, it was estimated that there were 750,000 elderly mentally ill residing in the more than 23,600 nursing homes in this country. Nursing homes are now the largest single setting for the institutional care of the mentally ill, exceeding the number of mentally ill in state mental institutions by some 600,000 (U.S. Department of Health and Human Services, 1981). Yet, as Talbott (1981: 700) has stated, "No nursing home in the country employs a full-time psychiatrist, and few offer any form of psychiatric rehabilitation, except periodic visits from psychiatric consultants, or employ mental health professionals."

OTHER FACTORS CONTRIBUTING TO DEINSTITUTIONALIZATION AND USE OF NURSING HOMES

Transfer of large numbers of mentally ill from state mental hospitals, most of whom went to nursing homes, was also facilitated by other factors such as introduction of psychotropic medications, development of community mental health programs, court decisions which gave patients the right to demand treatment in mental health facilities, as well as the right to refuse treatment, and the social and political climate of the times (Shadish and Bootzin, 1981b).

Psychotropic Medications

It is unlikely that significant reductions in mental hospital populations, irrespective of fiscal decisions and social forces, could have been initiated or sustained without psychotropic drugs, most especially the phenothiazines (Mechanic, 1986). Psychoactive drugs, such as thorazine, were helpful in blunting bizarre symptoms. It is only in the more recent past that the importance of high quality drug monitoring for the prevention and management of risk factors, such as tardive dyskinesia, has been stressed (Kane and Smith, 1982).

Community Mental Health Centers

As described in earlier chapters of this volume, in 1955 Congress established the Joint Commission on Mental Illness and Health to evaluate services for the mentally ill and to formulate a national mental health program. In 1961, the commission published *Action for Mental Health*, calling for an increased program of services, which led to the passage of the Mental Retardation Facilities and Community Mental Health Centers Construction Act of 1963 (Public Law 88–164). The goal was to reduce state hospital populations by 50 percent within two decades. Five essential services were to be provided: inpatient care, outpatient care, emergency treatment, partial hospitalization, and consultation and education. By the end of the 1970s, a total of approximately 760 federally funded community mental health centers had been established, the resident population of state and county mental hospitals had dropped to 140,000 from a high of 559,000 in 1955, and outpatient treatment was accounting for 73 percent of all mental health treatment episodes (Kramer, 1986). Nevertheless, a large percentage of discharged patients was being readmitted to state hospitals (albeit for shorter stays), and deinstitutionalization was being labelled reinstitutionalization (Goldman, Adams, and Taube, 1983), as large numbers of patients went directly from state hospitals to nursing homes. As Bachrach (1976) pointed out, deinstitutionalization largely ignored the needed custodial and asylum function of mental hospitals.

Changes in the Law

Changes in laws regarding civil commitment, the right to treatment, and the right to refuse treatment affected deinstitutionalization (Stone, 1975; Lamb and Mills, 1986). For example, in 1967 California adopted the Lanterman-Petris-Short Act, which specified that in order to be committed a person must be either dangerous or not have the capacity to care for himself. Also, length of treatment had to be determinate and brief, and committed persons were given rapid access to the courts and public defenders. Emphasis was placed on the rights of patients with little consideration given for their treatment needs. Even patients in need of hospitalization could not be kept long enough for appropriate medications to become effective. In 1971, the famous case of *Wyatt v. Stickney* established minimum standards for treatment of committed mentally ill, and the case of *O'Connor v. Donaldson* in 1975 gave nondangerous patients their freedom from commitment, especially when treatment was not being provided. As a result of good intentions without forethought, large ghettos of discharged patients, many of whom were homeless (Lamb, 1984), were created.

Social and Political Climate of Mid-Century America

Goffman (1961) has characterized mental hospitals as total institutions contributing to the breakdown of prior social roles and to fostering dependency.
The 1960s was a period in which custodial care in any institution was viewed
as untherapeutic and harmful to potential rehabilitation (Mechanic, 1986). During
the 1950s and 1960s, emphasis in psychiatry was on psychodynamic treatment,
but the growth of the inpatient population, which reached its peak in 1955, did
not permit intensive therapy, or sometimes any therapy, to flourish in mental
hospitals. Thus, the reform movement started by Dorothea Dix to build state
institutions to house the severely disturbed now gave way to a new wave of
well-intentioned reform, to release from these hospitals persons who were seen
as being denied optimal treatment.

The National Plan

Under the Carter administration, there were efforts to alter the statutory requirement categorizing nursing homes as ''mental institutions'' if 50 percent or
more of the patients had a psychiatric diagnosis. The National Plan for the
Chronically Mentally Ill (U.S. Department of Health and Human Services, 1980),
based on recommendations and data presented by the President's Commission
on Mental Health, resulted in the short-lived Mental Health Systems Act (Public
Law 96–398) of 1980, which subsequently was displaced by the state block
grants of the Reagan administration. Of all the recommendations made in the
National Plan, the only remnant was the continuation of the Community Support
Program, a federal program for the chronically mentally ill to provide comprehensive care through local case management (Talbott and Sharfstein, 1986).

The Alcohol, Drug Abuse, and Mental Health Services
Block Grant and the Gramm-Rudman-Hollings Balanced
Budget Act

Enacted in 1981 under the Omnibus Budget Reconciliation Act, the Alcohol,
Drug Abuse, and Mental Health (ADAMH) block grant essentially left planning
and implementation of community mental health services up to the states. As a
result of this legislation, any specific federal impetus through program design
was lost. States could now use block grant funds as they wished within fairly
wide parameters. Yet, federal funding for mental health decreased substantially
between fiscal years 1981 and 1988. Total funding for the constituent programs
in the ADAMH block grant declined by $54 million during this period, and
states did not entirely make up the substantial losses (see chapter 7 in this
volume).

In March of 1985, the Balanced Budget and Emergency Deficit Control Act
(Public Law 99–177), known as the Gramm-Rudman-Hollings Balanced Budget

Act, went into effect. The law called for reductions in federal spending in 1986 of $2 billion, including reductions in the block grant by withholding 4.3 percent of the 1986 appropriations (*Mental Health Services for the Elderly*, 1986). Federal contribution to Medicare, Medicaid, the Community Support Program, as well as other programs designed to help the elderly, was decreased.

Despite the efforts of those who worked on the National Plan in the 1970s and those who participated in the 1981 White House Conference on Aging (which focused on the delivery of mental health services to older adults), to this day nursing homes remain the primary institutional setting for the chronically mentally ill, but without the necessary incentives for appropriate treatment of these patients. The regulation requiring nursing homes not house over 50 percent of patients with psychiatric diagnoses (excluding organic mental conditions) for Medicaid reimbursement resulted in many mentally ill residents going undiagnosed and untreated.

PREVALENCE OF MENTAL ILLNESS IN NURSING HOMES

Determining prevalence of mental illness among nursing home residents is complicated by a number of factors. Some patients are transferred directly to nursing homes from mental hospitals and their likelihood of having a confirmed psychiatric diagnosis is high. Other individuals may enter the nursing home as a substitute to entering the mental hospital and may or may not have a confirmed diagnosis. Still others already residing in a nursing home may develop psychiatric illness and go undiagnosed. Determining prevalence requires that truly random samples of a large number of nursing homes be selected and patients interviewed by psychiatrists using established criteria for mental disorder such as those found in the American Psychiatric Association's *Diagnostic and Statistical Manual-III-Revised*. Studies that attempt to diagnose patients using information collected from the patients are seriously handicapped by the ability of older individuals who are often cognitively impaired to provide reliable data. Thus, up to half of a sample of patients may have to be excluded because they cannot communicate adequately. Despite the inherent problems, a number of surveys and studies have attempted to define the number of psychiatric patients in nursing home settings. It is little wonder that statistics vary greatly from lows of about 30 percent to well over 75 percent.

Until recently, data on the prevalence of mental illness in nursing homes had been lacking. The *National Nursing Home Survey of 1977* (1979), for example, gave only the number and percentage of residents who, when last examined, had a primary diagnosis of mental disorder or senility without psychosis, and the number of residents with a chronic mental disorder or senility. Only one primary diagnosis was recorded for each patient, though more than one condition could be listed by nursing staff. However, reimbursement policies of Medicaid would certainly mitigate against the tendency to give a primary diagnosis of a particular mental disorder. It was not until 1983 that organic mental syndrome could be excluded from the 50 percent limitation on persons with mental illness in nursing homes before Medicaid considered the facility an institution for mental disease and refused to pay for care. Therefore, it is reasonable to believe that the findings of the *National Nursing Home Survey* grossly underestimate the actual extent of mental illness in nursing homes. With this in mind, of the 1.3 million nursing home residents in 1977, about 514,000 were classified as purely physically ill, 72,000 as purely chronically mentally ill, 35,000 as having both physical and mental diagnoses, and 561,000 as senile with about three-quarters of these persons also having physical disorders. More than 7.6 percent of the mentally ill patients, compared with 1.6 percent of the physically ill patients, were younger than 45 years of age. A majority of them presented behavioral problems, such as agitation, abusiveness, or wandering. Chronically mentally ill residents were more likely to have long-term institutional involvement. They were more likely to have come from other health care facilities and were less likely to be discharged to the community once placed (Goldman, Feder, and Scanlon, 1986).

The first study designed specifically for the purpose of examining the extent of psychiatric illness in nursing homes was done in New York (Goldfarb, 1962). The study of 506 residents in nine long-term care facilities found that 87 percent had a psychiatric disorder. Fourteen years later, Teeter and associates (1976) reported that 85 percent of patients in two skilled nursing homes had significant psychiatric disorders and two-thirds of the disorders had not been diagnosed.

In a survey of nursing home residents in New York and Texas sponsored by the U.S. General Accounting Office (1982), records of 617 patients in a county multilevel facility and those of 240 patients in two proprietary nursing homes in Buffalo were reviewed; an additional 140 records from three nursing homes in Texas also were reviewed. The focus was to determine the prevalence of serious disorders that played a key role in institutionalization. Chronic psychotic illnesses of former state hospital patients and chronic brain syndrome were the most frequently diagnosed mental problems affecting over half of the residents. Only minimal psychiatric treatment was available to the former state hospital patients with almost no mental health treatment provided for the other mentally ill residents. Failure to accurately diagnose and treat emotional problems of nursing home residents has been found in other studies as well (Barnes and Raskind, 1981; Sabin, Vitug, and Mark, 1982). Miller and Elliott (1976), who examined the medical records of 100 patients consecutively admitted to two nursing homes, concluded that over 80 percent of all errors in primary diagnoses resulted from failure to correctly identify a disabling neurologic or psychiatric condition. This is particularly distressing since it is probable that many of these residents could be helped if, as a first step, proper diagnoses of their illnesses were made.

More recently, Rovner and associates (1986) studied a random sample of 50 residents from among 180 residents of a proprietary intermediate-care nursing home. What makes this study unique is that residents were examined by a psychiatrist to assess functional status, presence of chronic disease, psychiatric diagnosis, and degree of cognitive impairment using standardized clinical examinations of individuals. Results showed that 47 residents (94 percent) had a major psychiatric disorder, most often dementia (56 percent). Only one of the residents had a history of psychiatric hospitalization. Seventy-six percent had at least one behavioral problem, such as being disruptive, restless, noisy, and verbally and passively aggressive. Findings were consistent with other studies (Barnes and Raskind, 1981; Rovner et al., 1986) in terms of the prevalence of cognitive impairment. A limitation of this study was that the sample was a cohort of patients admitted from the date the nursing home opened and represented a heterogeneous mixture of residents with variable lengths of stay. In addition, whether a small sample of one nursing home is representative of others throughout the country cannot be determined. Nursing homes are known to vary geographically in patient characteristics, admission policies, lengths of stay, and other variables. However, one implication from the Rovner study is that the nursing home has become a long-term psychiatric facility in terms of its resident population, but appropriate diagnoses and treatment are lacking. Although many other sources would disagree, the *National Nursing Home Survey* (1979) suggests that the majority of the mentally ill in nursing homes are not there because of the transfer of large numbers of persons from state hospitals to nursing homes, illustrated by the fact that between the years 1973 and 1974 only 8 percent of nursing home admissions were from mental hospitals or other long-term specialty hospitals. However, poor record-keeping in nursing homes and the financial disincentives to diagnose mental illness accurately are likely to have resulted in underestimates of the problem (German, Shapiro, and Kramer, 1986). If the results of an in-depth look at the extent of mental illness in nursing homes, as reported by Rovner and associates (1986), are generalizable to other facilities, then one can conclude that the majority of nursing home residents have a diagnosable mental illness.

OUTCOMES OF PSYCHIATRIC PATIENTS IN NURSING HOMES

As an element of the mental health system, nursing homes provide primarily custodial care (Bootzin and Shadish, 1986). They are very much like the institutions that the deinstitutionalization movement had intended to eliminate. Moreover, nursing homes are geared to providing physical health care to the aged (Rosenfeld, 1978) and, partly as a result, many mental problems go undetected and sometimes worsen. For example, depression can be misdiagnosed as organic disease (Katon, 1984). However, if diagnosed properly, depression can be effectively treated. A survey and field study conducted by the Joint Information Service of the American Psychiatric Association and the National Association of Mental Health (Glasscote et al., 1976) explored the quality of care of mentally impaired older persons discharged or diverted from mental hospitals to nursing and board-and-care homes. Visits made to ninety-one facilities throughout the country found that nursing homes made little distinction in care on the basis of psychiatric diagnosis, and many depressed patients' illnesses went unnoticed and untreated. Lack of contact with the mental health system, lack of trained staff, lack of family involvement, and overplacement of patients fostered by federal regulations also were cited as problems. There is no reason to believe that conditions have drastically improved today.

Likewise, Dittmar and Franklin (1980) studied 497 patients placed in nursing homes who were matched with similar patients not discharged from hospitals in terms of age, sex, ethnic group, primary diagnosis, and length of hospital stay. They made an assessment as to whether the groups differed in physical, social, and psychological functioning. The purpose was to determine if state hospitals were transferring their more debilitated patients to nursing homes. Results showed, to the contrary, that patients retained in the hospital were functioning at a statistically significant lower level than those discharged to nursing homes. After three years, 15 medical social workers followed up on 317 of these matched pairs to determine their status. Results showed that the nursing home group, though functioning better at time of placement, was comparable to the state hospital group at the three-year follow-up. Moreover, those in the nursing homes were found to be receiving significantly fewer services than those in the hospitals.

In a Utah study (Schmidt et al., 1977), 680 psychotic and 475 nonpsychotic psychiatric patients placed in nursing homes through Medicaid were compared with patients identified as mentally retarded and "other" patients placed in nursing homes for a wide variety of physical problems, generally of a chronic degenerative type. About half of the psychotic patients and almost one-fifth of the nonpsychotic psychiatric patients came from the state hospital. Results showed that over time all groups of patients utilized more psychoactive medications and were less active, suggesting a custodial rather than a therapeutic environment. This conclusion was supported later by Shadish and Bootzin (1984), who found that nursing home care for 163 chronically ill psychiatric patients across twelve homes was custodial and institutional in nature with social integration of these patients generally low.

In regard to outcome of psychiatric patients placed in nursing homes, Linn and associates (1985) performed the first controlled study of nursing homes as an alternative to continued psychiatric hospitalization. Men (N-403) referred for nursing home placement from eight Veterans Administration (VA) medical centers were randomly assigned to community nursing homes, VA nursing care units, continued care on the same ward, or transfer to another psychiatric ward. Patients met defined criteria for schizophrenia or organic brain disease. Data were collected before random assignment and six and 12 months later, covering physical and mental function, psychopathology, mood, social adjustment, satisfaction with care, as well as drug use, characteristics of settings, and movement in and out of settings. Significant differences between settings were found in self-care, behavioral deterioration, mental confusion, depression, and satisfaction with care. Results were strikingly consistent, showing the group transferred to another ward doing better and the community nursing home group doing worse. Drug use did not differ from six months before entering the study or later between the settings. Cost showed a marked advantage for the community nursing home group. Thus the less costly community nursing home alternative must be viewed in the context of the nonmonetary costs of less favorable patient outcome.

Inappropriate drug usage, polypharmacy (i.e., multiple drug therapy), and altered pharmacokinetics (i.e., rate of drug absorbtion, distribution, excretion, etc.) are common problems in nursing homes (Zaske and Hunter, 1986). Ray, Federspiel, and Schaffner (1980) showed, for example, that a large number of nursing home patients, 43 percent of 5,902 patients across 173 nursing homes in Tennessee (U.S. General Accounting Office, 1982), were receiving anti-psychotic medications. The high percentage is suggestive of potential misuse, though without adequate knowledge of the patients' conditions or treatment plans, definitive conclusions cannot be drawn. Caution has been urged regarding both overmedicating and undermedicating in nursing homes (Kashgarian, 1980). Part of the problem is the tendency for prescriptions to be written "prn" or "as necessary." Nurses and aides then use their own discretion, and when the homes are understaffed and overburdened, patients are at risk for being improperly medicated. Unfortunately, this problem is exacerbated by the fact that the elderly are at great risk for suffering ill side-effects from medications due to their advanced age, declining health, and potentially hazardous drug interaction effects, the potential for which increases as the number of drugs prescribed increases. Surveys of SNFs have shown that the average patient receives six medications (U.S. Department of Health, Education, and Welfare, 1976). For these reasons, among others, special attention needs to be given to this population in prescribing and monitoring drug usage (Salzman, 1982). The evidence suggests that many nursing homes have significant problems in caring for psychiatric patients and that quality of psychiatric care can be compromised.

IMPROVING PSYCHIATRIC CARE IN NURSING HOMES

In regard to improving psychiatric care in nursing homes, several factors need to be considered. The nursing home originated as a place to care for very sick patients, even to the extent that it was considered a place where one was sent to die. Although this stereotype has been erased to a large extent, most nursing homes concentrate on providing for the patients' physical and medical needs. Thus, the paradox exists that nursing homes are medical in orientation, yet predominantly psychiatric in terms of their patient population. Staff are often underpaid, and there is high turnover. Staff have not been trained to care for psychiatric patients or to appreciate their special needs.

Lack of research into mental illness in nursing homes is a major problem. Harper (1986a) reported a total of only six studies supported by the National Institute of Mental Health from 1967 to 1980 on mental illness in nursing homes.

Over the last 15 years, however, the importance of assessing the quality of nursing home care has gained added recognition (Kahn et al., 1977), with some research linked to specific interventions and their outcomes (Beck, 1982). Studies concerning nursing home utilization (Liu and Manton, 1984), manpower needs (Kane et al., 1980), effects of innovative programming (Banziger and Roush, 1983), family involvement in care (Montgomery, 1982), and patient outcomes over time (Kane et al., 1983) have contributed information of potential benefit to nursing home patients.

Studies of the effects of staff training in nursing homes could lead to improved care. Stotsky (1967a) evaluated 16 nursing homes and 141 former state hospital patients to determine whether patient management and adjustment to community placement would be affected by intervention with nursing home staff. Residential stability for patients improved, with significant reduction in death and rehospitalization rates, though effects on psychiatric symptoms were negligible. Staff were enthusiastic about training and, coupled with enhanced residential stability, staff training was considered worthwhile. More recently, Linn, Linn, and Stein (1985) studied the effects of training staff in the psychosocial needs of terminally ill nursing home patients and the beneficial effect on both patients and staff. Patients were helped to feel less depressed and to have greater satisfaction with care, and staff increased their knowledge and skill in treating these patients. Though training staff in nursing homes has proven beneficial, ongoing support from administration is necessary if gains are to be sustained (Moses, 1982) and retraining is needed frequently because of high staff turnover.

Research focusing on nursing home nurses has been extremely limited. Wykle (1986) pointed out that nursing research has not dealt with the mentally ill in nursing homes. This lack cannot be surprising when one considers that an estimated 80 percent to 90 percent of the care provided to nursing home residents is provided by aides and orderlies with little or no training in working with the mentally ill (Hall, 1983). Linn, Gurel, and Linn (1977) showed that the more RN hours a home has, the better the quality of care provided to patients. Nevertheless, our society has yet to clearly define the level of nursing home quality it wants and is willing to pay for (Fottler, Smith, and James, 1981). Qualifications of staff and high staff turnover are problems that must be addressed to ensure continuity of care. In one state, 76 percent of the directors of nursing had less than a B.A. degree, which the American Nurses' Association now thinks is necessary for all graduated nurses (Barnes and Raskind, 1981). In a Salt Lake City study (Stotsky and Stotsky, 1983), almost 100 percent turnover of aides and 30 percent turnover of LPNs and RNs occurred in only three months. The study (Linn, Linn, and Stein, 1985) of ten nursing homes in Miami showed 60 percent of the nursing home staff were in the facilities less than one year. With the age group most likely to require institutionalization, those 75 and over, expanding at a greater rate than any other segment of the population, problems in providing adequate nursing care in nursing homes will worsen since shortages of RNs are expected (Lindeman, 1986).

Understanding the effects of environmental factors can help to alleviate some of the problems facing psychiatric patients. In a study of stress, coping, and survival, Lieberman and Tobin (1983) showed that the environment was crucial to the well-being of less "docile," or more mentally alert, institutionalized patients. Factors of importance included expressions of warmth and recognition by staff. Kruzich (1986), in studying the effects of deinstitutionalization on a group of mental patients placed in nursing homes, found that specific environmental factors have as much influence on residents' integration as do the residents' levels of physical and psychosocial functioning. Though an earlier study by Stotsky (1967b) suggested that it was the severity of the psychiatric patient's mental condition that predicted successful tenure in the institution, more recent studies (Simms, Jones, and Yoder, 1982; Stein, Linn, and Stein, 1986) have highlighted the importance of environmental factors, and particularly the quality of patient-staff interactions on patients' adjustments in, and perceptions of, the homes. As Faletti (1986: 181–182) stated,

One fundamental distinction we can make is that convalescent facilities have patients, whereas long-term care facilities have residents. While patients may be unaffected by the institutional, or hospital-like, aspects of their care environment (they will be leaving), residents are likely to, and should, view these same environmental factors in the context of 'home' and they are likely to react very differently.

Health, morale, self-esteem, and functioning are positively related to the extent that people can control their milieu (Huesman, 1978; Schulz and Hanusa, 1978). A major study (National Institute on Aging, 1979) found that patients who felt more in control over their move to a nursing home were more active after the move, and also reported improved physical and emotional well-being. The social climate of a nursing home, particularly the availability of events which can be predicted and controlled by the elderly themselves within the environment, has been shown to promote physical and psychological health (Schulz, 1976; Langer and Rodin, 1976). Thus, perceived control can be an important variable in explaining nursing home adjustment (Stein, Linn, and Stein, 1985).

Government regulation of nursing homes, particularly within the last twenty years, has contributed greatly to the improvement of the physical plant of many homes and the medical care of patients (Levey et al., 1973). However, as Kane and Kane (1980) have pointed out, institutions for the elderly need to be developed as dwelling places for those with chronic health problems. The long-term care person is in more need of a hospitable than a hospital environment. According to the *National Nursing Home Survey of 1977* (1979), the average length of nursing home stay is 2.6 years, with more than a quarter of all residents staying longer than three years. The effects of the nursing home environment, particularly as it can affect emotional disorders such as depression, have been well documented (Blazer, 1982). The work of Lemke and Moos and associates (Lemke and Moos, 1980; Moos, 1981; Moos et al., 1979; Moos and Lemke,

1979) has helped to make the objective assessment of institutional environments possible in considering such institutional factors as policy and program resources, physical and architectural resources, resident and staff resources, and social and environmental resources. Sherwood (1975) emphasized there is no evidence that one set of factors in the structure of institutional life can be deemed more important than any other in affecting patient behavior. The aged, particularly those who are psychiatrically impaired, are as sensitive to their environment as any other adults, if not more sensitive. The Omnibus Budget Reconciliation Act of 1987 contained numerous provisions for nursing homes, including a resident-centered outcome-oriented survey process. Residents would have direct input to state survey agencies regarding quality of care issues (Health Care Financing Administration, 1988).

ALTERNATIVE SETTINGS

It is clear that nursing homes have become the largest institutional caretakers of the mentally ill largely as a result of enabling legislation which made funds available for nursing home placement. And though the cost of care is less in nursing homes than in mental institutions, the quality of psychiatric care is poor or nonexistent. As the number of elderly increases in this country, the question must be asked whether nursing homes are the most appropriate places to house the mentally ill, particularly those who are ambulatory and have minimal or no physical illness. Furthermore, can emotionally disturbed persons who are currently residing in nursing homes be moved to alternative housing, and if so, should they be?

The tendency of society to isolate its deviant and dependent members undoubtedly has contributed to the institutionalization of many patients who probably could have functioned effectively in the community if appropriate aftercare programs, such as day treatment, had been readily available (Linn et al., 1979). Lack of an able and willing caregiver is a major reason for admission to and continued stay in a nursing home (Liptzin, 1986). Nursing home patients are more likely to be widowed or never married and without supportive kinship (Cohen, 1985). Although most of the persons now residing in nursing homes cannot live independently, probably as many as one-third of nursing home patients could be cared for at home or in a foster home if they had adequate support services (Eisdorfer and Stotsky, 1977). The nursing home has become a specialized way of meeting a basic human need for protective shelter for many elderly poor (Watson, 1986). The report *Toward a National Plan for the Chronically Mentally Ill* (U.S. Department of Health and Human Services, 1980) cited the lack of adequate and secure housing opportunities linked with support services as one of the major current needs of the chronically mentally ill. Research (Linn et al., 1977) has shown that alternative housing for the mentally ill, such as small foster care homes, can be more beneficial than continued mental hospital care. Yet the mechanisms for funding such alternative care are lacking. Moreover, there has not been a controlled study to determine whether mentally ill persons, once placed in nursing homes and perhaps living there for many months or years, would fare better if moved into protective community residences.

The debate continues as to whether state hospitals should be expanded and improved because deinstitutionalization has failed, or whether the community care system should be expanded because deinstitutionalization still can work (Gralnick, 1985). Moreover, with nursing homes now the largest repositories of the mentally ill, nursing home demonstration projects are in progress to develop less costly short-term rehabilitation programs for schizophrenic patients during exacerbation of their illness (Kraus, 1981). In essence, the nursing home can become a "mini" mental hospital, but is there a better solution?

No one can deny that there is a need for nursing homes to provide improved psychiatric care to their mentally disturbed patients. Even if community alternatives were found for all of the emotionally disturbed, less physically impaired, nursing home residents, there would still be a large number of emotionally disturbed residents who are too physically ill to live elsewhere. Cognitive disorders, depression, and disoriented behavior would still be prevalent in nursing homes. Ways of working with patients who wander (Snyder et al., 1978), improving patient cognition through environmental manipulation (Langer, Rodin, and Beck, 1979), interpersonal skill training for patients (Berger and Rose, 1977), and staff training (Barton, Baltes, and Orzech, 1980) are just some examples of ways to improve care in nursing homes. Moreover, there is an immediate need for finding ways to improve diagnosis of these disturbed patients (Sabin, Vitug, and Mark, 1982). It has been pointed out, for example, that the causes of intellectual impairment in the elderly may vary from case to case, involving conditions that can be cured, conditions that with our current state of knowledge show only a downhill course (such as Alzheimer's Disease), or conditions that can be ameliorated with treatment (National Institute on Aging Task Force, 1980). There is evidence that as many as 10 percent to 20 percent of all persons over sixty-five experiencing intellectual impairment have reversible conditions (Marsden and Harrison, 1979; Wells, 1978). Certainly, some of these impaired elderly reside in nursing homes.

The number of older persons requiring mental health services will increase drastically in the years ahead. It is well known that among community-dwelling elderly the incidence of psychosis and dementias increases substantially with age (U.S. Department of Health, Education, and Welfare, 1980). Moreover, studies estimate that about 10 percent of noninstitutionalized older persons have clinically diagnosable depression (Harper, 1986b). Discriminatory treatment of mental health services under the provision of Medicare must be reformed to reduce utilization of more costly and inappropriate forms of care, such as nursing homes. Up until 1988, only $250 was allowed per year for outpatient treatment of mental illness. This was revised slightly upward to $450 per year in 1988, and to $1,100 per year in 1989 (H.R. 3545-P.L. 100–203). It has been estimated that between 10 percent to 30 percent of elderly persons currently in nursing homes are there because they could not find adequate outpatient services (Morris and Youket, 1981). How can we keep people out of institutions and functioning in the community if we only pay for their care when they are hospitalized or placed in nursing homes?

To the present time, most of the expenditures for long-term care of the mentally ill have been for inpatient services. Though Title XX of the Social Security Act and Titles III and V of the Older Americans Act do fund community services, such as meals, transportation, senior centers, and board-and-care facilities, these funds have been woefully inadequate to meet the burgeoning demand. Without a wide range of supportive services, many older persons in need of long-term care will not be able to avoid institutionalization (Zawadski, 1984). For this reason, demonstration projects, such as the National Long-Term Care Channeling Project (a multi-state demonstration effort) and Access of Monroe County, New York (Eggert, Bowlyow, and Nichols, 1980), were established to determine whether an integrated system of providing services to persons at risk in the community would prevent institutionalization. In some cases, services were obtained through brokerage with existing agencies; in others, services were consolidated and provided directly by the demonstration project. The psychiatric health facility (PHF) (Moltzen et al., 1986), as established, for example, in California, was developed to provide acute, short-term crisis intervention for psychotic patients. Old motels, apartment houses, and community mental health centers became the sites for brief treatment of about nine days. Financial support was provided mainly through state funds. Some nursing homes were said to be considering conversion of part of their services to PHFs for short-term acute care. What the eventual outcome of these projects will be is uncertain, particularly since funds for social programs have been diminishing steadily. Fry (1983) emphasized the need, not so much for more study or data-gathering, but for advocacy on behalf of the elderly in want of housing and related services. As Lamb (1981: 108) points out in reviewing the needs of long-term patients, "The key omission is frequently a supportive living situation, without which these patients cannot survive in the community." He called for some kind of "semi-institutional" care such as supervised board-and-care and foster care homes.

SUMMARY

Though nursing homes now house more mentally ill persons than any other single setting, many persons are inappropriately placed in nursing homes. Government regulations and financial incentives have fostered the "reinstitutionalization" of patients, many of whom could have been cared for in the community if adequate planning for protective shelter and social services had occurred prior to hospital discharge. Moreover, some mentally ill now residing in nursing homes are there because they cannot obtain appropriate community support. Although there are calls for reforming the ways in which health services are provided and paid for, no one is quite sure what form these reforms will take in the future.

An amendment to the 1987 Omnibus Budget Reconciliation Act requires nursing homes to refuse admission to people suffering from mental retardation or mental illness (excluding Alzheimer's disease and related disorders). Moreover, by April of 1990 all such nursing home patients who have been in residence for less than 30 months will have to be moved. Inadequate community supports will likely render many of these people homeless. Diagnosis-related groups (DRGs) are likely to determine reimbursement for inpatient psychiatric care in general hospitals at some future time, further limiting the extent of care that can be paid for in the community. There will continue to be many physically ill people with moderate to severe emotional problems who need psychiatric care in nursing homes. One can only hope that further progress will be made in developing the nursing home as a teaching and research setting (Butler, 1981), since it is probably true that the way to quality care in the nursing home is through establishing an academic environment linked to the general health care system.

REFERENCES

Bachrach, L. L. 1976. *Deinstitutionalization: An Analytical Review and Sociological Perspective*. DHEW Publication No. (ADM) 76–351. Washington, D.C.: U.S. Government Printing Office.

Banziger, G., and Roush, S. 1983. Nursing Homes for the Birds: A Control-Relevant Intervention with Bird Feeders. *Gerontologist* 23: 527–531.

Barnes, R. F., and Raskind, M. A. 1981. DSM-III Criteria and the Clinicial Diagnosis of Dementia: A Nursing Home Study. *Journal of Gerontology* 36: 20–27.

Barton, E., Baltes, M. M., and Orzech, M. J. 1980. Etiology of Dependence in Older Nursing Home Residents during Morning Care: The Role of Staff Behavior. *Journal of Personality and Social Psychology* 38: 423–431.

Bassuk, E., and Gerson, S. 1978. Deinstitutionalization and Mental Health Services. *Scientific American* 238: 46–53.

Beck, P. 1982. Two Successful Interventions in Nursing Homes: The Therapeutic Effects of Cognitive Activity. *Gerontologist* 22: 378–383.

Berger, R. M., and Rose, S. D. 1977. Interpersonal Skill Training with Institutionalized Elderly Patients. *Journal of Gerontology* 32: 346–353.

Blazer, D. 1982. *Depression in Late Life*. New York: C. V. Mosby.

Bootzin, R. R., and Shadish, W. R. 1986. Assessment and Treatment in Nursing Homes: Implications for Research. In *Mental Illness in Nursing Homes: Agenda for Research*, eds. M. S. Harper and B. D. Lebowitz. Rockville, Md.: National Institute of Mental Health.

Bovbjerg, R. R., and Holahan, J. 1982. *Medicaid in the Reagan Era: Federal Policy and State Choices*. Washington, D.C.: Urban Institute.

Butler, R. N. 1981. The Teaching Nursing Home. *Journal of the American Medical Association* 245: 1435–1437.

Cohen, G. D. 1985. Mental Health Aspects of Nursing Home Care. In *The Teaching Nursing Home*, eds. E. L. Schneider, C. J. Wendland, A. W. Zimmer, N. List, and M. Ory. New York: Raven Press.

Dittmar, N. D., and Franklin, J. L. 1980. State Hospital Patients Discharged to Nursing

Homes: Are Hospitals Dumping Their More Difficult Patients? *Hospital and Community Psychiatry* 31: 251–254.

Eggert, G. M., Bowlyow, J. E., and Nichols, C. W. 1980. Gaining Control of the Long-Term Care System: First Returns from the Access Experiment. *Gerontologist* 20: 356–363.

Eisdorfer, C., and Stotsky, B. A. 1977. Intervention Treatment and Rehabilitation of Psychiatric Disorder. In *Handbook of the Psychology of Aging*, eds. J. E. Birren and K. W. Schaie. New York: Van Nostrand and Reinhold.

Faletti, M. V. 1986. Environmental Impact on Mental Health and Functioning in Nursing Homes: Implications for Research and Public Policy. In *Mental Illness in Nursing Homes: Agenda for Research*, eds. M. S. Harper and B. D. Lebowitz. Rockville, Md.: National Institute of Mental Health.

Fottler, M. D., Smith, H. L., and James, W. L. 1981. Profits and Patient Care Quality in Nursing Homes: Are They Compatible? *Gerontologist* 21: 532–538.

Fox, P. D., and Clauser, S. B. 1980. Trends in Nursing Home Expenditures: Implications for Aging Policy. *Health Care Financing Review* 2: 65–70.

Fry, W. R. 1983. Next Steps for the Elderly Deinstitutionalized Patient. *Psychiatric Quarterly* 55: 215–224.

German, P. S., Shapiro, S., and Kramer, M. 1986. Nursing Home Study of the Eastern Baltimore Epidemiological Catchment Area Study. In *Mental Illness in Nursing Homes: Agenda for Research*, eds. M. S. Harper and B. D. Lebowitz. Rockville, Md.: National Institute of Mental Health.

Glasscote, R. M., Beigel, A., Butterfield, A., Clark, E., Cox, B., Elpers, R., Gudeman, J. E., Gurel, L., Lewis, R., Miles, D., Raybin, J., Reifler, C., and Vito, E. 1976. *Old Folks at Homes: A Field Study of Nursing and Board and Care Homes*. Washington, D.C.: Joint Information Service.

Goffman, E. 1961. *Asylums: Essays on the Social Situations of Mental Patients and Other Inmates*. New York: Doubleday.

Goldfarb, A. 1962. Prevalence of Psychiatric Disorders in Metropolitan Old Age and Nursing Homes. *Journal of the American Geriatrics Society* 10: 77–84.

Goldman, H. H., Adams, N. H., and Taube, C. A. 1983. Deinstitutionalization: The Data Demythologized. *Hospital and Community Psychiatry* 34: 129–154.

Goldman, H. H., Feder, J., and Scanlon, W. 1986. Chronic Mental Patients in Nursing Homes: Reexamining Data from the National Nursing Home Survey. *Hospital and Community Psychiatry* 37: 269–272.

Gralnick, A. 1985. Build a Better State Hospital: Deinstitutionalization Has Failed. *Hospital and Community Psychiatry* 36: 738–741.

Hall, M. J. 1983. Mental Illness and the Elderly. In *Long-Term Care: Perceptions from Research and Demonstrations*, eds. R. J. Vosel and H. C. Palmer. Washington, D.C.: Health Care Financing Administration, DHHS.

Harper, M. S. 1986a. The Conference on Mental Health and Nursing Homes: An Agenda for Research in Mental Illness in Nursing Homes. In *Mental Illness in Nursing Homes: Agenda for Research*, eds. M. S. Harper and B. D. Lebowitz. Rockville, Md.: National Institute of Mental Health.

Harper, M. S. 1986b. Introduction. In *Mental Illness in Nursing Homes: Agenda for Research*, eds. M. S. Harper and B. D. Lebowitz. Rockville, Md.: National Institute of Mental Health.

Harrington, C., Newcomer, R. J., Estes, C. L., and associates. 1985. *Long-Term Care of the Elderly: Public Policy Issues*. Beverly Hills, Calif.: Sage.

Health Care Financing Administration. 1988. Medicare and Medicaid; Long-term care survey; Final Rule. *Federal Registrar* 22850–23101.

Huesman, L. R., ed. 1978. Learned Helplessness as a Model of Depression. Special issue. *Journal of Abnormal Psychology* 87.

Jazwieck, T., and Press, S. 1986. Federal Reimbursement for Long-Term Care of the Mentally Ill. In *Mental Illness in Nursing Homes: Agenda for Research*, eds. M. S. Harper and B. D. Lebowitz. Rockville, Md.: National Institute of Mental Health.

Kahn, K. A., Hines, W., Woodson, A. S., and Burkham-Armstrong, G. 1977. A Multidisciplinary Approach to Assessing the Quality of Care in Long-Term Care Facilities. *Gerontologist* 17: 61–65.

Kane, J. M., and Smith, J. M. 1982. Tardive Dyskinesia: Prevalence and Risk Factors 1959–1979. *Archives of General Psychiatry* 39: 473–481.

Kane, R., Solomon, D., Beck, J., Keeler, E., and Kane, R. 1980. The Future Need for Geriatric Manpower in the United States. *New England Journal of Medicine* 302: 1327–1332.

Kane, R. L., Bell, R., Riegler, S., Wilson, A., and Keeler, E. 1983. Predicting the Outcomes of Nursing Home Patients. *Gerontologist* 23: 200–206.

Kane, R. L., and Kane, R. 1980. The Nursing Home: Neither Home nor Hospital. In *Introduction to Health Services*, eds. S. J. Williams and P. R. Torrens. New York: John Wiley.

Kashgarian, M. 1980. On Drug Usage in Nursing Homes. *American Journal of Public Health* 70: 1217–1218.

Katon, W. 1984. Depression: Relationship to Somatization and Chronic Medical Illness. *Journal of Clinical Psychiatry* 45: 4–11.

Kramer, M. 1986. Trends of Institutionalization and Prevalence of Mental Disorders in Nursing Homes. In *Mental Illness in Nursing Homes: Agenda for Research*, eds. M. S. Harper and B. D. Lebowitz. Rockville, Md.: National Institute of Mental Health.

Kraus, R. T. 1981. A Nursing Home Model. In *The Chronic Mentally Ill: Treatment, Program, Systems*, ed. J. A. Talbott. New York: Human Sciences Press.

Kruzich, J. M. 1986. The Chronically Mentally Ill in Nursing Homes: Issues in Policy and Practice. *Health and Social Work* 11: 5–14.

Lamb, H. R. 1981. What Did We Really Expect from Deinstitutionalization? *Hospital and Community Psychiatry* 32: 105–109.

Lamb, H. R., ed. 1984. *The Homeless Mentally Ill: A Task Force Report of the APA*. Washington, D.C.: American Psychiatric Association.

Lamb, H. R., and Mills, M. I. 1986. Needed Changes in Law and Procedure for the Chronically Mentally Ill. *Hospital and Community Psychiatry* 37: 475–480.

Langer, E. J., and Rodin, J. 1976. The Effects of Choice and Enhanced Personal Responsibility for the Aged: A Field Experiment in an Institutional Setting. *Journal of Personality and Social Psychology* 34: 191–198.

Langer, E. J., Rodin, J., and Beck, P. 1979. Environmental Determinants of Memory Impairment in Late Adulthood. *Journal of Personality and Social Psychology* 27: 2008–2018.

Lemke, S., and Moos, R. H. 1980. Assessing the Institutional Policies of Sheltered Care Settings. *Journal of Gerontology* 35: 96–107.

Levey, S., Ruchlin, H. S., Stotsky, B. A., Kinloch, D. R., and Oppenheim, W. 1973. An Appraisal of Nursing Home Care. *Journal of Gerontology* 28: 222–228.

Lieberman, M. A., and Tobin, S. S. 1983. *The Experience of Old Age—Stress, Coping, Survival*. New York: Basic Books.

Lindeman, C. 1986. Manpower in Nursing Homes: Implications for Research. In *Mental Illness in Nursing Homes: Agenda for Research*, eds. M. S. Harper and B. D. Lebowitz. Rockville, Md.: National Institute of Mental Health.

Linn, M. W., Caffey, E. M., Klett, C. J., and Hogarty, G. 1977. Hospital versus Community Care for Psychiatric Patients. *Archives of General Psychiatry* 34: 78–83.

Linn, M. W., Caffey, E. M., Klett, C. J., Hogarty, G. E., and Lamb, H. R. 1979. Day Treatment and Psychotropic Drugs in the Aftercare of Schizophrenic Patients. *Archives of General Psychiatry* 36: 1055–1066.

Linn, M. W., Gurel, L., and Linn, B. S. 1977. Patient Outcome as a Measure of Nursing Home Care. *American Journal of Public Health* 67: 337–344.

Linn, M. W., Gurel, L., Williford, W. O., Overall, J., Gurland, B., Laughlin, P., and Barchiesi, A. 1983. Nursing Home Care as an Alternative to Psychiatric Hospitalization. *Archives of General Psychiatry* 42: 544–551.

Linn, M. W., Linn, B. S., and Stein, S. 1985. Impact on Nursing Home Staff of Training about Death and Dying. *Journal of the American Medical Association* 250: 2332–2335.

Linn, M. W., and Stein, S. 1982. Chronic Adult Mental Illness. *Health and Social Work* 54S–61S.

Liptzin, B. 1986. Major Mental Disorders/Problems in Nursing Homes: Implications for Research and Public Policy. In *Mental Illness in Nursing Homes: Agenda for Research*, eds. M. S. Harper and B. D. Lebowitz. Rockville, Md.: National Institute of Mental Health.

Liu, K., and Manton, K. G. 1984. The Characteristics and Utilization Pattern of an Admission Cohort of Nursing Home Patients. *Gerontologist* 24: 70–76.

Marsden, C. D., and Harrison, M. J. G. 1979. Outcome of Investigation in Patients with Presenile Mentia. *British Medical Journal* 2: 249–252.

Mechanic, D. 1980. *Mental Health and Social Policy*. 2nd ed. Englewood Cliffs, N. J.: Prentice-Hall.

Mechanic, D. 1986. The Challenge of Chronic Mental Illness: A Retrospective and Prospective View. *Hospital and Community Psychiatry* 37: 891–896.

Mental Health Services for the Elderly. Report on a Survey of Community Mental Health Centers, Vol. III. 1986. Action Committee to Implement the Mental Health Recommendations of the 1981 White House Conference on Aging. Washington, D.C.: U.S. Government Printing Office.

Miller, M. B., and Elliott, D. F. 1976. Errors and Omissions in Diagnostic Records on Admission of Patients to a Nursing Home. *Journal of the American Geriatrics Society* 24: 108–116.

Moltzen, S., Gurevitz, H., Rappaport, M., and Goldman, H. 1986. The Psychiatric Health Facility: An Alternative for Acute Inpatient Treatment in a Non-Hospital Setting. *Hospital and Community Psychiatry* 37: 1131–1135.

Montgomery, R. S. V. 1982. Impact of Institutional Care Policies on Family Integration. *Gerontologist* 22: 54–58.

Moos, R. H. 1981. Environmental Choice and Control in Community Care Settings for Older People. *Journal of Applied Social Psychology* 11: 23–43.

Moos, R. H., Gauvain, M., Lemke, S., Max, W., and Mehren, B. 1979. Assessing the Social Environments of Sheltered Care Settings. *Gerontologist* 19: 74–82.

Moos, R. H., and Lemke, S. 1979. *Multiphasic Environmental Assessment Procedure (MEAP): Preliminary Manual.* Palo Alto, Calif.: Social Ecology Laboratory, Stanford University and Veterans Administration Medical Center.

Moroney, R. M., and Kuntz, N. R. 1975. The Evaluation of Long-Term Care Institutions. In *Long-Term Care: A Handbook for Researchers, Planners and Providers*, ed. S. Sherwood. New York: John Wiley.

Morris, R., and Youket, P. 1981. The Long-Term Care Issues: Identifying the Problem and Potential Solutions. In *Reforming the Long-Term Care System*, eds. J. J. Callahan and S. S. Wallach. Lexington, Mass.: Lexington Books.

Moses, J. 1982. New Role for Hands-on Caregivers: Part-time Mental Health Technicians. *Journal of the American Health Care Association* 8: 19–22.

National Institute on Aging. 1979. Special Report on Aging. Publication No. 79–1907. Rockville, Md.: National Institute on Mental Health.

National Institute on Aging Task Force. 1980. Senility Reconsidered: Treatment Possibilities for Mental Impairment in the Elderly. *Journal of the American Medical Association* 244: 259–263.

National Nursing Home Survey of 1977. 1979. Publication No. (PHS) 79–1794. Washington, D.C.: U.S. Government Printing Office.

Ray, W. A., Federspiel, C. F., and Schaffner, W. 1980. A Study of Antipsychotic Drug Use in Nursing Homes: Epidemiologic Evidence Suggesting Misuse. *American Journal of Public Health* 70: 485–491.

Rosenfeld, A. H. 1978. *New Views on Older Lives. A Sampler of NIMH-Sponsored Research and Service Programs.* Rockville, Md.: National Institute of Mental Health.

Rovner, B. W., Kafonek, S., Philipp, L., Lucas, M. J., and Folstein, M. S. 1986. Prevalence of Mental Illness in the Community Nursing Home. *American Journal of Psychiatry* 143: 1446–1449.

Rubin, J. 1981. The National Plan for the Chronically Mentally Ill: A Review of Financing Proposals. *Hospital and Community Psychiatry* 32: 704–713.

Rubin, J. 1984. Developments in the Financing of Mental Health Care. In *The Chronic Mental Patient Five Years Later*, ed. J. A. Talbott. New York: Grune and Stratton.

Sabin, T. D., Vitug, A. J., and Mark, V. H. 1982. Are Nursing Home Diagnosis and Treatment Inadequate? *Journal of the American Medical Association* 248: 321–322.

Salzman, C. 1982. A Primer on Geriatric Psychopharmacology. *American Journal of Psychiatry* 139: 67.

Schmidt, L. J., Reinhardt, A. M., Kane, R. L., and Olsen, D. M. 1977. The Mentally Ill in Nursing Homes. *Archives of General Psychiatry* 34: 687–691.

Schulz, J. H. 1985. *The Economics of Aging*, 3rd ed. New York: Van Nostrand-Reinhold.

Schulz, R. 1976. Effects of Control and Predictability on the Physical and Psychological Well-being of the Institutionalized Aged. *Journal of Personality and Social Psychology* 33: 563–573.

Schulz, R., and Hanusa, B. H. 1978. Long-Term Effects of Control and Predictability-

Enhancing Interventions: Findings and Ethical Issues. *Journal of Personality and Social Psychology* 36: 1194–1201.

Shadish, W. R., and Bootzin, R. R. 1981a. Long-Term Community Care: Mental Health Policy in the Face of Reality. *Schizophrenia Bulletin* 7: 580–585.

Shadish, W. R., and Bootzin, R. R. 1981b. Nursing Homes and Chronic Mental Patients. *Schizophrenia Bulletin* 7: 488–498.

Shadish, W. R., and Bootzin, R. R. 1984. The Social Integration of Psychiatric Patients in Nursing Homes. *American Journal of Psychiatry* 141: 1203–1207.

Sherwood, S., ed. 1975. *Long-Term Care: A Handbook for Researchers, Planners, and Providers*. New York: Halsted Press.

Simms, L. M., Jones, S. J., and Yoder, K. K. 1982. Adjustment of Older Persons in Nursing Homes. *Journal of Gerontological Nursing* 8: 383–386.

Sirrocco, A., and Koch, H. 1977. *Nursing Homes in the U.S. 1972–1974: National Nursing Home Survey*. Vital and Health Statistics, Series 14, No. 17, DHEW Publication No. (HRA) 78–1812. Washington, D.C.: U.S. Government Printing Office.

Snyder, L. H., Rupprecht, P., Pyrek, J., Brekhus, S., and Moss, T. 1978. Wandering. *Gerontologist* 18: 272–280.

State Medicaid Manual: Part 4. 1983. Services Publication No. 45–4. Baltimore, Md.: Health Care Financing Administration.

Stein, S., Linn, M. W., and Stein, E. M. 1985. Patients' Anticipation of Stress in Nursing Home Care. *Gerontologist* 25: 88–94.

Stein, S., Linn, M. W., and Stein, E. M. 1986. Patients' Perceptions of Nursing Home Stress Related to Quality of Care. *Gerontologist* 26: 424–430.

Stone, A. A. 1975. The Right to Treatment—Comments on the Law and Its Impact. *American Journal of Psychiatry* 132: 1125–1134.

Stotsky, B. A. 1967a. A Systematic Study of Therapeutic Interventions in Nursing Homes. *Geriatric Psychology Monographs* 76: 257–320.

Stotsky, B. A. 1967b. A Controlled Study of Factors in the Successful Adjustment of Mental Patients to Nursing Homes. *American Journal of Psychiatry* 123: 1243–1251.

Stotsky, B. A., and Stotsky, B. S. 1983. Nursing Homes: Improving a Flawed Community Facility. *Hospital and Community Psychiatry* 34: 238–242.

Talbott, J. A. 1981. The National Plan for the Chronically Mentally Ill: A Programmatic Analysis. *Hospital and Community Psychiatry* 32: 699–704.

Talbott, J. A., and Sharfstein, S. S. 1986. Proposal for Future Funding of Chronic and Episodic Mental Illness. *Hospital and Community Psychiatry* 37: 1126–1130.

Taube, C. A., and Barrett, S. A., eds. 1983. *Mental Health, United States, 1983*. National DHHS Publication No. (ADM) 83–1275. Rockville, Md.: National Institute of Mental Health.

Teeter, R. B., Garetz, F. K., Miller, W. R., and Heiland, W. F. 1976. Psychiatric Disturbances of Aged Patients in Skilled Nursing Homes. *American Journal of Psychiatry* 133: 1430–1434.

U.S. Department of Health and Human Services. 1980. *Toward a National Plan for the Chronically Mentally Ill*. Report to the Secretary by the Steering Committee on the Chronically Mentally Ill. Washington, D.C.: U.S. Government Printing Office.

U.S. Department of Health and Human Services. 1981. *Care of the Mentally Ill in Nursing*

Homes. DHHS Publication (ADM) 81–1077. Washington, D.C.: U.S. Government Printing Office.

U.S. Department of Health, Education and Welfare. 1965. *Trends*, Part 1. Washington, D.C.: U.S. Government Printing Office.

U.S. Department of Health, Education, and Welfare. 1976. *Physician's Drug Prescribing Patterns in Skilled Nursing Care Facilities: Long-Term Care Facility Improvement Campaigns* (Monograph No. 2) Washington, D.C.: U.S. Government Printing Office, 1976.

U.S. Department of Health, Education and Welfare. 1980. *Mental Health and the Elderly*. Publication No. (OHDS) 80–20960. Washington, D.C.: U.S. Government Printing Office.

U.S. General Accounting Office. 1982. *The Elderly Remain in Need of Mental Health Services*. Publication No. (HRD) 82–112. Washington, D.C.: U.S. Government Printing Office.

Vladeck, B. C. 1980. *Unloving Care: The Nursing Home Tragedy*. New York: Basic Books.

Watson, W. H. 1986. Nursing Homes and the Mental Health of Minority Residents: Some Problems and Needed Research. In *Mental Illness in Nursing Homes: Agenda for Research*, eds. M. S. Harper and B. D. Lebowitz. Rockville, Md.: National Institute of Mental Health.

Wells, C. E. 1978. Chronic Brain Disease: An Overview. *American Journal of Psychiatry* 135: 1–12.

Wykle, M. H. 1986. Mental Health Nursing: Research in Nursing Homes. In *Mental Illness in Nursing Homes: Agenda for Research*, eds. M. S. Harper and B. D. Lebowitz. Rockville, Md.: National Institute of Mental Health.

Zaske, D., and Hunter, T. S. 1986. Polypharmacy and Altered Pharmacokinetics in Nursing Homes. In *Mental Illness in Nursing Homes: Agenda for Research*, eds. M. S. Harper and B. D. Lebowitz. Rockville, Md.: National Institute of Mental Health.

Zawadski, R. T. 1984. The Long-Term Care Demonstration Projects: What Are They and Why They Came into Being. In *Community-Based Systems of Long-Term Care*, ed. R. T. Zawadski. New York: Hawthorn Press.

12

Homelessness as a Public Mental Health Problem

IRENE SHIFREN LEVINE
and LORETTA K. HAGGARD

Perhaps no group of disabled people in the United States is as impoverished and underserved as the homeless mentally ill population. People who are homeless and mentally ill bear the cross of a dual disfranchisement, both from society and from service providers; mentally ill persons are often excluded from programs designed to serve the homeless, and homeless individuals are typically screened out from receiving services designed for the long-term, severely mentally ill (Levine, 1984b).

Across the country, though, a number of innovative programs are reaching out successfully to serve homeless mentally ill persons on the streets and in shelters. Many of these programs share a common approach and philosophy: they are grounded in the principles of the National Institute of Mental Health (NIMH) Community Support Program (CSP), a federal initiative designed to assist states and communities in addressing the mental health and social welfare problems of severely mentally ill persons (Turner and TenHoor, 1978; Turner and Shifren, 1979).

Since its inception in 1977, most states have come to embrace the Community Support Program approach to addressing the multiple service needs of severely mentally ill persons. Only in the last several years, however, as homelessness has grown into a phenomenon of national proportions, have mental health professionals begun to adapt the comprehensive CSP approach to serve homeless mentally ill persons. Mental health treatment alone has negligible value for an individual who is both severely mentally ill and homeless. Clearly, housing, health care, income support, and vocational assistance are also vitally important to successful care and rehabilitation. In fact, persons who are homeless and mentally ill require a far more comprehensive and intensive package of services than do other mentally ill persons who are fortunate enough to have homes and support from family, friends, or existing public and private programs.

This chapter will first provide an overview of research, sponsored by the National Institute of Mental Health, on the homeless mentally ill, focusing specifically on the service needs of the population. Second, the chapter will briefly trace the history of the federal Community Support Program, then explain how the community support approach can be adapted to meet the needs of homeless mentally ill persons. Specifically, it describes in some detail the five core services required to address the needs of this population comprehensively, and the qualitative manner in which these services must be provided. National consensus seems to be emerging regarding both short- and long-term approaches to reducing the problem of homelessness, and the role that the federal government must play in stimulating these changes. The chapter concludes with a discussion of the limitations of the Community Support Program model of care, in the absence of low-cost housing. No matter how innovative or comprehensive community mental health and social welfare services are, the successful rehabilitation and reintegration of homeless mentally ill persons into society hinges upon the availability of affordable housing.

OVERVIEW OF RESEARCH ON THE HOMELESS MENTALLY ILL POPULATION

A Profile of the Population

Delineating the boundaries and size of the homeless mentally ill population is no simple task. In the first place, definitions of "homelessness" vary widely from study to study and encompass a range of variables such as lack of shelter, income, social support, or affiliation with others. Bassuk (1983: 60) describes homelessness as "more than the lack of a home; it is a metaphor for profound disconnection from other people and social institutions." The Alcohol, Drug Abuse, and Mental Health Administration (ADAMHA) (1983: 1) defines homelessness as "both [the] lack of adequate and permanent shelter and [the] absence of community and social ties." According to these broad interpretations, the homeless population includes not only persons on the street, but also shelter residents and people boarded temporarily in welfare hotels.

Given such definitional ambiguities, it is difficult to precisely gauge the scope of the problem of homelessness. The two most frequently cited estimates of the number of homeless persons in the nation are 250,000–350,000 and 3 million. The first figure (250,000–350,000) represents the lowest estimated daily count of homeless persons used by the U.S. Department of Housing and Urban Development (HUD) in its controversial May 1, 1984, national report on the problem of homelessness (U.S. Department of Housing and Urban Development, 1984: 18). The second figure (3 million) represents an estimate, extrapolated from disparate local studies, that approximately 1 percent of the population lacks shelter at some point annually (U.S. Department of Health and Human Services, 1984: 2). Neither of these estimates is based on a systematic study or actual count of homeless persons in America. In fact, the wide discrepancy between the numbers suggests the extent of methodological problems that arise in attempting to define, locate, and count the homeless population. Moreover, critics sometimes accuse advocates of exaggerating the scope of the problem of homelessness in their competition for scarce human services resources, whereas governmental organizations are often accused of minimizing the extent of homelessness to conserve such resources.

In a 1985 report on homelessness, the U.S. General Accounting Office (1985: ii) noted that the problem has increased in recent years, "although there are no reliable data to identify how much it is increasing." A 1986 survey of mayors across the nation confirmed that the homeless population is increasing rapidly in size. On average, cities reported a 20 percent rise in the homeless population during 1986, based on heightened demands for emergency shelter and food (U.S. Conference of Mayors, 1986: 1).

As striking, perhaps, as the size or rate of growth of the homeless population, are changes in its composition. Homelessness, once a phenomenon exclusively of older, white, alcoholic males, is becoming "democratized." The number of homeless women and families has grown tremendously since the 1960s. For example, the number of families seeking emergency shelter in New York City grew by 24 percent just between July 1981 and July 1982, and increased another 200 percent by July 1983 (Hopper and Hamberg, 1984: 58). The 1986 U.S. Conference of Mayors survey reported that 28 percent of the homeless nationwide are families with children, and that 15 percent are single women (U.S. Conference of Mayors, 1986: 2). Racial and ethnic minorities represent another significant addition to the homeless population; often they predominate among shelter and street populations (Martin, 1987). The 1984 HUD survey revealed that 44 percent of shelter users nationwide are minorities, while only 20 percent of the total U.S. population are minorities (U.S. Department of Housing and Urban Development, 1984: 29).

Perhaps the most vulnerable and disabled members of the homeless population are severely mentally ill persons. Although there are no uniform national data on the homeless, a growing number of state and local studies consistently find that a significant proportion of the homeless suffer from long-term, severe mental illnesses, such as schizophrenia, manic-depressive illnesses, and depression.

Between 1983 and 1986 NIMH funded ten studies of homeless mentally ill persons (Bachrach, 1984; Spaniol and Zipple, 1985; Morrissey and Dennis, 1986). Each study employed different sampling techniques and diagnostic in-

Table 12–1
A Comparative Summary of Research on Homelessness and Mental Illness

Study Authors and Location	Sample Size	Percent with Prior Mental Hospitalization	Percent with Current "Serious Mental Illness"
Farr, Koegel, and Burnam, 1986 (Los Angeles)	379	27	28
Fischer et al., 1985 (Baltimore)	51	33	37
Ladner et al., 1986 (New York City)	8061		25
Morse et al., 1985 (St. Louis)	248	25	56
Mowbray et al., 1985 (Detroit)	75	26	61
Mulkern et al., 1985 (Massachusetts)	328	45	54
Rosnow, Shaw, and Concord, 1985 (Milwaukee)	237	42	40
Roth et al., 1985 (Ohio)	979	30	31

struments. Moreover, some studies focused on homelessness among the mentally ill, while others examined mental illness among the homeless. Although the comparability of these studies is thus limited, a summary of findings from eight completed studies is illuminating nonetheless and appears in Table 12–1.

One can anticipate differences in the prevalence of mental illness in different geographic samples, in shelter-based versus street populations, and in urban versus rural populations. For some who are homeless, mental illness is a contributing cause to their homelessness; for others, emotional distress is a consequence of their homelessness. Not surprisingly, in an era of deinstitutionalization with an emphasis on hospital diversion, some of those who are severely mentally ill have histories of hospitalization and others do not. Yet, despite discrepancies in the design and outcome measures of the NIMH-supported studies and other systematic surveys of the population, there is relative agreement that the severely mentally ill comprise a significant proportion (30–40 percent) of the homeless.

Factors in the Severely Mentally Ill Becoming or Remaining Homeless

A number of societal or contextual factors have contributed to the problem of homelessness in America. These include urban renewal and the lack of low-cost housing, unemployment, the complexity and discontinuity of our social service system, and the disintegration of the nuclear family. Each of these factors also contributes to homelessness among the mentally ill who, because of their disabilities, often have limited incomes and live in precarious socioeconomic circumstances. Historically, rooming houses provided a lower-priced alternative for those who could not afford larger apartment units. Unfortunately, between 1970 and 1980, about one million single-room units across the nation—nearly one-half of the total stock—were converted to other uses or destroyed (U.S. Department of Health and Human Services, 1984: 6). These reductions have severely limited housing opportunities for the mentally ill in the community.

The mentally ill are also at high risk of becoming or remaining homeless because of certain characteristics of their illness. A severely mentally disabled person generally has one or more functional problems, such as the inability to meet basic survival needs, difficulty with the tasks of daily living, extreme vulnerability to stress, the inability to develop or sustain social networks, and lack of motivation or ability to seek out the help of human service workers (Levine, 1984b: 8). Because the mentally disabled frequently do not have the skills to negotiate service systems in the community, they are often unable to secure welfare, Social Security benefits, or other entitlements for which they may be eligible.

It is important to note that the community also contributes to the severely mentally ill becoming or remaining homeless. The stigma against mentally ill persons is often manifest in community resistance that creates barriers and denies them access to opportunities for housing, jobs, and economic independence that might otherwise exist.

Finally, the implementation of deinstitutionalization without corresponding provision of sufficient community services clearly contributed to homelessness among the mentally ill. Over the past three decades, we have witnessed dramatic changes in the locus of mental health care that have come about because of changes in clinical practice, newly enacted legal mandates, and changes in public policy (particularly with respect to mental health care financing). In 1955, there were 559,000 psychiatric patients in state hospitals in this country; by 1980, the number had dropped to 132,000. The number is now below 120,000 (Levine and Stockdill, 1986: 7; chapter 13 in this volume).

The vast majority of severely mentally ill persons who have been discharged or diverted from state hospitals are not homeless, but rather live in an array of independent and supervised community residential settings. However, a number of mentally disabled persons do not have access to such living situations, basic life supports, and other human services essential for their ongoing care, treatment, and rehabilitation in the community. Instead they have been relegated inappropriately to nursing homes, substandard board-and-care homes, or single-room occupancy hotels—or are without homes altogether and living in emergency shelters, on the streets, or in local jails.

Because there have not always been adequate community funding, planning, and public support for the severely mentally ill, the success of deinstitutional-ization practices has varied significantly for different states, for different communities, and for different persons. This variation has led to a backlash against a policy that was never properly implemented and to calls for making civil commitment laws less restrictive. One common misperception, however, is that widespread deinstitutionalization of the mentally ill was the sole cause of homelessness. As we have said, though, homelessness is caused by a variety of economic and social dislocations, to which mentally ill people are particularly vulnerable. When affordable housing and income supports, as well as health and mental health care, are available in the community, homelessness does not have to be an outcome of deinstitutionalization.

Research Findings on Homeless Mentally Ill Persons

The ten NIMH-funded research studies collected basic descriptive information on the characteristics and service needs of the homeless mentally ill population. In July 1986 NIMH convened a meeting for these researchers to compare their findings, the most salient of which have been distilled by Morrissey and Dennis (1986):

1. All of the research studies agree that the homeless mentally ill are most commonly a multineed population, with substance abuse, physical and mental health problems, and vocational and social deficits. The New York City shelter study (Ladner et al., 1986) reports, for example, that 51 percent of homeless mentally ill persons have current physical health problems, and that 34 percent acknowledge regular past or present use of alcohol, heroin, or other drugs. Fischer and colleagues (1985) report in their Baltimore Epidemiologic Catchment Area study that the prevalence of drug and alcohol abuse among the homeless is two to three times greater than that of the general population.

2. Homeless mentally ill persons tend to have histories of residential instability, and currently have few housing options open to them; however, they do not move frequently between localities. The NIMH-sponsored study conducted in Ohio (Roth et al., 1985) found that over half of the sample of homeless mentally ill persons who were interviewed were either born in the county or had lived there for over a year.

3. A surprisingly large group of homeless mentally ill persons is involved with the criminal justice system. For instance, in the Baltimore study, homeless persons were more than twice as likely to have been arrested as domiciled adults (58 percent versus 24 percent). Forty-five percent of homeless mentally ill persons in the New York City shelter study had jail histories. The researchers agreed that individuals who become homeless are not inherently more prone to criminal behavior, but rather that the homeless life-style itself leads both to victimization and criminal involvements.

4. Homeless mentally ill persons are usually willing to accept assistance (Morse et al., 1985). However, service providers' perceptions of clients' needs

often differ from those of homeless mentally ill individuals. Clinicians tend to focus on the need for specialized mental health interventions, whereas homeless mentally ill people tend to emphasize the lack of basic housing and social supports. These differences in priorities may be wrongly interpreted by service providers as resistance to receiving help.

Although these findings are by no means definitive, they clearly suggest that homeless mentally ill persons suffer from severe health, mental health, residential, vocational, and social deprivation in many communities across the nation.

COMMUNITY SUPPORT SYSTEMS FOR THE HOMELESS MENTALLY ILL

The NIMH Community Support Program: An Overview

By the mid–1970s, the National Institute of Mental Health and others had documented the gaps and fragmentation in the existing service system for long-term, severely mentally ill persons. The Community Support Program, established in 1977, was the major federal response to redress these problems in care. CSP is a program of service demonstration grants to states premised on meeting the interrelated mental health and social welfare needs of severely mentally ill individuals. This approach departs from prior efforts to assist the mentally ill in the community in that it focuses on providing long-term treatment, care, and rehabilitation to persons with severe mental illnesses (Goldman and Morrissey, 1985).

The Community Support Program encourages state mental health agencies to establish a focal point of responsibility at both state and local levels for the severely mentally ill in order to make planning more responsive to their needs (Turner and Shifren, 1979; Stroul, 1986). The state mental health agency and its staff assist localities in developing community support systems (CSSs), which are defined as "networks of caring and responsible people committed to assisting mentally disabled individuals in meeting their needs and in developing their potentials without being unnecessarily isolated or excluded from the community" (National Institute of Mental Health, 1983:II).

CSP is a modestly funded federal demonstration that was not intended to support direct services. Rather, the program sought to stimulate a long-term process of systems reorientation and change that would make states and localities more responsive to the needs of the severely mentally disabled. While many communities have developed CSSs, financial constraints have limited the capacities of others to establish all the components of a comprehensive system or to serve the entire population. Moreover, because of scarce resources, most programs have been unable to extend outreach services to seriously mentally ill homeless people. In fact, in many communities, mental health professionals have only recently become aware of the prevalence of homelessness among the seriously mentally ill, and have just begun to acknowledge their responsibilities to these persons.

CSP guidelines specify that however a particular community arranges services, ten essential functions must be performed (Turner and Shifren, 1979):

1. Outreach, or "case finding," to inform clients of available services;
2. Provision of services to meet basic human needs (e.g., shelter, food, clothing, health and mental health care);
3. Comprehensive mental health care (e.g., screening and diagnosis, evaluation of treatment needs, prescription and appropriate medication management, individual and group counseling, and psychosocial rehabilitation);
4. Twenty-four-hour crisis assistance;
5. Comprehensive psychosocial services (e.g., day programs providing opportunities for vocational or skills training, supported work, socialization, leisure);
6. A range of rehabilitative and supportive housing options (e.g., crisis residences, halfway houses, group homes, foster family homes, supervised and independent apartments);
7. Backup support, assistance, consultation, and education to landlords, employers, neighbors, and families of the mentally ill;
8. Involvement of natural support systems (e.g., families, churches, voluntary agencies, businesses, neighborhood and community organizations) in assisting the population to meet its needs;
9. Grievance procedures and mechanisms to protect client rights; and
10. Case management (e.g., client identification and outreach, needs assessment, treatment and service planning, linkage with requisite services, monitoring of service delivery, and client advocacy).

The CSP approach thus assumes that the needs of severely mentally ill persons in the community extend beyond mental health treatment alone and must include a broad number and range of social supports.

The CSP Approach to Service Delivery for Homeless Mentally Ill Persons

Architects of the CSP program conceptualized community support systems as a generic planning tool for creating services and opportunities for severely mentally ill persons living in the community. Experience with the homeless subgroup of the CSP population, however, has suggested that there are five core elements of care that need to be specifically adapted in order to address the special needs of homeless mentally ill persons. Moreover, there are subtle, but significant, qualitative differences in methods of approaching and engaging this group. Intensity of effort, together with persistence and patience on the part of service providers, is perhaps the most salient characteristic of effective programs for the homeless mentally ill.

Outreach. As mentioned earlier, severely mentally ill persons are often not likely to seek out the assistance of mental health or human service professionals on their own, because of either lack of motivation or inability to establish and sustain rapport with such helpers (Test and Stein, 1979; Turner and TenHoor, 1978; Turner and Shifren, 1979). Among the homeless, the mentally disabled are probably least able to know where to find agencies, programs, and resources and are most vulnerable to the pressures created by too many questions and forms and long waits. The mentally ill, along with other frail and vulnerable populations, often never reach the doors of shelter, food, and service programs. Therefore, effective outreach to this population must occur in nontraditional settings such as shelters, soup kitchens, drop-in centers for the homeless, subway stations, or even the streets.

Outreach may be defined as "a service which increases the access of a homeless mentally ill individual to other needed treatments and services" (Intergovernmental Health Policy Project, 1987: 3). Trained outreach staff gradually develop rapport with homeless persons by approaching them in nonthreatening ways over periods of weeks and even months. Once they have built a relationship, outreach workers help clients to identify their needs and to make use of community resources, and may even accompany them to where the service is provided. At minimum, outreach workers must be able to perform the following activities:

- engage clients in a helping relationship (a process that can take up to several years of aggressive and persistent contacts and offers of assistance);
- assess clients' health, mental health, substance abuse treatment, housing, and social welfare needs;
- intervene in crisis situations (e.g., acute psychiatric episodes, health emergencies, or social welfare or personal crises); and
- refer clients to appropriate health, mental health, substance abuse treatment, housing, and social welfare agencies.

Many outreach programs also provide ongoing assistance to clients in meeting basic needs. Such assistance might include distribution of food and blankets, administration of psychiatric medication, or first aid for medical conditions not requiring hospitalization. Because of deficits in the existing service network for severely mentally ill persons, outreach programs for homeless mentally ill persons often are ambitious attempts to compensate for gaps in services. In essence, they have no waiting lists, no rejection criteria, and are services of last resort that must be elastic enough to provide care when no alternatives exist.

Case management. Many mentally ill persons living in the community are dependent on multiple community services, provided by multiple providers, and often multiple systems. Case management has been widely heralded as a solution to this fragmentation. Case management has been defined as "a method of fixing responsibility for systems coordination with one individual, who works with a given client in accessing necessary services'' (Levine and Fleming, 1986: i). As described earlier, the six generally accepted core components of case management are client identification and outreach, individual assessment, service planning, linkage with requisite services, monitoring of service delivery, and client advocacy.

According to an NIMH-sponsored study (Rog, Andranovich, and Rosenblum, 1987), effective case management for homeless mentally ill individuals must be ''intensive.'' That is, the case manager must invest more time and energy to meet the comprehensive needs of clients. Successful case management programs for the homeless mentally ill have small caseloads (15:1). Typically, these programs are not time-bound (not limited to fixed schedules or appointments), nor are they office-bound. Rather, effective case management for this population takes place in shelters, soup kitchens, and on the streets; it emphasizes aggressive outreach and requires a substantial investment of time and effort in preparing and educating clients to receive services and to live more independently. For example, case managers may assist clients directly in negotiating with landlords, learning to use public transportation, or applying for entitlement benefits.

Mental health treatment rehabilitation. Some homeless mentally ill persons shun traditional treatment settings because of histories of institutionalization in state hospitals, prior unsatisfying experiences with mental health programs, or unwillingness to acknowledge that they have a serious mental illness. They may also fear that if their illness is detected, they will be involuntarily committed.

Other homeless mentally ill persons have rejected traditional services because they feel that they will not receive the help they need. Ball and Havassy (1984) found significant discrepancies between the self-perceived needs of homeless persons who were repeatedly taken to psychiatric emergency rooms and the types of services provided by mental health caregivers. Homeless patients considered psychiatric services a strikingly low priority compared to their basic living needs.

In many instances, however, severely mentally ill homeless persons are denied access to mental health care. It is commonly thought that these individuals will automatically reject mental health services; this assumption is often used to justify the inertia of bureaucracies that are not eager to extend appropriate care to this population. Yet, as the NIMH studies found, homeless mentally ill people, in most cases, are willing to accept assistance in meeting their mental health needs.

Mental health personnel who provide care for this population must be sensitive to the unique circumstances of homeless persons and must be flexible, nonthreatening, and accessible. Initially, services may have to be offered ''in-vivo'' rather than in more traditional office settings.

Mental health treatment and rehabilitation services for homeless persons must include:

• psychiatric diagnosis and development of an appropriate treatment and service plan;
• prescription and appropriate medication management;
• detoxification and other drug/alcohol abuse treatments;

- individual and group counseling; and
- social and vocational rehabilitation programs, including so-called psychosocial day programs providing training in daily living skills, vocational assessment and training, supportive work, competitive employment, education, and/or recreation/social activities.

The mental health treatment/rehabilitation services needed by homeless mentally ill persons are really no different than those needed by mentally ill individuals with homes. In treating long-term, severe mental illnesses, one must remember the often cyclical nature of the illness. This almost inevitable series of ups and downs requires patience and enduring support on the part of service providers. Therapeutic progress is even further hampered and disrupted by the harsh living conditions in shelters and on the streets. Hence, treatment and rehabilitation programs must patiently attempt to enable clients to become as self-sufficient as possible, but not expect all clients to graduate permanently to independence.

Continuum of residential assistance. Many seriously mentally ill persons are homeless because of the lack of an appropriate number and range of community-based housing options (see chapter 10 in this volume). A February 1983 *Report on Federal Efforts to Respond to the Shelter and Basic Living Needs of Chronically Mentally Ill Persons* described how both shortages of affordable housing and the social stigma of mental health problems create barriers for mentally ill persons seeking housing (U.S. Department of Health and Human Services and U.S. Department of Housing and Urban Development, 1983). Additionally, the report noted how irregular funding patterns, unclear or antithetical legislation, restrictive eligibility determination criteria, planning and coordinating problems, and program inaccessibility all contribute to the use of substandard or inappropriate community living arrangements. Homeless mentally ill persons require a wide range of emergency, transitional, and long-term living situations with varying degrees of supervision and structure, as follows:

1. *Emergency shelter and drop-in centers.* Because the homeless mentally ill are not adequately served by the existing network of generic mental health, housing, and social service programs, emergency shelters and daytime drop-in centers are often the only alternative to the streets. They provide immediate protection from the elements, a refuge from the streets, and the opportunity for referral to specialized services.

Of course, the quality of life in these facilities varies greatly. Shelter capacities range from less than ten beds to several hundred; as their size increases, shelters become more anonymous, and their high client-staff ratios make it exceedingly difficult to personalize services to residents. Because large shelters usually house heterogeneous populations with multiple problems, staff are often unable to establish the intensive one-to-one relationships necessary to build trust and support with the severely mentally ill.

Most shelters are night operations and evict their guests after breakfast in the early morning. Drop-in centers often provide the only daytime refuge for homeless and homeless mentally ill persons. Drop-in centers are generally based in a locale where homeless people congregate or have easy access; frequently they occupy storefront space. They may offer counseling, vocational training, recreational activities, or simply a spot to rest during the day.

2. *Transitional housing.* Because of the nature of their mental disabilities and the paucity of appropriate residential options, it is often impossible to make permanent living arrangements for the homeless mentally ill during the short stay permitted at an emergency shelter. For this reason, emergency shelters need to be complemented by temporary residences that allow time for the homeless to receive more individualized assistance in making the physical and emotional transition from shelter to long-term housing. Transitional housing programs for the homeless mentally ill should provide or arrange for case management and mental health treatment/rehabilitation, and should assist residents in obtaining appropriate entitlement benefits and permanent housing.

3. *Long-term housing.* Due to the nature of their disabilities, severely mentally ill persons may require brief, and occasionally extended, periods of hospitalization to recover from acute episodes of illness. If the mentally ill person is living in a temporary residential treatment program with a long waiting list, the patient's bed may be given to someone else when he or she enters the hospital. If the patient has finally acquired an apartment, the termination of entitlement benefits during the hospitalization period may force the patient to give up that residence. These disruptive life situations often exacerbate the psychiatric problems of the mentally disabled.

Rules governing length of stay in residential settings coupled with the inability of the severely mentally ill to secure conventional housing at reasonable rents often propel them into a transient life-style, and lead to life on the streets. Long-term, *permanent* housing, linked to supportive services, is essential for the homeless mentally ill but is unavailable in many communities.

Of these three elements of a residential continuum, emergency shelter is most readily available to the homeless. Unfortunately, shelters no longer constitute a temporary service, since other low-cost housing resources are largely unavailable. Bassuk, Rubin, and Lauriat (1984) recognize that shelters have become a permanent, "institutionalized" feature of the service system.

The stability of a residence is a necessary (though not always sufficient) prerequisite to successful mental health interventions. Barrow and Lovell (1983) conducted a study of the Goddard Riverside outreach program for homeless mentally ill persons in New York City. They discovered a high correlation between successful housing/public assistance referrals and mental health referrals. Of those clients with successful housing referrals, 62 percent also had a successful mental health referral. Of those clients not referred to housing, 94 percent did not have a successful mental health referral. Barrow and Lovell admit that a causal relationship between decent housing and effective mental health treatment can only be inferred, not proven, but their discussions with outreach program staff "strongly suggest[ed] that stable housing and income are almost invariably secured before mental health referrals can be realistically undertaken'' (Barrow and Lovell, 1983, quoted in Baxter and Hopper, 1984: 117). Even the most supportive psychosocial services or intensive counseling cannot have much therapeutic value if the client subsists in a squalid shelter or on the street.

Staff training. Because of limited budgets and the unwillingness of many professionals to work with the homeless population, shelters and other service programs for the homeless frequently lack staff who have either professional training or expertise to deal with the overwhelming mental health needs of their clients. At minimum, staff of shelters, soup kitchens, drop-in centers, day programs, and transitional housing programs should receive didactic training that focuses on screening for a major mental illness; recognition of the symptoms of an acute psychiatric crisis; crisis intervention techniques; benefits and side effects of psychopharmacological treatments; and information about the full range of community resources.

Because of the high prevalence of substance abuse disorders among the homeless population (Mulkern and Spence, 1984a, 1984b), program staff also must learn about the special crises precipitated by drug abuse and excessive alcohol intake. Particularly common among young adult patients is the use of drugs and alcohol to ''self-medicate.'' Furthermore, staff should be trained to identify when a substance abuse problem is complicating a mental health disorder.

Other human service professionals, such as the police, nurses, family service workers, legal services workers, and librarians, frequently come into contact with homeless mentally ill persons as well. They too could benefit greatly from training concerning the symptoms and treatments of psychiatric illnesses among the homeless population.

Federal Assistance for the Homeless Mentally Ill Population

On July 22, 1987, the president signed Public Law 100–77, the Stewart B. McKinney Homeless Assistance Act. The broad provisions of the law include two grant programs specifically focused on the homeless mentally ill population. Section 611 of the law authorizes a ''Block Grant Program for Services to Homeless Individuals who are Chronically Mentally Ill.'' Section 612 authorizes ''Community Mental Health Services Demonstration Projects for Homeless Individuals who are Chronically Mentally Ill.'' These two programs of assistance to states require each of the five foregoing service components. Although the legislation is intended to provide emergency assistance to help the homeless, it is comprehensive and multifaceted in its approach. A comprehensive, community-based system incorporating outreach, case management, treatment/rehabilitation, a continuum of residential alternatives, and staff training offers promise for effectively serving homeless mentally ill persons.

A second piece of legislation, the ''Comprehensive State Mental Health Planning Act'' (Public Law 99–660), signed into law in October 1986, takes a longer-term approach. This law requires states to develop a comprehensive plan for community-based mental health and social welfare services for all long-term, severely mentally ill persons. The act aims to remedy the fragmentation of the mental health system that remains in the wake of deinstitutionalization. The act specifically requires that case management be provided to all severely mentally ill persons in each state, and that specialized services for the homeless mentally ill population be incorporated into the comprehensive plan.

Exactly how effective and far-reaching the mental health planning process will be is unclear. However, it is obvious that Congress is beginning to define a role for the federal government in leveraging state and local resources for comprehensive services to the homeless mentally ill, and in stimulating systemic changes within the mental health system. In fact, Public Law 100–77 states that "the Federal Government has a clear responsibility and an existing capacity to fulfill a more effective and responsible role to meet the basic human needs and to engender respect for the human dignity of the homeless."

HOUSING: PARAMOUNT NEED OF A DISABLED POPULATION

Unfortunately, neither the Community Support Program nor comprehensive federal demonstration programs for the homeless alone can resolve the problems of the homeless mentally ill. A residential continuum of emergency, transitional, and long-term housing is an integral part of a community support system, but the cost of developing such a continuum is enormous.

Healthy and mentally ill people alike are victims of a growing housing crisis. The supply of low-cost housing has dwindled precipitously in the last ten years. The U.S. General Accounting Office (1985) traces this decline to a variety of factors, including high interest rates, high property taxes, rent control, reduced federal subsidies for developers and tenants, redevelopment tax incentives, and greater profits accruing from nonresidential construction. The shortage of affordable residential facilities affects the availability of both specialized and non-specialized housing.

Because of their disabilities and high susceptibility to stress, severely mentally ill persons are more vulnerable than other low-income renters to displacement or eviction. As the National Coalition for the Homeless (1985: 7) so aptly recognizes, "the final and tragic development, which is further frustrating the chances for the homeless to find housing, is the pitting of one group of people who desperately need housing against another." In this stressful competition, the mentally ill are bound to lose out.

CONCLUSION

Homelessness is in part a public mental health problem. Between 30 and 40 percent of homeless people suffer from severe and disabling mental illnesses.

Few homeless persons in need of mental health interventions actually receive them. However, most homeless mentally ill persons express a willingness to receive assistance, especially if offered in a flexible, nonthreatening manner.

The Community Support Program template can be adapted to serve persons who are homeless and mentally ill. The advantage of the CSP approach over more traditional approaches to community mental health care is that it recognizes not only the mental health needs but also the extensive social welfare needs of severely mentally ill and homeless mentally ill individuals. Medications, supportive counseling, and psychosocial rehabilitation are not enough; severely mentally ill persons also need assistance in meeting their housing, income, vocational, social, and other needs.

Advocacy of community support systems must be tempered by a word of sober caution, however. Homelessness is not only a public mental health problem, but also an artifact of the nationwide low-cost housing shortage. As Goldman and Morrissey (1985: 730) say, we must not expect "that community support systems will solve the generic problems of homelessness in America." Community support systems mark a tremendous improvement over previous community mental health services, but their effectiveness depends upon the availability of non–mental health resources. Ultimately, the fate of homeless mentally ill persons depends upon the accessibility of both specialized and non-specialized residential alternatives. Sadly, right now the prospects for the development of either of these housing options seem remote.

ACKNOWLEDGMENT

The opinions expressed in this chapter are those of the authors and do not represent the official position of the National Institute of Mental Health. Portions of the chapter were drawn from I. S. Levine, A. D. Lezak, and H. H. Goldman, "Community Support Systems for the Homeless Mentally Ill," in *The Mental Health Needs of Homeless Persons*, ed. E. L. Bassuk. New Directions for Mental Health Services no. 30. San Francisco: Jossey-Bass, 1986.

REFERENCES

Alcohol, Drug Abuse, and Mental Health Administration (ADAMHA). 1983. *Alcohol, Drug Abuse, and Mental Health Problems of the Homeless: Proceedings of a Roundtable*. Rockville, Md.: Alcohol, Drug Abuse, and Mental Health Administration.

Bachrach, L. 1984. *Report and Analytical Summary of DHHS-Supported Researchers Studying the Homeless Mentally Ill*. Rockville, Md.: National Institute of Mental Health.

Ball, F. L. J., and Havassy, B. E. 1984. A Survey of the Problems and Needs of Homeless Consumers of Acute Psychiatric Services. *Hospital and Community Psychiatry* 35: 917–921.

Barrow, S., and Lovell, A. 1983. The Referral of Outreach Clients to Mental Health

Services: Progress Report for 1982–1983. New York: New York State Psychiatric Institute.

Bassuk, E. 1983. Addressing the Needs of the Homeless. *Boston Globe Magazine*, November 6, pp. 12, 60ff.

Bassuk, E., Rubin, L., and Lauriat, A. 1984. Is Homelessness a Mental Health Problem? *American Journal of Psychiatry* 141: 1546–1549.

Baxter, E., and Hopper, K. 1984. Shelter and Housing for the Homeless Mentally Ill. In *The Homeless Mentally Ill*, ed. H. R. Lamb. Washington, D.C.: American Psychiatric Association.

Farr, R., Koegel, P., and Burnam, A. 1986. *A Study of Homelessness and Mental Illness in the Skid Row Area of Los Angeles*. Rockville, Md.: National Institute of Mental Health.

Fischer, P., Shapiro, S., Breakey, W., Anthony, J., and Kramer, M. 1985. *Mental Health and Social Characteristics of the Homeless: A Survey of Mission Users*. Rockville, Md.: National Institute of Mental Health.

Goldman, H. H., and Morrissey, J. P. 1985. The Alchemy of Mental Health Policy: Homelessness and the Fourth Cycle of Reform. *American Journal of Public Health* 75: 727–731.

Hopper, K., and Hamberg, J. 1984. *The Making of America's Homeless: From Skid Row to New Poor, 1945–1984*. New York: Community Service Society.

Intergovernmental Health Policy Project of George Washington University. 1987. *Outreach Services for Homeless Mentally Ill People*. Rockville, Md.: National Institute of Mental Health.

Ladner, S., Crystal, S., Towber, R., Callender, B., and Calhoun, J. 1986. *Project Future: Focusing, Understanding, Targeting, and Utilizing Resources for the Homeless Mentally Ill, Elderly, Youth, Substance Abusers, and Employables*. Rockville, Md.: National Institute of Mental Health.

Lamb, H. R., ed. 1984. *The Homeless Mentally Ill*. Washington, D.C.: American Psychiatric Association.

Levine, I. S. 1984a. Homelessness: Its Implications for Mental Health Policy and Practice. *Psychosocial Rehabilitation Journal* 8: 6–16.

Levine, I. S. 1984b. Service Programs for the Homeless Mentally Ill. In *The Homeless Mentally Ill*, ed. H. R. Lamb. Washington, D.C.: American Psychiatric Association.

Levine, I. S., and Fleming, M. 1986. *Human Resource Development: Issues in Case Management*. College Park, Md.: Center of Rehabilitation and Manpower Services, University of Maryland.

Levine, I. S., Lezak, A. D., and Goldman, H. H. 1986. Community Support Systems for the Homeless Mentally Ill. In *The Mental Health Needs of Homeless Persons*, ed. E. L. Bassuk. New Directions for Mental Health Services, no. 30. San Francisco: Jossey-Bass.

Levine, I. S., and Stockdill, J. W. 1986. Mentally Ill and Homeless: A National Problem. In *Treating the Homeless: Urban Psychiatry's Challenge*, ed. B. E. Jones. Washington, D.C.: American Psychiatric Press.

Martin, M. 1987. *The Implications of NIMH-Supported Research for Homeless Mentally Ill Racial and Ethnic Minority Persons*. Rockville, Md.: National Institute of Mental Health.

Morrissey, J. P., and Dennis, D. L. 1986. *NIMH-Funded Research Concerning Homeless*

Mentally Ill Persons: Implications for Policy and Practice. Rockville, Md.: National Institute of Mental Health.

Morse, G., Shields, N. M., Hanneke, C. R., Calsyn, R., Burger, G., and Nelson, B. 1985. *Homeless People in St. Louis: A Mental Health Program Evaluation, Field Study, and Followup Investigation*. Rockville, Md.: National Institute of Mental Health.

Mowbray, C., Johnson, V., Solarz, A., and Combs, C. 1985. *Mental Health and Homelessness in Detroit: A Research Study*. Rockville, Md.: National Institute of Mental Health.

Mulkern, V., and Spence, R. 1984a. *Alcohol Abuse/Alcoholism among Homeless Persons: A Review of the Literature*. Rockville, Md.: National Institute on Alcohol Abuse and Alcoholism.

Mulkern, V., and Spence, R. 1984b. *Illicit Drug Use among Homeless Persons: A Review of the Literature*. Rockville, Md.: National Institute on Drug Abuse.

Mulkern, V., Bradley, V. J., Spence, R., Allein, S., and Oldham, J. E. 1985. Homelessness Needs Assessment Study: Findings and Recommendations for the Massachusetts Department of Mental Health. Boston.

National Coalition for the Homeless and SRO Tenants Rights Coalition. 1985. *Single Room Occupancy Hotels: Standing in the Way of the Gentry*. New York.

National Institute of Mental Health. 1983. *NIMH Definition and Guiding Principles for Community Support Systems*. Rockville, Md.

Rog, D., Andranovich, G., and Rosenblum, S. 1987. *Intensive Case Management for Persons Who Are Homeless and Mentally Ill: A Review of Community Support Program and Human Resource Development Program Efforts*. Rockville, Md.: National Institute of Mental Health.

Rosnow, M., Shaw, T., and Concord, C. 1985. *Listening to the Homeless: A Study of Homeless Mentally Ill Persons in Milwaukee*. Rockville, Md.: National Institute of Mental Health.

Roth, D., Bean, J., Lust, N., and Saveanu, T. 1985. *Homelessness in Ohio: A Study of People in Need*. Rockville, Md.: National Institute of Mental Health.

Spaniol, L., and Zipple, A. 1985. *NIMH-Supported Research on the Mentally Ill Who Are Homeless: A Second Meeting of Researchers Sponsored by the Division of Education and Service Systems Liaison, National Institute of Mental Health*. Rockville, Md.: National Institute of Mental Health.

Stroul, B. 1986. *Models of Community Support Services: Approaches to Helping Persons with Long-Term Mental Illness*. Rockville, Md.: National Institute of Mental Health.

Test, M. A., and Stein, L. I. 1979. Practical Guidelines for the Community Treatment of Markedly Impaired Patients. In *Community Support Systems for the Long-Term Patient*, ed. L. I. Stein. *New Directions for Mental Health Services*, no. 2. San Francisco: Jossey-Bass.

Turner, J. C., and Shifren, I. 1979. Community Support Systems: How Comprehensive? In *Community Support Systems for the Long-Term Patient*, ed. L. I. Stein. *New Directions for Mental Health Services*, no. 2. San Francisco: Jossey-Bass.

Turner, J. C., and TenHoor, W. 1978. The NIMH Community Support Program: Pilot Approach to a Needed Social Reform. *Schizophrenia Bulletin* 4: 319–348.

U.S. Conference of Mayors. 1986. *The Continued Growth of Hunger, Homelessness and Poverty in America's Cities: 1986.* Washington, D.C.

U.S. Department of Health and Human Services. 1984. *The Homeless: Background, Analysis, and Options.* Washington, D.C.

U.S. Department of Health and Human Services and U.S. Department of Housing and Urban Development. 1983. *Report on Federal Efforts to Respond to the Shelter and Basic Living Needs of Chronically Mentally Ill Persons.* Washington, D.C.

U.S. Department of Housing and Urban Development. 1984. *A Report to the Secretary on the Homeless and Emergency Shelters.* Washington, D.C.

U.S. General Accounting Office. 1985. *Homelessness: A Complex Problem and the Federal Response.* Washington, D.C.: U.S. Government Printing Office.

13

The Changing Role of the Public Mental Hospital

JOSEPH P. MORRISSEY

The thirty-five years from 1950 to 1985 encompass one of the most tumultuous and far-reaching periods of change in the history of mental health care in the United States. In little more than a generation the mental health service system was transformed from the near-monopoly of state and county mental hospitals as chief providers of psychiatric services to a greatly expanded, pluralistic array of public and private, inpatient and outpatient, institutional and community-based service providers. These changes resulted from a number of factors including psychosocial and legal reforms in the approach to institutionalization and treatment, the introduction and widespread use of psychotropic drugs, the growing availability of nursing homes and general hospital psychiatric services, changing attitudes of the public toward mental illness, and the increased financial support by the federal government for community-based mental health services (Bachrach, 1976; Klerman, 1982; Morrissey, 1982; Foley and Sharfstein, 1983; Brown, 1985).

Yet, even in this context of transformation and innovation, state mental hospitals continue today to serve a number of their historic functions, albeit in a reduced manner (Morrissey et al., 1980; Goldman et al., 1983). Inpatient care remains the dominant and most costly function of these facilities. They provide short-, intermediate-, and long-term custody and treatment, under both voluntary and involuntary (civil and criminal) legal statuses, to predominantly disadvantaged persons with the most severe chronic and acute mental disorders. As Goldman et al. (1983: 299) point out: ''It is the only inpatient mental health resource readily available (often as a last resort) for a large number of patients who have the most difficult problems, have failed in other treatment settings, or are considered 'inappropriate' (or 'unacceptable') for care elsewhere or are unable to afford it.''

The fact that state mental hospitals serve enduring functions does not mean that these institutions are monolithic or static in their organization and service programs, nor that their relationships with other parts of the mental health system will remain unchanged in the future. Indeed, state mental hospitals will face a set of challenges in the next few decades that will rival any in the past 150 years. To provide a perspective on these changes and challenges, this chapter will review the historical experience of public mental hospitals[1] in America, describe their current patterns of utilization, and discuss the social forces that will shape their roles in the years ahead.

HISTORICAL DEVELOPMENTS AND TRENDS

The history of public intervention on behalf of the mentally ill in America reveals a cyclical pattern of institutional reforms (Morrissey and Goldman, 1984; see also chapter 8 in this volume). The hallmark of each reform was a new environmental approach to treatment and an innovative type of facility or locus of care. The first cycle of reform, in the early nineteenth century, introduced moral treatment and the asylum (Grob, 1966; Rothman, 1971; Grob, 1973); the second cycle, in the early twentieth century, was associated with the mental hygiene movement and the psychopathic hospital (Sicherman, 1980; Rothman, 1980; Grob, 1983); and the third cycle, in the mid-twentieth century, spawned the community mental health movement and the community mental health center (Joint Commission, 1961; Musto, 1975; Foley and Sharfstein, 1983). Although each reform was the result of a unique set of sociohistorical circumstances, a number of striking parallels can be discerned in their goals, their evolution, and their outcomes.

Each reform began with the promise that early treatment in the new setting would prevent the personal and societal problems associated with long-term mental disability. However, the reforms were launched with little or no appreciation of the practical limits to which their core beliefs could be pushed. Consequently, each reform movement and its special facility flourished for a few decades and then faltered in the face of changing and unanticipated circumstances.

At first championed as a generic solution for the treatment of the mentally ill, each intervention ultimately proved viable only with acute or milder—not chronic—forms of mental disorder. In each cycle, early optimism soon faded into despair over the increasing numbers of chronic patients who were considered incurable and who began to accumulate in acute treatment settings. The public's reluctance to allocate sufficient resources for an ever-expanding population in need of mental health care, coupled with disappointment over the inability to meet exaggerated expectations, then led to a period of pessimism, retrenchment, and neglect—especially of the chronically ill.

The residue of each reform set the stage for the next generation of innovators, with little cumulative impact on the problems to which the reforms were addressed. By shifting attention from one locus of care to another, from community to institution and back again, and from isolated to centralized to decentralized services, each reform movement expanded and diversified the American mental health system into today's pluralistic patchwork of public and private, acute and chronic, voluntary and involuntary service settings. Yet each reform failed to prevent chronicity or to alter the care of the severely mentally ill in any fundamental way.

These reform cycles provide the sociohistorical context for understanding the origins, evolution, and persistence of public mental hospitals as a central component of the U.S. mental health service system. As the specifics of these reforms have been recounted in detail earlier in this volume and elsewhere, only the highlights of each reform will be noted here to set the stage for an analysis of recent trends and future prospects in the utilization of state mental hospitals.

Moral Treatment and the Asylum

The development of state-operated asylums in the early part of the nineteenth century represented the first formal system of public care for the mentally ill in this country (Grob, 1966; Caplan, 1969; Rothman, 1971; Grob, 1973). These facilities were founded during an era of social reform in response to the failures of "outdoor relief" and the practice of incarcerating the insane in local almshouses and jails. In contrast to the physical abuse, neglect, and ridicule that characterized these settings, the early asylums were championed as repositories of hope and humane care for the mentally ill. Under the aegis of "moral treatment," their superintendents claimed high rates of recovery for persons ill less than a year. Such hope for quick successes fueled the reformist zeal of social activists like Dorothea Dix (1971), whose lobbying efforts before state legislatures led to the proliferation of publicly supported asylums throughout the country. The optimism of this era soon dissipated, however, in the throes of massive waves of immigration, the related accumulation of large numbers of chronic patients, and a growing belief in the incurability of insanity.

What started out as a limited-purpose institution thus was transformed in the last half of the nineteenth century into a general-purpose solution for the social welfare burdens of a society undergoing rapid industrialization and stratification along social class and ethnic lines (Grob, 1973; Scull, 1977). The central purpose of public mental hospitals was defined by state legislatures in terms of custodial care and community protection; treatment was of secondary importance. With the death or retirement of the early moral therapists and the first group of hospital superintendents, the new generation of psychiatrists passively accepted the social role assigned to these institutions while attending to their own professionalism. In time, both hospital staff and local communities accepted as fact that the majority of patients committed to state institutions were destined to reside there for years. With overcrowding and staff shortages, the hospitals imposed a uniform custodial routine on all patients, leading to their institutionalization, or total dependency on the hospital (Wing, 1962; Gruenberg, 1974). Almost within a generation of their widespread introduction, therefore, the asylums were transformed from small, intimate, therapeutically oriented facilities to large, impersonal, custodially oriented warehouses, filled primarily with lower-class patients who suffered from a bewildering array of physical, mental, and social ills.

Mental Hygiene and the Psychopathic Hospital

Despite this seemingly irreversible course that state policies and programs supported, voices calling for institutional reform had not been completely silenced. By the late 1800s, neurologists, social workers, and lay reformers began to publicize some of the shortcomings of American psychiatry in an effort to break the stronghold of medical superintendents over the care of the insane (Quen, 1977; Sicherman, 1980). Therapeutic nihilism gave way to the optimism of a new scientific psychiatry associated with turn-of-the-century figures such as Adolf Meyer (Grob, 1983). The work of Meyer and his students, reinforced by the development of Freudian psychoanalysis, restored hope that the mentally ill could be effectively treated.

In 1909, Clifford Beers, a former mental patient who wrote about his experiences in the celebrated book *A Mind That Found Itself* (1908), enlisted the support of Meyer and William James, the Harvard philosopher and psychologist, to found the National Committee for Mental Hygiene (Dain, 1980). This reform organization revived notions about the treatability of mental disorder, especially by early intervention with acute cases. Mental hygienists advocated for a new generation of treatment facilities such as psychiatric dispensaries (outpatient clinics), child guidance centers, and "psychopathic hospitals," which were acute treatment or reception facilities affiliated with university training and research institutes.

However, these new facilities were unable to eliminate chronic mental illness. They provided high-quality care and evaluations, but most patients who needed extended care were shortly sent on to state institutions. As the movement matured, its original goal of improving the state asylums fell by the wayside. In its place, reformers began to champion the relevance of psychiatry in the care of the feebleminded, eugenics, control of alcoholism, management of abnormal children, treatment of criminals, prevention of prostitution and dependency, and the problems of industrial productivity.

Although the mental hygiene movement did little to alter the fundamental role of state institutions or their conditions, these facilities did undergo profound changes during these years (Grob, 1983). In 1890, New York passed the first State Care Act, which established the precedent for states to assume full financial responsibility and direct operational control over all county and municipal asylums. (The legislation also led to the name change of these institutions from state asylums to state mental hospitals.) Intended to provide fiscal relief and a remedy for the poor quality of care in local facilities, the longer-term consequences of this change led to a dramatic transformation in the demographic profile and length of stay of patients in state mental hospitals. County and local officials soon realized the advantages in redefining insanity to include aged and senile individuals. Transferring such patients from local almshouses to the state hospitals enabled the cost of their care to be shifted from local to state auspices. As a result, the hospitals were increasingly filled with an aged and senile population who required custodial care until life's end. Concomitantly, the almshouse declined in significance as a public institution. Throughout the first half of the twentieth century, then, state mental hospitals engaged in a vast holding operation. In the absence of specific treatments for mental disorders, they remained predominantly chronic care facilities providing long-term custody for the poor and disabled.

Community Mental Health and the Community Mental Health Centers

The first major break in this custodial pattern occurred in the aftermath of World War II. Media attention had focused on the rates of selective service rejection during the war for psychiatric reasons as well as the extent of psychiatric casualties associated with combat. The convergence of several factors stimulating renewed interest in prevention and new optimism for the treatment of mental illness heightened public awareness of this condition as a major public health problem and led to the infusion of new monies and resources. Psychiatrists returning from military service experimented with brief hospitalization and new psychosocial treatment techniques, and by the mid–1950s they were making extensive use of the new psychotropic medications. Innovative state hospitals opened aftercare clinics to serve increasing numbers of discharged mental patients and general hospitals opened acute psychiatric inpatient units. A new community mental health movement quickly took shape anchored on the belief that early intervention in a community setting could prevent chronicity and long-term disability, thereby rendering the state mental hospital obsolete.

Gradually, the federal government was drawn into a direct role in the financing and provision of mental health services. In 1946, the National Mental Health Act (Public Law 79–487) created the National Institute of Mental Health (NIMH) to stimulate research and extensive university-based training programs for desperately needed mental health manpower. The Mental Health Study Act of 1955 (Public Law 84–182) established the Joint Commission on Mental Illness and Health to evaluate national needs and resources with a view to recommending a national mental health program. The commission's final report, *Action for Mental Health* (Joint Commission, 1961), became the basis for the "bold new approach" adopted by President Kennedy in the Community Mental Health Centers Act of 1963 (Public Law 88–164), which called for the creation of an elaborate network of community mental health centers (CMHCs) which would provide a comprehensive array of treatment and preventive services in community settings.

The near-term accomplishments of the community mental health movement rivaled the successes once claimed for the early asylums. Between 1955 and 1980, for example, the resident population of state mental hospitals declined more than 75 percent, and since the mid–1960s more than 700 CMHCs serving catchment areas representing 50 percent of the U.S. population have been created. Upon closer scrutiny, however, it is clear that shifts in the locus of care did not solve the problem of chronic mental illness and its treatment. Indeed, many observers have argued that the centers exacerbated the plight of the chronic patient (Chu and Trotter, 1974; Bassuk and Gerson, 1978; Rose, 1979; Gruenberg and Archer, 1979).

These developments did have a tremendous impact on the number and mix of mental health service providers, however. In 1955, the resident census of state and county mental hospitals had reached its all-time high of 558,922 patients, but by 1975 it had been reduced to 193,436 patients, a decrease of 65 percent (Table 13–1; see, also, Figure 2–1 in this volume). In 1955, 77 percent of all mental health care episodes occurred on an inpatient basis and nearly two-thirds of these occurred in state and county mental hospitals. By 1975, however, only 28 percent of the episodes occurred on an inpatient basis and only one-third of these occurred in state and county mental hospitals (Table 13–2).

These figures, which seemingly indicate a large-scale shift in the locus of treatment from inpatient to outpatient services, more accurately represent a rapid expansion of the overall mental health services system. Between 1955 and 1975, total episodes of care presented through the mental health services system increased more than fourfold, including a twelvefold increase in the availability of community-based outpatient services alone. Most of this growth was associated with the expansion of ambulatory care in general hospital outpatient programs, community mental health centers, and other freestanding clinics. From all indications, the shift can be explained primarily by the entry into treatment of new populations of patients without prior contact with mental health services rather than by the engagement of the severely disturbed, long-stay clients released from state and county mental health hospitals (Goldman, Adams, and Taube, 1983). As a consequence, the relative role, or market share, of public inpatient institutions has diminished dramatically while their absolute role has endured, although in somewhat altered form (Goldman et al., 1983). In this connection, it is important to note that among inpatient episodes, state and county mental hospitals still predominate.

Deinstitutionalization of state and county mental hospitals proceeded through

Table 13-1
Number and Percent Change in Hospitals, Resident Patients, Admissions, and Additions to State and County Mental Hospitals, United States, 1950-1985

Year	Hospitals Number	Hospitals Percent Change	Resident Patients at End of Year Number	Resident Patients at End of Year Percent Change	Admissions During Year Number	Admissions During Year Percent Change	Additions[a] During Year Number	Additions[a] During Year Percent Change
1950	322	—	512,501	—	152,286	—	—	—
1955	275	−14.6	558,922	9.1	178,003	16.9	—	—
1960	280	1.8	535,540	−4.2	234,791	31.9	—	—
1965	290	3.6	475,202	−11.3	316,664	34.9	—	—
1970	315	8.6	337,619	−29.0	384,511	21.4	—	—
1975	313	−0.6	193,436	−42.7	376,156	−2.2	433,529	—
1980	276	−11.8	132,164	−31.7	—	—	370,344	−14.6
1985	279	1.1	116,136	−12.1	—	—	332,229	−10.3

Source: Data for 1950–1980 are adapted from Goldman, Adams, and Taube (1983); the data for 1985 are based on unpublished data from the Division of Biometry and Applied Sciences, National Institute of Mental Health.

[a]From 1950 to 1975 the National Institute of Mental Health collected information on inpatient admissions (admissions and readmissions) to state and county mental hospitals. Beginning in 1976 only information on number of *additions* is available. Additions differ from admissions because returns from leave and institutional transfers are included as well as admissions and readmissions.

two distinct phases (Morrissey, 1982). The timing and pace of each phase varied among the states, but nationally the first, or "benign," phase encompassed the period roughly from 1956 to 1965, and the second, or "radical," phase encompassed the period from about 1966 to 1975. The first phase was characterized by (1) the resurgence of active treatment programs and sharp reductions in length of stay, (2) a steady increase in annual admissions, and (3) small but steady decreases in the end-of-year resident patient census. Throughout this period, total admissions to state and county mental hospitals grew at the rate of 4 to 8 percent per year while the resident census declined at an annual rate of 1 to 3 percent. Cumulatively, the census decreases amounted to only 4 percent by 1960 and only 15 percent by 1965 (Table 13-1). Both figures are remarkable, nonetheless, in that they represented the first sustained decrease in the resident patient population of public mental hospitals in American history.

The operative policy during this first phase of deinstitutionalization emphasized "opening the back doors" of public mental hospitals for the early release of new admissions and for the placement of higher functioning long-stay patients in alternative housing and aftercare programs whenever appropriate arrangements could be found (Morrissey, 1982). The price of this policy was a high readmission rate for patients who could not make the transition back to community living in one step, but who needed periodic hospital stays to support their functioning in

Table 13-2
Inpatient and Outpatient Care Episodes in State and County Mental Hospitals and Other U.S. Mental Health Facilities, 1955–1985

Year	Total, All Facilities[b]	Inpatient Episodes[a]			Outpatient Episodes[a]		
		All Services	State and Co. Mental Hospitals	Other	All Services	State and Co. Mental Hospitals	Other
Number of Patient Care Episodes							
1955	1,675,352	1,296,352	818,832	477,520	379,000	—	—
1965	2,636,525	1,565,525	804,926	760,599	1,071,000	—	—
1970[c]	4,038,143	1,721,389	745,259	976,130	2,316,754	—	—
1975	6,409,447	1,791,171	598,993	1,192,088	4,618,276	332,518	4,285,758
1980[d]	6,161,555	1,720,392	499,169	1,221,223	4,441,163	169,165	4,271,998
1985[e]	6,868,230	1,860,302	459,374	1,400,928	5,007,928	198,904	4,809,024
Percent Distribution							
1955	100.0	77.4	48.9	28.5	22.6	—	—
1965	100.0	59.4	30.5	28.9	40.6	—	—
1970	100.0	42.6	18.5	24.2	57.4	—	—
1975	100.0	29.4	9.3	18.6	72.1	5.2	66.9
1980	100.0	27.9	8.1	9.8	72.1	2.7	69.4
1985	100.0	27.1	6.7	20.4	72.9	2.9	70.0

Rate Per 100,000 Population

1955	1,028	795	502	293	233	—	—
1965	1,376	817	420	396	559	—	—
1970	1,977	843	365	479	1,134	—	—
1975	3,033	847	283	564	2,185	157	2,028
1980	2,706	756	219	536	1,951	74	1,876
1985	2,956	799	198	603	2,155	86	2,070

Source: Data for 1955–1975 are from Goldman et al. (1983); the figures for 1980–1985 are unpublished data from the National Institute of Mental Health.

[a] Patient care episodes are defined as the number of residents in inpatient organizations at the beginning of the year (or the number of persons on the rolls of noninpatient organizations) plus the total additions to these organizations during the year. As additions involve a duplicated count of persons with more than one admission during the year, use of patient care episodes results in a duplicated count of persons.

[b] Includes inpatient and outpatient services of state and county mental hospitals, private mental hospitals, residential treatment centers for emotionally disturbed children, general hospital psychiatric services (non-VA), federally assisted CMHCs, and inpatient services only of VA hospitals. In order to present trends on the same set of facilities over this period, the following facilities are excluded from the episode counts: private psychiatric office practice, all psychiatric services offered by federal agencies other than the Veterans Administration (such as the Public Health Service, Indian Health Service, Department of Defense, and Bureau of Prisons), inpatient services at multiservice facilities not listed above, and all partial episodes.

[c,d,e] Figures for these years are based on 1971, 1981, and 1983, respectively.

the community. These readmissions, or revolving-door patients, contributed to the growth in annual admissions throughout the late 1950s and early 1960s (Table 13–1). Many clinicians willingly accepted this pattern of hospital use as the only way large numbers of patients could ever leave hospital wards.

The timing of the second or radical phase of deinstitutionalization also varied in different states, but nationally it began approximately in 1966. The operative policy during this phase emphasized "closing the front doors" of state and county mental hospitals as well as continuing the earlier "back door" policy for the accelerated release of both short- and long-stay patients to the community (Morrissey, 1982). The shift was occasioned by the coalescing of interests among community mental health advocates, civil libertarian reformers, and fiscal conservatives. These interest groups lobbied for the abrupt closure of state institutions and the transfer of patients to less restrictive and less costly community-based programs. Enactment of the Medicare-Medicaid amendments to the Social Security Act in 1965 also provided a fiscal incentive for state and county mental hospital authorities to place otherwise unreimbursable clients in nursing homes largely at federal expense (Morrissey and Goldman, 1984). Further, civil libertarian reforms in state commitment statutes placed limits on the use of these hospitals through the imposition of restrictive "dangerousness" criteria for admission and by mandating enriched institutional staffing and life-safety codes. State legislators were soon caught up in a general fiscal crisis associated with the economic downturn and "stagflation" of the early 1970s. They were receptive to census rundowns both to avoid the costs of bringing physical plants up to judicial or regulatory standards and to reduce the ever-rising annual appropriations for hospital operations (Robitscher, 1976).

These changes in policy toward the use of state and county mental hospitals led to a dramatic acceleration in the pace and character of deinstitutionalization. From 1966 through 1970 the annual resident census reduction jumped from 5 to 10 percent per year and was sustained at that level, on average, each year from 1971 through 1975. Whereas the census decline between 1960 and 1965 amounted to only 11 percent, it jumped to 29 percent for 1966–1970 and to 43 percent for 1971–1975 (Table 13–2). Cumulatively, the census decline by the end of the first phase of deinstitutionalization in 1965 amounted to only 15 percent, but by the end of the second phase in 1975, it had vaulted to 65 percent.

Annual admissions also started to decline during this second phase, and in 1970, for the first time in modern history, more patients were released than were admitted. This trend accelerated over the next several years. Deinstitutionalization efforts during this second phase also took on a decidedly different character than in the first phase. As Ernest Gruenberg (1982: 277, 280) has described it: "In each state mental hospital, directors vied for a better report on a dropping census. The states began to compete with one another for publicity, with one claiming to have dropped its census more than another. A falling mental hospital census became a fetish and an end in itself, without regard for the consequences to the patients."

The outcomes of this depopulation process are well known to even casual readers of the recent popular and professional literature. In the 1970s, thousands of patients were returned to communities across the country, where they often encountered the hostility and rejection of the general public and the reluctance of community mental health and welfare agencies to assume responsibility for their care (Bachrach, 1976; Morrissey and Goldman, 1984; Brown, 1985). For others, a process of *transinstitutionalization* occurred as many thousands of former patients came to reside in nursing homes, board-and-care homes, adult homes, and other institutional settings in the community (Morrissey, 1982; Brown, 1985). Still others have swelled the ranks of the urban homeless (Goldman and Morrissey, 1985; Morrissey and Dennis, 1986).

PUBLIC MENTAL HOSPITALS IN THE 1980s

There are no published reports which present up-to-date and comprehensive information on the structure and functioning of public mental hospitals in the various states. However, data from the national reporting program maintained by the NIMH (Redick et al., 1983) can be used to assemble a national or composite profile. Here we will focus on the capacity and volume of these hospitals; the social, demographic, and clinical characteristics of the patients served in this system; staffing patterns and types of treatments employed; and hospital financing. These data indicate that state mental hospitals continue to account for a substantial proportion of the total numbers of patients, staff, and dollars in the U.S. mental health system. In contrast to one of the prevailing myths in this field, the rapid expansion of community-based mental health and other protective systems since 1955 has diminished, but not supplanted, the role of state and county mental hospitals.

Capacity and Volume

During 1985, a total of 279 mental hospitals were operated by state mental health authorities in the United States. This compares to a total of 275 hospitals in 1955 when this system achieved its highest patient utilization and to 315 hospitals in 1970 at about the point that rapid deinstitutionalization was getting underway across the country. Since the resident patient population decreased by nearly 80 percent over the 1955–1985 interval, it is clear that the average size of these hospitals has undergone tremendous reductions as well. In 1981, the average daily census for all state mental hospitals was 122,073, with an average hospital size of about 440 patients; this contrasts with an average daily census of over 500,000 in 1955 and an average size of about 2,030 patients.[2]

Not only has the typical hospital become much smaller, but it also has become more specialized with a shorter average length of stay. Stimulated by the community mental health movement of the 1950s and 1960s, many hospitals initially developed or expanded outpatient and day-care services to accompany their

322   *The Community Mental Health Movement*

Table 13–3
Number, Percent Distribution, and Rate Per 100,000 Population of Resident Patients and Additions to State and County Mental Hospitals by Selected Primary Diagnoses, United States, 1984

Mental Disorder	Resident Patients Beginning of Year			Additions During Year		
	Number	*Percent*	*Rate*	*Number*	*Percent*	*Rate*
Schizophrenia-related	59,219	50.2	25.5	122,002	36.7	52.3
Alcohol-related	5,328	4.5	2.3	55,124	16.6	23.6
Drug-related	2,138	1.8	0.9	17,950	5.4	7.7
Affective Disorders	9,565	8.1	4.1	52,002	15.7	22.3
Organic Disorders	17,482	14.8	7.5	12,523	3.8	5.4
All Other	24,295	20.6	9.5	72,628	21.8	31.1
Total	118,027	100.0	49.5	332,229	100.0	142.4

Source: Unpublished data from the Division of Biometry and Applied Sciences, National Institute of Mental Health.

traditional inpatient programs. By 1982, however, only 91 of 277 hospitals (33 percent) offered outpatient services and 62 of 277 (22 percent) offered day treatment services. These figures represent a 50 percent reduction from the number of hospitals providing such services in 1970. The median stay for all annual admissions decreased from 41 days in 1970 to 23 days in 1980. Even so, public mental hospitals still accounted for nearly 44.6 million inpatient days in 1981, or 58 percent of all inpatient days for the entire mental health system.

Patient Characteristics

At the beginning of 1984 there were 118,027 resident patients in state mental hospitals and 332,229 additions during the year—i.e., direct admissions and readmissions as well as returns from leave and institutional transfers—for a total of 450,256 episodes of care. The additions profile is driven by current use patterns, whereas the resident patient profile reflects care patterns more typical of past decades. Taube, Thompson, and Rosenstein (1983), for example, estimate that about 40 percent of the end-of-year resident patient population was admitted during the year, while the other 60 percent had been admitted at a prior time and were hospitalized continuously during the current year. In 1980, approximately 80 percent of the total admissions to the state mental hospital system were readmissions. Over 58 percent were committed on an involuntary legal status, and 65 percent of total admissions were males. The diagnostic and age profiles of these patients are presented in Tables 13–3 and 13–4.

Schizophrenia and related conditions account for the majority of resident

Table 13–4
Number, Percent Distribution, and Rate Per 100,000 Population of Resident Patients and Additions to State and County Mental Hospitals, by Age Groupings, United States, 1984

Mental Disorder	Resident Patients Beginning of Year			Additions during Year		
	Number	Percent	Rate	Number	Percent	Rate
Under 18	6,214	5.2	9.9	18,240	5.5	29.1
18–24	12,605	10.7	43.7	61,313	18.5	214.7
25–44	43,150	36.6	62.8	172,590	51.9	247.5
45–65	27,586	23.4	61.9	63,387	19.1	142.0
65 and Over	28,472	24.1	103.6	16,699	5.0	60.2
Total	118,027	100.0	49.5	332,229	100.0	142.4

Source: Unpublished data from the Division of Biometry and Applied Sciences, National Institute of Mental Health.

patients (50.2 percent) followed by patients with organic disorders (14.8 percent). The additions diagnostic mix is a bit more varied. Schizophrenia still predominates (36.7 percent), but there are relatively few organic cases (3.8 percent) and many more patients with affective disorders (15.7 percent) and alcohol-related diagnoses (16.6 percent).

Notable differences are also present with regard to the age distribution of resident patients and additions. The general trend is for resident patients to be older than patient additions. The modal age category for both service categories is twenty-five to forty-four years but, whereas approximately 48 percent of the residents are older than forty-five years, only 24 percent of the annual additions are that old. Likewise, 24 percent of the additions are under age twenty-four, whereas only 16 percent of the residents are that young. These patterns are clearly visible in age-specific hospitalization rates per 100,000 population. For resident patients, the highest rate (103.6) is for the sixty-five and over age group, a figure which is nearly twice as large as any other age grouping. For additions, the highest rates are for the twenty-five to forty-four and eighteen to twenty-four age groups (247.5 and 214.7, respectively). In general, then, although the resident patient census of state mental hospitals still has a substantial elderly population, it is not being replenished at the same rate as in the years prior to deinstitutionalization. Today, patients entering state mental hospitals are much younger, and, as noted above, they are staying on average for much shorter lengths of time than in prior decades.

These overall trends mask the growth of a new long-stay population in many state systems, however. In 1979, NIMH staff commissioned a special sample study to identify the characteristics of these patients (Taube, Thompson, and Rosenstein, 1983). The findings indicated that about 60 percent of resident patients at a given point in time had been continuously hospitalized for at least one year. (Using 1985 data from Table 13–2, this amounts to about 69,700 patients.) Moreover, the survey revealed that these patients could be divided into three groups: *new long-stay patients* (41 percent of the total long-stay) who have been continuously hospitalized for one to five years, i.e., they have gained this status since deinstitutionalization began; *intermediate stay patients* (29 percent) who have been continuously hospitalized for five to nineteen years; and *old long-stay patients* (30 percent) who have been continuously hospitalized for twenty years or more, i.e., these patients have remained hospitalized in spite of efforts at deinstitutionalization.

The old long-stay group was found to be an aged schizophrenic population; almost 60 percent were over age sixty-five and 24 percent were over age seventy-five. (The long-term decline in the numbers of such patients in state mental hospitals has slowed markedly due to a reduced death rate in recent years.) Government programs were the primary source of payment for their care— Medicare (19 percent), Medicaid (21 percent), and other government funds (16 percent). About 40 percent of these patients were hospitalized in an involuntary legal status; the rest had been admitted on a voluntary basis or converted to voluntary status during their stay. These patients account for almost 20 percent of the annual state mental hospital days and over 13 percent of yearly expenditures. In 1979, their cost of care exceeded $25 billion and was growing at over $500 million a year in then-current dollars.

The new long-stay group was found to be similar to the old long-stay patients in a number of respects. Currently it is younger, but if it were to be hospitalized continuously for another 15 years, it will be similar in age distribution to the old long-stay group. However, there were some notable diagnostic differences between the two groups with new long-stay having more patients with organic and fewer with schizophrenic diagnoses. The latter differences were attributed to changes in diagnostic practices over the preceding twenty years (Taube, Thompson, and Rosenstein, 1983). The most striking finding of this study is the size of the new long-stay patient group, suggesting that the process of institutionalization in state mental hospitals, as determined by length of stay, goes on.

Two other characteristics underscore the social and economic circumstances of state mental hospital patients—marital status and source of payment. Only 21 percent of additions in 1980 were currently married, while 45 percent were never married and 34 percent were widowed, divorced, or separated (Manderscheid, Witkin, and Rosenstein, 1985: 45). Over half of male additions and one-third of female additions were among never-married patients. With regard to expected source of payment, nearly 47 percent of the admissions in 1980 had no payments for their care and another 18 percent were dependent upon government insurance programs. What these data suggest is that many in this patient group are socially isolated individuals who lack the resources needed to secure private sources of care.

Table 13–5

Number and Percent Distribution of Full-Time-Equivalent[a] Staff Positions in State and County Mental Hospitals, by Discipline, United States, 1982

Staff Discipline	Number	Percent
Professional Patient Care Staff	(48,224)	(25.3)
Psychiatrists	3,866	2.0
Other Physicians	2,012	1.1
Psychologists	3,196	1.7
Social Workers	6,276	3.3
Registered Nurses	15,613	8.2
Other Mental Health Professionals (B.A. and above)	9,179	4.8
Physical Health Professionals and Assistants	8,082	4.2
Other Mental Health Workers (less than B.A.)	75,940	40.0
Administrative, Clerical, Maintenance	66,102	34.7
Total Staff	190,266	100.0

Source: Manderscheid, Witkin, and Rosenstein (1985: 55).

[a]Full-time-equivalent (FTE) staff is computed as the total number of hours worked per week by full-time, part-time, and trainee staff divided by 40 hours.

Staffing and Treatment

In 1982, there were 190,266 full-time-equivalent staff positions in state mental hospitals (Table 13–5). Of this total, approximately 65 percent were allocated to direct patient care and 35 percent to administrative, clerical, and maintenance activities. Patient care staff, in turn, consisted of both professionals (25 percent) and nonprofessionals (40 percent). These figures represent a 15 percent decrease in total staff since 1972. Most of the overall decrease in the 1972–1982 period was accounted for by other mental health workers—those with less than a B.A. degree who function primarily as aides or attendants—(–24 percent), whereas the number of professionals increased significantly (+ 25 percent). Most of the latter increase was associated with physical health professionals and assistants (+ 74 percent) and other B.A. and above mental health professionals (+ 56 percent). Substantial increases also occurred for psychologists (+ 29 percent), social workers (+ 18 percent), and nurses (+ 17 percent). The two professional groups for which significant decreases occurred are psychiatrists (–12 percent) and other physicians (–18 percent), a decline that appears to be associated with a general decrease in medical school graduates entering psychiatry and with legal changes restricting the supply of foreign medical school graduates (Thompson, Checker, and Witkin, 1983).

Information is also available on the types of treatments that were received by the cohort of patient additions to state hospitals during 1980 (Table 13–6). Drug and individual therapy were the most commonly used treatments, involving about

Table 13–6
Number and Percent Distribution of Inpatient Additions to State and County Mental Hospitals, by Type of Treatment, United States, 1980

Type of Treatment	Number	Percent
Individual Therapy	235,822	63.9
Family/Couple Therapy	26,571	7.2
Group Therapy	184,155	49.9
Drug Therapy	240,620	65.2
Detoxification	53,310	15.8
Self-Care Skill Training	60,155	16.3
Social Skill Training	95,215	25.8
Activity Therapies	178,251	48.3
Other	87,465	23.7
Total 1980 Additions[a]	369,049	100.0

Source: Manderscheid, Witkin, and Rosenstein (1985: 49).

[a]Table entries exceed total additions as many patients received more than one type of treatment.

two-thirds of these patients. Group therapy and activity therapy were employed with about one-half of the patients. Self-care and social skill training were employed with less than one-quarter, but such treatments are much more prevalent for long-stay residents.

Finances

In 1983, expenditures by state mental hospitals amounted to $5.49 billion (Table 13–7). This amount represents 45 percent of total expenditures by mental health organizations in the United States and a per capita (civilian population) expenditure of $23.49 (Redick, Witkin, and Atay, 1987). About 78 percent of these funds were expended on staff salaries with the remainder allocated to other operating expenditures, depreciation, and contracts with other mental health organizations.

Government sources account for the bulk of these funds (94.5 percent). State government (69.1 percent) is the principal source of funding at $3.8 billion, primarily through legislative appropriations to the state mental health authorities. The federal government (23 percent) accounts for nearly $1.3 billion, primarily in the form of Medicaid and Medicare reimbursements. Local government (2.4 percent) and other sources make up the remaining funding. In contrast to most private mental health organizations, less than 2 percent of funding for state mental hospitals was derived directly from client fees.

THE RECURRING MENTAL HOSPITAL DEBATE

It is truly remarkable that, despite persistent criticism and opposition, state mental hospitals have endured for over 150 years in the United States. Indeed,

Table 13–7
Expenditures and Source of Funds (current dollars in thousands) for State and County Mental Hospitals, United States, 1983

Total Expenditures	Amount	Percent
Staff Salaries	4,304,973	78.4
Contracts with Other Mental Health Organizations	36,839	0.7
Other Operating Expenditures	948,922	17.3
Depreciation	88,667	1.6
Capital Expenditures	112,303	2.0
Total	5,491,473	100.0
Source of Funds	**Amount**	**Percent**
State Government		
Mental Health Agency Funds (excludes Medicaid)	3,372,783	61.8
Other State Funds	399,998	7.3
Federal Government		
Medicaid	990,825	18.1
Medicare	151,715	2.8
Other	112,119	2.1
Local Government	130,250	2.4
Contract Funds from Other Nongovernment Agencies	28,203	0.5
Client Fees		
Received Directly	90,121	1.7
Fees reverted to State	156,977	2.9
All Other	26,269	0.4
Total	5,459,460	100.0

Source: Redick, Witkin, and Atay (1987: 13, 22).

much of the past drama associated with the major cycles of reform in mental health care has involved the interplay between advocates and critics of the state hospital concerning its value on fiscal, therapeutic, and legal grounds. Although the specifics of the debate in each reform cycle were framed in terms of then-current practices, the fundamental or underlying issues have remained pretty much the same. In the following pages, I will focus on the post-deinstitutionalization era and present a brief synopsis of the major arguments (pro and con) advanced on behalf of the continued use of state mental hospitals.

The Case for Closing State Mental Hospitals

As described by Robert Okin (1983), former commissioner of both the Vermont and Massachusetts Departments of Mental Health, state mental hospitals are faced with a series of unremitting problems:

Physical structure. The physical plants of most state mental hospitals are antiquated, deteriorated, and inhospitable, and their architectural design is prison-like and inconsistent with modern treatment needs. Efforts to promote higher levels of patient functioning are undermined by the physical environment which "requires mass behavior and permits little differentiation and individual choice" (Okin, 1983: 578).

Isolation. Many state mental hospitals are isolated both geographically and programmatically. The nineteenth-century legacy of pastoral asylums has left many facilities in remote rural areas. This creates significant barriers for continuity of care between hospital and community programs and makes it difficult for families or other support networks to assist in a patient's return to community living.

Staffing. State hospitals often have chronic manpower problems both in the quantity and quality of their staff. Due to limited appropriations and low salary structures, they are forced to operate with much lower staffing levels than either private mental hospitals or general hospital psychiatric units while having to deal with the most difficult patients. These hospitals also have difficulty recruiting and retaining competent staff in all disciplines, but their nursing and psychiatric staffing problems are especially critical. A severe national nursing shortage disadvantages state hospitals, which cannot compete in salary and job conditions with other hospitals. Recent federal policy changes reducing the availability of foreign medical graduates and a general decline in psychiatric residency training have hit state hospitals especially hard (Thompson, Checker, and Witkin, 1983). The overall result is that "state hospital patients, who as a group need the highest level of psychiatric care, are forced to settle for the lowest" (Okin, 1983: 579).

Rehabilitative programs. The vocational and social rehabilitation programs that do exist in these institutions are understaffed, minimal, and often directed at "busy work" rather than skill enhancement to benefit patients in ways supportive of their functioning in the community.

Funding. Overall, state hospitals need a sizable infusion of funds to upgrade staffing and to modernize their physical plants. Yet it is unlikely that the necessary resources will be made available due to fiscal constraints on state governments, discriminatory practices in third-party reimbursement (both private and governmental) as regards state hospital care, competing resource claims from community programs, and the lack of ability by the state hospitals themselves to regulate caseloads commensurate with annual appropriations.

Bureaucratic constraints. State hospitals must work within a series of inflexible administrative constraints that undermine their ability to provide efficient and high-quality care. These include civil service controls over hiring and firing of personnel, job descriptions, and qualifications. Line-item budgets also severely hamper innovations and efficient use of appropriations to meet changing patient needs. Collective bargaining agreements and state purchasing requirements are other factors which hamper administrators and ultimately diminish the quality of care at state mental hospitals.

Referring to these several deficiencies, Okin (1983: 577) judges that "this situation is virtually unalterable and . . . most state hospitals are unlikely to yield in any substantial way to efforts at reform." He recommends that most state hospitals be completely replaced with a very different system in order to increase the likelihood that the lives of their patients will be substantially improved. Similar views have been expressed by many others in the past fifteen years (e.g., Talbott, 1978). Mendel (1976: 21) captures the essence of the antihospital movement in the following capsule assessment: "The [state] hospital as a form of treatment for the severely ill psychiatric patient is always expensive and inefficient, frequently antitherapeutic, and never the treatment of choice."

The Case against Closing State Mental Hospitals

Arguments against the closing of state mental hospitals have increasingly relied upon functionalist perspectives (Bachrach, 1976). This view recognizes that state hospitals do perform necessary and legitimate functions for which suitable alternatives do not exist at this time. Consequently, functionalists insist that state mental hospitals will endure for the foreseeable future (e.g., Lamb and Goertzel, 1972; Dingman, 1976; Rachlin, 1976; Morrissey et al., 1980; Craig and Laska, 1983; Goldman et al., 1983; Barton, 1983; Gralnick, 1985; Bachrach, 1986). Among the multiple functions served by these hospitals, several overlapping responsibilities are most often cited:

Back-up role. State mental hospitals continue to serve as the "facility of last resort" for the public and private mental health systems (Miller, 1981; Goldman et al., 1983; Rachlin, 1976; Shore and Shapiro, 1979). The argument is that the community mental health system as we know it today could not exist without having state hospitals to accept the failures, i.e., those patients for whom community care is not feasible at a particular point in their illness. As described by Barter (1980: 165), these cases include "chronic deteriorated patients, actively aggressive and assaultive patients, and some individuals suffering from a combination of mental and physical illness so severe as to tax local facilities. It is these individuals who vex most community programs and who consume enormous quantities of local treatment resources." Other hospitals and community services are thereby able to treat a selected target population and to refer the most difficult, least desirable, and most costly patients to state hospitals (Shore and Shapiro, 1979).

Community protection. State hospitals also insure public safety by removing from society individuals showing certain kinds of disruptive behavior. The many thousands of dangerous patients served in these facilities each year represent this function, as do the services provided to mentally ill offenders and to the courts in relation to insanity and incompetency proceedings (Steadman, Monahan, and Hartstone, 1982).

Custodial care. As indicated in the statistical profile of state mental hospitals presented earlier in this chapter, these facilities still have a sizable custodial care population (Taube, Thompson, and Rosenstein, 1983). As of 1985, as many as 41,000 residents had lengths of stay of five years or longer and nearly 20,000 had stays of twenty years or more. Many of these patients are elderly and chronically deteriorated persons who are unable to be placed in nursing homes due either to lack of space or to their own difficult and disturbed behavior. Others are persistently psychotic, or so disturbing and unmanageable that they "cannot and should not be discharged" (Pepper and Ryglewicz, 1985: 241), or both.

Treatment. State mental hospitals continue to provide acute treatment for many thousands of short-stay (less than 30 days) and intermediate stay (31–365 days) patients (Goldman et al., 1983). Most are involuntarily committed revolving-door admissions who fail to seek or accept community aftercare services. If these patients do enter the treatment system after discharge, they may discontinue involvement after an initial contact, eventually ending up in emergency rooms or inpatient units at general hospitals from which they will be quickly transferred to state facilities because their expected length of treatment or lack of insurance coverage makes them inappropriate for these settings. Some supporters of state mental hospitals argue that these facilities can play a unique role in the intensive treatment of severely mentally ill patients—such as children and adolescents, the elderly, and adults who have not responded to short-term treatment—who require specialized services not readily available elsewhere (Barton, 1983; Miller, 1981; Barter, 1980; Pepper and Ryglewicz, 1985).

Asylum and shelter. One of the historic functions served by state mental hospitals for many patients has been the provision of respite and temporary haven, as well as protection from victimization in the community setting. Although many commentators still see this as an enduring function of these hospitals (Bachrach, 1976; Dingman, 1976), its availability and access has diminished greatly in the past fifteen to twenty years. With civil libertarian reforms of commitment statutes and the concept of treatment in the least restrictive environment, gaining voluntary admission to state hospitals has become exceedingly difficult (Robitscher, 1976; Morrissey and Tessler, 1982). Indeed, the critique of deinstitutionalization that has been spurred by the problem of urban homelessness centers on the complaint that many former patients are unable to gain shelter and asylum at these facilities (Goldman and Morrissey, 1985; Appelbaum, 1987).

Latent functions. In addition to these patient care activities, a variety of other latent or secondary functions are often cited as relevant to the survival of and continuing need for state mental hospitals. Among these are the hospitals' role in clinical research and professional training (Dingman, 1976; Bachrach, 1976; Miller, 1981) as well as employment and economic support for surrounding communities (Goldman et al., 1983).

Toward a More Flexible Role for Public Mental Hospitals

There is a growing recognition that the future role of state mental hospitals will vary greatly from state to state and from community to community. Among the reasons for this are the varying character of patient populations in different hospitals, variations in the way communities want to use state hospitals, and the variability of community mental health alternatives both within and between states (Bachrach, 1986).

Pepper and Ryglewicz (1985) have described three different "ecological" and programmatic contexts that promote the role differentiation of state mental hospitals. In some communities, state hospitals are the *sole providers* of mental health care. This is typical in rural areas with low population densities and poor or nonexistent public transportation. Under these circumstances, state mental hospitals often provide a comprehensive service array including acute and long-term inpatient care and a full spectrum of rehabilitative and outpatient services. Sole provider status allows the hospitals the rare opportunity to develop treatment planning in a situation of full control and responsibility. Pepper and Ryglewicz point out that, in many instances, this potential is undermined by the reality that rural state mental hospitals are not up to date regarding either environmental conditions, treatment quality, or methods of care.

The opposite role emerges when the state mental hospital is *part of a fully developed system.* Here there is no burden to develop a full range of services but there also tends to be far less control over the treatment course of patients (especially if local communities provide general hospital inpatient psychiatric care as well). Under these circumstances, Pepper and Ryglewicz point out, state mental hospitals are frequently relegated to a backup role associated with a custodial rather than a rehabilitative orientation, and with severe resource problems.

Pepper and Ryglewicz also suggest a third approach that would employ the the state hospital as *an additional acute care hospital as well as a refuge for the residual long-term population.* This would allow for the development of specialty treatment units for intermediate and long-term care along with close collaboration and communication with community services to maintain continuity of care. One mechanism for realizing this more positive role is the "unified services" model implemented by these same authors in Rockland County, New York, that allows for staff and resource sharing between institutional and community programs (Pepper and Ryglewicz, 1983). Other models for integrating state hospitals and community agencies, both administratively and programmatically, have been described in the literature (see Talbott, 1983).

The implication of Pepper and Ryglewicz's analysis is that future roles of state mental hospitals will vary from one locality to another depending upon residual populations served and the level of development and integration of local services. As a consequence, the past unitary or monolithic image of the state mental hospital will become increasingly dated, making it difficult to generalize from a national perspective about the functions, utilization patterns, and performance levels of individual state systems (also see Bachrach, 1986).

FUTURE PROBLEMS AND PROSPECTS

The foregoing analyses make clear that state mental hospitals will continue to evolve and to adapt to changing national, state, and local circumstances. As

Goldman and Taube (1985) have pointed out, in principle as well as in practice, the issue is not whether individual state mental hospitals can be replaced (they can), but rather whether the general public, elected officials, and other mental health providers are willing to make the resource investments and organizational changes requisite to do so. Given the current limited efficacy of psychiatric treatments, the severe mental illnesses for the most part will remain chronic conditions, and both the public as well as persons with mental disorders will need many of the services now provided by the state mental hospitals. The issue, according to Goldman and Taube (1985: 29), "is not 'will they survive?' but 'can they provide quality services?' " during the period of time it will take to have their functions transferred to other facilities and settings. In the remainder of this chapter, a number of forces inside and outside the mental health arena that will influence the future course and direction of state mental hospitals will be highlighted.

Mental Health Financing

Funding issues have plagued state mental hospitals from their inception in America over 150 years ago. During the moral treatment era, the issue was the willingness of localities to support the per diem costs of housing and caring for the indigent insane. In the mental hygiene era, following state monopolization of asylum operation, the issue became the willingness of state legislatures to appropriate funds for minimal humane care in overpopulated and understaffed hospitals. In the community mental health era, the question initially was the willingness of the federal government to support new community services and income maintenance programs for the mentally ill, with state and federal authorities ultimately growing concerned about sorting out their respective responsibilities for acute as well as long-term care of the mentally ill. Given this history, it can be expected that the future roles and utilization of these institutions will continue to depend heavily on financing issues in the mental health and broader health arenas.

Current financing mechanisms for these institutions rely largely on state tax dollars and some federal reimbursements. State hospitals are denied full participation in federal health insurance reimbursements (inpatients aged twenty-one to sixty-four are excluded) and few of the hospitals' disadvantaged clientele are able to pay for their care directly. These long-standing financing constraints have now been exacerbated by federal policies which are increasing referrals from community agencies to the state hospitals (Goldman and Taube, 1985). These include stringent criteria for the receipt of Supplemental Security Income (SSI) and Social Security Disability Insurance (SSDI) payments by mentally ill persons, decertifications of substandard nursing home facilities, and Medicaid inpatient "caps" that limit days of hospitalization in community general hospitals. The impending introduction of prospective payment systems under Medicare for general hospital psychiatric care (Goldman et al., 1984) also raises the prospect that patients will be discharged "sicker and quicker," with referral to the state hospitals for intermediate- and long-term care. This could easily swell the population seeking care in these hospitals and, thereby, further diminish an already precarious resource base.

Demographic Trends

As the baby boom population (those persons born in the late 1940s and 1950s) continues to move through adulthood, the natural prevalence of major mental illnesses will result in greater demand for care in both hospitals and the community (Kramer, 1981). With other forces held constant, this development alone could significantly increase the numbers of persons with severe mental disorders that would be cycled through community programs and, predictably, into long-stay status in state institutions. Much current attention has focused on the "new young chronic population" (Pepper, Ryglewicz, and Kirshner, 1982; Bachrach, 1982) as a challenge to mental health providers, but inevitably this population will age into new "old chronics," thereby escalating demands for additional long-term care capacity in state hospitals or their surrogates.

Intrahospital Changes

A number of issues internal to state hospitals will also condition their future use and service delivery roles. Perhaps the most fundamental is that of leadership and "distinctive competence" (Selznick, 1957). With a few notable (but often transitory) exceptions (e.g., Morrissey et al., 1980), state hospitals have been relegated residual functions as the dumping ground for patients unwanted by other community agencies. The idea of "facility of last resort" has often proven to be a euphemism for low-grade custodial care. A major factor determining whether this role will be perpetuated or phased out is the quality of institutional leadership that emerges in individual hospitals. The challenge for such leadership is to negotiate a more positive role for the facility, thereby providing a basis for recruitment and retention of competent staff. One direction currently being pursued by a number of states in this regard is the development of linkages with university medical centers and other professional schools (Miller, 1981). Those hospitals advantaged by close proximity to a university medical complex may, therefore, have a much higher probability of surviving and developing a more positive treatment role as part of a community mental health services network.

Hospital-Community Integration

In most areas of the country, a dual system of public vs. private care still exists (Morrissey et al., 1980). This situation affects the resource base available for public mental health services, the problem of treatment continuity across the boundaries of the two sectors, and the case mix in various mental health agencies.

Much attention has focused on the charge that "the dollars have not followed the patients from institutions to community care" (e.g., Stein and Ganser, 1983), that both the public and private sectors are resource starved, and that the services required by the chronically mentally ill are not available in sufficient quantity or quality (Bachrach, 1986). Inevitably, then, those areas able to develop effective coordination, joint planning, and resource sharing between the regional state hospital and community programs will be better able to cope with resource scarcity and increased service demands than areas in which dual (and often antagonistic) systems persist.

Public Support and the Threat of Reinstitutionalization

There is both good news and bad news in the current state of public attitudes toward public mental hospitals. The good news is that organizations such as the National Alliance for the Mentally Ill (NAMI) are providing for the first time a strong consumer-based political advocacy and lobbying force to secure increased funding and support for the mentally ill (Hatfield, 1984). The bad news is that the public's image of the mental health system is still one of chaos and failure, especially with regard to deinstitutionalization and the homeless mentally ill (Goldman and Morrissey, 1985; Appelbaum, 1987; Morrissey and Dennis, 1986). How public confidence can be restored, and the extent to which additional resources can be secured for community-based programs, will have a significant impact on the role of state mental hospitals in the future. Already, there are signs that the public wants easier commitment statutes and a policy of "reinstitutionalizing" the mentally disabled (Elpers, 1987). Counter calls have also been made for mental health professionals, government agencies, and families of the mentally ill to launch a campaign against such reinstitutionalization, to educate the public and secure the resources necessary for adequate and comprehensive care, including public hospital facilities (Pepper, 1987). The success of these efforts will have profound implications both for the fate of public mental hospitals and the welfare of the chronically mentally ill well into the next century.

CONCLUSION

State mental hospitals no longer are the monolithic institutions studied by an earlier generation of social scientists in the 1940s and 1950s. They have taken on new functions and shed old ones with the movement of thousands of patients to alternative settings and the increasing specialization and differentiation of providers within the overall mental health system (Goldman and Skinner, 1987). Yet the historic functions of custody, control, and treatment largely persist. The present challenge for state mental hospitals is both to adapt to changing national policies and to find an appropriate ecological niche in their own local service delivery system. Individual hospitals that succeed in coping with these pressures will survive and even flourish in the years ahead, while those that fail to do so will be phased-out or absorbed into other structures.

ACKNOWLEDGMENTS

With approval, the section of this chapter entitled "Historical Developments and Trends" is drawn from the author's previously published writings on this subject in Morrissey, Goldman, and Klerman (1980), and in Morrissey and Goldman (1984).

NOTES

1. Throughout this chapter the terms "public mental hospital," "state and county mental hospital," and "state mental hospital" will be used synonymously.

2. Unless otherwise specified, all of the descriptive data in this section are based on tables presented in Manderscheid, Witkin, and Rosenstein (1985).

REFERENCES

Appelbaum, P. 1987. Crazy in the Streets. *Commentary*, 83: 34–39.

Bachrach, L. 1976. *Deinstitutionalization: An Analytical Review and Sociological Perspective*. DHEW Publication No. (ADM) 76–351. Washington, D.C.: U.S. Government Printing Office.

Bachrach, L. 1982. Young Adult Chronic Patients: An Analytic Review of the Literature. *Hospital and Community Psychiatry* 33: 189–197.

Bachrach, L. 1986. The Future of the State Mental Hospital. *Hospital and Community Psychiatry* 37: 467–474.

Barter, J. 1980. State Mental Hospitals as Domiciliary Care Facilities. In *State Mental Hospitals: Problems and Potentials*, ed. J. Talbott. New York: Human Sciences Press.

Barton, W. 1983. The Place, If Any, of the Mental Hospital in the Community Mental Health Care System. *Psychiatric Quarterly* 55: 146–155.

Bassuk, E., and Gerson, S. 1978. Deinstitutionalization and Mental Health Services. *Scientific American* 238: 46–53.

Beers, C. W. 1908. *A Mind That Found Itself*. 1st ed. New York: Longmans, Green.

Brown, P. 1985. *The Transfer of Care*. London: Routledge and Kegan Paul.

Caplan, R. 1969. *Psychiatry and the Community in Nineteenth Century America*. New York: Basic Books.

Chu, F., and Trotter, S. 1974. *The Madness Establishment*. New York: Grossman.

Craig, T., and Laska, G. 1983. Deinstitutionalization and the Survival of the State Hospital. *Hospital and Community Psychiatry* 34: 616–622.

Dain, N. 1980. *Clifford W. Beers: Advocate for the Insane*. Pittsburgh: University of Pittsburgh Press.

Dingman, P. 1976. The Alternative Care Is Not There. In *State Mental Hospitals: What Happens When They Close?*, eds. P. Ahmed and S. Plog. New York: Plenum.

Dix, D. 1971. *On Behalf of the Insane Poor*. Reprinted. New York: Arno Press.

Elpers, J. R. 1987. Are We Legislating Reinstitutionalization? *American Journal of Orthopsychiatry* 57: 441–446.

Foley, H., and Sharfstein, S. 1983. *Madness and Government: Who Cares for the Mentally Ill?* Washington, D.C.: American Psychiatric Press.

Goldman, H. Adams, N., and Taube, C. 1983. Deinstitutionalization: The Data Demythologized. *Hospital and Community Psychiatry* 34: 129–134.

Goldman, H., and Morrissey, J. 1985. The Alchemy of Mental Health Policy: Homelessness and the Fourth Cycle of Reform. *American Journal of Public Health* 75: 727–731.

Goldman, H., Pincas, H., Taube, C., Regier, D. 1984. Prospective Payment for Psychiatric Hospitalization: Questions and Issues. *Hospital and Community Psychiatry* 35: 460–464.

Goldman, H., and Skinner, A. 1987. Specialty Mental Health Services: Research on Specialization and Differentiation. Unpublished.

Goldman, H., and Taube, C. 1985. Mental Health Financing and the Future of the State Mental Hospital. *American Journal of Social Psychiatry* 5: 26–30.

Goldman, H., Taube, C., Regier, D., and Witkin, M. 1983. The Multiple Functions of the State Mental Hospital. *American Journal of Psychiatry* 140: 296–300.

Gralnick, A. 1985. Build a Better State Hospital: Deinstitutionalization Has Failed. *Hospital and Community Psychiatry* 36: 738–741.

Grob, G. 1966. *The State and the Mentally Ill: A History of Worcester State Hospital in Massachusetts, 1830–1920.* Chapel Hill, N.C.: University of North Carolina Press.

Grob, G. 1973. *Mental Institutions in America: Social Policy to 1875.* New York: Free Press.

Grob, G. 1983. *Mental Illness and American Psychiatry, 1875–1940.* Princeton, N.J.: Princeton University Press.

Gruenberg, E. 1974. The Social Breakdown Syndrome and Its Prevention. In *American Handbook of Psychiatry*, ed. S. Areti. 2nd ed., New York: Basic Books.

Gruenberg, E. 1982. The Deinstitutionalization Movement. In *Public Mental Health: Perspectives and Prospects*, eds. M. Wagenfeld, P. Lemkau, and B. Justice. Beverly Hills, Calif. Sage.

Gruenberg, E., and Archer, J. 1979. Abandonment of Responsibility for the Seriously Mentally Ill. *Milbank Memorial Fund Quarterly* 57: 485–506.

Joint Commission on Mental Illness and Health. 1961. *Action for Mental Health.* New York: Basic Books.

Hatfield, A. 1984. The Family Consumer Movement: A New Force in Service Delivery. In *Advances in Treating the Young Adult Chronic Patient*, eds. B. Pepper and H. Ryglewicz. *New Directions for Mental Health Services*, No. 21. San Francisco: Jossey-Bass.

Klerman, G. 1982. The Psychiatric Revolution of the Past Twenty-Five Years. In *Deviance and Mental Illness*, ed. W. Gove. Beverly Hills, Calif.: Sage.

Kramer, M. 1981. The Increasing Prevalence of Mental Disorder. Paper presented at the Langley Porter Neuropsychiatric Institute, San Francisco, Calif.

Lamb, H. R., and Goertzel, V. 1972. The Demise of the State Hospital—A Premature Obituary? *Archives of General Psychiatry* 26: 489–495.

Manderscheid, R., Witkin, M., and Rosenstein, M. 1985. Specialty Mental Health Services: System and Patient Characteristics—United States. In *Mental Health, United States 1985*, eds. C. Taube and S. Barrett. DHHS Publication No. (ADM) 85–1378. Washington, D.C.: U.S. Government Printing Office.

Mendel, W. 1976. The Case for Closing of the Hospitals. In *State Mental Hospitals: What Happens When They Close*, eds. P. Ahmed and S. Plog. New York: Plenum.

Miller, R. 1981. Beyond the Old State Hospital: New Opportunities Ahead. *Hospital and Community Psychiatry* 32: 27–31.

Morrissey, J. 1982. Deinstitutionalizing the Mentally Ill: Process, Outcomes, and New Directions. In *Deviance and Mental Illness*, ed. W. Gove. Beverly Hills, Calif.: Sage.

Morrissey, J., and Dennis, D. 1986. *NIMH-Funded Research Concerning Homeless Mentally Ill Persons: Implications for Policy and Practice*. Rockville, Md.: Division of Education and Service Systems Liaison, National Institute of Mental Health.

Morrissey, J., and Goldman, H. 1984. Cycles of Reform in the Care of the Chronically Mentally Ill. *Hospital and Community Psychiatry* 35: 785–793.

Morrissey, J., Goldman, H., Klerman, L., and Associates. 1980. *The Enduring Asylum: Cycles of Institutional Reform at Worcester State Hospital*. New York: Grune and Stratton.

Morrissey, J., and Tessler, R. 1982. Selection Processes in State Mental Hospitalization. In *Social Problems and Public Policy*, ed. M. Lewis. Greenwich, Conn.: JAI Press.

Musto, D. 1975. Whatever Happened to Community Mental Health? *Public Interest* 39: 53–79.

Okin, R. 1983. The Future of State Hospitals: Should There Be One? *American Journal of Psychiatry* 140: 571–581.

Pepper, B. 1987. A Public Policy for the Long-Term Mentally Ill: A Positive Alternative to Reinstitutionalization. *American Journal of Orthopsychiatry* 57: 452–457.

Pepper, B., and Ryglewicz, H. 1983. Unified Services: A New York State Perspective. In *Unified Mental Health Systems: Utopia Unrealized*, ed. J. Talbott. *New Directions for Mental Health Services*, No. 18. San Francisco: Jossey-Bass.

Pepper, B., and Ryglewicz, H. 1985. The Role of the State Hospital: A New Mandate for a New Era. *Psychiatric Quarterly* 57: 230–251.

Pepper, B., Ryglewicz, H., and Kirshner, M. 1982. The Uninstitutionalized Generation: A New Breed of Psychiatric Patient. In *The Young Adult Chronic Patient*, eds. B. Pepper and H. Ryglewicz. *New Directions for Mental Health Services*, No. 14. San Francisco: Jossey-Bass.

Quen, J. 1977. Asylum Psychiatry, Neurology, Social Work, and Mental Hygiene: An Exploratory Study in American History. *Journal of the History of the Behavioral Sciences* 13: 3–11.

Rachlin, S. 1976. The Case against Closing of State Hospitals. In *State Mental Hospitals: What Happens When They Close?*, eds. P. Ahmed and S. Plog. New York: Plenum.

Redick, R., Manderscheid, R., Witkin, M., and Rosenstein, M. 1983. *A History of the U.S. National Reporting Program for Mental Health Statistics*. DHHS Publication No. (ADM) 83–1296. Rockville, Md.: National Institute of Mental Health.

Redick, R., Witkin, M., and Atay, J. 1987. Expenditures and Sources of Funds for Mental Health Organizations, United States, 1983. *Statistical Note No. 180*. Rockville, Md.: Division of Biometry and Applied Sciences, National Institute of Mental Health.

Robitscher, J. 1976. Moving Patients Out of Hospitals—In Whose Interest? In *State*

Mental Hospitals: What Happens When They Close?, eds. P. Ahmed and S. Plog. New York: Plenum.

Rose, S. 1979. Deciphering Deinstitutionalization: Complexities in Policy and Program Analysis. *Milbank Memorial Fund Quarterly* 57: 429–460.

Rothman, D. 1971. *The Discovery of the Asylum: Social Order and Disorder in the New Republic*. Boston: Little, Brown.

Rothman, D., 1980. *Conscience and Convenience: The Asylum and Its Alternatives in Progressive America*. Boston: Little, Brown.

Scull, A. 1977. *Decarceration: Community Treatment and the Deviant—A Radical View*. Englewood Cliffs, N.J.: Prentice-Hall.

Selznick, P. 1957. *Leadership in Administration*. Evanston, Ill.: Row, Peterson.

Shore, M., and Shapiro, R. 1979. The Effects of Deinstitutionalization on the State Hospital. *Hospital and Community Psychiatry* 30: 605–608.

Sicherman, B. 1980. *The Quest for Mental Health in America, 1880–1917*. New York: Arno Press.

Steadman, H., Monahan, J., and Hartstone, E. 1982. Mentally Disordered Offenders: A National Survey of Patients and Facilities. *Law and Human Behavior* 6: 31–38.

Stein, L., and Ganser, L. 1983. Wisconsin's System for Funding Mental Health Services. In *Unified Mental Health Systems: Utopia Unrealized*, ed. J. Talbott. *New Directions for Mental Health Services*, No. 18. San Francisco: Jossey-Bass.

Talbott, J. 1978. *The Death of the Asylum*. New York: Grune and Stratton.

Talbott, J. 1985. The Fate of the Public Mental Health System. *Hospital and Community Psychiatry* 36: 46–50.

Talbott, J., ed. 1983. *Unified Mental Health Systems: Utopia Unrealized. New Directions for Mental Health Services*, No. 18. San Francisco: Jossey-Bass.

Taube, C., Thompson, J., and Rosenstein, M. 1983. The "Chronic" Mental Hospital Patient. *Hospital and Community Psychiatry* 34: 611–615.

Thompson, J., Checker, A., and Witkin, M. 1983. The Decline of State Mental Hospitals as Training Sites for Psychiatric Residents. *American Journal of Psychiatry* 140: 704–707.

Wing, J. 1962. Institutionalism in Mental Hospitals. *British Journal of Social and Clinical Psychology* 1: 38–51.

Part 5
Financing, Legal, and Service System Issues

14

Mental Health Insurance

M. SUSAN RIDGELY
and HOWARD H. GOLDMAN

Financing of mental health care is not an issue original to the 1980s and its climate of cost containment, diagnostic related groups (DRGs), mandated insurance benefits, and Medicaid cutbacks. The present financing system evolved in tandem with the historical cycles of reform in the care of the mentally ill (see chapters 5, 8, and 13 in this volume), acting as both cause and effect of new directions in programs and practice. Future policy decisions on how mental health care will be financed, particularly for the chronically mentally ill, will continue to shape the structure of the mental health system. A brief review of how financing of the mental health system has developed and influenced the provision of care coupled with an analysis of current issues and trends in mental health insurance allows us a glimpse at what the future may hold.

EVOLUTION OF FINANCING OF THE MENTAL HEALTH SYSTEM

Origins of the Mental Health System

Before the nineteenth century, such mental health services as existed were provided in private facilities. When a patient's personal finances were exhausted, two primary recourses were available: appeal to charitable organizations for support of care, or become the ward of an undifferentiated welfare institution such as an almshouse. Over time, a more complex system of care for the mentally ill was developed, including public facilities as the response to failure of the "private market" in the early nineteenth century. The private system remained one of "fee-for-service," while the new public system was funded by "categorical resources," i.e., the government was directly responsible for providing the services.

By the start of the twentieth century, authority and responsibility for the care of the chronically mentally ill had become centralized in the hands of state government. Beginning in the 1830s, state governments built asylums for the mentally ill, but local governments were expected to pay for patient care. However, at the turn of the century, a series of state care acts placed all responsibility for the care of the mentally ill poor in the hands of state government. This caused a large-scale shift of patients, especially the elderly, out of almshouses and into state mental hospitals. Almost as soon as specialized private and public mental health facilities had come into existence, then, they were further specialized socially to serve different populations (on the basis of race, religion, and social class) and functionally to meet different treatment needs (acute care, long-term care, voluntary hospitalization, and involuntary hospitalization). Through "historic accident and social purpose" (Goldman and Skinner, 1987: 2), certain functions became concentrated in certain facilities. Public hospitals cared for the most disturbed and disadvantaged patients.

The Introduction of Health Insurance

This two-class system of financing mental health care persisted until the 1930s when the concept of health insurance evolved. Insurance is an arrangement for transferring and distributing risk. A number of individuals agree to pay a small definite cost periodically in the form of premiums for a guarantee that they will be compensated in the event of a large loss. Those who escape such loss subsidize the unfortunate few who do not. A successful insurance plan is one able to balance the premiums and the expenditures.

The advent of insurance coverage for inpatient health care in the 1930s largely ignored mental health services. The expansion of general hospital services for the insured middle classes did not include psychiatric care until the early 1950s, when inpatient mental health benefits were first made available in insurance policies (Goldman, Sharfstein, and Frank, 1983: 489). At that point there was some erosion of the functional division between public and private hospitals, but the poor still tended to be served in public general hospitals when not relegated to state and county mental hospitals and Veterans Administration (VA) medical facilities.

By the 1950s, outpatient treatment had become an important component of the mental health service system. Like inpatient care, however, it was available primarily to those who could afford it. Those with the needed resources could receive high-intensity treatment like psychotherapy. The poor received less-individualized, lower-quality treatment in public dispensaries and state and county mental hospitals. This distinction was reinforced by prevailing opinion suggesting that psychotherapy was a suitable treatment only for the well-to-do, articulate client.

In an effort to make the health care system more egalitarian, public health insurance was established in the 1960s. The introduction of Medicare and Medicaid provided resources for the poor, the elderly, and the disabled to pay for care in the private, fee-for-service sector. Additionally, creation of a network of federally funded, typically privately operated community mental health centers (CMHCs) across the country was an attempt to "hybridize" the system, i.e., to blur the boundaries of the two-class system of care. CMHCs proliferated along with psychiatric units in general hospitals partly because of the expanded availability of third-party payment.

Yet the introduction of third-party funders also created a complicated set of financial and service arrangements in health care, particularly within the mental health sphere. The system of mental health financing was only partially hybridized because of the large, well-developed system of public services that was already in place. Partial hybridization allowed private facilities to release patients into public care when these patients were too sick, too difficult to handle, or chronically ill and costly. Thus, although the line between public and private is more blurred today than at the turn of the century, an essentially two-class system of care remains.

The Problem of Mental Health Benefits in Insurance

In general, insurance coverage for treatment of mental disorders is inferior to coverage for somatic illnesses. Discriminatory coverage for mental disorders in insurance is evident in the fact that only 12 percent of the payment for treatment of mental illness comes from private insurance dollars, as contrasted with 25 percent of the payment for the treatment of general medical conditions.

Why is the coverage for mental disorders so underdeveloped in private insurance? One reason is that until recently patients and their families were not held liable for the costs of care provided in public mental hospitals. Insurance subscribers, as well as insurers, had little incentive to cover services that were already financed through another system (Hustead et al., 1985: 184). Today's economic and political forces have diminished the resources available for publicly provided care, however, and many previously public functions are being transferred to the private sector.

Special problems also exist in insuring for mental health. Generally, three issues are raised. First are definitional questions which arise from the absence of universally accepted notions of the nature and proper treatment of mental disorders. As Muszynski et al. (1985: 16) have put it, "A broken leg presents clearly defined conditions of disorder and treatment; a 'broken mind' raises a host of questions about observable disease, necessary and appropriate treatment, and reliable prognosis.'' Physicians must be able to convince insurers that their choice of treatments is ''medically necessary'' and appropriate, but this is not always easy to do in treating the mentally ill.

Second, and compounding this definitional problem, is the stereotype of psychiatric treatment as mere ''self-fulfillment'' for the ''worried well'' rather than medical treatment for persons with a severe or disabling illness. Paradoxically, others view persons with mental disorders as incurable and therefore consider treatment a waste of public and private resources. Some commentators have related this pessimistic outlook to the fact that most of those with severe psychopathology are individuals at the bottom of the socioeconomic scale (Sharfstein, 1978: 1186).

Finally, the insurance industry is a highly competitive one that keeps a sharp eye on consumer demand. The features offered in a benefit plan must appeal to the largest number of potential enrollees. Unfortunately, when insurers look at patterns of employee preferences as shown by enrollment trends and market research, demand for such features as dental and vision benefits far outweighs demand for mental health benefits. Consumers of mental health services and their families have generally not proven effective advocates in their own behalf, and others simply do not anticipate becoming mentally ill. In sum, poor coverage for mental health problems stems from the lack of predictability, effectiveness, and accountability of costs (Muszynski et al., 1985: 16).

The financial risk assumed by insurers who do cover mental health services is affected by two major factors: *moral hazard* and *adverse selection*. *Moral hazard* refers to the temptation for subscribers to use health care services because their insurance will subsidize the cost. For example, someone with coverage for psychotherapy may opt for more extensive (and expensive) treatment than someone without insurance. Insurers attempt to reduce moral hazard through copayments, deductibles, and limits. Yet, given that utilization increases when the effective price of services is lowered by insurance, significant policy questions arise: Does the higher use by those with free or subsidized care constitute overuse or does the lower use by those without such benefits reflect underuse? Will underuse mean an increase in costs for mental health and other health services down the line due to continued impairment?

Adverse selection refers to the risk that any particular insurance plan will attract and accumulate a disproportionate share of sick and ''high users'' in the plan, threatening its economic viability. Many insurers feel that the provision of comprehensive mental health benefits will make their plan susceptible to such adverse selection (and higher costs) and that low-risk subscribers, not wanting to subsidize these high risks, will opt out for a cheaper plan. To combat this problem, insurers like to avoid providing mental health benefits altogether, or provide those of the lowest common denominator that a large segment of consumers would demand. Adverse selection is certainly a risk, but many feel that the problem is overstated by insurers. Advocates for mandated mental health benefits believe that forcing all insurers to a minimum level of benefits would flatten, or equalize, the competitive field while, at the same time, improving the availability of mental health benefits.

The Costs of Mental Health Care

A review of the costs of care for mental illnesses gives insight into the demand they place on overall health care resources. In the most comprehensive study to date, Frank and Kamlet (1985) have estimated the direct costs of diagnosis, treatment, and rehabilitation of the mentally ill. These estimates include the costs in the specialty mental health sector (i.e., specialized providers, such as psychiatric hospitals, clinics, and practitioners), the general medical sector (i.e., general medical and surgical hospital beds, emergency and ambulatory care departments, and nursing homes), and the human service system (i.e., other caregivers, such as welfare departments and the schools), providing a view of both the total burden and the distribution of resource use.

Using their high estimate of direct costs for 1980, Frank and Kamlet (1985) report that the direct costs of mental health care, approximately $20 billion, accounted for roughly 7.7 percent of direct costs for all health care in the United States in that year. The specialty mental health sector handled 54 percent of the direct costs, the general medical sector 31 percent, and the human services sector the remaining 15 percent. Both the mental health sector and the general medical sector spent a considerable proportion of their resources on hospital care (48 percent and 46 percent respectively). Proportions of total expenditures for nursing home care were also comparable, at 7.5 percent and 9 percent respectively for these two sectors.

A modest amount of growth in real costs for mental health care occurred in the period from 1971 to 1980, at approximately 1.7 percent per year. This contrasts with the average annual growth rate in general health care costs of 3.6 percent for the same period (Frank and Kamlet, 1985: 166).

For whom are these costs incurred? Of the approximately $20 billion in direct costs attributed to the care and support of mentally ill patients in 1980, more than 50 percent was spent on the 15–20 percent of patients treated in the specialty mental health sector. Many of these patients are the chronically mentally ill who, consistent with the more disturbed nature of their illnesses, consume a disproportionate share of the health care resources targeted to the overall population of mentally ill individuals. In addition to these direct costs, another $3.7 billion was spent in income transfer payments such as disability payments and housing and food subsidies.

Who Pays for Mental Health Services?

In addition to direct public support through grants and legislative appropriations, today an elaborate system of third-party funding mechanisms—both public and private—finances the care and support of the mentally ill through disability payments and through reimbursement for services in institutional and noninstitutional settings (Figure 14–1). Significant disparities exist in what different levels of government pay for mental health care vs. general medical care. "Total federal [health care] expenditures for mental health account for only 4% of total federal health care expenditures. . . . [while] state 'categorical' dollars account for over 30% of mental health care costs, compared to 12% of general medical costs" (Goldman, Sharfstein, and Frank, 1983: 489).

The public sector continues to provide the mainstay of financing for mental health care, although it should be noted that the expected principal payment source for mental health care in the specialty sector does vary according to the type of facility. According to National Institute of Mental Health (NIMH) data, commercial insurance was the most frequently reported principal payment source for inpatient admissions (under age sixty-five) to private psychiatric hospitals (65.2 percent) and for psychiatric admissions to nonpublic general hospitals (48.9 percent). By contrast, commercial insurance was the anticipated payment source for only 10.9 percent of admissions to state and county mental hospitals (Manderscheid et al., 1985). Again, the two-class system of care is apparent.

Private insurance, the mainstay of financial support for specialty mental health care in the private sector, is the form of insurance coverage held by a majority of the insured population of the United States. According to the U.S. Bureau of the Census, at the end of 1983, 82 percent of the civilian, noninstitutionalized population was covered by private health insurance (U.S. Bureau of the Census, 1983). While widespread access to health insurance should help defray the governmental costs of providing care, restrictive benefit levels for mental illnesses mean that even those privately insured face the prospect of requiring publicly financed or publicly provided care at some time in their lives. Patterns of coverage for different kinds of mental health services will be outlined and discussed further later in the chapter.

GENERAL PUBLIC POLICY ISSUES

Equity

Equity and *parity* are two important concepts in understanding the debate over the financing of mental health care. *Equity* is a fundamental goal of an egalitarian society and, in the current context, means that health services should be "accessible, available and utilized by patients according to illness and need, not according to income, insurance coverage, race, geographic locale, age, sex, education or other characteristics unrelated to need" (Goldman, Sharfstein, and Frank, 1983: 488). However, evidence of the continued two-class system of care in both the inpatient and outpatient sectors obviously suggests that accessibility, availability, and utilization of psychiatric services continue to be determined by social status, income, and third-party coverage.

Figure 14–1
Mental Health Care Financing Resources

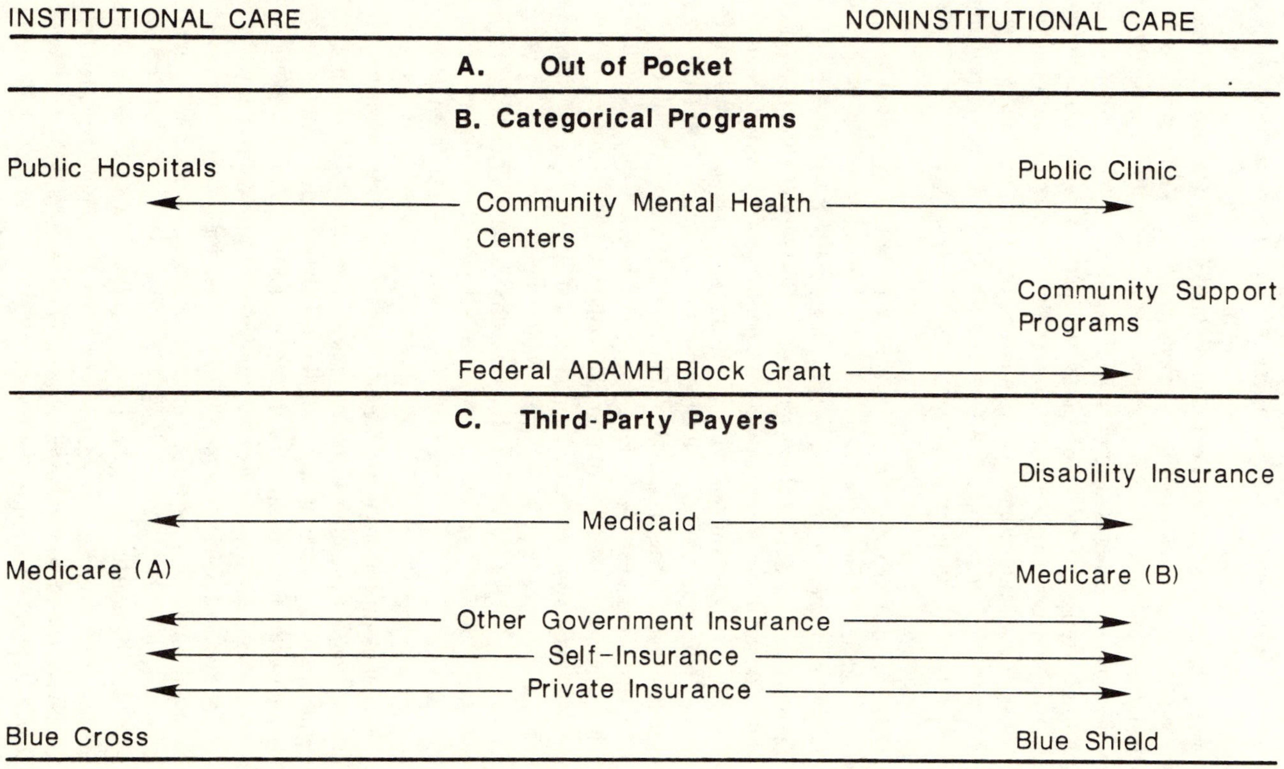

INSTITUTIONAL CARE   NONINSTITUTIONAL CARE

A. Out of Pocket

B. Categorical Programs

Public Hospitals ⟶ Community Mental Health Centers ⟶ Public Clinic

Federal ADAMH Block Grant ⟶ Community Support Programs

C. Third-Party Payers

Medicare (A) ⟶ Medicaid

Medicare (A) ⟶ Other Government Insurance ⟶ Disability Insurance

⟶ Self-Insurance

⟶ Private Insurance ⟶ Medicare (B)

Blue Cross ⟶ Blue Shield

Parity

Parity means that mental health services should be as accessible and available as general health services to those who need them. There should be no additional barriers (financial or otherwise) to the use of mental health services. Historically, mental health services have not been covered by health insurance on a par with general medical services. Special limits were imposed on the benefits available to persons with mental disorders both because of the expectation of public responsibility (the existence of a large tax-financed public system of care), and because of the "moral hazard" concept that increased use would result from lowering out-of-pocket costs through insurance coverage. Both of these concerns have some basis in reality, but their legitimacy as excuses for perpetuating the present underdevelopment of mental health insurance has been exaggerated (Goldman and Taube, 1988).

Parity implies that the same rules should apply to the distribution of resources for mental health care as for general medical services, but it does not necessarily imply that all mental health services will be covered without limits. Limits are imposed on resource allocations for most medical services; they have been applied arbitrarily and unfairly in some cases. A policy of parity would require evaluating the medical necessity, availability of alternatives, and the moral hazard of specific services before determining the allocation of resources. The allocation principles applied to psychiatric services should be those that apply to all other categories of services. For example, if long-term psychotherapy appears to be responsive to the price-lowering effect of insurance (when compared to some other outpatient service), then some increase in patient cost-sharing should be considered (if resources are scarce.) The same cost-sharing should apply to other medical services that appear to be equally price responsive. This is not the case in most insurance policies. As regards coverage for outpatient mental health services, for example, copayments are usually higher, and there often are limits on the number of visits.

Recent modifications in Medicare benefit design related to Alzheimer's disease (and related organic brain disorders) show some movement toward partial parity. Reimbursement guidelines for Medicare Part B were modified to distinguish between visits for "medical management" and visits for psychotherapy. Office visits for medical management will now be reimbursed on a par with ambulatory care of nonpsychiatric patients, whereas those for psychotherapy are subject to the usual limitations for treatment of patients with mental disorders (Goldman, Cohen, and Davis, 1985).

Parity as a policy can cut both ways, however. At the same time that special restrictions on the use of mental health services should be lifted, special protections or resources that currently work in favor of mental health services would also disappear. Parity in insurance benefits may lead to curtailed grant support by government for public facilities, such as public hospitals and community mental health centers. It may also remove certain exemptions from mainstream financing policies such as psychiatric services have enjoyed under Medicare's Prospective Payment System (PPS). Under a policy of strict parity, Medicare would have to reimburse the care of a psychiatric patient in a specialized unit of a general hospital in an identical fashion to routine care for a patient in a general medical or surgical bed, i.e., according to the application of stringent average cost criteria under a specified diagnostic related group (DRG). At this time, Medicare's DRG system has not been extended to psychiatric hospitals and all psychiatric units in general hospitals, although such a change is possible.

Controlling Utilization and Costs

For those who seek expanded mental health benefits in insurance policies, controlling utilization and the cost of care are major issues. As part of the contemporary so-called revolution in reimbursement practices for health care, major payers are increasingly involving themselves directly in the pursuit of cost containment. Deciding precisely who will be covered, for what services, in which settings, and under what review mechanisms are decisions that have to be made in an attempt to stem the rapid rise of health care costs in this country. In 1950, national health expenditures accounted for only 4.4 percent of the country's Gross National Product (GNP); by 1982, health expenditures equaled more than 10 percent of the GNP. Between 1971 and 1982, health expenditures increased from $83.3 billion to $322.4 billion dollars, an average annual increase of 13.1 percent (American Medical Association, 1985). Even though health care spending slowed some in the mid–1980s, the American Medical Association projects that health care expenditures will reach $700 billion in 1990 and will account for 12.3 percent of the GNP.

Current solutions for braking these runaway costs will be discussed later. Regardless of the specifics, however, attempts to control use (including utilization review and quality assurance programs) must determine "the necessity, appropriateness, and efficiency of the use of medical services, procedures, and facilities" (Muszynski et al., 1985: 59).

One of the major issues related to utilization is the balance between the need and demand for services. Perceptions are that mental health services are basically discretionary services for which the demand will disappear as the price goes up. The experience of major insurers (such as Blue Cross and Blue Shield/Federal Employees Health Benefits Program) and various studies of demand for mental health services in the 1980s appeared to confirm that view (Sharfstein and Taube, 1982: 1427; Frank and McGuire, 1986). However, further analysis shows that these "demand" studies examined annual use by aggregating a variety of mental health services into a single dependent variable. Differences in demand for various types of services are not clear, making further research necessary to determine which services are responsive to price and, hence, hold the potential for "moral hazard" (Goldman and Taube, 1988).

Perhaps a bigger challenge to informed benefit design is to define guidelines for what constitutes acceptable practice in mental health, as well as the range of acceptable variations, so as to distinguish medically necessary from discretionary care. In this process, mental health professionals must be willing to alter their practice behavior if they are to qualify for reimbursement. And the system as a whole must face the difficulty of balancing the needs of patients against the need to control costs.

Some commentators question whether the emphasis in policymaking should be on the potential for over-utilization by the many or the reality of over-utilization by the few. National data indicate that 10 percent of users of ambulatory mental health services are responsible for 50 percent of total expenditures. An effective mechanism to control costs arguably should focus on these high users. Case management and clinical review of this subset of cases may go further toward limiting use, and thus costs, than toward limiting shorter episodes of care with high deductibles and steep copayments (Goldman and Taube, 1988). A policy that focuses on limiting excessive use rather than erecting financial barriers to the initiation of treatment could control costs and increase access, thereby satisfying insurance principles as well as promoting public health.

Limiting mental health benefits in insurance by the use of cost sharing and caps on total visits and dollars is a demand-side control. These mechanisms are designed to discourage unnecessary use by reducing the incentive to seek services. Prospective payment, by contrast, is a supply-side strategy. It controls costs and utilization by limiting the supply of services through establishment of supplier risk-sharing (McGuire, forthcoming). Both mechanisms are effective in limiting use; both mechanisms also create problems. They may be used in combination to maximize benefits and minimize risks.

Because the current emphasis is on containing and reducing costs, questions are being raised about the effect of new financing mechanisms on quality of care. For example, considerable concern exists that prospectively determined rates for mental health care will simply not be sufficient to provide adequate treatment, resulting in undertreatment in the name of efficiency. Under this arrangement, providers who have assumed the burden of the poorer, severely disabled, treatment-resistant patients will be placed at enormous financial risk, and some who perform the most important (and costly) functions will fail. Too, because the mental health service system is functionally differentiated, specialty facilities are vulnerable to systematic risk due to their likelihood of admitting more costly patients.

Recent evidence on the impact of Medicare's Prospective Payment System shows that hospitals can and do respond to incentives (Taube et al., 1988; Jencks and Goldman, 1987). What is not yet clear, however, is the effect on the patients. The philosophy that more treatment is always better is no longer acceptable. The question now is, How little is too little?

FINANCING OF MENTAL HEALTH CARE IN THE 1980s

With the recent decline of direct grant support from governmental sources (see chapter 7 in this volume), any discussion of the financing of mental health care in the 1980s must focus on two key issues: the development of mental health benefits in private and public insurance, and cost containment, specifically, cost containment aimed at the development of alternatives to traditional fee-for-service payment. Fee-for-service payment is widely regarded as having contributed to, if not having produced, the skyrocketing inflation in health care costs. Alternative mechanisms for payment focus on having the providers of services share the risk of costs in order to modify or regulate their behaviors.

The Availability of Mental Health Benefits in Insurance

Current coverage in private insurance. In the most comprehensive overview to date of private indemnity insurance programs, Brady, Sharfstein, and Muszynski (1986) analyzed annual survey data collected by the U.S. Bureau of Labor Statistics (BLS) from 1979 to 1984 to examine both the current level of insurance benefits for mental disorders and changes in these benefit levels over time. The BLS Level of Benefits Survey is a yearly study of fringe benefits offered by medium and large firms in the private sector. Over 22 million full-time employees are included. The authors warn that the results of the study are biased toward a favorable view of mental health benefits because medium and large firms usually have more comprehensive coverage than smaller companies (Brady, Sharfstein, and Muszynski, 1986: 1277).

Ninety-nine percent of all BLS Survey participants offered insurance coverage for inpatient psychiatric care, but fewer than half had coverage for inpatient psychiatric care equal to their coverage for other illnesses. In fact, this "parity" percentage declined from 58 percent of participants covered on an equal basis in 1981 to 48 percent covered on an equal basis in 1984. Limitations on days of care have remained relatively constant but the researchers found a discernible increase in the prevalence of separate dollar limits on psychiatric benefits (from 15 percent of employers with dollar caps in 1981 to 24 percent of employers with caps in 1984). As inflation erodes the buying power of the dollar, such dollar caps become an increasingly significant limit on the quantity of services covered by insurance.

The "Blues" (Blue Cross and Blue Shield) had a smaller percentage of plans with parity than commercial insurers. Employees with hospital benefits insured by commercial carriers were more than twice as likely (63 percent vs. 30 percent) to have plans with parity between benefits for mental disorders and for general medical care than those insured by the Blues.

Coverage for care in institutions that specialize in the treatment of mental illness was provided to less than a third of those surveyed in 1984. This was, however, an increase from the 21 percent of those covered in 1981.

Ninety-six percent of all survey participants had coverage for some type of outpatient psychiatric treatment, but 89 percent of all participants had limitations on that coverage which were separate from the limitations on coverage for other illnesses. This percentage of participants with less than parity is up from 82 percent in 1981. The majority of employees were subject to more than one restriction, for example, an annual limit on visits, a limit on dollars per visit, and lifetime limits on dollars and visits. As with inpatient coverage, limits on number of visits remained fairly constant while the percentage of employees with dollar limits increased markedly.

In sum, while mental health insurance benefits were available to the vast majority of employees surveyed in 1984, that coverage lacked depth. According to the researchers, "most psychiatric care expenses are not covered, since often short-term and acute care is covered but longer-term and catastrophic care is not" (Brady, Sharfstein, and Muszynski, 1986: 1278). Interestingly, this indicates that most of the coverage provided in current private indemnity insurance fails to address the broad goal of insurance—to cover against potential significant loss. The result is that not only are the poor and uninsured at risk, but there is a growing crisis for the middle class. Expenses arising from serious or chronic mental illness may find them inadequately insured (Brady, Sharfstein, and Muszynski, 1986: 1278).

Current coverage in public insurance. Medicaid and Medicare are the two primary insurance plans in the public sector. Developed in the 1960s, these programs were aimed respectively at giving the poor and the elderly and disabled the opportunity to purchase health care services in the private sector. Each features freedom of choice of providers.

The Medicaid program is a federal-state program providing subsidy of medical care for the poor. The benefit levels and restrictions vary from state to state. In the early 1980s, many states began to impose limits on inpatient stays in general hospitals. These took two general forms: limits on the length of reimbursable stay per admission and limits on daily allowable charges. Ten states limited the former while nine states lowered the daily rates of reimbursement. During 1982 and 1983, most states adopted changes that limited the allowable length of stay in general hospitals to between twelve and fifteen days (Sharfstein, Frank, and Kessler, 1984: 213). This reduction in Medicaid benefits often led to the dumping of patients from general hospitals to state mental hospitals after the new limits were reached (Frank and Lave, 1985). Other Medicaid changes since 1980 have placed limits on outpatient treatment, limiting the ability to substitute outpatient for inpatient care for Medicaid beneficiaries (Sharfstein, Frank, and Kessler, 1984: 215).

Medicare is a federal program of reimbursement to hospitals and medical providers for services rendered to the elderly and disabled. Unlike Medicaid, there is no means test for eligibility for Medicare, which is part of the federal social security system. Medicare also places strict limits on reimbursement for mental health services. Inpatient stays in beds currently included under the Prospective Payment System (i.e., some nonexempt psychiatric units and general medical/surgical beds used for psychiatric care in general hospitals) are limited by the appropriate DRG. Those currently exempt from PPS must still live within reimbursement limits set by the Tax Equity and Fiscal Responsibility Act of 1982. Outpatient mental health services had been limited since 1965 to a dollar cap of $500 per year with a 50 percent co-payment. The Omnibus Budget Reconciliation Act of 1987 (Public Law 100–203) increased the outpatient limit to $2200 per year over the next two years (retaining the 50 percent co-payment), but exempted from any limits brief visits for the medical management of patients requiring monitoring or changes in psychotropic drugs. In addition, the Act introduced a partial hospitalization benefit.

Public insurance plans also discriminate in other ways when it comes to mental health coverage. For instance, the Medicaid program does not cover inpatient care for beneficiaries aged twenty-two to sixty-four in specialty mental hospitals labeled as Institutions for Mental Disease (IMD). Not only are state mental hospitals affected, but nursing homes are as well. Any nursing home with more than 50 percent of its residents carrying a diagnosis of nonorganic mental disorder may be denied Medicaid reimbursement.

Besides imposing general use limits and restrictions on certain types of facilities, public insurance programs are also biased toward particular types of care. As a result, the needs of many mentally disabled patients often go unmet. For example, Medicare is biased toward acute inpatient care in that coverage for ambulatory services is extremely limited yet inpatient coverage is comparatively generous. Some observers believe, therefore, that it may be necessary to differentiate between medically necessary long-term treatment and custodial care that may legitimately be excluded from insurance coverage in order to have reimbursement for at least some of the care required by the chronically mentally ill. The determining factor would not be the chronic nature of the illness but, rather, whether "active treatment" is provided. A good case can be made that there should not be different benefits for chronic mental illnesses and for chronic somatic diseases, such as heart disease and diabetes, that also require continuing or intermittent care on an inpatient or outpatient basis (Hustead et al., 1985: 185).

Mandated mental health benefits. Efforts to expand the availability of mental health insurance aim at increasing parity and improving equity. However, the absence of insurance is not the only or necessarily the worst barrier to obtaining good mental health care. For this reason, mandated benefit plans are not the only answer to this problem, and some believe that mandates may not even be a good answer.

According to the *American Psychiatric Association State Issues Handbook* (1987), the first mandate bill was passed into law in 1971. Since that time twenty-four other states have adopted some form of mandate legislation. Mandate legislation can take two forms: mandates to offer coverage or make it available at the policyholder's option, and mandates to provide coverage.

Advocates believe that state laws mandating the inclusion of a minimum package of mental health benefits will accomplish several goals, including spreading the cost of mental health care more equitably between the public and private sectors; spreading the risk of cost across a wider spectrum of the population; and addressing the problem of adverse selection. In short, insurers would no longer be competing on the basis of different levels of benefits. Unfortunately, the minimums established in the law can quickly become "the ceiling as well as the floor" so that insurance plans with a higher level of benefits find it in their interest to conform to the minimum or, again, face adverse selection by high mental health benefit users. These mandates, then, while insuring some coverage, may have a negative effect on the availability of comprehensive coverage. Additionally, insurers aggressively resist the imposition of mandates, arguing that costs in mandate states have escalated (McGuire and Montgomery, 1981). There is reason to believe, however, that these higher costs will soon reach a plateau. McGuire (1981) reports that, in the experience of the federal employee Blue Cross and Blue Shield plan, introduction of broad mental health benefits led to an initial jump in costs, followed eventually by stability in the percentage of health costs accounted for by mental health services. Sharfstein and Taube (1982: 1429) interpret this pattern to indicate that mental health costs can be "predictable, stable, and limited."

Because of the ceiling/floor danger in mandated mental health benefit legislation, advocates often find themselves turning back to the legislature in subsequent years with efforts aimed at increasing the level of mental health benefits in the mandate legislation, raising questions about the effectiveness and longevity of mandate provisions.

Gaps in insurance coverage. Gaps caused by inadequate benefits represent lack of depth of coverage and may, additionally, deny appropriate coverage to whole groups of the population.

As mentioned previously, special limits, copayments, and deductibles have been included in insurance policies due to the assumption that mental health care is discretionary and subject to overuse when the price of services is lowered by insurance. This assumption of moral hazard ignores the diversity of mental health services, however, and the diversity of need of those who use them. Unfortunately, research on the demand for mental health services is in its infancy, and differentiation of discretionary from medically necessary use is not yet clear. In the meantime, visit and dollar limits fall equally upon all mentally ill patients without distinguishing the truly disabled from the well but discontented.

The population that stands out as most disadvantaged under current benefit plans of the majority of private and public insurance policies is the chronically mentally ill. This is an important at-risk group considering that approximately 43 percent of the estimated $20 billion a year in direct costs for mental disorders are expended on behalf of chronically mentally ill persons (Goldman, 1986: 6).

These patients are the most severely affected by mental disorder and yet, ironically, the insurance system often underwrites the least desirable treatment for their illnesses. Medicare and most private insurance plans favor high skill, medically oriented treatment benefits, excluding from coverage maintenance and custodial care services as well as lower intensity alternatives such as psychosocial rehabilitation. This occurs even though small-scale controlled studies have shown the effectiveness and economy of such treatments compared to hospitalization. Additionally, most benefit plans exclude services (such as home health care and respite care) to aid the families of chronically mentally ill patients. Families often act as the primary caretakers and their ability to keep a mentally ill family member in the community is a main line of defense against costly institutionalization (Talbott and Sharfstein, 1986: 1128).

Prospective Payment of Providers: Alternative Mechanisms, Controls, and Incentives

Cost-containment efforts have been spurred by government action at the federal and state levels and by private business, the major payers for health care. Customary attitudes about health care, patterns of service delivery, and financing arrangements are under scrutiny and revision.

The federal government, which is responsible for paying 43 cents of every health care dollar, has focused its efforts on prospective payment for Medicare and has proposed taxation of employer contributions to employee health insurance. State governments, for their part, have moved to restrict eligibility for, and coverage of, services under Medicaid. Some states have also set up all-payer hospital rate setting systems to contain hospital costs. Private business has sought to reduce employee health insurance costs by shifting costs to their employees (increasing copayments and deductibles) and by promoting alternatives such as Health Maintenance Organizations (HMOs) and Preferred Provider Organizations (PPOs). Some analysts have already questioned whether sustained efforts to contain costs may succeed in reining in the high inflation rate of health care services at the expense of posing serious risks for access and quality (Goldman and Sharfstein, 1987: 627).

Under retrospective reimbursement the provider of care receives payment after the fact based either on actual costs or allowable charges. Under a prospective payment system, by contrast, rates are established in advance according to a specified unit of payment. In this way, rates are fixed and not affected by actual costs. Fixed rates offer an incentive for the provider to deliver the needed care at the lowest possible cost. The provider must absorb any excess of incurred costs over the rate, but if actual costs fall below the rate, the provider is rewarded with the surplus.

The Medicare PPS and mental health. In 1983 Congress enacted the Prospective Payment System for hospital reimbursement under Medicare. The system was predicated on the idea that variations in resource use among hospitals were due to one of two factors: patient need and efficiency. The factor of patient need would be controlled for by the use of diagnosis related groups corresponding to national averages for all patients within a certain category of presumed need. Efficiency would then be rewarded and inefficient hospitals would find themselves faced with financial losses.

In mental health services, however, there are other factors operating. Patterns of use and cost between facility types may reflect functional differentiation as well as differences in efficiency. Research has shown dramatic differences in the cost of care based on facility type (due to patient variables and case mix), provider type (due both to provider preferences and efficiency), and state (due to differences in systems of care) (Goldman and Skinner, 1987: 6). DRGs cannot predict resource use for mental health care and thus, at least for the time being, psychiatric facilities have remained exempt from PPS (with the exception of "scatter beds" in general medical facilities). What is also clear from this research is that in all cases specialty mental health care is more expensive than mental health care provided in a general medical setting, even when adjusted for DRGs. Whether the specialized nature of such services or patient need or both may justify the additional cost is a question for further research (Goldman and Sharfstein, 1987: 627).

PPS does not currently cover most psychiatric facilities, but it has had impact on the mental health system. Inferred from the Frank and Lave (1985) Medicaid data, Medicare's emphasis on shorter stays and less treatment has likely produced an increase in the number of transfers of Medicare patients to state mental hospitals and other long-term care facilities. Any facility without control over its admissions and discharges thus becomes a target for dumping. Under these conditions, other hospitals may thrive while state mental hospitals face additional financial risk.

Finally, questions have been raised about the general effectiveness of PPS in reducing health care costs. While costs per hospitalization have been reduced, this saving may be offset by higher readmission rates (Rupp, Steinwachs, and Salkever, 1984: 456). Capitation, a financing arrangement discussed below, addresses this potential "revolving door" problem.

Alternative delivery systems: HMOs, PPOs, and mental health care. HMOs and PPOs are referred to as alternative delivery systems because "they are an alternative to traditional office or group practice, and they combine different clinical as well as organizational and economic models of health care delivery" (Muszynski et al., 1985: 22). As these alternative systems continue to gain acceptance with enrollees, further growth is expected.

Capitation is a method of payment for services in which the health care provider receives a fixed amount for each person served per time period without regard to the number or nature of services provided. In this way, capitation addresses for the insurer both the problem of a high number of episodes of care as well as the cost of an individual episode. HMOs are an example of capitation financing.

HMOs receive a predetermined, prepaid capitated rate for each of their voluntarily enrolled members. They agree to provide a fixed range of comprehensive services in exchange for the fixed payment. Members of the HMO may not use non-HMO providers. All HMOs have some sort of utilization review or quality assurance mechanism (Muszynski et al., 1985: 22). Regarding acute hospital care, HMOs are intrinsically concerned with minimizing lengths of stay, but because HMOs are also responsible for total health care (within the fixed range of contracted services), it is not to their advantage simply to decrease lengths of stay and provide less treatment. Since they will be financially at risk if less treatment now means more impairment and higher service utilization later, they must also consider the long-term impact of the care they provide.

A survey of 205 HMOs nationwide undertaken by Levin, Glasser, and Roberts (1984) assessed the status of mental health benefits in HMOs. Ninety-four percent offered mental health benefits as part of their basic coverage. Fifty-seven percent provided thirty days of inpatient care per person per year (80 percent of this group did so without additional copayments). Seventy-seven percent of those responding offered the federally mandated minimum of twenty outpatient visits per year. (This mandate was a part of the legislation establishing standards for qualified HMOs, i.e., those eligible for federal benefits. There was no mandate for inpatient coverage.)

Comparison with coverage in standard insurance shows that HMOs are as likely to restrict coverage of mental health services as other insurance plans. Additionally, the probability of access to specialty mental health providers may be diminished by the HMO's primary physician gatekeeper, whose function is to decide, and indeed limit, how much tertiary care should be provided or purchased. Finally, HMOs generally focus on acute care and lack provisions for treating chronically mentally ill patients (Flinn, McMahon, and Collins, 1987: 255). For these reasons, HMOs, rather than representing an improvement in organization and delivery of mental health care, may expose mentally ill members to financial risk.

Preferred Provider Organizations generally consist of groups of independent providers who have agreed to provide health care at a reduced rate by contract with a given payer such as a major employer or insurance carrier. Enrollees are not required to use these identified providers, but they have the incentive of cost savings to do so. When opting for a PPO provider, enrollees may receive, for example, first-dollar coverage or a higher rate of reimbursement than when choosing a non-PPO provider. The benefit to the payer is usually a provider discount of 10 percent to 20 percent below customary charges. PPOs typically have some type of utilization review whose purpose is to control use, balancing quality and economy (Muszynski et al., 1985: 24).

Few data are available on mental health benefits in PPOs. In a 1985 telephone survey of twenty-three members of the American Association of Preferred Provider Organizations, Altman and Frisman (1987) found that all reimbursed on a fee-for-service basis. For thirteen of the twenty-three organizations, provider fees were discounted. Typical benefit plans involved some combination of deductibles and copayments. Levels of cost sharing varied. Some deductibles were waived when subscribers used the PPO providers. All twenty-three PPOs provided outpatient services, and twenty-one also provided inpatient psychiatric treatment. Some of the PPOs specifically excluded certain services.

This study is not a conclusive review of PPOs nationwide. Even within the organization surveyed, the researchers chose a special study group (i.e., those in the directory of PPOs who cited mental health services or mental health professionals) and did not attempt to sample the membership randomly (Altman and Frisman, 1987: 359). Nevertheless, the survey raises questions about PPOs and mental health care. In addition to the issue of formal benefit restrictions, other concerns center on the role utilization review may play in determining how much care is necessary for a particular patient. Some fear increased liability for providers in cases where care is terminated prematurely (Altman and Frisman, 1987: 359), while others express concern that patients will be undertreated.

Capitation for high-risk groups. During the past few years policymakers have been considering, and, indeed, the federal government has been experimenting with, capitation arrangements for high-risk groups such as Medicaid- and Medicare-eligible persons. Capitating payment for such a clientele has in turn raised the issue of the need for "risk-adjusted capitation rates," that is, a plan membership fee based on the health status of the enrollee. HMOs for the general population have not faced this problem because enrolling patients through employers has given them some guarantee that their prospective enrollees are in general reasonably healthy, functioning individuals. Just the opposite is true of high-risk groups, however. These proposed capitation plans face unknown risks due to age, preexisting disabilities, poverty, and other factors (Lehman, 1986: 9).

Developing a formula to compute adjusted rates of this type may not be feasible at this time, and yet applying capitation financing to the care of the chronically or episodically mentally ill requires just such an effort (Lehman, 1986: 9). Capitation offers the hope of flexibility and the substitution of more appropriate for less appropriate services. Yet it does not, in and of itself, guarantee adequate coverage.

SCENARIOS FOR THE FUTURE

Changes in both the financing and structure of the mental health system are ongoing. Today as in the past, it is sometimes difficult to differentiate cause and effect. Based on prior experience, however, it is possible to set out several scenarios for how the mental health system is likely to be influenced by the ongoing evolution of health care financing. With cost containment continuing as the key policy direction in health care financing and health care delivery, the structure of the mental health system will clearly be altered.

One scenario for the future is that mechanisms such as prospective payment will lead to dehybridization of the current system and reemergence of the old two-class system with sharp demarcation of the private and public sectors. As private facilities find themselves at financial risk because of patients whose care outstrips revenues, these patients will be transferred to public facilities. This dumping phenomenon will even shift patients who have public insurance from out of the sphere of private providers into the already fully developed, publicly operated system. Obviously, those with chronic mental illnesses will be among the first to be identified as bad risks in the private care system because of their need for longer or more frequent hospitalizations.

An alternative scenario is that public and private sectors of mental health care will remain but will assume different functions. In some states there has already been a shift in this direction, with private facilities delivering acute care services and public facilities providing long-term care.

A third scenario suggests that attempts to lower costs in the public sector may lead to the privatization of all mental health care. Public facilities may be essentially eliminated with public resources used to fund private facility care and treatment of those who could not otherwise afford services. Private facilities would be funded by out-of-pocket payments by those who could afford it, by private insurance for those employed, by public insurance, and by a series of contracts for the indigent. Benefits under such an insurance scheme might cover the full array of mental health services on a par with general health benefits. It is more likely, however, that some services (e.g., inpatient care and office visits for medical management) would be funded on a par, while other services (e.g., psychotherapy and partial hospitalization) might have separate limits. If the state mental hospital, the mainstay of the public system, no longer existed, the private sector would be forced somehow to assume its role.

Such a scenario poses several questions and problems for policymakers. For example, how will the chronically mentally ill, those most devastated by mental disorder, fare in such a system? Will a two-class system evolve *within* the private sector? Will some private facilities take only patients who can pay out of pocket or have adequate insurance coverage with other private facilities serving those patients with inadequate funding? Will private facilities have ghetto wards for the indigent that bear little resemblance to the private-pay wards?

The danger exists that a fully privatized system might ultimately result in failure of the market, much as it did in the 1830s, when the need for public asylums first arose. A very elaborate public system of care could once again emerge if another market failure occurs. While some may see this as a disastrous repetition of history, others consider it the only way the United States will establish a national health service as a matter of national social policy.

Mental health financing policy must be enlightened by mental health services and economics research. Recognizing the diversity of needs and services, we must find financing mechanisms to match. This poses both a challenge and an opportunity in the design of insurance coverage for persons with mental disorders. We must take special care to protect severely mentally ill persons who have the greatest need and incur a disproportionate share of the costs. It will be difficult to balance our desire for equity, quality, and controlled costs.

ACKNOWLEDGMENT

Portions of the sections of this chapter entitled "Evolution of Financing of the Mental Health System" and "Scenarios for the Future" and Figure 14–1 are drawn with permission from Howard Goldman (1987), "Financing of the Mental Health System," *Psychiatric Annals* 17: 580–585.

REFERENCES

Altman, L., and Frisman, L. 1987. Preferred Provider Organizations and Mental Health Care. *Hospital and Community Psychiatry* 38: 359–362.

American Medical Association. 1985. *The Environment of Medicine: Report of the Council on Long Range Planning and Development*. Chicago.

American Psychiatric Association. 1987. *American Psychiatric Association State Issues Handbook*. Washington, D.C.

Brady, J., Sharfstein, S., and Muszynski, I. 1986. Trends in Private Insurance Coverage for Mental Illness. *American Journal of Psychiatry* 143: 1276–1279.

Flinn, D., McMahon, T., and Collins, M. 1987. Health Maintenance Organizations and Their Implications for Psychiatry. *Hospital and Community Psychiatry* 38: 255–262.

Frank, R., and Kamlet, M. 1985. Direct Costs and Expenditures for Mental Health Care in the United States in 1980. *Hospital and Community Psychiatry* 36: 165–168.

Frank, R., and Lave, J. 1985. The Impact of Medicaid Benefit Design on Length of Hospital Stay and Patient Transfers. *Hospital and Community Psychiatry* 36: 749–753.

Frank, R. and McGuire, T. 1986. A Review of Studies of the Impact of Insurance on the Demand and Utilization of Specialty Mental Health Services. *Health Services Research* 21: 241–265.

Goldman, H. 1986. Financing Long-Term Psychiatric Care. *Business and Health* March-April: 5–7.

Goldman, H. 1987. Financing of the Mental Health System. *Psychiatric Annals* 17: 580–585.

Goldman, H., Cohen, G., and Davis, M. 1985. Economic Grand Rounds: Expanded Medicare Outpatient Coverage for Alzheimer's Disease and Related Disorders. *Hospital and Community Psychiatry* 36: 939–942.

Goldman, H., and Sharfstein, S. 1987. Are Specialized Psychiatric Services Worth the Higher Cost? *American Journal of Psychiatry* 144: 626–628.

Goldman, H., Sharfstein, S., and Frank, R. 1983. Equity and Parity in Psychiatric Care. *Psychiatric Annals* 13: 488–491.

Goldman, H., and Skinner, A. 1987. Specialty Mental Health Services: Research on Specialization and Differentiation. Unpublished.

Goldman, H., and Taube, C. 1985. Mental Health Financing and the Future of the State Mental Hospital. *American Journal of Social Psychiatry* 4: 26–30.

Goldman, H., and Taube, C. 1988. High Utilizers of Ambulatory Mental Health Services: Implications for Practice and Policy. *American Journal of Psychiatry* 145: 24–28.

Hustead, E., Sharfstein, S., Muszynski, I., Brady, J., and Cahill, J. 1985. Reductions in Coverage for Mental and Nervous Illness in the Federal Employees Health Benefits Program, 1980–1984. *American Journal of Psychiatry* 142: 181–186.

Jencks, S., and Goldman, H. 1987. Implications of Research for Psychiatric Payment. *Medical Care Supplement* 25: S42–S51.

Lehman, A. 1986. Capitation Payment and Mental Health Care: A Review of the Opportunities and Risks. *Hospital and Community Psychiatry* 38: 31–38.

Levin, B., Glasser, J., and Roberts, R. 1984. Changing Patterns in Mental Health Service Coverage. *American Journal of Public Health* 74: 453–458.

Manderscheid, R., Witkin, M., Rosenstein, M., Milazzo-Sayre, L., Bethel, H., and MacAskill, R. 1985. Specialty Mental Health Services: System and Patient Characteristics—United States. In *Mental Health, United States, 1985*, eds. C. Taube and S. Barrett. DHHS Publication No. (ADM) 85–1378. Washington, D.C.: U.S. Government Printing Office.

McGuire, T. 1981. *Financing Psychotherapy: Costs, Effects, and Public Policy*. Cambridge, Mass.: Ballinger Press.

McGuire, T. Forthcoming. Financing and Reimbursement for Mental Health Services. *Health Services Research*.

McGuire, T., and Montgomery, J. 1981. *Mandated Mental Health Benefits in Private Health Insurance Policies: A Legal and Economic Analysis*. New Haven: Yale University Center for Health Studies, Institute for Social and Policy Studies.

Muszynski, I., Brady, J., Walsh, J., Roberts, H., and Sharfstein, S. 1985. *An Economic Survival Manual for Private Practice Psychiatrists*. Washington, D.C.: American Psychiatric Press, Inc.

Rupp, A., Steinwachs, D., and Salkever, D. 1984. The Effect of Hospital Payment Methods on the Pattern and Cost of Mental Health Care. *Hospital and Community Psychiatry* 35: 456–459.

Sharfstein, S. 1978. Third Party Payers: To Pay or Not To Pay. *American Journal of Psychiatry* 135: 1185–1188.

Sharfstein, S., Frank, R., and Kessler, L. 1984. State Medicaid Limitations for Mental Health Services. *Hospital and Community Psychiatry* 35: 213–215.

Sharfstein, S. and Goldman, H. 1989. Financing the Medical Management of Mental Disorders. *American Journal of Psychiatry* 146: 345–349.

Sharfstein, S., and Taube, C. 1982. Reductions in Insurance for Mental Disorders: Adverse Selection, Moral Hazard, and Consumer Demand. *American Journal of Psychiatry* 139: 1425–1430.

Talbott, J., and Sharfstein, S. 1986. A Proposal for Future Funding of Chronic and Episodic Mental Illness. *Hospital and Community Psychiatry* 37: 1126–1130.

Taube, C., Goldman, H., Burns, B., and Kessler, L. 1988. High Users of Outpatient Mental Health Services: Definition and Characteristics. *American Journal of Psychiatry* 145: 19–23.

U.S. Bureau of the Census. 1983. *Economic Characteristics of Households in the United States: Fourth Quarter 1983*. Washington, D.C.: U.S. Department of Commerce.

Wells, K., Manning, W., Jr., Duan, N., Newhouse, J., and Ware, J. 1986. Use of Outpatient Mental Health Services by a General Population With Health Insurance Coverage. *Hospital and Community Psychiatry* 37: 1119–1125.

15

Legal Issues in Mental Health Care: Current Perspectives

INGO KEILITZ

Beginning in the 1960s, the plight of mental patients—especially those warehoused in large, public institutions with inadequate professional staff, little or no treatment, and deplorable living conditions—became a civil rights issue of the first order (Brakel, Parry, and Weiner, 1985). Aggressive legal advocacy led to the widespread adoption of legal safeguards for involuntary mental patients resembling the due process guarantees of the criminal justice model. During the late 1960s and early 1970s, mental health law emerged as an identifiable discipline, overlapping with the traditional fields of psychiatry, law, psychology, sociology, and philosophy. Marking this emergence, the Mental Health Law Project, a public interest law firm at the center of much mental health litigation then and now, was formed in 1972; the first casebook in mental health law appeared in 1974 (Brooks, 1974); and professional organizations concerned with mental health law issues established divisions, each with its own journal, focusing on legal issues in mental health care.

In the last twenty-five years, mental health law has flourished as a rapidly growing field of scholarship and practice. Dozens of journals and hundreds of books devoted exclusively to mental health law have produced a burgeoning literature (Shah, 1981: 219–220). "Rivers of ink, mountains of printers' lead, and forests of paper" have been expended on the topic of the insanity defense alone (Morris and Hawkins, 1970: 176). Indeed, today it would be difficult for mental health professionals, administrators, and practitioners alike to avoid the confluence of mental health and the law.

This chapter describes a decided shift which has occurred in recent years in the underlying approach, guiding formula, or pattern of inquiry in mental health law, from an emphasis on ideology and doctrine to empiricism and pragmatism. I describe this shift, which I regard as a sign of the maturing of this field of specialization, in general terms. The major portions of the chapter then explore its impact in six areas of interaction between the legal and mental health systems: (1) involuntary civil commitment, (2) compulsory outpatient treatment, (3) the insanity defense, (4) competency to stand (criminal) trial, (5) treatment refusal by mental health patients, and (6) mental health malpractice. Much of the material in these sections draws on the work of me and my colleagues at the National Center for State Courts' Institute on Mental Disability and the Law. The chapter concludes with some observations about implications of the shift for public policy, mental health service delivery, and research.

PRAGMATISM AND EMPIRICISM OVER IDEOLOGY AND LEGAL DOCTRINE

Walter Lippmann (1927: 18) observed that "we do not first see, and then define, we define first and then see." Aggressive legal advocacy on behalf of mental patients during the 1960s and early 1970s was fueled by clashing ideologies that defined the paradigm governing what we "saw." ("Paradigm" as used here refers to the general structure and mode of inquiry used to frame a problem and identify solutions.) Logic and reason were applied in the service of such self-evident native principles as individual freedom, privacy, and human dignity, on the one hand, and the abstract ideas of helping others, the general welfare, and the needs of an organized society, on the other hand. These values and ideologies defined and made us see what *ought* to be. At the heart of this enterprise, which involved a clash of philosophies, values, and professional ideologies, were difficult questions about the proper balance between the need for legal safeguards against improper commitment—which would delay and complicate treatment—and the need to allow mental health and social service professionals sufficient discretion and autonomy in their decision making—which might endanger the civil liberties of involuntary patients. Yet most observers readily agreed that existing laws, particularly concerning the rights of mental patients and the essential obligations of the state, needed to be reformed to eliminate the horrors of insane asylums and to curtail the mistreatment of mental patients.

By the mid–1970s, most states had established laws providing significant substantive rights and entitlements to involuntary mental patients resembling the due process guaranteed criminal defendants (e.g., the right to a lawyer, a judicial hearing, the right to notice, and so forth). Reform was advocated and implemented according to the paradigm that was then the stock-in-trade of the legal scholar, advocate, and, to a lesser degree, the social philosopher: A social ill was brought successfully to public attention; the question "What ought to be?" was addressed by the application of rational analysis to self-evident, albeit abstract, principles and concepts; and, finally, new rights and entitlements were afforded mental patients who were subjected to state coercion.

This emphasis on reforming the "law on the books" dominated the practice and development of mental health law throughout the mid–1970s. Many academic psychiatrists, psychologists, and sociologists joined ranks with legal scholars in analyzing the substantive and procedural law formally governing criminal defenses based on mental aberration, competency to stand trial, involuntary civil commitment, civil competency, tort liability of mental health professionals, and other legal issues. Though mental health program directors, mental health professionals, mental patients and their families often had difficulty reconciling the abstractions of legal doctrine and rational analysis with their own daily needs and activities, for the most part they deferred to contending medical and legal professionals, whose positions owed much to ideology and varying territorial interests.

Without negating the success of this paradigm in tackling what have been referred to as "first-generation" issues in mental health law (Wexler, 1981: 257–261)—tighter commitment standards, procedural safeguards, durational limits on confinement, and deinstitutionalization—many observers began to question the utility of the governing paradigm by the early 1980s. First, successful litigation and legal reform had spawned a host of "second-generation" issues that did not yield easily to the use of the paradigm. Ideology was seen as largely irrelevant to understanding the wide gap between the "law on the books" and the "law in practice" (Shah, 1981: 255). Second, in many ways the paradigm did not fit well the realities facing the public mental health system: a dramatic decline in the number of patients residing in large public hospitals; an increase in the number of chronically mentally ill persons who were poor, uninsured, or underinsured; a burgeoning homeless population; the transinstitutionalization of mentally ill patients from public hospitals to other institutions including nursing homes, jails, and temporary shelters; a critical shortage of adequate community-based mental health care and related social services; escalating costs of all human services at a time of increased pressures to control expenditures; and continued prejudice against and fear of mentally disabled persons among the general public.

So it was that the predominant question "What ought to be?" began to give way to the questions "What actually is?" and "What can be?" Ideology, doctrine, and theory surrendered ground to pragmatism and empiricism. This shift in governing paradigms, which will be discussed in this chapter in the context of a number of areas of mental health law, has significant consequences for mental health. Not only does it alter the questions that are asked, but the shift inevitably brings into the conversation the great majority of mental health professionals who are not lawyers, legislators, legal scholars, or social philosophers.

INVOLUNTARY CIVIL COMMITMENT

Involuntary civil commitment is the legal, medical, and psychosocial process—operating at the confluence of the mental health, public safety, justice,
and social service systems—whereby an individual alleged to be mentally ill and
dangerous to self or others and in need of treatment is forced into involuntary
mental health care, presumably for his or her own good and the good of others.
The ways in which this authority is exercised reflect different combinations of
legal criteria which establish the situations and characteristics of persons who
may become subject to commitment, as well as the obligations of the state to
function as the protector of society.

Today, involuntary civil commitment is usually the last resort used by family
members, law enforcement officers, mental health and social service professionals, and judicial officers for providing treatment and care to individuals who
are either unwilling or unable to receive such services voluntarily. Decision
making requires a balance among three complex and often competing societal
interests: those of the individual, the family, and the state. First and foremost,
the individual has an interest in being left alone. Even if compelling reasons
exist for infringing on his or her privacy and freedom, the individual maintains
an interest in being treated fairly, honestly, and as humanely as possible. Second,
the family, as well as the individual's friends, acquaintances, and the community
in which he or she lives, have an interest in providing the individual the care
and treatment that he or she may desperately need but is unwilling or unable to
seek voluntarily. Families may also have an interest in lightening the often
overwhelming burden that a failure to provide professional treatment and care
to their loved ones may entail. Finally, the state, as the protector of society, has
two essential interests: first, to protect its citizenry from dangerously mentally
disabled persons and to care for its sick and helpless; second, to carry out its
obligations and duties as efficiently and economically as possible. What should
be clear is that a perfect balance among the interests of the individual, the family,
the community, and the state in involuntary civil commitment may not be possible, because the process involves competing moral values, political ideologies,
and different approaches to decision making.

During the last three decades, intense debate and controversy have centered
on the factors that commitment courts are legally required to consider in deciding
whether or not a person is a proper subject for involuntary civil commitment.
These factors make up the standards, criteria, or tests for involuntary civil
commitment, factors that many consider the core of commitment laws. They
include mental illness; present or future dangerousness to self, others, or property;
a likelihood that the person will suffer substantial mental or physical deterioration
in the future; impaired capacity to make informed decisions about treatment and
care; the probability of successful treatment and care; and the availability of
alternatives to involuntary civil commitment. Reflecting the long-standing dominance of abstract legal doctrine over pragmatism and empiricism, much of the

history of involuntary civil commitment in the United States has been a working and reworking of these formal legal tests for commitment, with relatively little regard to whether the different tests make any difference in actual practice.

The November 1986 publication of the National Center for State Courts' "Guidelines for Involuntary Civil Commitment" signaled a new direction. Based on a five-year research project of the National Center's Institute on Mental Disability and the Law, and two years of hard work by a national task force composed of prominent mental health, justice, and law enforcement experts, as well as representatives of citizen and advocacy groups, the guidebook contains fifty guidelines with detailed commentaries and reference notes for use in making involuntary civil commitment as fair and workable as possible.

Departing from the tradition of past initiatives to reform involuntary civil commitment (Parry, 1986), the "Guidelines" does not advocate a particular legal standard for commitment to be applied in all jurisdictions, but instead recommends the careful application of extant standards prescribed by state statutes. The National Task Force on Guidelines for Involuntary Civil Commitment, the group that formulated the "Guidelines," expressed the concern that the calibration of a statutory standard for commitment may have been overemphasized and due consideration of the conscientious administration of those standards underemphasized (National Center for State Courts, 1986: 493–497). The Task Force agreed that an overemphasis on the particular wording and the ideological underpinnings of states' commitment criteria may have prevented attention and valuable resources of the mental health, justice, public safety, and social service systems from being applied instead to improve procedure and practice.

A basic premise of the "Guidelines" is that the tendencies to view complexities of the involuntary civil commitment process in abstract, polar terms—e.g., personal liberties versus treatment needs, doctors versus lawyers, the legal model versus the medical model, or the police power of the state versus its *parens patriae* function—are stultifying and counterproductive. Perhaps theoretically and historically useful, such dichotomies do not fit the realities facing the public mental health system today and are at odds with signs pointing to a virtual breakdown of that system (e.g., the emergence of a dual system of care for the poor and for those who can afford to pay). Rather than focus on the "law on the books," where most of the debate about civil commitment has centered, the "Guidelines" directs attention to the process of involuntary civil commitment, its organization and structural arrangements, and its everyday administration, that is, the "law in practice." Involuntary civil commitment is defined as a process that, though operating within the general framework of legal principles, legislation, and court decisions, is shaped and adjusted by a host of extralegal factors identified with the workings of the various components of the mental health, justice, public safety, and social service systems including hospitals, community mental health centers, social service agencies, courts, law enforcement agencies, bar associations, advocacy groups, and legislatures. Accordingly, the main task set for improvement of the process is not further analysis of legal doctrine and a resulting press for legal reform, but rather the description of the actual characteristics of the commitment process, the identification of "trouble spots," and the development of promising solutions inspired by empirical research.

Because commitment processes throughout most of the country are fragmented and uncoordinated, the "Guidelines" encourages continuity and better coordination of the interrelated tasks and events for which the various components of the systems assume responsibility, as well as increased communication and cooperation among those responsible for administering the processes. The first three guidelines set the stage for this to occur. Guideline A1 (National Center for State Courts, 1986: 421–423) calls for the creation of interdisciplinary "community coordinating councils" made up of representatives of the components of the mental health, social service, and justice systems involved in involuntary civil commitment. It urges that meetings of the councils become the forum for discussion of informal, expedient solutions to the many systemic problems that arise in the commitment process. To ensure that available mental health and related services in the community are known to those responsible for administering involuntary civil commitment, Guideline A2 (National Center for State Courts, 1986: 423–425) recommends, in part, the preparation and distribution of a comprehensive, up-to-date directory of those services. Finally, to contribute to much needed understanding of the actual operation of involuntary civil commitment, as well as to improve the quality of the process, Guideline A3 (National Center for State Courts, 1986: 425–426) urges that involuntary civil commitment be subjected to vigorous ongoing research and program evaluation.

A suggested role of local community coordinating councils is the encouragement and support of research and systematic evaluation by local, state, and national researchers and research organizations. The noted emphasis on pragmatism and empiricism, and the themes of continuity, coordination, communication, and cooperation, recur throughout the "Guidelines." It may well be that the major value of the "Guidelines" is the redefinition of the "problem" of involuntary civil commitment, which no longer is viewed primarily as a legal issue to be solved by the application and reform of legal doctrine. This relatively narrow definition, appropriate during the 1960s and 1970s when aggressive legal advocacy was necessary to establish the rights of mental patients, is now receding in prominence and giving way to issues of implementation and programmatic outcome.

OUTPATIENT INVOLUNTARY CIVIL COMMITMENT

Dissatisfaction with inflexible involuntary civil commitment laws that sometimes make it too hard to get a person into the hospital and too easy for them to get out, the perceived failures of deinstitutionalization including an alarming number of homeless mentally ill persons, and the "revolving door" syndrome of repeated brief inpatient hospitalizations followed by relapse after discharge have all spawned an interest in compulsory *outpatient* treatment and care. The attention paid to coerced treatment and care in the community has expanded the fiercely debated issue of the criteria for involuntary psychiatric hospitalization to a much wider frame of reference to include the permissible scope of involuntary treatment and care in noninstitutional settings (Bonnie, 1986).

Simply put, involuntary outpatient civil commitment is the process whereby an allegedly mentally ill and dangerous person is forced to undergo mental health treatment or care in an outpatient instead of an institutional setting. Although procedures authorizing commitment to outpatient treatment have been on the books in almost all states for many years in the form of requirements to commitment to the "least restrictive alternative" and provisions for conditional release from hospitalization (Keilitz and Hall, 1985), involuntary outpatient commitment appears to have become the new battleground for ideological clashes between civil libertarians on the one side, and families and mental health professionals on the other. At the center of the fierce debate are questions about what ought to be, i.e., whether the permissible scope of legally coerced treatment should extend to noninstitutional settings, whether outpatient commitment is really a *more* restrictive alternative, and whether outpatient involuntary civil commitment is going to "widen the net" of social control and be invoked against persons who would otherwise be left alone. Empirical and practical questions of whether involuntary outpatient commitment *can* be achieved (whether it ought to be or not), and *if* it can be achieved, by what mechanisms and to what effects, have been secondary. In the following preamble to its "Guidelines for Involuntary Civil Commitment," the National Center for State Courts (1986: 497) urged caution in the use of less restrictive alternatives to compulsory hospitalizations, such as involuntary outpatient commitment, whenever such use may be appropriate:

Involuntary outpatient commitment, whereby a court orders mental health care and related social service in lieu of institutionalization, should be used cautiously, because its goals are questionable and its implementation is problematic. Administration of involuntary outpatient commitment as part of a general civil commitment scheme requires much more of the mental health-justice system than was required in times when a court order to commitment invariably meant institutionalization.

Caution was urged because, like many other abstract legal concepts (Shah, 1981: 225–256), the translation of involuntary outpatient commitment into fair and workable practices is fraught with difficulties. Most of these difficulties are suggested by a consideration of the sharp differences between commitment to self-contained institutions, where complete responsibility for all treatment decisions and supervision of patients rests with mental health professionals in those institutions, and commitment to fragmented community-based facilities with limited capabilities for case management, patient supervision, treatment monitoring, review of compliance with court requirements, and so forth. The difficulties enumerated in the National Center's "Guidelines" (1986: 499, 513) include:

1. uncertainties about whether state laws and local rules authorize court orders to involuntary mental health care and related social services in the community;
2. serious questions of policy, professional attitudes, and practice regarding the obligation of community-based mental health programs to accept involuntary patients ordered to undergo outpatient treatment and care by a court;
3. few organizational structures, procedural mechanisms, and limited resources for the supervision of outpatients and the monitoring of their compliance with the conditions of an involuntary outpatient commitment order;
4. the lack of standards and procedural mechanisms for reviewing and for certifying respondent's compliance with an outpatient treatment program; and
5. the lack of procedural mechanisms whereby commitment courts and mental health professionals could impose sanctions or remedies for respondent's noncompliance with a court order or with the terms of release from an institution under an outpatient commitment order.

Other related difficulties and problems likely to be confronted in the implementation of involuntary outpatient civil commitment include:

6. because of lack of resources, an understandable (though not laudable) disinclination by community mental health centers to accept, treat, and adequately monitor indigent chronically mentally ill and potentially dangerous patients in outpatient programs (Miller and Fiddleman, 1984);
7. the variability of social supports for outpatients (Hiday and Goodman, 1982), including adequate housing and transportation to and from outpatient settings;
8. political and fiscal barriers to a smooth transfer from care in institutions to care in the community; and
9. the threat of increased liability realized by community-based mental health facilities in providing compulsory outpatient treatment and care.

Undoubtedly, the use of legal coercion for treatment and care in the community will receive more careful and systematic attention in the next few years. Empirical questions are many. What are the histories and characteristics of involuntary outpatients as compared to involuntary inpatients? How are they selected? By whom? What are the structural, operational, administrative, and fiscal characteristics of compulsory outpatient programs? Are outpatient programs successful in terms of clinical efficacy, social protection, patient functioning, service utilization, family satisfaction, and other outcomes when compared to voluntary programs and simple release? Seen in the context of the operational problems enumerated above, the answers to these questions are central to the ongoing development of public policy regarding compulsory outpatient treatment.

THE INSANITY DEFENSE

The June 21, 1982, acquittal of John Hinckley by reason of insanity ignited swift and vociferous public outrage. The legislative response to the public indignation over defendants like Hinckley "beating their rap" and the related fear that thousands of insanity acquittees are being released to the community was equally swift. A total of thirty-three states made changes in their laws governing the insanity defense during the Hinckley trial and its aftermath (Callahan, Mayer, and Steadman, 1987; Keilitz and Fulton, 1984). Although the heat of the debate has abated in the last five years, the insanity defense remains one of the most controversial issues in mental health law. The observations made by Goldstein (1967: 20) more than twenty years ago remain valid today:

The insanity defense is caught up in some of the most controversial, ideological currents of our time. The direction it takes depends, essentially, upon the place in social control one assigns to the criminal law as it competes with other methods of regulation by the state, to each of the themes underlying the criminal law, to the confidence one has that the mentally ill offender can be identified and treated, and the importance one attaches to the idea of blame. However difficult it has been in the past to find one's way among considerations of this sort, events are conspiring to make the problem even more complex.

The insanity defense is rooted in the fundamental concept of Anglo-American jurisprudence that holds criminal behavior punishable only when it is blame-worthy. The insanity defense and its procedural apparatus define the extent to which persons accused of crime may be relieved of criminal responsibility because of serious mental disorder which substantially impairs his or her knowledge or appreciation of the wrongful act (cognition) or his or her behavioral controls (volition).

Much like the preoccupation with the tests for involuntary civil commitment discussed earlier in this chapter, the modern history of the insanity defense has been primarily one of periodic calibration of the standard of criminal responsibility. For the most part, the prevailing standards have all turned on two excusing conditions that are embodied in contemporary criminal law and are as old as the writings of Aristotle, namely, *ignorance* of fact or of law and an uncontrollable *compulsion* to act contrary to law and morality (Moore, 1984: 460). These two excusing conditions, ignorance and compulsion, if caused by mental illness, make up the contemporary tests for legal insanity.

The oldest and most venerable test is the McNaughtan test, stemming from the 1843 English case of Daniel McNaughtan who, intending to assassinate the British prime minister Sir Robert Peel, mistakenly shot and killed Peel's secretary, Edward Drummond. Evidence presented at the trial established that McNaughtan was suffering from what today might be characterized as paranoid schizophrenia. The jury returned a verdict of not guilty by reason of insanity (Moran, 1981).

The McNaughtan test turns on the ignorance of the accused about the nature of his or her own actions. Essentially, a defendant will be acquitted by reason of insanity under the test if the defense establishes three requirements: disease of the mind; defect of reason causally related to the disease; and lack of knowledge about the act itself, its legality or morality. By the end of 1985, twenty-five states employed a version of the McNaughtan test (Callahan, Mayer, and Steadman, 1987: 56).

The McNaughtan test does not exculpate defendants who knew that their actions were morally wrong or illegal but who, as a result of mental disorder, were unable to control their actions. Attempts to broaden the McNaughtan test by incorporating impairments in a defendant's ability to control his or her behavior led to the development of the "irresistible impulse test." Generally speaking, under this test an accused is not criminally responsible if, because of mental illness, he or she could not exercise proper control over unlawful actions (Goldstein, 1967: 90). In the 1950s, the American Law Institute (ALI) developed a test which sought compromise among the previously developed tests including the McNaughtan and irresistible impulse tests, that were considered to be either too narrowly or too broadly formulated. Under the ALI test,

A person is not responsible for criminal conduct if at the time of such conduct as a result of mental disease or defect, he lacked substantial capacity either to appreciate the criminality (wrongfulness) of his conduct or to conform his conduct to the requirements of the law. (American Law Institute, 1962: 74)

Approximately twenty states employed some version of the ALI test at the end of 1985 (Callahan, Mayer, and Steadman, 1987: 56).

The newest test to dominate scholarly debate brings full circle the search for the best formulation in determining an accused person's criminal responsibility. In 1983 the American Bar Association (ABA) endorsed a test for criminal responsibility that echoes the 1983 McNaughtan test's reliance on cognitive incapacity (Keilitz, 1987). While the ABA rejected altogether the volitional prong of the ALI test (the principal difference between the ALI test and the McNaughtan test), it retained the more "modern" wording of its cognitive prong by replacing the familiar McNaughtan phrase "know the nature and quality" with the word "appreciate." Thus, under the Appreciation test, a person is not responsible for criminal conduct if, at the time of such conduct, that person was unable to *appreciate* the wrongfulness of such conduct. On the basis of logic and reason— not empirical data—the ABA argued that the language of the Appreciation test is preferable to both the McNaughtan and the ALI test because the former takes into better account all aspects of a defendant's mental and emotional functioning and is in better concert with current clinical knowledge (American Bar Association, 1984: 323–335). However, one must wonder whether, as Shah (1981: 244) has noted, "all this obsessing over the subtle nuances of words and their meaning and interpretations makes very much actual difference." One can question whether changes in the language of the insanity test really matter in terms of a lawyer's decision to try a case in front of a jury or the actual frequency of insanity acquittals, for example. Notwithstanding the apparent reasonableness of various theories and assertions, in the absence of reliable, detailed data, the empiricist position requires an attitude of skepticism.

Although it is probably prudent not to be overly optimistic about what empirical research on its own can do to help solve social problems, replacing some of the dogma with hard data may well refresh the dialogue about the insanity defense. Wexler (1984: 25) undoubtedly expressed the sentiments of many observers when he noted that it is "tiring—even embarrassing—to be arguing in 1984 whether we should return to the M'Naghten [*sic*] Rule of 1843 or to the rule of an even earlier era."

However modest, there have been signs within the last five years that scientific findings about the operation, administration, and outcome of the insanity defense have begun to inform public policy and compete with the influence wielded by the long tradition of legal scholarship. Empirical research on the insanity defense has been of two types. The first is descriptive, addressing such questions as how many and what types of defendants plead insanity, how often they are successful, how long those acquitted by reason of insanity are detained in a hospital compared to how long they would have been imprisoned had they been found guilty, and how likely acquittees are to repeat crimes. Much of this research has been conducted by Steadman and his colleagues (see, e.g., Steadman, 1985; Steadman and Braff, 1983) and has often been called into service to counter misconceptions about the insanity defense. Today, few commentaries on the insanity defense fail to acknowledge at least some of the conclusions of this empirical research, namely, that the insanity defense is seldom raised, and even more infrequently successful; that most insanity defendants are not murderers who commit random acts of violence; that the great majority of insanity cases reflect agreement, rather than disagreement, among mental health experts' testimony, not a "circus" of conflicting testimony; and that insanity acquittees rarely go free immediately after trial (Keilitz and Fulton, 1984). Even if this descriptive research on the insanity defense were entirely consistent across jurisdictions—which it is not— its value to policymakers would be limited because it does not address the major question that is the focus of policy debate: What difference does the reform of the insanity defense make?

The second type of empirical research on the insanity defense addresses this basic question and therefore holds greater promise for affecting public policy. It is concerned with understanding and evaluating the effects of changes in the insanity defense, especially major statutory reforms. Relatively little research of this type yet exists, though its potential significance for public policy has been acknowledged (Keilitz, 1987; Callahan, Mayer, and Steadman, 1987).

Four major questions about the *outcomes* of changes in the insanity defense deserve close empirical attention. First, does the reform measure curtail the use of the insanity defense? That is, does it decrease the size of the class of defendants pleading and succeeding with insanity defenses? Second, does it lengthen or shorten the period of time that insanity acquittees spend in confinement? Third, even if the reform does not curtail the use of the insanity defense, does the reform alter the composition of the class? For example, does it reduce the number of crimes of homicide for which the defense of insanity is raised? Fourth, does the reform reduce the "trouble" that this class of defendants causes the criminal justice and mental health systems before, during, and after trial? For example, will insanity cases be easier to prosecute and harder to defend?

These questions are central to widespread concerns about the insanity defense. Despite frequently made arguments that deliberation of reform proposals must turn on strictly legal and normative grounds, assumptions about the empirical consequences of the insanity defense lie at the heart of most changes in policy and practice. In the past, reforms of the insanity defense have been based largely on untested assertions and polemics instead of on actual experience and experimentation resulting in hard data. Yet such a sterile, out-of-context approach may have brought us to a point of intellectual stagnancy. At least one commentator has been struck by the fact that "suggestions for reform seem invariably to fall on one side or the other of the standard philosophical, legal, and psychiatric arguments" (Wexler, 1984: 17).

COMPETENCY TO STAND TRIAL

Competency to stand trial is an issue usually addressed at the threshold of criminal proceedings. It concerns a defendant's capacity to assist in his or her defense and understand the criminal process. By contrast, insanity, or lack of criminal responsibility, concerns the mental state of a criminal defendant at the time of the commission of the alleged crime. A criminal defendant may be considered mentally fit to participate in the criminal process, but following a trial, the same defendant may be found not criminally responsible for his or her acts. Conversely, criminal defendants adjudged incompetent cannot be put to trial, though once restored to competency, they may be tried and held responsible for criminal actions.

The doctrine of incompetency to stand trial, establishing the "nontriability" of a defendant found mentally unfit to stand trial, is the law's most far-reaching provision for criminal defendants who may have mental disorders. While the insanity defense, the focus of intense debate and media attention, affects a small few, the threshold issue of a criminal defendant's competency to stand trial affects a much larger number of defendants. For every criminal defendant found to be insane, at least a hundred are determined to be incompetent to stand trial (Steadman et al., 1982: 33).

The prohibition against subjecting a mentally incompetent defendant to a criminal trial stems from the common law ban against trials in absentia, that is, when the accused is not present at trial. The accepted legal test for competency to stand trial follows from the U.S. Supreme Court decision in *Dusky v. United*

States (1960). The Dusky test is whether the defendant has "sufficient present ability to consult with his lawyer with a reasonable degree of rational as well as factual understanding of the proceeding against him" (*Dusky v. United States*, 1960: 402).

Principles of fundamental fairness and notions of common humanity underlie the need to suspend a criminal trial against an accused who is found to be unable to participate meaningfully in criminal proceedings. First, the accuracy of the criminal proceedings demands a certain level of competence in criminal defendants in order to acquire the facts of the case. This is particularly crucial when the accused may be the only person, other than the complainant, who has direct knowledge of the facts and circumstances of the alleged crime. Second, the protections afforded by due process of law depend on a defendant's ability to exercise his or her rights in the criminal process, including the right to choose and assist legal counsel, to confront accusers, and to act as a witness on his or her own behalf. Third, notions of common humanity would be offended and the integrity and dignity of the legal process undermined by the trial of an incompetent defendant. Fourth, the objectives of punishment would not be served by the criminal sentencing of a defendant who fails to comprehend punishment and reasons for its imposition.

In practice, judges routinely tend to approve motions for forensic mental health examinations for competency to stand trial even though such motions do not relate to real concerns about the competency of a client. Instead, such motions often are used as the only available legal device whereby a defense attorney or a court can obtain mental health care for mentally disordered defendants who are charged with minor crimes (Gutheil and Appelbaum, 1982; Roesch and Golding, 1980). In such circumstances, theory obviously departs from practice.

Today, throughout the country, increasing numbers of transient, poor, homeless, and mentally disordered individuals are straining the resources of law enforcement agencies, the courts, and all of the other human services. More often than not, the charges and complaints—sometimes called "junk charges"— that bring these individuals into contact with the criminal justice system are minor (e.g., trespassing, being drunk in public, or failing to pay for a meal). The great need for an array of social services for these individuals, e.g., mental health treatment, drug rehabilitation, food and shelter, is typically grossly disproportionate to the seriousness of the misdemeanor offenses committed by them. Meloy (1985: 382–385) has characterized this general patient type as follows:

The . . . type is called the "sunshine chronic," an individual who is schizophrenic, has a lengthy but misdemeanor criminal history, and is often booked on charges such as trespassing, petty theft or defrauding an innkeeper. This individual has a long history of noncompliance with medication and is usually quite content to live as a transient. He has slowly drifted to the bottom of the socioeconomic ladder, but knows how to "survive on the street." He is most likely to abuse alcohol. When the inpatient program has first

contact with him, he is usually psychotic, gravely disabled, and harmless. He has no
contact with family or relatives, and has usually never been married.

   In many jurisdictions, a large number of individuals like the "sunshine
chronic" described by Meloy are ostensibly referred by the courts for forensic
mental health examinations of competency to stand trial but, in fact, they are
being referred for other reasons that have little to do with fitness to stand trial
per se (Gutheil and Appelbaum, 1982: 263–264). Judges and defense attorneys
may use the competency issue as a vehicle for "criminally" committing the
defendant to a state hospital or other inpatient facility. As a result, defendants
may spend a considerable amount of time in a forensic treatment facility undergoing long-term observation and examination to determine competency or, alternatively, they may receive treatment aimed at restoration of competency. An
individual arrested on petty charges who, if convicted of those charges, would
probably spend no more than a few days in jail, may be denied bail and a speedy
trial because the competency referral is being used to hold the defendant for the
well-intentioned (albeit extralegal) purpose of providing mental health treatment
that is either otherwise unavailable or that the defendant would not accept voluntarily. Of course, the competency referral may be misused for less benevolent
purposes such as the social control of certain socioeconomic and racial groups.
   Some observers blame the misuse of the competency concept by the courts
on restrictive civil commitment statutes that have left large numbers of severely
ill, but presently nondangerous, persons in the community with no means for
the state to provide treatment. Paradoxically, based on the benevolent intent of
providing misdemeanor defendants with mental health treatment and care—even
if only for short periods of time and even in jail if necessary—judges and attorneys
(often with the encouragement of some families of severely mentally ill persons)
have used the issue of incompetency to stand trial as the only available means
to keep mentally disordered defendants *in* the criminal justice system rather than
to divert them *from* the criminal justice system as was intended by the concept.
   As was pointed out in the earlier discussions of involuntary civil commitment,
outpatient commitment, and criminal responsibility, it should be clear that in
questions of competency to stand trial there are also important distinctions between pronouncements of law that are primarily *prescriptive* (telling people how
they should behave and how things ideally *ought* to be) and a *descriptive* approach
(describing events and behaviors as they actually occur). This again points out
the gap between legal fiction and fact (Feeley, 1976). As suggested in the
following quotation by Professor David B. Wexler, the exploration of the actual
antecedents (e.g., reasons for referrals for competency examinations), operation
and administration (e.g., inpatient or outpatient competency examination), and
actual consequences (e.g., treatment in jail versus release without treatment) of
raising the issue of incompetency to stand trial may be far more interesting and
important than the abstract rules of law.

[V]arious incentives (fiscal or otherwise) that are purposely or often intentionally built into the criminal commitment system, and the consequences that flow from those incentive patterns, are generally of far more interest and importance than are the tests for determining whether one is incompetent to stand trial, not guilty by reason of insanity, and so forth. (Wexler, 1981: 118)

TREATMENT REFUSAL

Parry (1986: 334) recently lamented that at the height of our sophistication in mental health law, we seem to be grounded in a number of intractable problems such as "simultaneous litigation that advocates for the right to services and the right to refuse services without rationally or effectively demarking the lines between the two." Much that has been written about refusal of care and treatment (for a recent review, see Rapoport and Parry, 1986) has centered on the nature and scope of mental patients' legal right to exercise this option. With some notable exceptions (e.g., Gutheil and Appelbaum, 1982: 91–139; Appelbaum and Hoge, 1986), commentators on the topic typically begin with a discussion of the legal grounds for the right to refuse treatment in common law, state statutes, and the Constitution. This may include extended legal analyses of a potpourri of constitutional arguments about the First Amendment rights to freedom of speech, Fourth Amendment rights to freedom from illegal search and seizure, Eighth Amendment rights to freedom from cruel and unusual punishment, Fourteenth Amendment rights to due process and to equal protection, the right to privacy, and the right to treatment in the least restrictive setting. Deductive logic is then applied to derive from these abstract concepts or principles a right to treatment that somehow strikes a balance among the varying interests of the individual, the family, the community, and the state. In such an exercise, personal values are critical, whether they are made explicit or not.

Meanwhile, questions with important practical implications remain unanswered. For example, given the opportunity, how many mental patients actually refuse treatment? What types of treatments, in what settings, are refused and why? What are the characteristics of refusers as compared to patients who comply with the treatment and care offered to them? What is the natural history, as well as the clinical and social consequences, of treatment refusal? What are the responses to treatment refusal by individual treatment providers and the mental health delivery system as a whole? Roth and Appelbaum (1982) have noted that, unfortunately, the right to refuse treatment has generated far more questions than reliable, empirical answers. Appelbaum and Hoge (1986) recently reviewed the results of the few published and unpublished studies of refusal of antipsychotic medication by psychiatric inpatients. They succinctly summarized the current state of knowledge about refusal of treatment:

Short-term refusal is frequent, but long-term refusal rare. Refusers are likely to be sicker than accepting patients, but it is unclear if they are legally incompetent. Over the short term, many refusers do poorly in the hospital, but if ultimately treated, they do at least as well as other patients. Finally, patients' refusals are usually not upheld, with the vast majority of refusal patients being treated, at least initially, over their objections. (Appelbaum and Hoge, 1986: 95)

Though studies of treatment refusal are limited in number and embody certain methodological flaws (Appelbaum and Hoge, 1986: 87), their contribution to the debate is informative and refreshing. Clearly, more and better research is needed.

MALPRACTICE LIABILITY

> In every house where I come I will enter only for the good of my patients;
> keeping myself far from all intentional illdoing and all seduction . . . .
>
> —Hippocrates
> *The Physician's Oath*

Malpractice, in legal terms, is an action in tort, a noncriminal wrong committed by one individual against another. It is considered a negligent tort when a mental health professional damages a patient or a client to whom that professional owes a duty to care. Four basic elements need to be established to sustain a claim of malpractice: (1) a relationship existing between the patient/client and the mental health professional that creates a duty to care; (2) a negligent breach of that duty defined by some external standard of professional care; (3) demonstrable harm to the patient/client (a mental health professional will not be liable for damages, even for a grossly negligent act, unless some harm ensues); and (4) causation, i.e., the negligent act must be the "proximate cause" of the harm.

The most common categories of malpractice actions against mental health professionals involve sexual activity between patients and therapists, misdiagnoses (or failures to diagnose) mental disorder that causes or is likely to cause harm to the patient or others (e.g., attempted suicide, suicide, homicide, and damage to property), negligent use of somatic treatments (e.g., use of the wrong or improper dosage of medication), and failure to warn others of potentially dangerous patients (Gutheil and Appelbaum, 1982: 150–157). Notwithstanding unprecedented media attention focused on the "litigation explosion," the "liability insurance crisis," and our "litigious society," the threat of malpractice liability often seems more imagined than real (Daniels and Martin, 1986; Bales, 1987). The factual basis for assertions regarding the wide scope of malpractice is shaky at best.

According to Gutheil and Appelbaum (1982: 144), psychiatrists are the least frequently sued medical specialists. Among the approximately 26,000 psychologists who hold malpractice insurance policies through the American Psychological Association's Insurance Trust, 940 had suits *filed* against them between 1982 and 1986 (Goodstein, 1986). Compared to physicians, psychologists have a lower chance of being sued for malpractice and pay less for malpractice insurance. According to the American Psychological Association's Insurance Trust, members of the American Psychological Association have only a 0.5 percent chance of being sued for malpractice, while members of the American Medical Association have a 26 percent chance. A psychologist pays an annual premium of $450 for $1 million of liability coverage; a physician pays $25,000 (Bales, 1987).

No doubt, malpractice claims against mental health professionals will continue to rise, no less than claims against firemen, police officers, municipal employees, baseball coaches, and lawyers, this being the nature of our litigious society. Also, it is likely that increased litigation will continue to refine the concept of mental health malpractice, potentially creating new grounds for suits against mental health professionals. However, as noted by Gutheil and Appelbaum (1982: 178), this state of affairs justifies neither despair nor nihilism. A number of relatively simple, practical measures based in common sense should go a long way toward prevention of malpractice suits: adherence to professional standards, staying within one's area of competence and expertise, consultation with colleagues, documentation of procedures and treatment decisions, clarification of all relevant procedures with patients, obtaining informed consent, written permissions, and releases from patients, checking treatment histories, and avoidance of physical contact (Bales, 1987).

Ironically, by giving in to a perceived threat of liability, by practicing what has been referred to as "defensive" mental health care, and by abandoning common sense, a mental health professional may, in fact, be exposed to *increased* liability. Consider the situation of a mental health professional employed by an inpatient facility that has admitted an involuntary patient on an emergency basis and has detained that person pending a judicial hearing on involuntary civil commitment some time in the future. Three days after admission, the mental health professional determines that the person has become relatively stable and, in any event, no longer meets the statutory requirements for involuntary civil commitment. Assuming that the professional has clear statutory authority to release the person at any time (a provision in most states), and the statutory criteria for commitment in fact no longer apply, the question is, Should the mental health professional release the individual immediately, perhaps risking a third-party suit for negligent release, or detain the person until the commitment court orders release? Arguably, the therapist who detains an involuntary patient pending the outcome of a judicial hearing, knowing full well that the patient no longer meets involuntary commitment criteria, is as vulnerable to claims of false imprisonment, an intentional tort, as he or she is vulnerable to a claim of improper release causing harm to a third party.

Unfortunately, as in other areas of mental health law, very little reliable empirical data exist regarding the frequency of mental health malpractice claims, judgments, awards, and final payments. Large monetary awards for damages in mental health malpractice cases are newsworthy and visible but probably tell an incomplete story because they do not represent a random sample of suits. Anyone can initiate a lawsuit against anyone else for reasons that need not be valid. Many suits are dropped or simply abandoned without further actions by the mental health professional as defendant. Still more are dismissed before trial. Even when a malpractice claim is proven, the trial court's judgment and award for damages may not be the final judgment upon appeal to a higher court.

Amid abundant charges and countercharges as to who should be blamed for the malpractice crisis–negligent health care providers, lax professional regulations, poor management of the insurance industry, a tort system in desparate need of repair, greedy lawyers, or inefficient courts–one thing is painfully clear. Too little is known about key matters regarding malpractice, even so fundamental an issue as whether a professional liability crisis exists at all. Who sues whom and for what reasons? Who makes what types of malpractice claims (e.g., sexual misconduct, neglect in suicide cases, failure to warn, fraud, or bad faith) against whom (public or private individuals, classes of mental health providers, number of defendants in a case, etc.)? What is the nature of the malpractice claims resolution process? What are the "disputing behaviors"? Are there discernible trends or patterns over time? What are the immediate and intermediate outcomes, and the ultimate consequences of this process on individual mental health providers, the helping profession as a whole, as well as the provision of mental health services to patients? What are the actual effects (or likely effects) of potential changes in the malpractice resolution system (e.g., a limitation on the scope of liability, a cap on the size of damage awards, arbitration, and pretrial investigation and screening panels)? An understanding of the crisis in mental health malpractice awaits answers to such questions as these.

CONCLUSION

This chapter traces what this author believes has been an important shift in the last five years in the paradigm governing inquiry and implementation in six important areas of mental health law: involuntary civil commitment, compulsory outpatient treatment and care, the insanity defense, competency to stand (criminal) trial, treatment refusal, and mental health malpractice. The emphasis is on the nature and the content of the shift, not on a thorough review of the development of the six areas themselves. (The interested reader will find an excellent review of these and other areas in mental health law in *The Mentally Disabled and the Law*, by Brakel, Parry, and Weiner [1985].)

My discussion of the nature of this shift from an emphasis on legal doctrine and ideology to empiricism and pragmatism does not pretend to offer a systematic, comprehensive analysis. Instead, my perceptions are largely impressionistic and based on or inspired by the work of me and my colleagues on the interaction of the mental health system and the civil, criminal, and juvenile law over the last ten years. It is worth noting, however, that this same shift has been discerned by others (e.g., Shah, 1981: 257–258) and can be viewed as part of a larger movement in law toward greater emphasis on social science (Loh, 1984; Monahan and Walker, 1985) and what has been referred to as the "sociology of law" (Friedman and Macaulay, 1969; Melton, 1987).

Perhaps more difficult than describing the current shift in orientation is discerning its causes and antecedents. No doubt, it reflects a more pragmatic temper and greater impatience with legal abstractions among those who are relatively late entrants into the field, for example, family self-help advocacy groups. The shift may also be attributed to a growing realization among academic scholars and legal advocates that it is reckless to advocate reform based on their professional values and ideologies if they do not know and cannot tell if such reform will achieve its goals or simply evoke more litigation (Bok, 1983). The single-minded manner in which reforms were advocated and implemented may have demonstrated the "rule of the instrument" (Kaplan, 1964): The handyman whose tool box contains only one tool will approach every job the same way. If that tool happens to be a hammer, he may have considerable success in hanging a picture, but he is unlikely to get much return business repairing watches.

What does the shift in the governing paradigm in mental health law mean to mental health policymakers, program administrators, and practitioners? To recapitulate briefly, it will allow more mental health professionals who are involved in mental health law interactions, but who are not legal scholars, lawyers, or legislators, into the conversation about positive change. (Indeed, what is there to do within the old paradigm except litigate, legislate, or advocate for reform of mental health law on the books?) Second, the shift will cause a redefinition of the problem and the terms of inquiry in mental health law. Questions about "what is" and "what can be" are taking precedence over the question "what ought to be?" For example, if improvement of the involuntary civil commitment process is seen as a human resource management problem, instead of strictly a legal issue viewed in terms of rights and entitlements, the natural consequence would be an attempt to break down the process into a series of tasks and events for which the various components of the mental health, public safety, justice, and social service systems share responsibility. Trouble spots in the process—much more likely to occur as duties are transferred across, instead of within, components and systems—could be identified and various corrective measures evaluated.

Perhaps most important, not only for mental health professionals but for the sake of progress in mental health law and its administration, is that increasing attention to empiricism and pragmatism will build capacities for new knowledge. Whether a discipline is vital or stagnant often is said to be gauged by how far and often it must reach back into its own history to find answers, and how long it clings to those answers even when they are found wanting. Although we certainly should not expect the redefinition of the terms of inquiry to deliver quick and final answers to some of the seemingly intractable problems in mental health law, it can help untangle some of the complexities, downscale the problems, and guide improved policy and practice.

REFERENCES

American Bar Association. 1984. *Standing Committee on Association Standards for Criminal Justice Mental Health Standards*. Chicago.

American Law Institute. 1962. *Model Penal Code* (Section 4.01, Proposed Official Draft).

Appelbaum, P. S., and Hoge, S. K. 1986. Empirical Research on the Effects of Legal Policy on the Right to Refuse Treatment. In *The Right to Refuse Antipsychotic Medication*, eds. D. Rapoport and J. Parry. Washington, D.C.: American Bar Association.

Bales, J. 1987. A Few Smart Habits Cut Malpractice Risks. *APA Monitor* 18(9): 39.

Bok, D. C. 1983. The Flawed System of Law Practice and Training. *Journal of Legal Education* 33: 570–585.

Bonnie, R. J. 1986. Mental Disability Law Crosses a New Frontier: A Review of Recent Developments. *Developments in Mental Health Law* 6: 21–23, 40–42.

Brakel, S. J., Parry, J., and Weiner, B. 1985. *The Mentally Disabled and the Law*. 3rd ed. Chicago: American Bar Association.

Brooks, A. 1974. *Law, Psychiatry and the Mental Health System*. Boston: Little, Brown.

Callahan, L., Mayer, C., and Steadman, H. H. 1987. Insanity Defense Reform in the United States—Post-Hinckley. *Mental and Physical Disability Law Reporter* 11: 54–59.

Daniels, S., and Martin, J. 1986. Jury Verdicts and the "Crisis" in Civil Justice. *Justice System Journal* 11: 321–348.

Dusky v. United States, 362 U.S. 402 (1960).

Feeley, M. 1976. The Concept of Laws in Social Science: A Critique and Notes on an Expanded View. *Law and Society Review* 10: 497–523.

Friedman, L. M., and Macaulay, S. 1969. *Law and the Behavioral Sciences*. New York: Bobbs-Merrill.

Goldstein, A. S. 1967. *The Insanity Defense*. New Haven: Yale University Press.

Goodstein, L. D. 1986. Across My Desk (opinion). *APA Monitor*, August.

Gutheil, T., and Appelbaum, P. S. 1982. *Clinical Handbook of Psychiatry and the Law*. New York: McGraw-Hill.

Hiday, V., and Goodman, R. R. 1982. The Least Restrictive Alternative to Involuntary Hospitalization, Outpatient Commitment: Its Use and Effectiveness. *Journal of Psychiatry and Law* 10: 81–96.

Kaplan, A. 1964. *The Conduct of Inquiry*. Scranton, Penn.: Chandler.

Keilitz, I. 1987. Researching and Reforming the Insanity Defense. *Rutgers Law Journal* 37: 289–322.

Keilitz, I., and Fulton, J. P. 1984. *The Insanity Defense and Its Alternatives: A Guide for Policymakers*. Williamsburg, Va.: National Center for State Courts.

Keilitz, I., and Hall, T. 1985. State Statutes Governing Involuntary Outpatient Civil Commitment. *Mental and Physical Disability Law Reporter* 9: 378–397.

Lippmann, W. 1927. *Public Opinion*. New York: Macmillan.

Loh, W. D. 1984. *Social Research in the Judicial Process: Cases, Readings, and Text*. New York: Russell Sage Foundation.

Meloy, J. R. 1985. Inpatient Psychiatric Treatment in a County Jail. *Journal of Psychiatry and Law* 13: 377–396.

Melton, G. B. 1987. Bringing Psychology to the Legal System: Opportunities, Obstacles, and Efficacy. *American Psychologist* 42: 488–495.

Miller, R. D., and Fiddleman, P. B. 1984. Outpatient Commitment: Treatment in the Least Restrictive Environment. *Hospital and Community Psychiatry* 35: 147–151.

Monahan, J., and Walker, L. 1985. *Social Science in Law: Cases and Materials*. Mineola, N.Y.: Foundation Press.

Moore, M. S. 1984. *Law and Psychiatry: Rethinking the Relationship*. New York: Cambridge University Press.

Moran, R. 1981. *Knowing Right from Wrong: The Insanity Defense of Daniel McNaughtan*. New York: Free Press.

Morris, N., and Hawkins, G. 1970. *The Honest Politician's Guide to Crime Control*. Chicago: University of Chicago Press.

National Center for State Courts. 1986. Guidelines for Involuntary Civil Commitment. *Mental and Physical Disability Law Reporter* 10: 409–514.

Parry, J. 1986. Civil Commitment: Three Proposals for Change. *Mental and Physical Disability Law Reporter* 10: 334–338.

Pasewark, R. A., Pantel, M. L., and Steadman, H. J. 1979. Characteristics and Dispositions of Persons Found Not Guilty by Reason of Insanity in New York State, 1971–1976. *American Journal of Psychiatry* 136: 655–660.

Rapoport, D., and Parry, J. 1986. *The Right to Refuse Antipsychotic Medication*. Washington, D.C.: American Bar Association.

Roesch, R., and Golding, S. L. 1980. *Competency to Stand Trial*. Urbana, Ill.: University of Illinois Press.

Roth, L. H., and Appelbaum, P. S. 1982. What We Do and Do Not Know about Treatment Refusals in Mental Institutions. In *Refusing Treatment in Mental Institutions: Values in Conflict*, eds. A. E. Doudera and J. T. Swazy. Ann Arbor, Mich.: AUPHA Press.

Shah, S. 1981. Legal and Mental Health Interactions: Major Developments and Research Needs. *International Journal of Law and Psychiatry* 4: 219–270.

Steadman, H. J. 1985. Empirical Research on the Insanity Defense. *Annals of the American Academy of Political and Social Science* 477: 58–71.

Steadman, H. J., and Braff, J. 1983. Defendants Not Guilty by Reason of Insanity. In *Mentally Disabled Offenders*, eds. H. J. Steadman and J. Monahan. New York: Plenum Press.

Steadman, H. J., Monahan, J., Hartstone, E., Davis, S. K., and Robins, P. C. 1982. Mentally Disordered Offenders: A National Survey of Patients and Facilities. *Law and Human Behavior* 6: 31–38.

Wexler, D. B. 1981. *Mental Health Law: Major Issues*. New York: Plenum Press.

Wexler, D. B. 1983. The Structure of Civil Commitment: Patterns, Pressures, and Interactions in Mental Health Legislation. *Law and Human Behavior* 7: 1–18.

Wexler, D. B. 1984. An Offense-Victim Approach to Insanity Defense Reform. *Arizona Law Review* 26: 17–25.

16

Administrative and Service Provision Issues

JEANETTE M. JERRELL
and S. LEE JERRELL

To complement the discussion of mental health policy development in the United States that appears in Part 3 of this volume, our emphasis in this chapter will be primarily on the manner in which community mental health centers have formulated and carried out internal "business" strategies, usually in response to government directives or legislative actions relating to broader public policy issues. The purpose of this chapter, then, is to describe, analyze, and discuss the major service delivery and administrative issues currently faced by community mental health centers. To accomplish this goal, current policy issues must be understood in terms of the changing context experienced by these local centers since their inception in the 1960s. Thus, our approach will be, first, to employ an "industry analysis" framework which provides an overview of the major driving forces within the business environment of local mental health centers, and then to apply an "organizational analysis" framework which examines the way local centers have adjusted their operations and policies to achieve a successful "fit" with this changing environmental context.

CONCEPTUAL FRAMEWORK

Every organization establishes service or product goals for itself based on its primary mission and then seeks to achieve these goals through its management decisions and policies. Indeed, historically, formulating and implementing a strategy for operating local mental health organizations was fairly straightforward. A great many of these organizations began operations as single-service child guidance clinics or ambulatory service units in local hospitals which offered specific treatment services to local residents. The single-service, limited market was gradually augmented by increased service volume, variations in services such as those aimed at slightly different client groups, or movement into adjacent geographical areas as demand for service increased.

As long as the environmental context surrounding mental health services remained relatively stable with only gradual evolution over time, business strategy also remained essentially unchanged from year to year, allowing for minor fine-tuning of administrative practices and gradual changes in service provision. Under these stable and predictable conditions, the successful fitting of the mental health organization to its environment was not difficult. Practices proving effective could be standardized over a period of time while those that proved ineffective could be avoided, eliminated, or remediated. When this stability shifted in favor of a rapid policy, regulatory, and fiscal revolution, however, the luxury of incremental improvement gave way to extreme pressures to quickly find new patterns of service mix and administration to fit the new context of the organization. The major administrative and service provision issues now confronting mental health organizations relate to the difficult choices they face in trying to achieve a new equilibrium or strategic fit which will allow the organization to survive, maintain its operations, and grow under rapidly changing circumstances.

The concept of strategic fit has two components: *environmental fit*, i.e., relating the services provided to external demands and constraints, and *operating fit*, i.e., relating services to organizational structure and management practices which enable effective performance (Thompson and Strickland, 1987: 97, 131–132). Dimensions of environmental fit include those things that

government regulators and funding sources *require;*

clients *need;*

stakeholders in local community advocacy or public groups *want;*

third-party payors *reimburse;* and

local competition *constrains.*

Dimensions of internal or operating fit include those things that

organizational structures *facilitate;*

scope, volume, and diversity of operations *encompass;*

monetary, staff, and facility resources *allow;*

personnel *practice;* and

management policies *guide.*

To operate effectively in a changing environmental context, mental health organizations need to understand what services are in demand in the environment and the major forces affecting the delivery of these services, which of these services their organization is capable and desirous of providing, and how to organize to best deliver the chosen services. Understanding why a particular local mental health center is behaving in a certain manner necessitates, in turn, an appreciation of these same driving forces and their impact on local centers. Our starting point, then, is gaining a thorough grasp of the major changes and driving forces in the mental health industry which affect delivery of services.

THE ENVIRONMENTAL CONTEXT OF THE 1960s AND 1970s

This section traces environmental changes in the mental health industry in the 1960s and 1970s and identifies the major federal forces which shaped the initial organization and operations of local mental health service systems. In contrast to earlier chapters in Part 3 of this volume which focused on the structural and systems aspects of public policy change, the discussion of mental health policy development here is directed toward its distinctive administrative implications. A later section will provide a parallel discussion of the 1980s and emphasize both the new influence of state governments in this period and dramatic changes within the private mental health services sector.

Prior to the 1960s, public mental health services were offered primarily in state hospitals. Reductions in the state hospital patient population were initiated in the 1930s as an effort to save resources during the depression; however, the deinstitutionalization process did not gain momentum until mental health practitioners introduced short-term intensive treatment techniques after World War II and lengths of stay were further reduced by the introduction of antipsychotic and antidepressant medications in the 1950s (Morrissey and Goldman, 1984). By the 1960s, many state mental institutions had also developed ambulatory services, which offered crisis intervention, partial hospitalization, and aftercare, and had established networks of decentralized services in the 1960s. Outpatient care was generally available through a limited number of private psychiatric practitioners or through child guidance clinics.

Major economic incentives for expanding and diversifying local mental health services appeared between 1963 and 1981, when federal funding was made available under the Community Mental Health Centers Act of 1963 (Public Law 88–164). The legislation contained two explicit goals: (1) the treatment and rehabilitation of the mentally ill within the community, and (2) the promotion of mental health generally. These goals were to be accomplished through the development of community mental health centers (CMHCs), which merged prevention ideology and acute treatment and consultation philosophies, on the one hand, with the service mix of the state hospital-based ambulatory centers, on the other, to produce an integrated services model promoting continuity of patient care throughout an episode of illness. Federal guidelines required local centers to expand their service mix to provide a comprehensive array of services within a designated local catchment area in order to qualify for funding. However, there was no clear mandate for community-based centers to coordinate their efforts with state hospitals or to care for the chronically ill persons being discharged from state institutions. As a result, mental health centers primarily served new client populations in need of acute services and failed to meet the continuing care needs of those discharged from public mental hospitals (Bassuk and Gerson, 1978; Chu and Trotter, 1974).

As previously discussed in chapter 6, between 1965 and 1979 the Community Mental Health Centers Act was amended several times, progressively expanding the federal role in mental health services funding and provision. The 1965 amendments (Public Law 89–105) authorized funding for staff. The 1975 amendments (Public Law 94–63) expanded the number of required services from inpatient, outpatient, partial hospitalization, emergency, and consultation/education to include follow-up, children's services, services for the elderly, transitional halfway houses, screening for the courts, alcohol and drug services, and emergency services on a twenty-four-hours-a-day, seven-days-a-week basis. The 1975 revisions of the CMHC Act also mandated cooperation between state mental hospitals and local centers to improve care for chronically ill patients, but still did not address these patients' social welfare and housing needs. In response to criticism of the federal role in the deinstitutionalization process, the National Institute of Mental Health (NIMH) allocated funds in 1978 under its Community Support Program to nineteen state authorities for pilot projects designed to initiate a more systematic approach to care of the chronically mentally ill through the development of a community-based network of crisis, psychosocial rehabilitation, supportive living and working arrangements, and case management services to augment mental health treatment.

ADMINISTRATION OF CMHCs IN AN ERA OF FEDERAL CONTROL

The major service and administrative issues facing CMHCs during the first fifteen years of the program concerned their rapid startup and the continuing demand to rapidly expand service programs and administrative control mechanisms, such as information and evaluative systems. Early concerns in the community mental health field focused primarily on attempting to delineate the rationale, mission, and proper functions of community mental health centers, and on dealing with problems of supplying adequate human resources to deliver community-based services in the late 1960s and early 1970s. In their review of trends in the community mental health literature published between 1965 and 1976, Lounsbury et al. (1978) found that 21 percent of these articles focused on training and staffing issues such as using professional and nonprofessional staff, while another 8 percent discussed administrative issues, such as organizing center services, planning for new services, and needs assessment.

As the community mental health ideology became more established and more communities applied for grant funds, advocacy groups coalesced around specific underserved target groups such as children, minority populations, and the elderly. As the field matured, then, administrative and service concerns shifted to a focus on issues of delivering clinical services to these special target groups, for example, child abuse, death and dying, severe medical problems, and cultural differences to be considered in services for specific minority populations. Programs representing alternatives to hospitalization and aftercare for patients who were being discharged from inpatient facilities were being implemented, and there was beginning to be a distinct movement away from a more traditional clinical approach toward psychosocial rehabilitation. Consultation services also were a primary focus of attention, reflecting the concern of mental health professionals for linking community resources, providing skills training to non–mental health staff, and community development in general (see Lounsbury et al. [1978] or issues of the *Community Mental Health Journal*).

By the late 1970s, the administrative and service issues faced by local mental health centers grew increasingly diverse. A larger percentage of the articles in *Community Mental Health Journal* concentrated on clinical services issues, including rural programs, recidivism and dropout rates, continuity of care, peer review, and services to special target groups such as sex offenders, the mentally retarded, and juvenile offenders. After the 1975 amendments to the CMHC Act, centers were under growing pressures to develop management information systems and to use up to 2 percent of their budgets to evaluate their programs. Thus in the late 1970s, many of the articles published in the *Community Mental Health Journal* provided examples of program evaluation techniques, as well as emphasizing administrative issues such as the development of management information systems, the role of governing boards, and the development of performance measures. Staffing issues of primary concern were the roles of professional versus nonprofessional staff in service delivery and in services aimed at special target groups, job satisfaction among community-based staff, and the exodus of psychiatrists from CMHCs. Only a few articles focused on funding issues, marketing, or relations with the local business community, which would dominate the professional concerns of CMHCs in the 1980s. The predominant administrative issue for local centers concerned the impact on local services of "graduating" from federal funding (Naierman et al., 1978; Woy, Wasserman, and Weiner-Pomerantz, 1981).

THE ENVIRONMENT OF THE 1980s

In 1981 a major policy and funding shift occurred when Congress passed the Omnibus Budget Reconciliation Act (Public Law 97–35), consolidating federal categorical funds for services in mental health, alcoholism and alcohol abuse, and drug abuse into one block grant. The act provided that most CMHCs initially funded prior to fiscal year 1982 would continue to receive some portion of each state's allotment for as many years as they would have been eligible for basic staffing or operations support when first funded; however, the amount of the award to each center was not guaranteed. Federal funding levels for the programs included in the block grant dropped a total of about 20 percent for fiscal year 1982. Under block grant legislation, centers were required to provide only five mental health services—outpatient, emergency, partial hospitalization/day treatment, screening, and consultation/education. State authorities acquired considerable discretion in designating special target groups.

For their part, state authorities have differed greatly in the handling of their new responsibilities under the block grants based to some extent on previous orientation toward the federal model of local services development. Funding under the CMHC Act had flowed directly from the federal government to the local centers, intentionally bypassing state mental health authorities (Windle and Scully, 1976). During this period, some states already had community-based mental health agencies in operation and proceeded to maintain fiscal and operational control over existing agencies while establishing a parallel system of federally funded centers within their states. Others relied on direct federal support to develop centers throughout the state. A third group of states remained completely autonomous and developed centers without federal support or input. Such interstate differences in the establishment of community mental health services, and in the extent to which federal support was used to build the state service system, play an important role in the structure of community programs and are important determinants of current attitudes of state mental health departments toward local mental health centers. For example, those states that kept some fiscal and operational control over the CMHC program seem to have developed a stronger sense of ownership of CMHCs. In these states, the current program more predictably reflects individual state policies on deinstitutionalization and community care.

In a study of the changes occurring in state mental health systems following the initiation of block grants to states, Jerrell and Larsen (1985b) found that state mental health authorities were shifting state general revenue funding to replace declining federal resources for community-based services, and that major portions of state funding for local services were being redirected exclusively toward chronically and severely disabled clients in the community. Furthermore, regulatory policies were in the process of change as well. States have imposed additional accountability mechanisms in contracts with local centers, new administrative guidelines and performance indicators are being instituted for annual program reviews, and reimbursement mechanisms are being expanded to cover a broader array of services for the chronically or severely disabled. States still differ substantially in the percentage of the mental health budget allocated to community-based programs compared to the percentage assigned to institutional programs (Mazade, Glover, and Lutterman, 1984). However, most state mental health authorities report that, since the block grants were initiated, funding of community services has demonstrated a slight but steady increase or has at least remained stable relative to state hospital funding (Larsen and Jerrell, 1986). Funding gains, although small in most states, have depended on strong lobbying from both local and state authorities, thus demonstrating the commitment of state legislative and mental health authorities to building and maintaining a viable community-based system. In these ways, states are assuming more direct control over funding, service priorities, and accountability and regulatory procedures.

Concomitant with these changes in the public mental health setting, the number and variety of community-based services in the system as a whole continue to expand dramatically (Regier, Goldberg, and Taube, 1978). These facilities include county and private psychiatric hospitals, general hospital psychiatric units, Veterans Administration (VA) psychiatric centers, residential treatment centers for children adolescents, freestanding outpatient and partial hospitalization facilities, as well as a plethora of licensed mental health practitioners treating clients through individual or group practices. In addition to these specialty mental health units, many nursing facilities, board-and-care homes, and halfway houses offer care to mentally ill patients. As Klerman (1985: 585) has noted, the current pluralism, diversity, and deinstitutionalization in mental health care contrast sharply with the tightly organized care offered chiefly through state institutions prior to the middle of the twentieth century. The meaning of these environmental changes for CMHCs is clear: competition for resources—including clients, staff, revenues, and community backing—substantially increased for many centers and became a significant force in center management.

CHANGES IN SERVICE PROVISION

The major policy issues confronting CMHCs in making changes in service operations following implementation of block grants concern the emphasis of state authorities on certain high-priority target groups, i.e., the most severely and chronically disabled, improving efficiency and accountability, and trimming the community-based mental health system to conform to funding cutbacks.

Following the shift to state control in 1981, a core group of services offered by CMHCs, and targeted for increased attention under previous amendments, have continued to grow. As found in a multiyear study by Cognos Associates of seventy-one centers located in fifteen states, these include case management services, community residential programs, and partial hospitalization/day treatment services (Jerrell and Larsen, 1986). Most current increases in public mental health services are aimed primarily at chronically mentally ill clients who have been discharged from state institutions. Deinstitutionalization policies and funding changes at the federal and state levels have encouraged local mental health centers to increase their attention to this target group. An equally important target group of clients for these services are severely ill young adults with chronic disabilities who have not been treated in state institutions but who are frequently treated in inpatient units of local hospitals. Often these clients are also substance abusers in addition to being verbally abusive or even violent, a combination that presents problems for staff who are unaccustomed to dealing with such problems.

The third target group receiving increased attention at the local level is severely disabled children and adolescents. Many centers were reporting increased development of partial care programs financed through expanded third-party reimbursement regulations, additional contracts with local schools and juvenile justice authorities for assessment and treatment services, and additional funding from local and state social service agencies for prevention and treatment of child abuse.

An emphasis on continuity of care is evident in the substantial improvements reported in case management programs. Related changes include better needs assessments; more extensive collaboration between state institutions, local hospitals, and CMHCs, and greater cooperation among staff from different agencies; closer case monitoring; increased assignment of clients to specific staff caseloads, and increased home visits and casework with families. Staff time devoted to case management activities and, in some states, funding for this purpose have increased as well.

To complement these changes, the continuum of services for the severely and chronically disabled has been expanded to include more psychosocial rehabilitation programs, and residential alternatives. Expansions in community residential services involve an increased number of beds or the addition of residential facilities to the array of local service options, including halfway houses, lodge programs, shared apartments, group homes, beds in private homes, and other projects funded by the Department of Housing and Urban Development (HUD). Funding for these expansions in some states comes from the use of Community Support Program monies or block grant funds to expand community residential programs, or from HUD grants for community housing arrangements to supplement state allocations.

Increased attention to chronic clients has also caused a major reorientation in outpatient programs. Aftercare efforts with deinstitutionalized clients are moving into a maintenance phase, supplemented by community residential and emergency services. Publicly funded services to less severely impaired clients are being curtailed because of policy and funding limitations. As an alternative, many centers are trying to increase services to mildly distressed private clients; however, the volume associated with these clients is not yet equivalent to the numbers of total clients lost in recent years. While current conditions may be leading in some locales to a dual system of mental health care—one set of services oriented toward the most severely disabled indigent clients, and other services designed along a private practice model and aimed at paying clients— this development is evident only in about 20 percent of the centers studied by Jerrell and Larsen (1985a) and does not appear to represent a major trend. Rather, it could be viewed as one of several ways that local centers may be adapting to changes in their local service markets while trying to maintain a broad array of services and clientele.

The transformation of inpatient services may be another sign of the challenge centers face as they try to move from a dependency on public funding to a different client mix with the goal of generating additional revenues. The attention currently being directed toward community-based inpatient services reflects a growing awareness among centers that inpatient units must yield much-needed cash from private-pay clients in order to help subsidize center operations. Available inpatient beds often are not being used to capacity, especially in communities experiencing increased competition from private, for-profit hospitals. A further complicating factor for local mental health centers is the tendency of some states to use empty state hospital beds for inpatient clients rather than keeping those clients in the community, a practice resulting in the loss of accompanying Medicare payments to local inpatient units run by mental health centers and a reduction in the monies available to subsidize local center operations.

Services experiencing the greatest cutbacks since 1981 are consultation/education, prevention, and program evaluation. The preventive orientation envisioned for CMHCs was to be fulfilled through consultation efforts to other human service professionals, through public education efforts, and through the delivery of prevention services to augment direct treatment services. These services were mandated under previous federal legislation but are currently de-emphasized under federal and state guidelines. Consultation and education services have been terminated at many centers for lack of support and funding. Because the current mission of CMHCs has been narrowly defined under state control and cutbacks have occurred in most services, very few outreach efforts are being made except where targeted toward the severely disturbed. Prevention efforts continue to be pursued in drug and alcohol programs and in rural areas where direct service models are less feasible as financial cutbacks take place. In the Jerrell and Larsen (1984a) study, center directors also reported that many of these outreach efforts are now being offered as marketing ploys, i.e., to raise public interest in certain clinical conditions or treatments, thus improving the center's visibility in the community and advertising its services to potential client groups.

Program evaluation has also been de-emphasized recently in favor of activities assessing fiscal and treatment accountability and efficiency. Program evaluation activities that once were centralized and assigned to specialized staff have been reassigned to clinical program directors and, in some cases, integrated with quality assurance reviews. Centers in some states are not required to conduct program evaluations since the state mental health authority annually reviews their performance. In these cases, responsibility for evaluation of local treatment programs has been transferred to the state and integrated into fiscal or clinical administrative functions. These changes usually are not described as decreases but as reorganizations. Evaluation activities that are being maintained in local agencies usually are conducted for specific contracts, to support market analyses for new services, or to conduct cost-effectiveness or productivity studies. These evaluation activities continue only in larger centers where such functions are well developed and can be supported from administrative overhead.

Staffing changes occurring during the past several years reflect these same service directions and target groups. Reductions in clinical staff have been instituted primarily in response to funding cutbacks or changing client needs. Staff who have not been laid off have been reassigned to different functions, e.g., clinical supervisors demoted to clinicians, or reassigned certain functions of jobs performed by lost staff. Not uncommonly, clients have been added to clinicians' caseloads. By the mid–1980s, staffing reductions seemed to have stabilized and some staff were even being added for new programs, such as services for young adult chronics, initiated as a result of state policy changes. Differential turnover rates are apparent for various clinical disciplines. The trend toward decreasing involvement of psychiatrists in local mental health centers appears to have reached a plateau in the mid–1980s, but increasingly psychologists are leaving CMHCs to establish private practices in those states where reimbursement for their services has been expanded. The number of social workers and nurses remains fairly constant, as does the number of mental health workers. These changes in staffing probably reflect changes in service delivery, and shifts in the types of professional skills required to serve changing client needs. Apparently, center administrators are using different strategies to manage human resources. Rather than instituting general layoffs, they are retaining staff with necessary credentials as one means of attracting third-party payments or are using part-time and contract staff to fill temporary staffing needs, rather than hiring permanent staff and incurring overhead expenses for benefit packages and salary scales. Strategies for coping with new environmental demands for efficiency include conducting staff performance and productivity reviews, and reassigning staff to serve different client groups. However, other strategies such as hiring more part-time staff or consultants, who are a cheaper labor source but who have less commitment to the long-term goals and work of the center, may eventually undermine a center's viability and performance.

Given the extensive reduction in overall level of services and staffing during the past few years, questions about sustained service quality have been raised. In the Larsen and Jerrell study (1986), centers reported an increase in the number of quality assurance studies conducted. Many state authorities and third-party payers are requiring better monitoring of service quality, which is a powerful impetus for increased attention to these issues. This finding is particularly important in view of the decline in senior staff along with declining resources for staff development and supervision. Times of limited resources usually mean that programs such as staff development are reduced as part of an effort to limit administrative overhead. Certainly the status of quality assurance activities is still unclear, and given the drastic reductions in program evaluation efforts, questions concerning efficacy of services remain unanswered as well.

Most centers have had to substantially review current service programs in relation to agency priorities, with the goal of expanding selected services to maximize return on investment. Specific strategies include developing programs for special target groups, expanding services funded by first- and third-party payers, and maintaining government-supported services. Various forms of group treatment are also being used more frequently. For the most part, centers are staying closely aligned with state funding priorities except where the payoffs are immediate, e.g., diversifying service operations to capture new sources of revenues. A common pattern of services diversification involves obtaining contracts to provide specific services, e.g., employee assistance program contracts with business organizations to offer screening and counseling services for employees with chemical dependencies or mental health problems, and contracts for screening with local corrections agencies. More comprehensive services are also being provided in contracts with other human service agencies, contracts with health organizations and the VA, and in providing community educational programs.

CHANGES IN ADMINISTRATION

In general, although most centers seem to have successfully weathered the transition from federal to state authority, funding for CMHC services is shrinking, resulting in sizable cutbacks in their scale of operations (staff, amount of service, and fiscal resources). In the sample studied by Jerrell and Larsen (1984a,b; 1985a,b; 1986), the percentage of CMHC revenues coming from direct, federal sources, including CMHC grants and block grants, decreased from 34 percent in 1969 to 21 percent in 1978 to only 2 percent in 1984. At the same time, direct state revenues, which had remained fairly constant at 30 and 40 percent until block grants were instituted, rose to 50 percent of total revenues by 1984. Revenues from local and other government sources fluctuated between 10 percent and 15 percent of total center revenues between 1969 and 1984. The largest percentage increase in revenues came from client fees and third-party payers, with revenues from these sources doubling from 16 percent to 32 percent, primarily due to federal/state Medicaid reimbursements. While the source of government revenues has changed dramatically from the federal to state level, the overall proportion of direct government revenues has remained fairly constant, between 60 and 70 percent of total revenues despite considerable policy shifts. Revenues from nongovernment sources rose slightly from an average of 4 percent in 1980 to 8 percent in 1984.

Business strategies designed to enhance fiscal and administrative control mechanisms have been a major focus of local centers since 1982 (Jerrell and Jerrell, 1987). Specific business strategies include assessing the cost of individual services, developing accounting and record-keeping systems, implementing better management information systems to monitor resources, installing a third-party billing system, and analyzing accounts receivable. For many local centers, personal computer technology has enabled administrative staff to make substantial improvements in these business procedures and to fine-tune many aspects to contain costs and push for more efficient operations. State authorities are requiring more exact tabulations of performance indicators such as units of service provided by types of clients, unduplicated client counts, and better accounting procedures for tracing expenditures. Business strategies requiring staff involvement include incorporating therapists in fee collection, tightening financial screening procedures, and improving communication with middle managers.

Governing boards representing the citizens of the community were required under the original federal CMHC legislation. Later versions of the legislation dropped this requirement, allowing the size, composition, and function of the board to change. As a result, the role of the citizen governing board or advisory board is in transition. In 1982, immediately following the policy shift and decreased role of the federal government, many boards increased representation from local business and financial organizations. Many center directors made a concerted effort to involve their newly revamped governing boards more in financial and policy decisions, in hopes of improving internal business practices and garnering additional local support. While there is still considerable diversity among centers in this area, many boards continue to be moderately to very influential in setting general policy. They are less involved, however, in determining service priorities. Involvement in lobbying state and local officials on behalf of the center was a role originally intended under categorical grants to be filled by community governing boards. In the mid–1980s community governing boards apparently are serving as a liaison between the agency and the community only on a limited basis, if at all. Governing boards clearly have come to play an oversight role, perhaps to satisfy state laws regarding corporations. Seldom do they function as representatives of the center to local or state leaders.

A related service system issue for CMHCs is citizen participation. During the 1970s this concept was a key issue in the CMHC amendments. Besides having community groups represented on the governing board of CMHCs, citizens were supposed to be increasingly involved in program reviews and evaluations to ensure that services were appropriate and accessible to special target groups of clients. Without specific guidelines from state authorities, citizen participation is virtually being ignored in current CMHC operations. Executives are more concerned with being responsive to funding sources and enlisting the backing of local advocacy groups to accomplish this goal rather than with involving citizens in management and policy initiatives. The emphasis is on making operations more efficient, not more democratic.

Under current circumstances, the executive director of most CMHCs has many more audiences and stakeholders to attend to since direct federal support was terminated. The external forces perceived by administrators today as most significant for CMHCs are state funding, state policy and regulations, and the availability of other sources of funding. Other factors such as pressure from local sources and community perceptions of the center are of relatively little influence. Executive contacts with the state mental health authority are now very frequent, often occurring on a weekly basis, as are contacts with primary health care organizations, the criminal justice system, and community human service groups. Contacts with public agencies usually involve budget hearings at the local and state levels rather than the direct lobbying of legislators or county officials, or meetings with public advocacy groups.

During the past few years, development of more efficient center operations has been a driving force. By contrast, establishing linkages with outside organizations that could help the agency move toward increased effectiveness has received less attention. Despite compelling payoffs for establishing and maintaining interorganizational linkages—e.g., growth, efficiency, and risk reduction—there are many reasons why linkages are difficult to establish and are avoided, such as lost autonomy, higher administrative costs, and agency incompatibility. The adjustments centers have made to external factors generally are narrowly focused and aimed primarily at securing resources for the survival of the organization. To accomplish this, centers have built positive working relationships with their state mental health authorities and placed increased emphasis on building linkages with those other human service agencies that not only supply clients but offer new sources of funding as well.

An issue discussed frequently since the termination of direct federal funding is the extent to which the federal definition of catchment areas is being continued. The catchment area definition continues to prevail in most state systems except where the consolidation of catchment areas, or the combination of services at a regional level, has been perceived as being more efficient. In some states, these changes in service areas essentially have opened the door for other health and human services agencies to compete with mental health centers for clients.

Competition from proprietary facilities or private practitioners is an increasing concern to center directors. An important survival issue for centers is whether they can afford to stay closely aligned with state priorities and still offer a comprehensive range of services. Some observers feel that unless centers offer different sets of services, attracting different sources of revenue, they cannot continue. Consequently, some centers are providing different services to public and private clients. Under this dual system, revenues received from private-pay clients can offset losses in publicly funded services. The need to diversify the center's service operations and fiscal base places an additional burden on managers to plan for new service markets and to balance limited staff time for delivering current services with the need to market new services. Further, the emphasis on efficiency and accountability requires that the reimbursement potential of services be considered.

Many administrators see diversification of service operations as a means of bolstering fiscal viability in order to subsidize public operations, retain high level staff, and avoid becoming narrow local institutions. Yet as centers develop new services and begin to specialize their structures, new administrative complexities arise which vie for limited resources and may tax the management capabilities of these organizations. For example, some centers are creating alternative, parallel service operations, including offering services at sites other than those where public clients are served, or reassigning staff to treat clients when services are reimbursable by third-party payers. Obviously, these changes consume fiscal and administrative resources so that centers must generate income beyond the expenses actually incurred for these operations. While center administrators making choices of this kind deny that they result in changes detrimental to the public component of their operations, they also acknowledge that these changes are riskier than simply conforming to cutbacks and remaining essentially a public agency.

SUMMARY AND CONCLUSION

To portray the major organizational issues currently facing CMHCs, we have examined the types of changes in service and administrative operations that government regulations and funding sources have required from local centers, as well as the ways that increasing pressures imposed by a competitive environment have influenced internal operations. We also considered the ways that local centers have been reorienting their service operations and administrative practices to achieve an environmental fit between external demands and service operations, and an operational fit between management structure or functioning and service operations. It is now in order briefly to summarize the factors and issues highlighted in the industry and organizational analysis and to describe those policy matters of continuing concern to CMHCs.

The shift from federal to state authority and fiscal control has meant that local centers must become more closely aligned with new perceptions of their mission, new priorities for their service activities, and new guidelines for their administrative operations. To conform to these changing directives, CMHCs have adjusted to a much more narrowly defined scope for their publicly funded operations: only certain target groups are funded, a less comprehensive array of services is offered, total revenues are shrinking, and human resources are being cut back or changed.

Client needs are also changing. More indigent, homeless, deinstitutionalized, or severely disturbed, "acting-out" clients are being treated (Jerrell and Larsen, 1986). To provide the necessary services for these clients, different staff skills and training are required than may be available among existing CMHCs whose mission and orientation have changed drastically over the last decade. Rather than serving a high percentage of mildly distressed, middle-class clients, centers are being forced by state policies to redirect their programs and staff towards those most in need and, in some cases, to make a conscious commitment to continue to serve these less severely disabled clients through parallel service operations.

Stakeholders in local community advocacy or public interest groups do not always want what state authorities have mandated for the state-supported system. Today, center directors are much less attuned to local demands unless a sizable portion of their revenues are from local sources. This funding does not have to emanate from local government sources but can be from private patients who choose to use the CMHC instead of other private mental health providers. If there are enough resources in the local market or environment, center directors usually devote attention to meeting these needs and demands for service, otherwise they turn their attention to the survival needs of the organization and seek support elsewhere.

The fiscal situation in many states is adequate, since most are increasing the range of services for severely disabled clients reimbursed by Medicaid (Jerrell, Larsen, and Moore, 1985). In addition, many states have enacted legislation requiring minimal mental health coverage by third-party payers (Jerrell, Larsen, and Moore, 1985). However, as other not-for-profit and for-profit providers move into local service markets, even these larger pies have to be split more ways. Therefore, centers are under intense pressure to keep pace with competing health care organizations, which have begun to encroach on the centers' operations and to make claims on possible sources of fiscal support. Center directors vary considerably in their perceptions of the impact of these new competitive forces and in their previous experience and ability to deal with such pressures.

In general, organizational structure in local CMHCs has changed minimally. When external resources were considerable, specialization of staff clinical and administrative functions was important. Now, middle managers and program supervisors increasingly are reverting to dual clinical and administrative roles, and clinical programs more often are staffed with generalists who can treat a broad array of clients. More centers are experimenting with parallel organizational structures to maintain their direct government contracts *and* to continue capturing third-party reimbursements. Yet these initiatives often are very taxing for executives and business managers to maintain. Nonetheless, these modifications in CMHC structure seem to facilitate the service changes being implemented to meet environmental demands.

The scope, volume, and diversity of CMHC service operations have greatly diminished, although some centers are attempting to maintain a more comprehensive array of services than is currently supported by direct government funding. Almost all preventive and outreach services consistent with the former community mental health ideology, strictly defined, have either been terminated, severely curtailed in response to funding requirements, or transformed into marketing or promotional activities to increase the visibility of the center to potential client groups. Dual care systems are developing in some centers but these developments are not perceived by those responsible as having adverse effects on the publicly supported mental health system. Such changes in internal service and administrative operations are directly related to cutbacks in monetary, staff, and facility resources. Activities which would forge closer linkages between CMHCs and other local health and human service agencies are concerned primarily with maximizing revenue sources, channeling clients who can be served in other agencies toward these services, and resolving continuity of care problems. Less central is an attempt on the part of the CMHCs to play a pivotal role in establishing a comprehensive local service system.

While these aspects of CMHC operation and administration now seem to have reached a point of relative stability following the tumultuous national policy changes in 1981, several difficult organizational and public policy issues remain which promise to challenge the CMHC system into the next decade: a definition of its primary mission and clientele, maintenance of adequate fiscal resources, and the use of quality control as a mechanism to balance efficiency and cost-control considerations, on the one hand, and effective service operations, on the other.

REFERENCES

Bassuk, E., and Gerson, S. 1978. Deinstitutionalization and Mental Health Services. *Scientific American* 238: 46–53.

Chu, F., and Trotter, S. 1974. *The Madness Establishment*. New York: Grossman.

Jerrell, J. M., and Jerrell, S. L. 1987. Selecting the Proper Management Strategy. *Community Mental Health Journal* 23: 19–29.

Jerrell, J. M., and Larsen, J. K. 1984a. Mental Health Center Adaptation in a Changing Environment. *Administration in Mental Health* 12: 133–144.

Jerrell, J. M., and Larsen, J. K. 1984b. Policy Shifts and Organizational Adaptation: A Review of Current Developments. *Community Mental Health Journal* 20: 282–293.

Jerrell, J. M., and Larsen, J. K. 1985a. How Community Mental Health Centers Deal with Cutbacks and Competition. *Hospital and Community Psychiatry* 36: 1169–1174.

Jerrell, J. M., and Larsen, J. K. 1985b. Policy and Organizational Changes in State Mental Health Systems. *Administration in Mental Health* 12: 184–191.

Jerrell, J. M., Larsen, J. K., and Moore, D. 1985. *Changes in the Internal Functioning of Community Mental Health Organizations*. Technical Report 85–3. Los Altos, Calif.: Cognos Associates.

Jerrell, J. M., and Larsen, J. K. 1986. Community Mental Health Services in Transition—Who Is Benefiting? *American Journal of Orthopsychiatry* 56: 78–88.

Klerman, G. L. 1985. Trends in Utilization of Mental Health Services: Perspectives for Health Services Research. *Medical Care* 23: 584–597.

Larsen, J. K., and Jerrell, J. M. 1986. *Factors Affecting the Development of Mental Health Services: Final Report*. Los Altos, Calif.: Cognos Associates.

Lounsbury, J. W., Roisum, K. G., Pokorny, L., Sills, A., and Meissen, G. J. 1978. An Analysis of Topic Areas and Topic Trends in the *Community Mental Health Journal* from 1965 through 1977. *Community Mental Health Journal* 15: 267–276.

Mazade, N., Glover, R., and Lutterman, T. 1984. *Revenues and Expenditures for State Mental Health Programs*. Washington, D.C.: National Association of State Mental Health Program Directors.

Morrissey, J. P., and Goldman, H. H. 1984. Cycles of Reform in the Care of the Chronically Mentally Ill. *Hospital and Community Psychiatry* 35: 785–793.

Naierman, N., Haskins, B., Robinson, G., Zook, C., and Wilson, D. 1978. *Community Mental Health Centers: A Decade Later*. Cambridge, Mass.: Abt Books.

Regier, D. A., Goldberg, I. D., and Taube, C. A. 1978. The De Facto U.S. Mental Health Services System: A Public Health Perspective. *Archives of General Psychiatry* 35: 685–693.

Thompson, A. A., and Strickland, A. J. 1987. *Strategic Management: Concepts and Cases*. 4th ed. Plano, Texas: Business Publications.

Windle, C., and Scully, D. 1976. Community Mental Health Centers and the Decreasing Use of State Mental Hospitals. *Community Mental Health Journal* 12: 239–243.

Woy, J. R., Wasserman, D. B., and Weiner-Pomerantz, R. 1981. Community Mental Health Centers: Movement Away from the Model? *Community Mental Health Journal* 17: 265–276.

17

Preventive Services in Mental Health

RAYMOND P. LORION
and LaRUE ALLEN

Had this volume been written a decade ago, it is unlikely that a chapter on prevention would have been included. Although the goal of preventing emotional and behavioral disorders was being conceptualized at the time, there was little scientifically accepted evidence of its programmatic feasibility. Without substantive evidence of the concept's viability as a service delivery option, the only real policy issue at the time was whether scarce research dollars should be spent pursuing such evidence.

Those advocating such expenditures (e.g., Kessler and Albee, 1975; Kelly, 1977) were frequently confronted by the argument that interventions could not be developed in the absence of an adequate etiological understanding of the disorders to be affected (Cummings, 1972; Lamb and Zusman, 1979; Sanford, 1972). In response, prevention advocates argued that the nation's mental health needs vastly exceeded existing or potential treatment resources (Albee, 1959, 1967). Moreover, they noted, available evidence raised doubts that existing mental health interventions were even effective for the segments of the population suffering most from serious emotional disorder (Hollingshead and Redlich, 1958; Lorion, 1978; Myers and Bean, 1968; Srole et al., 1962). Finally, they reminded their critics of the public health axiom that no disease had ever been controlled by treatment but only through preventive efforts.

Importantly, the debate over the relevance of prevention for the nation's mental health policies was on the agenda of the President's Commission on Mental Health convened during the Carter administration. The commission's final report argued convincingly for the benefits to be gained through the development of viable preventive interventions and recommended that requisite funding be made available (President's Commission on Mental Health, 1978).

The commission's recommendations were legislatively translated into the Mental Health Systems Act of 1980 (Public Law 96–398). Unfortunately, this law was rescinded shortly after President Ronald Reagan took office. Significantly, however, two of its key prevention provisions were retained: the establishment of a coordinating office within the National Institute of Mental Health (NIMH), and a mandate to develop a core of preventive intervention research centers (PIRC) throughout the nation. Implementation of those provisions gave rise to unprecedented levels of federal funding for the development of preventive interventions during the five-year period from 1982 to 1987 (U.S. Department of Health and Human Services, 1984, 1985, 1986). Additionally, legislation—the Alcohol and Drug Abuse Amendments of 1983 (Public Law 98–24)—was passed mandating that the Alcohol, Drug Abuse, and Mental Health Administration (ADAMHA) establish an agency-wide coordinating office to oversee the development of prevention research programs targeted to reducing the prevalence of alcohol, drug abuse, and mental health problems among the nation's citizens.[1] Thus, early in the decade of the 1980s requisite structures and resources were provided to stimulate the development of preventive intervention research and the implementation of resulting programs.

As will be described below, these efforts led to substantial gains in our scientific understanding of the design and evaluation of preventive interventions. Of equal importance, they created a momentum for such research and for programming. Consequently, activities related to the prevention of emotional and behavioral disorders were sought and funded at local and state, as well as federal, levels.

From a concept whose application was uncertain, then, the idea of preventing mental health disorders has become the impetus behind a major national movement. Unquestionably, the evidence available thus far does not justify the conclusion that all mental health disorders can be controlled through prevention. At the same time, however, doubters can no longer argue that the goal is unachievable for some forms of dysfunction, as evidence presented later in this chapter will confirm.

DEFINING A POSITIVE PREVENTIVE OUTCOME

What constitutes a positive preventive outcome? Obviously, measured reductions in the incidence and prevalence rates of a disorder would apply. We would also suggest that a form of preventive success may be achieved if the onset of a problem can be postponed long enough to allow the development of individual competencies or environmental supports needed to resist or moderate serious forms of dysfunction. For example, delaying the initiation of alcohol or drug use until late adolescence is not equivalent to avoiding such use entirely, but it is preferable to having such use begin in early adolescence.

The definition of a preventive outcome must also be flexible enough to reflect the consequences of avoiding emotional and behavioral ripple effects. These effects can occur, for example, to other family members when an adolescent becomes a substance abuser or when a parent experiences a serious affective disorder. Thus, we would propose that the concept of a preventive outcome include the potential for documenting and evaluating both direct and indirect effects.

As noted, early in its history the field of prevention justified its existence on the basis of an as yet largely unrealized potential. At the present stage of prevention, however, its defenders can and should document that potential by referring to the results of systematic evaluations of preventive interventions. In presenting this evidence, we will limit our discussion to three interrelated problem areas: adolescent pregnancy, developmental delay and academic failure in children reared in high-risk families, and substance abuse.

These problems were selected for several reasons. First, they represent high prevalence dysfunctions whose associated costs mandate their political consideration. Second, their interrelationship exemplifies a distinct characteristic of emotional and behavioral disorders; that is, they often share common etiological pathways, and attempts to influence the prevalence of one frequently affect the others. This quality of interdependence has significant implications for assessing evaluative findings relevant to preventive interventions. Its appreciation is also important in determining the costs and benefits of such interventions.

Finally, these problems were selected because they exemplify the link between targeting developmental processes occurring during childhood and adolescence and the maximization of benefits from preventive interventions. Unfortunately, some individuals are at risk for any and all of these negative outcomes. Which might be prevented depends, in large part, on when intervention takes place. Thus, the importance of calculating the cost of *not* preventing an outcome should also be appreciated. Failure to prevent an early dysfunction becomes truly costly if it catalyzes a continuing sequence of subsequent disorder.

The point to be emphasized in this chapter is that policymakers must appreciate that both the early successes and the early failures of preventive interventions are likely to have snowballing effects which may not be immediately recognized and whose costs are difficult to compute. When positive, however, such effects may be the true gold which results from mining the prevention vein.

Before considering what is currently known about the effects of preventive interventions and the consequent policy implications of that evidence, it is important to provide a taxonomy for such interventions. Definitional precision is needed because the multiple connotations associated with terms relevant to prevention (Cowen, 1983) have frequently blurred the salience of findings (Lorion,

1985). It is also important that programmatic differences among these interventions be appreciated and appropriately exploited.

PREVENTIVE INTERVENTIONS: A RANGE OF MENTAL HEALTH SERVICES

Two taxonomic systems have been offered to categorize preventive interventions. The first adopts the classic public health distinction among primary, secondary, and tertiary interventions (Caplan, 1964). The second involves an "operational classification" system recently proposed by Gordon (1983). Because each system highlights distinct aspects of such interventions, their structures will be presented and contrasted.

Public Health Typology

The public health concept of prevention is related to the control of physical diseases such as malaria. Public health focuses on decreasing the rate of occurrence of diseases in a population or a whole community rather than on curing diseases once they have begun (Caplan, 1964). In public health thinking disease can be interrupted in one of four ways: (a) strengthen the person who may get the disease (host inoculation), (b) remove the cause of the disease (the pathological agent), (c) remove the mechanisms by which the disease is spread, and (d) change the environment to reduce the chances that host and pathological agent come together (Bloom, 1984).

Prevention (particularly primary prevention) in the community mental health setting has the same potential to interrupt the course of disorders in multiple ways. These include interventions focused on the host, the pathological agent (stress, for example), or the environment (social support as an antidote to stress, for example) (Albee, 1982).

The American Public Health Association (1962) has identified six categories of preventable mental disorders, all of known etiology. Intervention strategies for these diseases represent the mix of host inoculation, environmental manipulation, and control of the disease itself or its spread which may be required to achieve effective prevention (Bloom, 1984; Rickel and Allen, 1988). The six disease categories are poisoning, infections, genetic disorder, nutritional deficiency, physical injury of the nervous system, and general systemic disorders such as toxemia during pregnancy. A closer look at two of these causes will illustrate variations in methods of interrupting the course of disease.

Preventable diseases caused by poisoning may result from the intentional or accidental ingestion of poison in many forms, including drugs, solvents, and industrial toxins, and can lead to chronic brain syndromes. One prevention strategy requires that the host's life-style be altered in order to avoid the poisoning agent. Another preventive strategy is to change the environment to reduce the chances that host and pathological agent make contact. This can be accomplished by making the poisoning agents unavailable, for instance, by removing lead paint from window sills so that children cannot ingest the lead by chewing on the sills.

The second example concerns diseases caused by infections such as rubella and syphilis during the fetal period, or measles and influenza during childhood. Most of these diseases can be prevented through strengthening the host (the child) with inoculations, or by treating the mother for fetally transmitted diseases, thus removing the pathological agent.

Tertiary prevention. Caplan (1964) was among the first to propose adoption of the public health triad to distinguish efforts to prevent emotional disorders. Within that system, "tertiary" prevention efforts refer to activities initiated after a disorder occurs to reduce the intensity and sequelae of symptoms. Tertiary efforts seek to minimize the level of disability resulting from disorder. They include rehabilitation programs designed to enable one to resume premorbid activities and to avoid recidivism. Examples within mental health would include day hospital programs to assist the chronically mentally ill to cope with the demands of independent living; the use of peer support groups following hospitalization for addiction to alcohol or drugs; and the inclusion of "booster sessions" within time-limited psychotherapy regimens.

It should be noted that the effectiveness of all tertiary preventive interventions may not be reflected in reductions in the prevalence of targeted disorder (Bloom, 1984). In fact, because they minimize disability, such programs may extend the life of the chronically impaired (e.g., by protecting the deinstitutionalized mentally ill from life-threatening situations) and thus increase the overall number of cases in the population. Tertiary efforts do not necessarily remove chronic conditions. In many cases, they enable individuals to cope more effectively with the consequences of those conditions than they otherwise could have. As discussed below, assessing the benefits-to-costs ratios of such interventions must therefore include consideration of factors such as the quality of life of their recipients.

Secondary prevention. Public health practitioners define secondary prevention programs as interventions applied to individuals who have begun to display symptomatic manifestations of a disorder. Involving the planned combination of early detection/case-finding and focused interventions, such programs seek to reduce the period of morbidity by arresting further symptomatic development and returning the individual to effective functioning. As noted by Bloom (1984: 197), "Secondary prevention efforts are preventive only in that systematic early case-finding brings with it the possibility of reducing the duration of the disorder."

In effect, within the classic public health definition, secondary prevention refers to rapid and efficient application of treatment. Insofar as that treatment achieves its goals, prevalence is reduced because of the removal of cases from the overall group affected by the disorder. For example, by intervening at the onset of an acute psychotic episode, one would seek to minimize the intensity and duration of psychotic symptoms. Similarly, the judicious application of psychological first-aid and crisis intervention techniques can significantly reduce the duration of emotional dysfunction (Slaikeu, 1984). Such techniques have been effectively applied to affective disorders, phobic reactions, and even some characterological problems (Koss and Butcher, 1986).

Some confusion has resulted from mental health researchers' use of the term *secondary prevention* to refer to two distinct kinds of interventions (Cowen, 1973). In addition to the public health definition of early treatment, the term has referred to programs applied to individuals who manifest incipient forms of dysfunction that presumably, if ignored, would evolve into diagnosable disorder. The term *early intervention* has frequently been applied to such secondary preventive interventions.

A widely cited and replicated example of prevention via early intervention is the Primary Mental Health Project (Cowen et al., 1975). This program involves the identification of primary grade children deemed at risk for subsequent disorder based on teacher ratings of their academic readiness, emotional maturity, and ability to control aggressive impulses. Selected children are assigned to a non-professional ''child-aide'' who is trained and supervised to assist these children to remediate deficits in the assessed areas of functioning. Multiple evaluations have confirmed this project's positive impact on academic and behavioral functioning (e.g., Lorion, Cowen, and Caldwell, 1974; Cowen et al., 1979; Cowen, 1980).

According to this alternate definition, secondary prevention efforts involve programs designed to select (through the application of sensitive screening procedures) individuals who display either precursor conditions which antecede diagnosable dysfunction, or developmental lags which predict subsequent dysfunction. Typically but not necessarily, such interventions are targeted to children and have as their defined goal the remediation of the noted deficit. Interventions of this kind are usually quite distinct from established treatments because the needs of their recipients are less serious than those of treatment recipients.

Silver, Hagin, and Karlen (1988) provide an excellent example of this distinction in their ''Search and Teach'' program, which uses a screening strategy to identify kindergarten children whose reading-related perceptual skills are significantly delayed. These children are then assigned to structured perceptual training programs. The program's efficacy is reflected in the number of program children who acquired grade-appropriate reading skills. Because the intervention occurs soon after school entry, many participating children did not fall so far behind that they met the criteria for certification of a ''specific learning disorder'' and thus neither required nor received formal special education remedial services.

In highlighting the distinction between these two forms of secondary preventive interventions, we do not intend to suggest that they are mutually exclusive. Rather we hope to convey the range of alternative strategies which have been attempted for the purpose of responding early. In each case, recipients of secondary preventive interventions must display either an indicant of dysfunction or evidence of an antecedent to dysfunction. In either situation, the intervention is targeted to individuals who meet programmatic criteria, and effectiveness is measured, at least in part, by the demonstrated reduction or removal of those very criteria.

In the case of early treatment, the prevalence rate of a disorder will be affected because the period of time when a diagnosis is applicable will be shortened. By comparison, early intervention affects the incidence rate of a disorder because, if intervention is effective, the antecedent dysfunctions will not evolve to the point of meeting diagnostic criteria. Because the reduction of the incidence rate of a disorder is also the defining goal of "primary prevention" strategies, it should be apparent that the distinction between primary and secondary prevention, as applied by mental health researchers, at times represents merely a difference in the means by which a common end is pursued.

Primary prevention. "Primary prevention" refers to interventions designed to reduce the prevalence of disorder in the population by avoiding its onset, that is, by lowering the incidence rate. Unlike the strategies described thus far, primary prevention interventions are not targeted to specific individuals *qua* individuals. Rather, the intervention is addressed to segments of the population typically selected because they have been determined epidemiologically to be at enhanced risk for the occurrence of a disorder. Targeting, for a majority of primary prevention interventions, has been defined in terms of such population or subgroup characteristics following the general assumption that intervention must occur prior to onset of the process leading to disorder (Cowen, 1986; Lorion, 1987a; Lorion, Price, and Eaton, 1987).

It should be noted that many indicants used to define "risk" and to infer increased likelihood of an ongoing pathogenic process are also found in the general population but do not always predict subsequent disorder (Lorion, 1987a; 1989). Thus, the undeviating sequential model of etiology applied to many viral illnesses has limited value for understanding the development of emotional and behavioral conditions (Bell, 1986; Kohlberg, La Crosse, and Ricks, 1972; Sameroff and Chandler, 1975; Sameroff and Fiese, 1988). A transactional model of behavior helps explain this discrepancy. According to this framework, combinations of individual and environmental/situational factors must be simultaneously present in order for the developmental process to be maintained and evolve in a positive or negative direction.

An important implication of the transactional model is that the capacity to alter outcomes—preventing the pathogenic process from reaching full symptomatic expression—can exist not only at the outset but for some period of time thereafter. Mental health specialists would do well to recognize this expanded opportunity to influence measured incidence rates. And public policies relevant to the support of prevention programs and prevention research must be made consistent with the complexity of underlying etiological mechanisms.

Primary preventive interventions are often conceptualized in terms of the three nonoverlapping categories of disease prevention, health promotion, and health protection (Price and Smith, 1985). Disease prevention can only occur when a disorder has a known etiology, and so, for psychiatric disorders, has relatively limited use when compared to medical disorders. Health promotion, however, can occur in the absence of a disease of known etiology, and consists of interventions having a positive but nonspecific effect on health. Activities such as stress reduction belong to this category. Finally, health protection is a public health mechanism which seeks to reduce the number of health hazards in the environment through public regulatory activities. Examples in mental health would be controlling the availability of drugs and alcoholic beverages, teaching adolescent mothers child-rearing skills, and regulating the use of child restraint to protect against head injuries in vehicular accidents.

Gordon's Prevention Typology

Although not originally linked to the transactional framework, Gordon's (1983) alternative taxonomy for preventive interventions is consistent with its tenets. Because the classic public health triad did not, in his view, easily apply to emotional and behavioral disorders, Gordon suggested that preventive interventions be classified instead according to their recipient and target specificity. For example, he proposed that interventions aimed at the population at large be labeled "Universal." This category would include such activities as public service announcements against alcohol and drug abuse; the use of brochures or other media to assist parents in interacting positively with their children; and the addition of social skills training within a primary grade curriculum.

Alternatively, interventions may be designed specifically for application to segments of the community at known risk for disorder due to demographic or situational characteristics epidemiologically associated with dysfunction. Gordon labels such interventions "Selected." Examples would include programs for children in families with a mentally ill or substance abusing parent; children from low-income single-parent families; and programs to assist the recently separated to adjust to the adaptive demands of that life event.

Finally, preventive interventions can be designed to respond to the needs of those presenting early indices of dysfunction. Such programs are labeled "Indicated" by Gordon. Examples presented above for early treatment and early intervention forms of secondary preventive interventions apply here. This category requires the use of screening or early detection procedures to determine those individuals appropriate for the intervention. As with either form of secondary prevention, Indicated interventions are designed to respond directly to the functional index used to determine an individual's eligibility. Effectiveness is thus defined both in terms of the reduction or elimination of that indication of dysfunction and in terms of evidence that more serious problems do not develop.

Admittedly, Gordon's categories do not differ dramatically from those of the public health triad. Universal interventions represent one approach to the achievement of primary prevention goals, that is, reducing the incidence rate of a disorder. Selected interventions may also result in a reduction in incidence, although they are targeted at epidemiologically defined high-risk groups rather than the population at large. And Indicated interventions, as noted, can refer to early intervention procedures and thus also lead to incidence reduction. They may involve, as well, the application of early treatment strategies and, in that way, have an impact on prevalence by reducing the duration of symptoms.

Gordon's focus on the recipient rather than the intended outcome—incidence vs. prevalence reduction—encourages prevention specialists to examine directly the balance between the risk assigned to an intervention's recipient and the iatrogenic potential of that intervention. As noted elsewhere (Lorion, 1987b), the potential of preventive interventions to have negative consequences for their recipients must be appreciated. Gordon's typology highlights this potential. For example, he explains that Universal interventions must be so designed that, at worse, their impact is neutral. He argues that this is necessary since one can neither control nor even identify which members of the population have received them. For that reason, procedures must be carefully designed not to initiate potentially harmful changes, for example, in parental behavior, interpersonal relationships, or substance involvement.

Because recipients of Selected interventions have a higher probability of experiencing emotional or behavioral disorder than the general population, it is reasonable to tolerate an increased risk of inadvertent harm regarding such interventions, provided a greater corresponding possibility of benefit also exists. Gordon proposes further that, since the recipients of Indicated interventions already display dysfunctional signs or symptoms, additional intensity and "problematic specificity" are justified in their cases. Thus, Gordon's approach highlights the importance of intentionally matching the known risk of participants with the potential risk of positive and negative outcomes of participation.

Gordon's typology and benefit-cost estimates. Another noteworthy contribution of Gordon's system is that it acknowledges directly the links among the intervention to be delivered, the associated cost per individual served, and the savings expected through the achievement of the preventive goals. Thus, Universal interventions are least likely to produce detectable short-term reductions in the occurrence of disorder. Given this fact and the large number of potential recipients, Gordon notes that it is important that the "per unit" cost be low. Such interventions should require minimal direct professional involvement and make use of efficient media approaches to communicate the intended message. Insofar as possible, Universal approaches should be incorporated within existing social service systems (e.g., classroom curricula, public health programs, preschool day-care programs) and require minimal programmatic changes. Associated costs would then primarily involve the preparation of materials.

By comparison, the per-unit cost of Selected interventions increases somewhat because the heightened intensity of the intervention is likely to require increased professional input and some direct contact between recipients and intervention staff. Highest per-unit cost will occur for Indicated interventions. In such instances, it must be ascertained directly that recipients are currently experiencing dysfunction. Contact with intervention staff is typically an essential aspect of responding to that dysfunction. In such cases, intervention costs can be compared directly to the costs of subsequently treating the dysfunction and the associated economic costs such as lost or reduced productivity.

Application of benefit-cost estimation procedures to the assessment of preventive interventions has been rather limited thus far. In large part, this reflects the evolving status of such interventions and the relative newness of analyses of this kind. Their analytic value, however, will be evident in our descriptions of several interventions targeted to children born in high-risk families.

EXEMPLARY PREVENTIVE INTERVENTIONS

Three interrelated problems—adolescent pregnancy, developmental delays and academic failure in children born in high-risk families, and substance abuse—provide a focus for describing in greater depth the nature and potential impact of preventive interventions relevant to mental health.

Avoidance of Adolescent Pregnancy

The importance of designing and implementing interventions to prevent adolescent pregnancy cannot be overstated. Approximately five million teenage females and seven million teenage males are sexually active (Johnson and Rosenbaum, 1986). At age fifteen, 20 percent of all teens report having experienced sexual intercourse; by age sixteen, the proportion increases to 33 percent. Over 40 percent of seventeen-year-olds report being sexually experienced. Overall, 60 percent of female teenagers and 70 percent of males report having had sexual intercourse (Zelnik, Kantner, and Ford, 1981). As a by-product of these levels of sexual activity, fourteen-year-old females become pregnant at the rate of more than 5 per 1,000. For young women between fifteen and seventeen years old, the rate soars to 62 per 1,000. Furthermore, one of every eight births to teens under the age of eighteen is *not* a first birth (Johnson and Rosenbaum, 1986).

The long-range consequences of early births to adolescent mothers present a bleak picture: significant increases in maternal mortality and nonfatal maternal complication rates, especially among young, poor, and black adolescents (Alan Guttmacher Institute, 1981). Young mothers are disproportionately prone to discontinue their educations (Moore and Burt, 1982). Those who seek work find limited employment opportunities with less prestige and lower salaries than those available to peers who postponed childbearing (Card and Wise, 1978). The impact of adolescent childbearing radiates to the offspring as well. Frequently, babies born of these mothers suffer from low birth weights and concomitant medical and other complications (Alan Guttmacher Institute, 1981).

Each of these possible outcomes represents significant potential costs to society to support, treat, employ in low-skill jobs, or educate through belated, labor-intensive efforts. Thus dollars spent on preventing first or subsequent pregnancies to teen mothers represent primary prevention efforts in health, education, and labor force participation.

In 1980, the Ford Foundation and the U.S. Department of Labor began Project Redirection (Polit and Kahn, 1985). By 1983, 900 pregnant and parenting teens were enrolled in four projects managed by community agencies. A key purpose of the program is to motivate teens to use a broad range of educational, employment, family planning, and health care services, many of which are already available in the community. When a teen enters the program, she is assigned to an older volunteer who acts as a role model and helps her locate and use services. Only when services are not otherwise available in the community does the program step in to provide them.

Project Redirection participants are interviewed when they join the program and then again one year later and at a two-year follow-up. Results are compared to carefully matched control group members who live in communities where Project Redirection is unavailable. After the first year, the program's preliminary data indicated that 52 percent of the Project Redirection teens (as opposed to 40 percent of those in the comparison group) have held a job. Among those who dropped out of school before pregnancy, 49 percent of the Project Redirection participants, versus only 20 percent of those in the comparison group, were in school or had received a high school degree. Teens in Project Redirection also showed a lower rate of subsequent (after enrollment in the program) pregnancies than those in the comparison group (16.8 percent versus 22.4 percent).

Schools have also proved an excellent setting for implementing preventive interventions to reduce the occurrence and consequences of adolescent pregnancy. One exemplary program was conducted in a school system in St. Paul, Minnesota, in which a multidisciplinary team—social workers, nurses, and physicians—provided students with pregnancy diagnosis, screening for sexually transmitted diseases, birth control information, and prenatal care (Edwards et al., 1980). More than three-quarters of the students used the services, with one in four getting birth control assistance. Positive outcomes included both increased use of contraceptives as well as reduced rates of pregnancies in schools which implemented the program.

Schinke and his associates (Barth, Schinke, and Maxwell, 1983; Gilchrist and Schinke, 1983) have demonstrated the applicability of a cognitive behavioral approach to the prevention of teen pregnancies. It appears that knowledge of birth control methods alone is not sufficient to guarantee either their use or their correct use. Interpersonal, communication, and social support skills are necessary for increasing teens' effective use of contraceptives (Schinke, 1984). For that reason, Schinke developed a pregnancy prevention curriculum with both cognitive and behavioral components which could be provided over a semester through fourteen one-hour sessions. Fifty-three high school sophomores and juniors, none of whom had experienced pregnancy, were randomly assigned to one of four experimental and control groups.

Group leaders were trained male and female social workers who engaged participants in discussions of the mechanics and human values involved in sexual activity. Leaders also discussed elements of social problem solving, including problem specification, generating options for addressing the problem, and choosing which option to implement. These steps were applied in behavioral exercises in which youths role-played conversations with family members and peers on topics such as birth control and intercourse. Additional behavioral practice was encouraged through the weekly contracts negotiated between participating youths and group leaders. In these, the teens promised to apply their new learning in their natural ecologies.

Evaluation findings showed that post-test scores were higher for prevention group than for control subjects on a measure of reproductive and contraceptive knowledge. Prevention group youths were also better able than controls to score well on problem-solving tests and on behavioral performance of problem-solving skills. Follow-up evaluations were conducted six, nine, and twelve months after the end of the program. Encouragingly, intervention subjects showed fewer incidences of unprotected intercourse, more habitual use of birth control, and more positive attitudes toward delaying pregnancy than did nonprogram subjects (Gormally, 1982; Schinke, 1984).

The programs described here all illustrate the potential for effectively applying preventive interventions to the problem of teen pregnancy. We believe that priority should be given to their use *before* an adolescent ever becomes pregnant. In that way, the broadest array of health benefits can be derived by the adolescent, and the largest number of negative consequences (e.g., limitations in educational gains and occupational options) avoided. Failure at this point, however, does not preclude other preventive interventions. Pregnant adolescents can become involved in programs designed to support them medically and psychologically during the prenatal period. Preventive programs are also available to assist pregnant adolescents to gain the knowledge and skills needed to avoid subsequent pregnancies. Finally, as described in the section which follows, interventions are available that respond simultaneously to recognized health risks of the adolescent mother and her offspring.

Reducing the Risk of Developmental Delay in Children from High-Risk Families

Considerable attention has been paid to the application of preventive interventions to children reared in high-risk families, which include some of the longest existing and most extensively evaluated interventions. Four specific programs will be described as examples of how interventions applied early in the development of such children can have a profound impact on the subsequent course of their lives. Programs are presented in the order in which they become involved with the family, from the prenatal to the preschool period.

Olds's (1988) "Prenatal/Early Infancy Project" focuses on the offspring of low-income adolescent mothers. To prevent maternal and child health problems frequently associated with poverty, this project engages the mother during the second trimester of pregnancy. Prenatal health care is provided to mothers who participate in home visits provided by public health nurses. Nonparticipating controls receive health care but are not visited. During the visits, the nurses provide the mothers with information on fetal and infant development, parenting behavior, and appropriate dietary practices to use during pregnancy. Other topics include career and educational planning, family planning, child-rearing techniques, and child health care.

Nurse-visited mothers reported healthier diets and reductions in their use of tobacco. They also had fewer premature babies and fewer complications with the delivery than their nonparticipating peers. Continued contact with these mothers for two years after birth revealed that members of the nurse-visited group were much less likely than their counterparts to abuse their children, to employ physical punishment and severe restrictions, and to experience child-care difficulties. Additional positive consequences of the intervention included increases in the number of nurse-visited mothers who completed school, obtained employment, ceased receiving welfare payments, and postponed subsequent pregnancies. The overall findings for this project suggest that the implementation of a fairly intense program during the critical prenatal period and its continuation during the child's initial months of life can have substantial benefit for both mother and child. At the very least, it appears that reductions can be anticipated in rates of prematurity, subsequent adolescent pregnancy, and child abuse. Arguably, the societal costs avoided by not having to respond to the victims of these problems are sufficient to defray the nurse visitation program. To the benefits side of the equation one can also add the savings associated with mothers completing their education and becoming economically independent.

Pierson's (1988) "Brookline Early Education Project" is also initiated with families during pregnancy. Unlike Olds's program, however, this involvement continues throughout the preschool period. Program components include making available to parents innovative educational and support programs to assist them in understanding and applying child-rearing techniques, monitoring the health status of children, and providing an organized prekindergarten experience for the child. Pierson's evaluation documented educational gains for participating children that continue at least through the second grade. Cost-benefit analysis also revealed that while the most costly version of the program is needed for economically disadvantaged families, less costly versions can be useful for low- and middle-income participants.

Ramey's (1988) "Carolina Early Intervention Program" engages similarly at-risk families when their children reach six weeks of age. Essential components of this program include a highly structured day-care program with an organized parent support program. Like the Pierson project, Ramey's program continues its involvement with the children throughout the preschool period. Participating children are involved in a planned sequence of experiences designed to optimize their cognitive, motoric, intellectual, and social development. It should be noted that children are selected for this project based on evidence of the mother's mental retardation. Using a rigorous randomized-groups evaluation design, Ramey and his colleagues have found that program children entered school with significantly higher intellectual functioning than comparable nonprogram children. In fact, many program children performed at or above grade level from the outset, and their educational advantage appeared to continue throughout their primary grade experience. In contrast, many of the control children displayed significant developmental lags from the beginning of school entry; many, in fact, met the criteria for certification as educationally handicapped.

Admittedly, Ramey's project is quite expensive given the close attention that each child receives throughout the preschool period. For example, if transportation is an obstacle for involving a child in the program, it is provided at no cost. Further, materials are made available for use in the home. Yet savings gained by omitting the preschool program are easily exceeded by the costs of providing services for children who could need special education classes throughout their academic careers—and additional social services that might be needed throughout their lives.

Johnson's (1988) "Houston Parent-Child Development Project" involves the at-risk families when the child is between the ages of one and three. During this period, if at all possible, *both* parents participate in a highly structured parent training program designed to inform them about child rearing and to provide a supportive network of similar parents for dealing with children's developmental problems. Participating children displayed higher levels of academic and behavioral functioning than their demographically comparable peers and these differences appear to be sustained over many years. Importantly, positive consequences can also be found for other members of the families who participated in this intervention.

Finally, Schweinhart and Weikart's (1988) "High Scope/Perry Preschool Program" deserves careful attention by policymakers. This project focuses its intervention during the period just prior to school entry, between a child's third and fourth birthday. As in many of the programs described thus far, participating families experienced the combination of a structured prekindergarten program and a parent education and support component. To date, the original cohort of participants has been followed for nineteen years. In addition to confirming the positive academic advantages for participating children, Schweinhart and Weikart report that these children displayed less antisocial behavior, less involvement with substances, and higher levels of high school graduation and subsequent employment. Moreover, the direct assessment of the program's benefit-cost ratio revealed that the program returned between $3 and $6 for each $1 of service delivery costs.

These programs provide vivid examples of demonstrably effective and currently applicable strategies to prevent long-term emotional and behavioral problems in the children of high-risk families. Not to consider the widespread dissemination of such strategies represents, in our view, ill-considered national health care policy. Admittedly, these programs would add immediately to an already unacceptably high deficit with little offsetting savings. The benefits of such programs, however, would begin to appear as the children born to high-risk families experience improved development of their physical, cognitive, and emotional capacities, as they begin their educations with less serious deficits and disadvantages, and as they avoid the sequelae of conduct disorder, academic failure, and early involvement with alcohol and drugs. Early development programs are not inexpensive. They may, however, be much less expensive than not providing them (Lorion, 1989).

Prevention of Substance Abuse

Except for AIDS, the nation's number one health concern at present appears to be substance abuse, particularly among youths. The basis for such concern is unquestionably real (Johnston, O'Malley, and Bachman, 1986). One out of every six children in seventh grade has used marijuana. By age eighteen, more than 90 percent of all high school seniors have tried alcohol; 45 percent of the boys and 28 percent of the girls will be drinking heavily. Nearly 60 percent will have tried marijuana, and nearly one of ten will be using that drug regularly. Alcohol, drugs, or both are involved in the majority of cases of adolescent mortality from automobile accidents and suicide. Reportedly, nearly one-half of adolescent pregnancies were conceived after one or both partners had used alcohol or drugs. Substances are increasingly involved in gang war homicides, and in a significant percentage of robberies and assaults by adolescents.

Increasing attention is being paid to preventive approaches to substance abuse because of both the physical dangers associated with such use and the limited success of treatment once addiction has occurred (Rickel and Allen, 1988). For the most part, preventive interventions have combined the determination of risk factors for identifying those more likely to become abusers, and the implementation of procedures to reduce those risks. Since many of the cited risk factors for the various substances overlap, it has been suggested that there is a youth subculture that is more likely to participate in all forms of substance abuse (Blount and Dembo, 1984). Frequently identified risk factors for substance abuse include the adolescent's attitudes toward substance use, personality factors such as impulse control, and an array of familial, social, and academic correlates.

Substance abuse prevention efforts have attempted to influence the presence of abused substances (the agent), the settings where use occurs (the environment), and the user or potential user (the host) (Schinke and Gilchrist, 1985). Examples of agent interventions include legal controls, such as changing the minimum drinking age, police sweeps to reduce the availability of drugs, and the strict enforcement of laws against possession, sale, and use. Environmental efforts have included the use of media, such as the "Just say no!" campaign, family interventions, or community activities to replace potential substance-related activities. At this point, national drug abuse prevention campaigns are in their infancy (Bandy and President, 1983). Little solid scientific evidence is available to support their preventive impact, although early findings seem promising (Flay and Sobel, 1983; Rhodes and Jason, 1987).

The most effective interventions to date have focused directly on adolescents. Such strategies seek to foster cognitive and behavioral abilities which could help those in this age group avoid substance use. Many programs occur within the school setting. Some have been targeted to substance use generally, whereas others have focused on specific substances. Early preventive intervention efforts toward smoking tobacco, for example, emphasized the health risks. Underlying these knowledge-based approaches is the assumption that providing youths with information about the health risks of smoking will result in the development of negative attitudes toward smoking and thus a lesser likelihood of engaging in the practice. While health educators in the United States still utilize this approach, there is little evidence of its effectiveness (Rhodes and Jason, 1987). Young adolescents may readily admit to smoking, yet may not label themselves as "smokers." They would not, then, expect to experience the health consequences that affect "smokers."

Recent advances in school curricula which focus on the social factors motivating smoking and on the short-term physiological consequences of smoking have reported improved success. Murray et al. (1984) report on a school-based program with approximately 7,000 seventh-grade students in Minnesota school districts. Mostly white, male and female youths were involved from all socio-economic levels and both rural and urban areas. The most effective deterrents of the initiation of adolescent smoking were (1) same-age peer leaders teaching specific skills for resisting social pressures to smoke; and (2) presentation of the physiological consequences of smoking. These positive findings were not found for students who were already smoking cigarettes. In fact, the program did not even decrease their smoking. These results exemplify the importance of early intervention when attempting to address substance-related problems.

Several programs highlight the usefulness of teaching social skills as a means of preventing smoking (Covington, 1981; Schinke and Gilchrist, 1985). Aspects of such programs include social problem solving, self-instruction, and interpersonal communication procedures that center specifically upon situations dealing with potential tobacco use and peer pressure (Schinke and Gilchrist, 1985). Several authors (Covington, 1981; Greenberg and Pollack, 1981) point out that, in order for such interventions to be effective, they must work within the naturally occurring motivations and cognitive abilities of adolescents. Interventions should therefore address the immediate, direct advantages of not smoking, according to the adolescents' own value systems (Greenberg and Pollack, 1981). They must be directed to issues of personal competency, social desirability, self-consciousness before classmates, peer pressures, and needs for affiliation and autonomy.

Botvin and Tortu (1988) report compelling evidence for the "Life Skills Training" program as a means of preventing the onset of tobacco use and, to a lesser extent, involvement with other substances. The program combines a knowledge-based intervention with specific exercises to help junior-high youths develop basic personal and social skills in order to enhance their sense of personal control. Its focus extends beyond substance-related situations to assisting young adolescents in dealing with a range of anxiety-arousing events characteristic of this developmental period. Through the program, participants learn ways to manage anxiety, to develop positive peer relationships, to make independent judgements about substance use, and to understand the implications of involvement with drugs. If needed, additional sessions are provided to participants during grades 8 and 9. Early results of a series of evaluation studies confirm the positive preventive consequences of this comprehensive intervention. At present, large-scale trials are underway to determine its generalizability to a broad array of population subgroups.

Because the negative results of knowledge-based smoking prevention programs were obtained in alcohol and drug prevention programs as well (Bandy and President, 1983), other affectively and behaviorally oriented programs have been tried. For example, a drug prevention program entitled "Ombudsman" has been disseminated to school settings throughout the nation (Kim, 1981). Ombudsman involves a three-phase approach in which program instructors work with regular classroom teachers, health teachers, and guidance counselors in providing the program to adolescents. Phase 1 consists of exercises to foster increased self-awareness regarding the adolescents' value systems. Phase 2 teaches participants group skills, including improving communication, decision-making, and problem-solving abilities. Phase 3 requires students to apply these skills and insights by planning and implementing a related outreach project within their school or community. Several replications support the conclusion that this program is more effective with elementary than junior high school children, that the addition of the program staff's assistance increases the effectiveness of teacher involvement, and that providing strict factual information about drugs *and* developing related skills can lead to improved attitudes and decisions regarding the use of drugs.

Another program developed in response to the ineffectiveness of purely educational drug prevention programs is the Alternatives Approach (Cook et al., 1984; Dohner, 1972). This is a school-based educational program that combines affective and behavioral components, with the central idea behind the program being that individuals use and abuse drugs because of the rewards and pleasures drugs provide. It is assumed that drugs fill certain social, psychological, and physiological needs, so attempts are made to fill these needs with alternative, healthier activities. Although a wide variety of activities have been suggested as alternatives, from athletics to meditation, it is difficult to find those salient enough to outweigh the immediate effects of drugs.

In summary, prevalence information indicates that the problem of substance abuse is a serious, continuing one which has thus far resisted many approaches to its prevention and treatment. A preventive focus appears most reasonable due to the physiological dangers involved, as well as the difficulty in treating addictive behaviors. Preventive efforts have occurred through legal controls on the substances, media campaigns, public service announcements, family interventions, and community activities. Most programs, however, have been implemented through direct efforts to reach adolescents at school. Initial programs that offered educational information regarding substance use showed few positive results. Therefore, more recent programs have attended to broader areas, such as emotional and behavioral components, which center more specifically on the adolescent's own motivations, needs, and level of cognitive development.

Prevention of alcohol and drug involvement in youth is complicated by some confusion about what is to be prevented. At various times the focus has shifted from "use" to "misuse" to "abuse." Each represents very different preventive goals with major policy implications. The broadest sweep would occur if the avoidance of initiation of alcohol and drug involvement is the goal. As noted, such use occurs in a majority of the adolescent population by age eighteen. To achieve significant reductions in the percentage of youth who have "ever used" would require the dissemination of very comprehensive interventions (e.g., Botvin's "Skill Training" or Kim's "Ombudsman") and, specifically with respect to alcohol use, the consistent and predictable enforcement of laws related to the sale, purchase, and consumption of alcohol by minors. We would suggest that the serious consequences of alcohol use by adolescents mandate a national drug abuse prevention effort beginning with the important substances of tobacco and alcohol.

Available prevalence data indicate that the majority of those who try substances discontinue use on their own (Johnston, O'Malley, and Bachman, 1986). For this reason, some have called for preventive interventions directed to the problem of misuse (levels of use which place one at risk for physical or psychological dependence), or abuse (dependence or addiction). The logic is that only those who misuse are at risk for abuse. This position cannot, in our opinion, be considered reasonable. It ignores the serious consequences of even limited use by youth, the uncertain (at best) impact of interventions once use has started, the possible rapid progression from limited to extensive use, and the unwillingness of many users to become involved in substance-related programs. It is, therefore, far too risky to condone "limited" use on the part of any segment of youth on the assumption that only a minority of individuals will actually need programs to prevent abuse. The pursuit of such programmatic savings strikes us as unacceptable health policy.

POLICY AND PROGRAM ISSUES

Funding, Reimbursement, and Other Obstacles

Despite federal policy and professional actions, the Community Mental Health Centers Act of 1963 did not produce a significant increase in preventive activities in the mental health field. One survey conducted in the late 1970s sought to determine the commitment to primary prevention among community mental health centers (CMHCs) in a three-state area (Klein and Goldston, 1977). The median amount of staff time spent on prevention programs was reported to be 5 percent. The comparable figure for secondary prevention activity was 10 percent. Major barriers to prevention programming included funding problems, community acceptance, lack of knowledge and skills, difficulties in evaluation, competition with direct services, limited number of staff, lack of administrative or staff interest and support, and difficulties in setting goals and priorities for prevention. Most of these problems persist today in the prevention field, and their resolution poses a challenge to future public policy development.

Because fees typically are paid only for traditional treatment services, CMHCs face pressures to provide even more treatment and less prevention programming in the 1980s, when federal cutbacks for social programs are the norm. Thus funding problems, insufficient staff, and competition with direct services are likely to escalate in limiting the availability of preventive interventions unless alternative prevention strategies are developed.

Before funding assistance is sought from charitable organizations or private industry, however, existing prevention programs must undergo rigorous evaluations that demonstrate convincingly their cost-effectiveness (Price and Smith, 1985). Such evidence is gradually accumulating for some programs, yet even more attention must be placed on sound evaluations able to reveal each intervention's "bang for the buck." Practitioners need the support of researchers who can translate the theory of evaluation research into the actual practice of prevention program assessment (Lorion, 1983). For their part, policymakers must set aside the funds needed to underwrite this applied research.

The clientele served by some programs poses another kind of barrier to the expansion of prevention efforts under public auspices. For example, children, the largest minority group in the country and a common focus of prevention activities, confront the same obstacles to policy change as do other minority groups (Westman, 1979). As a minority, they lack the clout which accrues to groups having large numbers of vocal and influential members. They cannot directly articulate their needs, and are dependent on systems (e.g., schools) which historically have resisted change. Moreover, children's needs often conflict with the needs of other interest groups (e.g., parents and teachers), and many who make policy regarding children have only limited knowledge of their needs. Other disadvantaged groups that are the target of prevention programs, such as racial minorities and female-headed families, face similar difficulty when competing for resources in the political realm.

Identifying Target Populations

Prevention programs may be administered to groups of people identified in several ways. Bloom (1984), for example, explains that prevention programs may be thought of as community-wide, milestone, or high-risk programs.

Community-wide, or Universal, interventions are available to all residents within a specific geographic area. Washington, D.C.'s "Beautiful Babies Right From the Start" is a community-wide media program to reduce the number of disorders that originate during the fetal period by involving pregnant women in an eighteen-month intervention program. By contrast, for milestone approaches, every individual in a population who reaches a certain hurdle is a member of the target group. The milestones include critical life transitions such as being fired, becoming a parent for the first time, or going away to college. Illustrative programs include outplacement counseling for fired employees, orientation programs for entering college students, and buddy systems for children who enter a new school midway through the academic year. Finally, high-risk programs focus on populations rather than events. For example, children of alcoholics, children with chronic illnesses, and minority children are all groups who are vulnerable to mental disorders. Interventions, such as stress reduction programs for presurgical children, can reduce the chances that members of these high-risk groups manifest a disorder.

No single method for identifying recipients of preventive interventions is clearly superior. Community-wide and milestone programs are expensive because many of the people who get the program will not need it. As is true with the distribution of other resources in our society, those most likely to avail themselves of milestone or community-wide interventions are frequently those least in need. Critical flaws also undermine the high-risk approach to identifying clients of prevention programs. Individuals who are at risk are usually overidentified in terms of the number who would actually develop a problem without preventive intervention. At the same time, the mere labeling of a person as being high-risk can have profoundly disturbing effects and can actually increase risk (Hobbs, 1975).

Probably the most cost-effective method for identifying client populations in terms of optimized gain and minimized risk is one that combines the labeling approach with a "take-all-comers" approach. Establishing a milestone program for those entering high school, and then further screening entrants using one or more risk indices, is an example. Use of multiple-risk criteria in an already selected population of needy individuals decreases the chances of labeling children unnecessarily. Reduction of a milestone population through the additional use of person-centered risk criteria likewise decreases the number who receive intervention, and therefore the total cost.

Risk Assessment

Risk is a key concept in epidemiology because determining who is at risk for illness enables improved tracking and prevention. For preventive interventions, identifying risk factors allows for the most efficient use of program resources in that programs can target those individuals most in need (Hough, 1985).

Risk factors are usually placed in one or two categories depending on when they occur relative to the onset of symptoms. The first category is predisposing factors. These occur from several months to years before the appearance of symptoms. Such factors can be further subdivided into those which can be modified and those which are, by their very nature, unmodifiable: gender, social class, and ethnicity (Allen and Britt, 1983); age, early history of mental disorder, and a family history of mental disorder (Hough, 1985). Women, for example, appear to be more prone to depression than men, adolescents more prone to pathological reactions to loneliness than adults, and the offspring of schizo-phrenics more prone to the development of psychotic symptoms than their counterparts from "normal" families.

Other predisposing risk factors are modifiable, or avoidable. Typically, these include events which occur early in life that increase the chances for later disorder. Early home environment and personality are two such factors which can be altered through early intervention. Most of the interventions described for children from high-risk families would be included in this category. As another example, children with low self-esteem can be involved in programs that increase their self-esteem and render them more resilient in the face of stressors.

Other modifiable risk factors include demographic variables such as education, occupation, income, and marital status. These can be altered through microlevel interventions such as social support intervention, and macrolevel interventions such as a national full employment policy. One may blunt their impact by increasing individuals' ability to deal with the risk factors without changing the individuals' status. Thus if people with higher incomes are generally more resilient than those with lower incomes, one can, of course, attempt to increase the income level of at-risk individuals. Alternatively, one might intervene by teaching low-income people to use available funds optimally, and to capitalize on available coping resources such as social support or personal assertiveness.

Precipitating risk factors occur just before the onset of symptoms. By definition they are assumed to trigger this onset. Investigation into the role of life events as precipitants of disorder has accelerated appreciation of their significance in the etiology of mental disorders (Dohrenwend et al., 1974). Researchers are also actively investigating life strain, daily stress, and macroenvironmental traumas as precipitating factors in mental illness (Hough, 1985).

The literature on life events consistently indicates that some events, whether singly or in close temporal proximity with other events, place individuals at considerable risk for emotional disorder. Events such as divorce in the family, bereavement, or immigration, are significant stressors. Several implications for the design and implementation of prevention programs follow from research on life events (Hough, 1985). First, populations can be taught to anticipate stress in order to avoid becoming overwhelmed. Second, the level of social competence in populations can be increased to strengthen their resilience. Children starting junior high school, for instance, can be taught survival skills beforehand which will reduce the anxiety associated with the school transition. Third, interventions can be designed to help at-risk individuals alter their perceptions of risk factors and consequently lower their estimations of the possible stressful impact of events. Fourth, programs to teach specific coping techniques have been designed for at-risk groups such as newly divorced or newly bereaved people (e.g., Bloom and Hodges, 1988).

Prevention Advocacy and Social Reform—An Uncertain Boundary

Prevention specialists need to make a commitment to generating the kinds of information that will aid decision making by policymakers. Prevention advocates need also to gain a better understanding of what social policy is and how it is shaped by popular sentiment, cultural traditions, and customs, among other forces (Sarason and Doris, 1979; Westman, 1979). A brief history of policymaking in one area, adolescent pregnancy control, illustrates the diversity of factors which can influence the policymaking process.

At the federal level, adolescent pregnancy is a relatively recent priority. A landmark year was 1970, which saw the enactment of the Family Planning Services and Population Research Act (Public Law 91–572) providing federal support for family planning services to teens and other age groups in the population. In 1978, the Adolescent Health, Services, and Pregnancy Prevention and Care Act (Public Law 95–626) created the first federal program specifically concerned with teen pregnancy. Then, in 1981, Congress established funding for "Adolescent Family Life Projects" aimed at controlling the problems of premarital sex and unwanted pregnancy among adolescents. Intervention by the federal government occurred about twenty years after the peak number of births to teens indicated the existence of a serious national problem (Vinovskis, 1981). Reasons for this lag between awareness of the problem and federal efforts to deal with it may provide clues about the period of time it could take for governmental action to respond to current social problems.

An early obstacle to effective federal response to high birthrates among women aged fifteen to nineteen, which reached 97.3 per 1,000 in 1957, was the uncertainty surrounding birth control techniques at the time. Many had just become available and were considered experimental and potentially hazardous, even for mature women. For this and other reasons, providing birth control to teens was (and remains) extremely controversial and very unpopular with many segments of society. Moreover, the social costs of teen pregnancy had not reached their current crisis proportions.

In the 1970s, impetus for legislative action increased as changes in adolescent sexual behavior became a matter of increasing concern. Factors stimulating calls of action included evidence that among teens (a) sexual activity increased (Zelnik and Kantner, 1978); (b) the number of abortions increased (Alan Guttmacher Institute, 1981); (c) out-of-wedlock births increased; and (d) the number of mothers keeping their infants rather than giving them up for adoption rose (Vinovskis, 1981).

Federal response to the problem of adolescent pregnancy prevention is currently impeded by controversy over several key factors which could serve as ingredients in a well-formulated prevention solution. Most pertinent research concurs with the view that family involvement can attenuate some of the negative outcomes of teen childbearing. What policymakers need, however, is research which clarifies the precise role that families should play in adolescent pregnancy prevention programs (Everett, 1984).

In a similar vein, debate continues over whether abortion should be included in a federally funded comprehensive teen pregnancy program. Although abortion is clearly a significant adolescent birth control method, federal Medicaid funds do not support abortion-related activities at present except in certain narrowly defined circumstances. Opponents of abortion, like opponents of family planning in general, argue that these are ineffective ways of dealing with teen pregnancy and that the very availability of such techniques increases the percentage of sexually active teens, leading to increased pregnancy rates. This casual link has not been supported by research (Chilman, 1983).

In the debate over sex education, both sides agree that sex education must reach teens before they become sexually active (Baldwin, 1982). Disagreement occurs, however, over who, the schools or the family, should provide this education. Opponents of school-based programs claim that they increase adolescent sexual activity by giving implicit approval to such activity. Proponents argue that failure to use the schools to ensure teens are provided with information on birth control impedes the prevention of pregnancies (Scales, 1981). As yet, comprehensive evidence is unavailable about the relative effectiveness of home-based vs. school-based sex education as a preventive strategy (Moore and Burt, 1982). In this and other ways, insufficient understanding of approaches for preventing unwanted teenage pregnancies remains a serious deficiency in the 1980s that obstructs the design of effective policy solutions. Nonetheless, the great psychological, social, and economic risks of teen pregnancy require public action beyond the provision of prenatal and postnatal services.

CONCLUSION

The past two decades have been most fruitful for the science and practice of mental health prevention. Initially, prevention specialists had to plead for federal support to confirm the mental health field's capacity to design programs which would reduce the prevalence of emotional and behavioral disorder. Limited though such support was, it allowed for the development of demonstrably effective interventions. Appropriately, a considerable proportion of that effort has intervened with children and adolescents. By responding early, it is now possible to change in a positive manner the anticipated developmental course of children born to high-risk families or vulnerable to high-risk activities (e.g., adolescent pregnancy and substance use). We know that the negative consequences of such vulnerabilities can now be avoided or reduced. We also know that in doing so we affect the lives not only of the direct recipients of preventive services but also of other members of their families, their peers, and significant others in their environments.

Yet preventive interventions are not free. Difficult decisions about the allocation of limited human service dollars will have to be made. Funds expended in response to current needs cannot be used to reduce future need. Benefit-cost analyses are persuasive but alone cannot dictate the choice between trying to maintain an inadequate treatment system and trying to develop a comprehensive federal prevention program. Presently, it seems that the de facto policy is to underfund each, thereby allowing neither to meet its potential. More importantly, current funding policies have resulted in treatment and prevention practitioners becoming competitors rather than collaborators (Albee, 1986).

The alternative recommended by the present authors is for policy to reflect current realities regarding the effectiveness of different preventive interventions. Funds need to be made available to begin the systematic dissemination of demonstrably effective interventions on a national basis. Large-scale preventive trials need to be supported in order that the dissemination process include the capacity to modify these interventions for diverse settings and populations. The lag between start-up and profits, however, must be recognized by policymakers. To assume that promised savings in direct care costs will occur immediately would be shortsighted. In many cases, five to ten years will be required before significant reductions in prevalence will be reliably reported.

Massive reductions in direct care costs resulting from prevention programs should not be expected in the short-run, therefore. Still, as reflected in the evidence reviewed in this chapter, the expectation that greater investment in mental health prevention will in time yield significant beneficial returns both to society and to the individuals served can now be supported by data rather than mere promise.

NOTE

1. The senior author served as the Acting Associate Administrator of ADAMHA for Prevention between 1983 and 1984. Dr. Morton Silverman was subsequently appointed to that position and served in that capacity from 1984 through 1987. A legislated responsibility of the incumbent is to prepare an annual report to Congress describing the nature and extent of prevention-related activities carried out throughout ADAMHA.

REFERENCES

Alan Guttmacher Institute. 1981. *Teenage Pregnancy: The Problem That Hasn't Gone Away*. New York.

Albee, G. W. 1959. *Mental Health Manpower Trends*. New York: Basic Books.

Albee, G. W. 1967. The Relation of Conceptual Models to Manpower Needs. In *Emergent Approaches to Mental Health Problems*, eds. E. L. Cowen, E. A. Gardner, and M. Zax. New York: Appleton-Century-Crofts.

Albee, G. W. 1982. Preventing Psychopathology and Promoting Human Potential. *American Psychologist* 37: 1043–1050.

Albee, G. W. 1986. Advocates and Adversaries of Prevention. In *A Decade of Progress in Primary Prevention*, eds. M. Kessler and S. E. Goldston. Hanover, N.H.: University Press of New England.

Allen, L., and Britt, D. W. 1983. Social Class, Mental Health and Mental Illness: The Impact of Resources and Feedback. In *Preventive Psychology: Theory, Research and Practice*, eds. R. D. Felner, L. A. Jason, J. N. Moritsugu, and S. S. Farber. New York: Pergamon.

American Public Health Association. 1962. *Mental Disorders: A Guide to Control Methods*. New York.

Baldwin, W. H. 1982. Trends in Adolescent Contraception, Pregnancy and Childbearing. In *Premature Adolescent Pregnancy and Parenthood*, ed. E. R. McAnorey. New York: Grune and Stratton.

Bandy, P., and President, P. A. 1983. Recent Literature on Drug Abuse Prevention and Mass Media: Focusing on Youth, Parents, Women and the Elderly. *Journal of Drug Education* 13: 255–271.

Barth, R. P., Schinke, S. P., and Maxwell, J. S. 1983. Psychological Correlates of Teenage Motherhood. *Journal of Youth and Adolescence* 12: 471–487.

Bell, R. Q. 1986. Age-Specific Manifestations in Changing Psychosocial Risk. In *Risk in Intellectual and Psychosocial Development*, eds. D. C. Farran and J. D. McKinney. New York: Academic Press.

Bloom, B. L. 1977. *Community Mental Health: A General Introduction*. Monterey, Calif.: Brooks/Cole.

Bloom, B. L. 1984. *Community Mental Health: A General Introduction*. 2nd ed. Monterey, Calif.: Brooks/Cole.

Bloom, B. L., and Hodges, W. F. 1988. The Colorado Separation and Divorce Program: A Preventive Intervention Program for Newly Separated Persons. In *Fourteen Ounces of Prevention: A Casebook for Practitioners*, eds. R. H. Price, E. L. Cowen, R. P. Lorion, and J. Ramos-McKay. Washington, D.C.: American Psychological Association.

Blount, W. R., and Dembo, R. 1984. Personal Drug Use and Attitudes toward Prevention among Youth Living in a High Risk Environment. *Journal of Drug Education* 14: 207–224.

Botvin, G., and Tortu, S. 1988. Preventing Adolescent Substance Abuse through Life Skills Training. In *Fourteen Ounces of Prevention: A Casebook for Practitioners*, eds. R. H. Price, E. L. Cowen, R. P. Lorion, and J. Ramos-McKay. Washington, D.C.: American Psychological Association.

Caplan, G. 1964. *Principles of Preventive Psychiatry*. New York: Basic Books.

Card, J., and Wise, L. 1978. Teenage Mothers and Teenage Fathers: The Impact of Early Childbearing on the Parents' Professional Lives. *Family Planning Perspectives* 10: 199–205.

Chilman, C. S. 1983. *Adolescent Sexuality in a Changing American Society*. New York: John Wiley.

Cook, R., Lawrence, H., Morse, C., and Roelh, J. 1984. An Evaluation of the Alternatives Approach to Drug Abuse Prevention. *International Journal of the Addictions* 19: 767–787.

Covington, M. V. 1981. Strategies for Smoking Prevention and Resistance among Young Adolescents. *Journal of Early Adolescence* 1: 349–356.

Cowen, E. L. 1973. Social and Community Interventions. *Annual Review of Psychology* 34: 423–472.

Cowen, E. L. 1980. The Wooing of Primary Prevention. *American Journal of Community Psychology* 8: 258–284.

Cowen, E. L. 1983. Primary Prevention in Mental Health: Past, Present, and Future. In *Preventive Psychology: Theory, Research and Practice*, eds. R. D. Felner, L. A. Jason, J. N. Moritsugu, and S. S. Farber. New York: Pergamon Press.

Cowen, E. L. 1986. Primary Prevention in Mental Health: Ten Years of Retrospect and Ten Years of Prospect. In *A Decade of Progress in Primary Prevention*, eds. M. Kessler and S. E. Goldston. Hanover, N.H.: University Press of New England.

Cowen, E. L., Orgel, A. R., Gesten, E. L., and Wilson, A. B. 1979. The Evaluation of an Intervention Program for Young School Children with Acting-Out Problems. *Journal of Abnormal Child Psychology* 7: 381–396.

Cowen, E. L., Trost, M. A., Lorion, R. P., Dorr, D., Izzo, L. D., and Issacson, R. V. 1975. *New Ways in School Mental Health: Early Detection and Prevention of School Maladaptation*. New York: Human-Sciences.

Cummings, E. 1972. Primary Prevention—More Cost Than Benefit. In *The Critical Issues of Community Mental Health*, ed. H. Gottesfeld. New York: Behavioral Publications.

Dohner, V. A. 1972. Alternatives to Drugs: A New Approach to Drug Education. *Journal of Drug Education* 2: 5–22.

Dohrenwend, B., Dohrenwend, B. S., Gould, M. S., Link, B., Neugebauer, R., and Wunsik-Hitzig, R. 1974. *Mental Illness in the United States*. New York: Praeger.

Edwards, L. E., Steinman, M. E., Arnold, K. A., Hakanson, E. Y. 1980. Adolescent Pregnancy Prevention Services in High School Clinics. *Family Planning Perspectives* 12: 6–14.

Everett, B. 1984. Adolescent Pregnancy. *Washington Report*, Society for Research in Child Development Newsletter. 1: 1–12.

Fairweather, G. W., and Tornatzky, L. 1976. *Experimental Methods for Social Policy Research*. New York: Pergamon.

Flay, B. R., and Sobel, J. L. 1983. The Role of Mass Media in Preventing Adolescent Substance Abuse. In *Preventing Adolescent Drug Abuse: Intervention Strategies*, eds. T. J. Glynn, C. G. Leukfeld, J. P. Ludford. National Institute on Drug Abuse, Research Monograph 47. DHHS Publication No. (ADM) 83–1280. Washington, D.C.: U.S. Government Printing Office.

Gilchrist, L. D., and Schinke, S. P. 1983. Counseling with Adolescents about Their Sexuality. In *Adolescent Sexuality in a Changing American Society*, ed. C. S. Chilman. New York: John Wiley.

Gordon, R. S. 1983. An Operational Classification of Disease Prevention. *Public Health Reports* 98: 107–109.

Gormally, J. 1982. Evaluation of Assertiveness: Effects of Gender, Rater Involvement, and Level of Assertiveness. *Behavior Therapy* 13: 219–225.

Greenberg, J. A., and Pollack, B. 1981. Motivating Students Not To Smoke. *Journal of Drug Education* 11: 341–359.

Hobbs, N. 1975. *The Futures of Children*. San Francisco: Jossey-Bass.

Hollingshead, A. B., and Redlich, F. C. 1958. *Social Class and Mental Illness*. New York: John Wiley.

Hough, R. L. 1985. Psychiatric Epidemiology and Prevention: An Overview of the Possibilities. In *Psychiatric Epidemiology and Prevention*, eds. R. L. Hough, P. A. Gongla, V. B. Brown, and S. E. Goldston. Los Angeles: University of California, Neuropsychiatric Institute.

Johnson, D. L. 1988. The Houston Parent-Child Development Project. In *Fourteen Ounces of Prevention: A Casebook for Practitioners*, eds. R. N. Price, E. L. Cowen, R. P. Lorion, and J. Ramos-McKay. Washington, D.C.: American Psychological Association.

Johnson, K., and Rosenbaum, S. 1986. *Building Health Programs for Teenagers*. Unpublished manuscript, Children's Defense Fund.

Johnston, L. D., O'Malley, P. M., and Bachman, J. G. 1986. *National Trends in Drug Use and Related Factors among American High School Students and Young Adults, 1975–1986*. National Institute on Drug Abuse. DHHS Publication No. (ADM) 87–1535. Washington, D.C.: U.S. Government Printing Office.

Kelly, J. G. 1977. The Search for Ideas and Deeds That Work. In *Primary Prevention of Psychopathology, Vol. I: The Issues*, eds. G. W. Albee and J. M. Jaffe. Hanover, N.H.: University Press of New England.

Kelly, J. G., Snowden, L. R., and Munoz, R. F. 1977. Social and Community Interventions. *Annual Review of Psychology* 28: 323–361.

Kessler, M., and Albee, G. W. 1975. Primary Prevention. *Annual Review of Psychology* 26: 557–591.

Kim, S. 1981. An Evaluation of the Impact of an Ombudsman Primary Prevention Program on Student Drug Abuse. *Journal of Drug Education* 11: 27–36.

Klein, D. C., and Goldston, S. 1977. *Primary Prevention: An Idea Whose Time Has Come*. Washington, D.C.: U.S. Government Printing Office.

Kohlberg, L., La Crosse, J., and Ricks, D. 1972. The Predictability of Adult Mental Health from Childhood Behavior. In *Manual of Child Psychopathology*, ed. B. B. Wolmen. New York: McGraw-Hill.

Koss, M. P., and Butcher, J. N. 1986. Research on Brief Psychotherapy. In *Handbook of Psychotherapy and Behavior Change*, eds. S. L. Garfield and A. E. Bergin. New York: John Wiley.

Lamb, H. R., and Zusman, J. 1979. Primary Prevention in Perspective. *American Journal of Psychiatry* 136: 12–17.

Lorion, R. P. 1978. Research on Psychopathology and Behavior Change with the Disadvantaged: Past, Present and Future Directions. In *Preventive Psychology: Theory, Research and Practice*, eds. R. D. Felner, L. A. Jason, J. N. Moritsugu, and S. S. Farber. New York: Pergamon Press.

Lorion, R. P. 1983. Evaluating Preventive Interventions: Guidelines for the Serious Social Change Agent. In *Preventive Psychology: Theory, Research and Practice*, eds. R. D. Felner, L. A. Jason, J. N. Moritsugu, and S. S. Farber. New York: Pergamon Press.

Lorion, R. P. 1985. Environmental Approaches and Prevention: The Dangers of Imprecision. In *Beyond the Individual: Environmental Approaches and Prevention*, eds. A. Wandersman and R. Hess. New York: Haworth.

Lorion, R. P. 1987a. Methodological Challenges in Prevention Research. In *Preventing Mental Disorders: A Research Perspective*, eds. J. A. Steinberg and M. M. Silverman. National Institute of Mental Health. DHHS Publication No. (ADM) 87–1492. Washington, D.C.: U.S. Government Printing Office.

Lorion, R. P. 1987b. The Other Side of the Coin: The Potential for Negative Consequences of Preventive Interventions. In *Preventing Mental Disorders: A Research Perspective*, eds. J. A. Steinberg and M. M. Silverman. National Institute of Mental Health: DHHS Publication No. (ADM) 87–1492. Washington, D.C.: U.S. Government Printing Office.

Lorion, R. P. 1989. *Protecting the Children: Strategies for Optimizing Emotional and Behavioral Development*. New York: Haworth Press.

Lorion, R. P., Cowen, E. L., and Caldwell, R. A. 1974. Problem Types of Children Referred to a School-Based Mental Health Program: Identification and Outcome. *Journal of Consulting and Clinical Psychology* 42: 491–496.

Lorion, R. P., and Felner, R. E. 1986. Research on Mental Health Interventions with the Disadvantaged. In *Handbook of Psychotherapy and Behavior Change*, eds. S. L. Garfield and A. E. Bergin. 3rd ed. New York: John Wiley.

Lorion, R. P., and Lounsbury, J. W. 1981. Conceptual and Methodological Considerations in Evaluating Preventive Interventions. In *Innovative Approaches to Mental Health Evaluation*, eds. W. R. Tash and G. Stahler. New York: Academic Press.

Lorion, R. P., Price, R. H., and Eaton, W. W. 1987. The Prevention of Child and Adolescent Disorders: From Theory to Research. In *Project Prevention*, ed. American Academy of Child and Adolescent Psychiatry. Washington, D.C.

Moore, K., and Burt, M. 1982. *Private Crisis, Public Costs: Policy Perspectives on Teenage Childbearing*. Washington, D.C.: Urban Institute.

Moynihan, D. 1985. *Family and Nation*. New York: Harcourt Brace Jovanovich.

Murray, M. M., Johnson, C. A., Luepker, R. V., and Mittalmark, M. B. 1984. The Prevention of Cigarette Smoking in Children: A Comparison of Four Strategies. *Journal of Applied Social Psychology* 14: 274–288.

Myers, J. K., and Bean, L. L. 1968. *A Decade Later: A Follow-Up of Social Class and Mental Illness*. New York: John Wiley.

Olds, D. 1988. The Prenatal/Early Infancy Project. In *Fourteen Ounces of Prevention: A Casebook for Practitioners*, eds. R. H. Price, E. L. Cowen, R. P. Lorion, and J. Ramos-McKay. Washington, D.C.: American Psychological Association.

Pierson, D. E. 1988. The Brookline Early Education Project. In *Fourteen Ounces of Prevention: A Casebook for Practitioners*, eds R. H. Price, E. L. Cowen, R. P. Lorion, and J. Ramos-McKay. Washington, D.C.: American Psychological Association.

Polit, D. F., and Kahn, J. R. 1985. Project Redirection: Evaluation of a Comprehensive Program for Disadvantaged Teenage Mothers. *Family Planning Perspectives* 17: 150–155.

President's Commission on Mental Health. 1978. *Report to the President*, Vol. II. Washington, D.C.: U.S. Government Printing Office.

Price, R., and Smith, S. S. 1985. *A Guide to Evaluating Prevention Programs in Mental Health*. Washington, D.C.: U.S. Government Printing Office.

Ramey, C. 1988. The Caroline Early Intervention Program. In *Fourteen Ounces of Prevention: A Casebook for Practitioners*, eds. R. H. Price, E. L. Cowen, R. P. Lorion, and J. Ramos-McKay. Washington, D.C.: American Psychological Association.

Rhodes, J. E., and Jason, L. A. 1987. *Preventing Substance Abuse among Children and Adolescents*. New York: Pergamon Press.

Rickel, A. U., and Allen, L. 1988. *Preventing Maladjustment from Infancy through Adolescence*. Newbury Park, Calif.: Sage.

Sameroff, A. J., and Chandler, M. J. 1975. Reproductive Risk and the Continuum of Caretaking Casualty. In *Review of Child Development Research*, Vol. 4, eds. F. D. Horowitz, M. Hetherington, S. Scarr-Salapatek, and G. Siegel. Chicago: University of Chicago Press.

Sameroff, A. J., and Fiese, B. 1988. Conceptual Issues in Prevention. In *Project Prevention*, eds. D. Shaffer and I. Phillips. Washington, D.C.: American Academy of Child and Adolescent Psychiatry.

Sanford, N. 1972. Is the Concept of Prevention Necessary or Useful? In *Handbook of Community Mental Health*, eds. S. E. Golann and C. E. Eisdorfer. New York: Appleton-Century-Crofts.

Sarason, S. 1983. Psychology and Public Policy: Missed Opportunity. In *Preventive Psychology*, eds. R. D. Felner, L. A. Jason, J. N. Moritsugu, and S. S. Farber. New York: Pergamon.

Sarason, S., and Doris, J. 1979. *Educational Handicap, Public Policy and Social History*. New York: Free Press.

Scales, P. 1981. Sex Education and the Prevention of Teenage Pregnancy: An Overview of Policies and Programs in the United States. In *Teenage Pregnancy in a Family Context: Implications for Policy*, ed. T. Ooms. Philadelphia: Temple University Press.

Schinke, S. P. 1984. Preventing Teenage Pregnancy. In *Progress in Behavior Modification*, Vol. 14, eds. M. Herson, R. M. Eisler, and P. M. Miller. New York: Academic Press.

Schinke, S. P., and Gilchrist, L. D. 1985. Preventing Substance Abuse with Children and Adolescents. *Journal of Consulting and Clinical Psychology* 53: 596–602.

Schweinhart, L. J., and Weikart, D. P. 1988. The High/Scope Perry Preschool Program. In *Fourteen Ounces of Prevention: A Casebook for Practitioners*, eds. R. H. Price, E. L. Cowen, R. P. Lorion, and J. Ramos-McKay. Washington, D.C.: American Psychological Association.

Silver, A. A., Hagin, R. A., and Karlen, A. L. 1988. Prevention of Learning Disorders. In *Project Prevention*, eds. D. Shaffer and I. Phillips. Washington, D.C.: American Academy of Child and Adolescent Psychiatry.

Slaikeu, K. A. 1984. *Crisis Intervention: A Handbook for Practice and Research*. Boston, Mass.: Allyn and Bacon.

Srole, L., Langer, T. S., Michael, S. T., Opler, M. K., and Rennie, T.A.C. 1962. *Mental Health in the Metropolis: The Midtown Manhattan Study*. New York: McGraw-Hill.

U.S. Department of Health and Human Services. 1984. *Prevention Activities of the Alcohol, Drug Abuse, and Mental Health Administration: Fiscal Year 1983 Report to Congress*. Rockville, Md.: Alcohol, Drug Abuse, and Mental Health Administration.

U.S. Department of Health and Human Services. 1985. *Prevention Activities of the Alcohol, Drug Abuse, and Mental Health Administration: Fiscal Year 1984 Report to Congress*. Rockville, Md.: Alcohol, Drug Abuse, and Mental Health Administration.

U.S. Department of Health and Human Services. 1986. *Prevention Activities of the Alcohol, Drug Abuse, and Mental Health Administration: Fiscal Year 1985 Report to Congress*. Rockville, Md.: Alcohol, Drug Abuse, and Mental Health Administration.

Vinovskis, M. A. 1981. An Epidemic of Adolescent Pregnancy? Some Historical Considerations. *Journal of Family History* 6: 205–230.

Westman, J. C. 1979. *Child Advocacy*. New York: Free Press.

Zelnik, M., and Kantner, J. F. 1978. Sexual Activity, Contraceptive Use and Pregnancy among Metropolitan-Area Teenagers, 1971–1979. *Family Planning Perspectives* 12: 230–237.

Zelnik, M., Kantner, J. F., and Ford, K. 1981. *Sex and Pregnancy in Adolescence*. Newbury Park, Calif.: Sage.

Part 6

Planning for Mental Health Services

18

Needs Assessment Techniques

PHILLIP M. MASSAD
and BARRIE E. BLUNT

Perhaps one of the most difficult jobs facing mental health professionals in the United States today is the planning of mental health service delivery. At least three simultaneous trends have contributed to the increasing complexity and importance of this task. First, as pointed out in earlier chapters on block grants and contemporary issues in mental health administration, the onus of service planning has been shifting from the national government to state and local governments. Second, and related to this development, there have been reductions in federal resources with which to maintain existing services (Massad, Sales, and Sabatier, 1983). And third, numerous state and local governments have found it necessary to curtail a variety of services, not only because of reductions in federal resources, but also because of indigenous fluctuations in their own revenues and expenditures (Bahl, 1982).

One of the combined effects of these trends is a growing interest in needs assessment techniques. Indeed, the delivery of services must now, more than ever before, be targeted to specifically identified individuals and groups having documented need (Blunt, 1986). Budgetary hearings at the executive and legislative levels commonly require the presentation of empirical data as a basis for deciding how to allocate funds, and consequently, agency personnel must respond with systematic procedures for the determination of mental health needs.

The purpose of this chapter is to familiarize the reader with needs assessment techniques used by mental health professionals in responding to this evolving situation. The emphasis is not on providing a how-to guide but rather a review of key issues surrounding the selection and application of different methods. In this process we will first introduce the concept of mental health need and then consider alternative strategies used to determine such needs, particularly at the community level. We then focus on two needs assessment techniques that, owing to aspects of the present budgetary and public policy environment, have received substantial attention in the recent literature. We close by considering directions for future work in mental health needs assessment and the planning of services.

MENTAL HEALTH NEED AND TECHNIQUES FOR ITS ASSESSMENT

"Need" and "assessment" are difficult concepts to define. According to Kahn (1969: 63), need includes a "view of what an individual or group requires in order to play a role, meet a commitment, [or] participate adequately in a social process." In mental health planning, a condition of true need, however defined, is generally considered as a perceived requirement for the receipt of services.

The assessment of mental health need, then, involves the determination of who meets the requirements for services. As Stewart (1979) suggests, there is a range of techniques that might be used to identify these prerequisite conditions. Such procedures may vary in providing different information about needs and, thus, can be used either in combination with each other to form a comprehensive assessment, or by themselves to assess particular aspects of a given situation.

Starling (1979) suggests that needs assessment take place at the beginning of the planning process. He outlines a model in which the identification of needs is followed by policy formulation, then policy adoption, program operations, and finally, evaluation. This model is similar to others in that it defines need (or problem) identification as fundamentally important to the development of sound policy (note also Jones, 1977).

A detailed conceptualization of mental health "needs," and the corresponding techniques for assessing such needs, has been outlined by Bradshaw (1977). Bradshaw suggests four types of need: (1) normative need, being that which an expert defines; (2) felt need, consisting of input from an actual population; (3) expressed need, or the actual use of services; and (4) comparative need, determined by examining personal attributes associated with mental illness and then locating those characteristics in the population. Correspondingly, there are a number of techniques used to assess these types of mental health needs. Five of the most commonly used approaches are the key informant, community forum, community survey, rates-under-treatment, and social indicator approaches.

The key informant approach relies on the views of experts in the community (e.g., clergymen, public health nurses, mental health service providers, etc.) as an indication of normative need and the services that should be developed to meet this need (Warheit, Bell, and Schwab, 1977). One advantage of this approach is that any decision outcomes are based on the views of those individuals who would "know best" what service needs exist and how they might be met. As Cagle (1984) has suggested, however, the success of this approach depends on the ability of the policymaker to meld a variety of viewpoints into a coherent package and, further, on the ability of the informants to go beyond the normal or traditional ways of conceptualizing need and service delivery.

The community forum approach measures felt need by encouraging community residents to participate in public meetings where they can voice their views concerning desired services (Warheit, Bell, and Schwab, 1977). This approach is appealing because it helps the planner identify issues and concerns unique to the community within which services are being considered. Additionally, citizen involvement in the planning process may help to insure effective implementation. This procedure has the same problem associated with the key informant approach; that is, success is contingent upon the above noted abilities of the policymaker to achieve a meaningful synthesis of opinions expressed and informants to step beyond normal ways of conceptualizing need and service delivery. Also, there is the concern that a given forum may not constitute a representative group of citizens.

The community survey approach indexes both felt and comparative need by canvassing individuals to determine their attitudes toward services, their demographic characteristics, and their own mental health status (Goldstein, Zautra, and Goodhart, 1982; Murrell, Brockway, and Schulte, 1982). Unlike other methods, the survey technique seeks to establish contact with a representative segment of the citizenry and then to gear service planning to the identified preferences and requirements. As with the foregoing approaches, the survey technique has the disadvantage of possible sampling biases and the subjectivity of assimilating such information into a plan of action. Additionally, a special concern here is the quality of the survey instrument and the inherent difficulty of developing valid and reliable measures of mental illness and health, a subject discussed in chapter 3 on psychiatric epidemiology.

The rates-under-treatment approach employs the number of individuals already seeking treatment (i.e., utilization rates) in an attempt to discern expressed need (Hagedorn, 1977; Zautra and Simons, 1978). This procedure also has a number of advantages and disadvantages which we will discuss shortly.

The social indicator approach to needs assessment is based on the notion that certain sociodemographic variables are highly correlated with need for mental health services (Hagedorn, 1977). This approach measures comparative need by attempting to provide an estimate of the number and location of individuals in the service area fitting a recognized demographic profile associated with a need for mental health services. The strengths and limitations of this approach will also be discussed at length later in this chapter.

Of the five techniques outlined above, the latter two, the rates-under-treatment and the social indicator approaches, have received growing attention in the literature. Both approaches may be attractive to planners due to their apparent objectivity and amenability to quantification. Furthermore, relative to the other approaches which each require the collection of original data, rates-under-treatment and social indicators are more cost-effective in that they involve the secondary analysis of existing data. Since researchers often couple both techniques in examining mental health needs (e.g., Beshai, 1984; Ford and Schmittdiel, 1983; Goldstein, Zautra, and Goodhart, 1982), we will discuss issues relevant to the two approaches as used separately and in combination with each other. We believe that both rates-under-treatment and social indicators are techniques worthy of serious consideration by the mental health planner, but they are not without their own drawbacks, of which potential users should have a solid understanding.

NEEDS ASSESSMENT THROUGH SECONDARY DATA ANALYSIS

Rates-Under-Treatment: Strengths and Limitations

As used to estimate mental health needs and plan for services, the rates-under-treatment approach has received a variety of criticisms. It has been asserted that current utilization of services does not adequately identify unmet needs in that there may be many individuals who need treatment but do not choose to obtain services (Goldstein, Zautra, and Goodhart, 1982; Royse and Drude, 1982; Stewart, 1979). Also, utilization rates may underestimate service needs by not identifying special populations which need and desire services but for whom services are unavailable (Hagedorn, 1977). Furthermore, the rates-under-treatment approach does not typically account for needs being met by multiple service providers because it relies primarily on utilization data from a specific community mental health center and thus may exclude private practitioners or other local providers (e.g., juvenile services, church-sponsored groups, etc.). This clearly has the potential of misleading the researcher who is trying to define overall need for services in a specified community. Finally, some commentators have asserted that use of services may have less to do with true needs than with clients' perception of needs, or consumer demand (Murrell, Brockway, and Schulte, 1982).

In addition to the foregoing conceptual issues, a number of procedural problems have surfaced in empirical research on the rates-under-treatment approach. For example, the definition of utilization has varied from one study to the next. Different researchers have defined it as: (1) unduplicated patient contacts, (2) total number of patient contacts, and (3) the availability of psychiatric beds across time periods ranging from one week to three years. Clearly, further research is needed to examine how such different definitions affect the prediction of service use.

Another problem is the diverse units of analysis used in previous studies. In this regard, census tracts, counties, and catchment areas have all been examined. Accordingly, it is conceivable that conclusions from studies using either counties or catchment areas may differ from those relying on census tracts in relating indicators to use because of greater sample heterogeneity in geographically larger units of analysis.

Despite the above-mentioned difficulties with the rates-under-treatment approach, there are several reasons to argue for further application and refinement of this technique as a means for determining expressed need. First, utilization rates have been and will continue to be a major source of information for allocating resources and planning for mental health services. Indeed, given recent budgetary constraints and corresponding reductions in the development of new services, the importance of existing utilization in the planning process has increased. Put quite simply, in a time of cutbacks, policymakers often base funding decisions on present-use patterns (Blunt, 1983). Furthermore, and also as a result of resource limitations, mental health planners may be less likely or less able to conduct other, more complicated forms of needs assessments than would be the case when financial resources are more plentiful.

Second, legislative decision makers are responsive to straightforward estimates of need such as utilization projections (Massad, Sales, and Sabatier, 1983). Although other types of assessments are necessary for a comprehensive needs estimate, projections of utilization data tend to be viewed seriously by legislative membership. Such estimations of service use provide information in developing budgets for services, examining the effects of previous and present policies on use, and in providing the most cost-effective type and amount of resources, both in personnel and capital projects (Moore et al., 1967).

Third, there is growing evidence that utilization rates are, in fact, closely related to the level of psychiatric impairment and distress, negative affect, and quality of community life as these qualities have been measured by alternative methodologies (Goldstein, Zautra, and Goodhart, 1982; Zautra and Simons, 1978). In addition, an association appears to exist between utilization and community members' opinions regarding their general level of health and depression (Warheit, Holzer, and Robbins, 1979). Hence, utilization may be indicative, at least at a minimum level, of several dimensions of need for services in a particular community.

Fourth, an examination of utilization rates alone can do much in helping specific treatment programs, training of personnel, and determining staffing patterns. For example, knowing the number of individuals with particular types of presenting problems (e.g., affective disorders, anxiety disorders, etc.) may suggest a need to provide staff with supplemental training programs to enhance their expertise accordingly. The same information may call for developing or expanding specific treatment regimes such as group activities or parental workshops.

An examination of utilization patterns across time and geography may also be valuable to the mental health planner and administrator in developing manpower strategies (note Hagedorn, 1977, and Yates, 1979, for a discussion of such strategies). For example, cyclical, but regular, demand for various problems may indicate that the mental health administrator should employ part-time staff during specific peak periods, rather than maintaining a fixed number of personnel at all times. In a like manner, the inspection of utilization patterns across different locations may suggest that certain numbers and types of personnel should be assigned differentially to urban, rural, central, satellite, or other type of site.

Social Indicators: Strengths and Limitations

Social indicators may be defined as "aggregate measures of community characteristics typically taken from official reports" (Goldstein, Zautra, and Goodhart, 1982: 275). The assumption underlying the use of such indicators in planning mental health services is that certain subpopulations characterized by specific attributes (e.g., low income, divorce, etc.) may be considered at high risk of experiencing mental health problems and in greater need of services relative to individuals not possessing these attributes (Dohrenwend and Dohrenwend, 1974; see also chapter 17 in this volume).

In estimating mental health service need, the use of social indicators has received increased attention across various disciplines over the last decade. There are several reasons for this development. First, epidemiologists have now compiled much research data in their examination of possible relationships between social indicators and mental disorders (e.g., Dohrenwend and Dohrenwend, 1974; Schwab, Warheit, and Fennel, 1975; Weissman and Klerman, 1978). Second, there has been considerable interest in the use of social indicators to identify individuals and groups needing services, and the types of services appropriate to a given community (e.g., Bachrach and Zautra, 1980; Ciarlo, 1980; Goldstein, Zautra, and Goodhart, 1982; Warheit, Bell, and Schwab, 1977). Third, professionals have expressed interest in using social indicators as a means of cost-effective planning in the delivery of mental health services (Greenspan and Sharfstein, 1981; Graves et al., 1985; Yates, 1979, 1980; Cagle, 1984).

Evidence of this heightened interest in understanding relationships between social indicators and mental disorders has been reflected in the Mental Health Demographic Profile System (MHDPS). This system, compiled by the National Institute of Mental Health (NIMH), describes a service area population through the use of selected demographics. Based on social indicators previously found to be associated with a need for mental health services, this system can be quite beneficial for the planner who faces the task of determining service need for a given area (Hagedorn, 1977; Rosen, 1977; Rosen et al., 1979).

The MHDPS was designed to facilitate community planning and incorporates numerous demographic items from the U.S. Census (Goldsmith et al., 1981). The items allow delineation of residential areas in which people have similar characteristics (e.g., life-style and social rank) and, thus, provide the researcher with an opportunity to make inferences regarding community needs. Life-style is measured using indices such as family status, and social rank uses indices such as economic status. In addition, the system includes indicators such as community stability and ethnicity.

Epidemiologists commonly use the MHDPS to assist practitioners in examining relationships between various indicators, on the one hand, and the incidence and prevalence of mental disorders across different geographic sectors (e.g., catchment area, census tract) on the other. Thus, by examining community demographics, epidemiologists can identify groups of people who are considered (epidemiologically) at high risk of needing mental health services. Consequently, programmatic decisions can be made with community needs more clearly in mind.

One problem associated with the social indicator approach is the source of information, most frequently, the census. Although these data are generally considered to be reliable, as is the case with all secondary sources, reliability is not assured (Royse and Drude, 1982). Another problem is that social indicator data are available most frequently at the census-tract level. This means that conclusions or inferences can only be drawn about geographic groupings and not about individuals. Finally, social indicators are not direct, but indirect, measures of need, a point which we will clarify later in the chapter.

A Combination of Approaches

Some commentators have considered the possibility of using the rates-under-treatment and social indicator approaches in concert with each other (e.g., Cagle, 1984; Goldstein, Zautra, and Goodhart, 1982; Hall, 1988; Hall and Royse, 1987; Zautra and Simons, 1978). The primary reason has been to identify the main users of services, as described by a cluster of social indicators (e.g., race, income, etc.), and then to discern relationships between community demographics and service use. In addition, this information can, of course, be used to create indices of expressed and comparative needs, as well as providing more comprehensive information to the mental health planner than might be the case when examining sets of data (e.g., utilization patterns and client-community demographics) in isolation. For example, in attempting to identify community needs, a combination of approaches allows the mental health planner to look for demographic patterns of service users, in comparison to community demographics, across variables such as diagnosis, duration of treatment, and outcome.

Data generated from this combination of approaches may also be helpful in addressing such issues as attrition, staffing patterns, and even the structuring of the therapeutic process itself. In regard to attrition, for example, if the incidence of dropouts were related to certain demographic characteristics, treatment regimes for certain demographic profiles and presenting problems might be structured in such a manner as to counteract any discernible underlying factors (e.g., attitudinal, motivational, etc.) that might be associated with such a trend.[1]

In regard to staffing patterns, an analysis of social indicators and previous utilization rates might assist the administrator in predicting future client demand according to type and severity of problems. For example, a composite analysis of social indicators and service rates across time may reveal that individuals possessing certain demographic attributes and/or presenting problems use services differentially. In fact, current research suggests an emerging profile of high users of services, at least in certain settings (i.e., high users of medical services are likely to be high users of psychiatric services) (Friedman and West, 1987).

As a further example, an analysis of such information might reveal that during the school year a clinic receives an abundance of referrals for children having an attentional deficit, most of whom come from lower socioeconomic families. Consequently, the clinic director may want to plan workshops focusing on suggestions for dealing with the particular type of disorder in conjunction with the demographic class in which it is represented. This and the foregoing examples are, of course, only illustrative and are intended to be suggestive of an array of possible uses of social indicator information in planning mental health services. As always, the warrant is for more data.

The treatment process also has the potential of being altered by identifying relationships between social indicators and utilization patterns. For example, some commentators have discussed specializing therapeutic techniques with lower-class, unsophisticated clients (e.g., Heitler, 1976). Ultimately, the use of different preparatory remarks, type of interventions, and pacing of therapy, among other aspects, across client subgroups may be prescribed as a function of the potential interactions between social indicators and service use.

In addition, the analysis of relationships between indicators and utilization could help to determine if services are actually reaching individuals targeted as being at high risk for mental illness. This is known as examining the "geographic and demographic accountability" of a service area (Bachrach and Zautra, 1980). Indeed, because most mental health programs are mandated to serve poorer community areas (geographic accountability), as well as clients characterized by certain demographics (demographic accountability), analyses examining the type and location of clients can address concerns about accountability of either type (Brown, 1976; Dohrenwend and Dohrenwend, 1974).

Finally, and in relation to planning services, it seems clear that the identification of indicators that are associated with both mental illnesses and the use of services may help in estimating various aspects of unmet need. Specifically, such information might be used to identify persons in the community who are not receiving services but are in some specified way similar to current clients, and outreach programs might thus be appropriately targeted. It should be noted, of course, that individuals in the community who resemble clients demographically do not necessarily require treatment.[2]

To date, empirical results examining relationships between indicators and utilization have been inconsistent. There are at least four reasons for this inconsistency. First, studies have found different social indicators to be related to service utilization. In other words, the set of indicators selected for correlation with service utilization has varied. This concern is not inherently problematic to the rates-under-treatment method, but it is an important practical issue for the researcher who is trying to determine which social indicators to use in actually planning for mental health services. Furthermore, even when indicators are constant from one study to the next, their operational definitions may differ. For example, poverty level may be defined in a variety of ways, each of which might affect the outcome of analysis. Hence, it is difficult to make definitive conclusions across studies.

Second, the extent to which indicators actually correlate with utilization varies. Statistically significant relationships have been found in some studies but not in others (Bachrach and Zautra, 1980; Banziger, Smith, and Foos, 1982; Cagle, 1984; Goldstein, Zautra, and Goodhart, 1982; Zautra and Simons, 1978; Bloom, 1968; Faris and Dunham, 1960; Klee et al., 1967; Koran and Meinhardt, undated; Rowitz and Levy, 1968; Slem, 1975).

Third, the interaction between demographic and nondemographic factors has been overlooked by previous researchers in their efforts to isolate relationships between indicators and utilization. Type of diagnosis, for example, may interact with social indicators in a way that reduces the correlation between demographic variables and utilization (Bloom, 1968; Rowitz and Levy, 1968; Slem, 1975). Indeed, the use of social indicators to predict rates-under-treatment in the previously cited studies accounted for only about half of the total variance in the dependent variable. Thus, there may be nondemographic variables that mediate the relationship between indicators and utilization rates which, if isolated, could enhance the predictive equation between these data. (Trainor, Boydell, and Tibshirani, 1986).

Finally, an underlying assumption in most of the research in this area is that fluctuations in the demographic profile of a service area across years will not significantly affect correlations with utilization patterns. Empirical analyses have relied predominantly on the U.S. Census, which is collected in ten-year intervals, even though service-use data may have been gathered several years prior to, or after, the census. It is quite possible that indicators related to service use at one time do not maintain the same relationship at another time. For example, as occupational pressures on women have increased in recent decades, the relationship between sex and occupation, on the one hand, and utilization, on the other, may have changed in a relatively short period of time. Thus, although these variables may remain integral components of a comprehensive needs equation, their proportional contribution to the assessment of need could change within very few years. It is reasonable to assume that the change in relationship between demographic variables and use of services over time is incremental and, thus, virtually inconsequential from one year to the next; however, as indicated above, the social indicator data commonly used are not collected on a yearly basis, but rather are provided by the census encompassing a ten-year unit of time. Accordingly, if the social indicator approach is to be utilized as a basis for actual prediction of, and correlated with, service use in the making of relevant policy decisions, it is essential that this assumption be tested.

FUTURE DIRECTIONS

In this chapter we have attempted to provide a brief overview of needs assessment techniques with particular emphasis on the rates-under-treatment and social indicator approaches. In addition, we have summarized the strengths and limitations of these approaches and tried to point out areas of potential research as indicated by gaps in the literature. It may be beneficial to elaborate briefly on these latter points.

The various methodological issues already noted could be addressed in one comprehensive study. Service utilization by type of service (e.g., mental health, alcohol, and drug) and diagnosis (e.g., affective disorder, substance abuse, etc.) could be incorporated in an analysis with both client and community demographics to discern the interaction between indicators and use. Simultaneously, utilization could be operationalized in a number of different ways (e.g., total cases, new cases, hours of utilization, etc.) to examine how such definitions may affect the predictive efficacy of a regression equation. Likewise, the unit of analysis could be varied (e.g., individual, census tract, and catchment area) to explore any predictive consequences.

The assumption that the demographic profile of a service area remains relatively static across years and the feasibility of developing a time-based model employing demographics to project future use rates could also be examined in a single study. Although census data do not permit such an analysis, annually collected consumer data (available through market research firms) afford a unique opportunity to examine how relationships between demographics and service use might change on an annual basis. If consistent and statistically significant relationships were established across time, a model could be generated to predict future use rates based on trends in community demographics.

Despite the advantages of using needs assessment data in the planning of services and the potential rewards of future studies, some researchers have questioned whether decision makers actually employ this information in planning for services (Richman, Boutilier, and Harris, 1984; Wutchiett et al., 1984). Indeed, the role of social science information in the policy process in general has been a subject of long standing controversy (see Massad, Sales, and Acosta, 1983). This is an important question that goes far beyond the scope of this chapter. Clearly, however, the use of needs assessment information in general, and social indicator and utilization approaches in particular, cannot be presumed, even in light of what seems to be a renewed interest in such technologies within state mental health policy. Hence, the efficacy of meeting mental health service needs becomes dependent on the extent to which policymakers are willing to base decisions on needs assessment information and on the ability of mental health practitioners to carry out identified system changes. In this chapter we have sought to show that attempts to determine mental health service needs in a community are a start, if only a start, in the direction of more sophisticated policy planning.

NOTES

1. Identifying the possible mediating variables is, of course, an empirical venture. Nevertheless, there are enough data in the psychological literature concerning certain demographic groups and special treatment needs that could generate training programs for staff members in how to address attrition if related to certain demographic attributes and presenting problems (e.g., Bonner and Everett, 1986).

2. Service utilization rates can be considered an expression of need within the context of the *existing* service delivery system (Goldstein, Zautra, and Goodhart, 1982). Utilization rates provide information for only the number of individuals actually receiving treatment at specific times. Consequently, utilization rates do not reflect a need for potential, nonexistent services, or the demand for services which may be currently unmet.

REFERENCES

Bachrach, K. M., and Zautra, A. 1980. Some Uses of Client and Census Records in Community Mental Health Planning. *American Journal of Community Psychology* 8: 365–378.

Bahl, R. 1982. The Fiscal Health of State and Local Governments: 1982 and Beyond. *Public Budgeting and Finance* 2: 5–21.

Banziger, G., Smith, R. K., and Foos, D. 1982. Economic Indicators of Mental Health Service Utilization in Rural Appalachia. *American Journal of Community Psychology* 10: 669–686.

Beshai, N. 1984. Assessing Needs of Alcohol-Related Services: A Social Indicators Approach. *American Journal of Drug and Alcohol Abuse* 10: 417–427.

Bloom, B. L., 1968. An Ecological Analysis of Psychiatric Hospitalizations. *Multivariate Behavioral Research* 3: 423–463.

Blunt, B. E. 1983. *The Oklahoma Department of Mental Health: A Case Analysis of Community Service Delivery and Funding in the Oklahoma City Mental Health Catchment Areas*, Oklahoma House of Representatives.

Blunt, B. E. 1986. The Determination of Service Gaps in a Community Mental Health System. *Administration in Mental Health* 13: 285–286.

Bonner, B. L., and Everett, F. L. 1986. Influence of Client Preparation and Problem Severity on Attitudes and Expectations in Child Psychotherapy. *Professional Psychology: Research and Practice* 17: 223–229.

Bradshaw, J. 1977. The Concept of Social Need. In *Planning for Social Welfare: Issues, Models and Tasks*, eds. N. Gilbert and H. Specht. Englewood Cliffs, N.J.: Prentice-Hall.

Brown, B. S. 1976. Critical Issues for Community Mental Health. *Journal of Social Welfare* 3: 7–21.

Cagle, L. T. 1984. Using Social Indicators to Assess Mental Health Needs: Lessons from a Statewide Study. *Evaluation Review* 25: 417–452.

Ciarlo, J. A. 1980. *Statistical Needs Assessment Models for Colorado: A Working Paper*. Technical Report, Mental Health Systems Evaluation Project, University of Denver, Colorado.

Dohrenwend, B. P., and Dohrenwend, B. S. 1974. Social and Cultural Influences on Psychopathology. *Annual Review of Psychology* 5: 417–452.

Faris, R.E.L., and Dunham, H. W. 1960. *Mental Disorders in Urban Areas: An Ecological Study of Schizophrenia and Other Psychoses*. New York: Hafner.

Ford, W. E., and Schmittdiel, C. J. 1983. Predicting Alcoholism Service Needs from a National Treatment Utilization Survey. *International Journal of the Addictions* 18: 1073–1084.

Friedman, M. J., and West, A. N 1987. Current Need Versus Treatment History as Predictors of Use of Outpatient Psychiatric Care. *American Journal of Psychiatry* 144: 355–357.

Goldsmith, H., Unger, E., Windle, C., Shambaugh, J., Rosen, B. 1981. *A Typological Approach to Doing Social Area Analysis*. DHEW Publication (ADM) 81–262. Washington, D.C.: National Institute of Mental Health.

Goldstein, J., Zautra, A., and Goodhart, D. 1982. A Test of the Utility of Social Indicators for Behavioral Health Service Planning. *Social Indicators Research* 10: 273–295.

Graves, S. C., Leff, H. S., Natkins, J., and Bryan, J. 1985. A System for Allocating Mental Health Resources. *Administration in Mental Health* 13: 43–68.

Greenspan, S. I., and Sharfstein, S. S. 1981. Efficacy of Psychotherapy—Asking the Right Questions. *Archives of General Psychiatry* 38: 1213–1219.

Hagedorn, H. 1977. *A Manual on State Mental Health Planning*. DHEW Publication No. (ADM) 77–473. Washington, D.C.: National Institute of Mental Health.

Hall, G. B. 1988. Monitoring and Predicting Community Mental Health Centre Utilization in Auckland, New Zealand. *Social Science and Medicine* 26: 55–70.

Hall, O., and Royse, D. 1987. Mental Health Needs Assessment with Social Indicators: An Empirical Case Study. *Administration in Mental Health* 15: 36–46.

Heitler, J. B. 1976. Preparatory Techniques in Initiating Expressive Psychotherapy with Lower-Class, Unsophisticated Patients. *Psychological Bulletin* 83: 339–352.

Jones, C. O. 1977. *An Introduction to the Study of Public Policy*, 2nd. ed. North Scituate: Duxbury Press.

Kahn, A. J. 1969. *Theory and Practice of Social Planning*. New York: Russell Sage Foundation.

Klee, G. D., Spiro, E., Bahn, A. K., and Gorwitz, K. 1967. An Ecological Analysis of Diagnosed Mental Illness in Baltimore. In *Psychiatric Epidemiology and Mental Health Planning*, eds. R. R. Monroe, G. D. Klee, and E. B. Brody. Psychiatric Research Report No. 22. Washington, D.C.: American Psychiatric Association.

Koran, L. M., and Meinhardt, K. Undated. Social Indicators in Statewide Mental Health Planning. Unpublished manuscript.

Massad, P. M., Sales, B. D., and Acosta, E. 1983. Utilization of Social Science Information in the Policy Process: Can Psychologists Help? In *Advances in Applied Social Psychology*, eds. R. F. Kidd and M. J. Saks. Hillsdale, N.J.: Lawrence Erlbaum.

Massad, P. M., Sales, B. D., and Sabatier, P. 1983. Influencing State Legislative Decisions. In *Annual Review of Applied Social Psychology*, Vol. 4, ed. L. Bickman. Beverly Hills, Calif.: Sage.

Moore, D. N., Bloom, B. L., Gaylin, S., Pepper, M., Pettus, C., Willis, E. M., and

Bahn, A. K. 1967. Data Utilization for Local Community Mental Health Program Development. *Community Mental Health Journal* 3: 30–32.

Murrell, S. A., Brockway, J. M., and Schulte, P. 1982. The Kentucky Elderly Need Assessment: Concurrent Validity of Different Measures of Unmet Need. *American Journal of Community Psychology* 10: 117–132.

Richman, A., Boutilier, C., and Harris, P. 1984. The Relevance of Socio-Demographic and Resource Factors in the Use of Acute Psychiatric-In-Patient Care in the Atlantic Provinces of Canada. *Psychological Medicine* 14: 175–182.

Rosen, B. M. 1977. *A Model for Estimating Mental Health Needs Using 1970 Census Socioeconomic Data.* DHEW Publication (ADM) 77–63. Washington, D.C.: National Institute of Mental Health.

Rosen, B. M., Lawrence, L., Goldsmith, H. F., Shambaugh, J. P., and Windle, C. D. 1979. *Mental Health Demographic Profile System Description: Purpose, Contents, and Sampler of Uses.* DHEW Publication (ADM) 79–263. Washington, D.C.: National Institute of Mental Health.

Royse, D., and Drude, K. 1982. Mental Health Needs Assessments: Beware of False Promises. *Community Mental Health Journal* 18: 97–106.

Rowitz, L., and Levy, L. 1968. Ecological Analysis of Treated Mental Disorders in Chicago. *Archives of General Psychiatry* 19: 571–579.

Schwab, J. J., Warheit, G. J., and Fennel, E. B. 1975. An Epidemiological Assessment of Needs and Utilization of Services. *Evaluation* 2: 65–67.

Slem, C. M. 1975. *Community Mental Health Need Assessment: The Prediction of Census Tract Utilization Patterns Using the Mental Health Demographic Profile.* Unpublished Ph.D. dissertation. Detroit: Wayne State University.

Starling, G. 1979. *The Politics and Economics of Public Policy.* Homewood, Ill.: Dorsey Press.

Stewart, R. 1979. The Nature of Needs Assessment in Community Mental Health. *Community Mental Health Journal* 15: 287–295.

Trainor, I., Boydell, K., and Tibshirani, R. 1986. Short-term Economic Change and Utilization of Mental Health Facilities in a Metropolitan Area. *Canadian Journal of Psychiatry* 32: 379–383.

Warheit, G. J., Bell, R. A., and Schwab, J. J. 1977. *Needs Assessment Approaches: Concepts and Methods.* DHEW Publication (ADM) 77–472. Washington, D.C.: National Institute of Mental Health.

Warheit, G. J., Holzer, C., and Robbins, L. 1979. Social Indicators and Mental Health Planning: An Empirical Case Study. *Community Mental Health Journal* 15: 94–103.

Weissman, M. M., and Klerman, G. L. 1978. Epidemiology of Mental Disorder: Emerging Trends in the United States. *Archives of General Psychiatry* 35: 705.

Wutchiett, R., Egan, D., Kohaut, S., Markman, H. J., and Pargament, K. I. 1984. Assessing the Need for Needs Assessments. *Journal of Community Psychiatry* 12: 53–60.

Yates, B. T. 1979. How to Improve, Rather Than Evaluate, Cost-Effectiveness. *Counseling Psychology* 8: 72–75.

Yates, B. T. 1980. *Improving Effectiveness and Reducing Costs in Mental Health.* Springfield, Ill.: C. C. Thomas.

Zautra, A., and Simons, L. S. 1978. An Assessment of a Community's Mental Health Needs. *American Journal of Community Psychology* 6: 351–362.

19

Mental Health System Strategic Planning

DAVID GOODRICK

Mental health systems presently confront a strategic imperative. At risk are the past decade's significant advances in cost-effective community-based treatment of serious mental disorders. With shrinking resources and expanding service demands, the infrastructures of many mental health systems are increasingly under stress. Mental health services today exist in an environment of interacting threats and opportunities: greater competition for scarce human service resources, expanding knowledge about psychosocial and biomedical treatment, increasing recognition of the consequences of runaway inpatient costs, and expanding information and skills to serve persons experiencing serious mental illness in their communities. Service systems also confront environmental turbulence as a result of increasing challenges and rates of change in reimbursement mechanisms, client populations, funding, legislative influence, and social expectations. These sources of intensifying complexity and uncertainty have several implications.

First, mental health service system stakeholders (consumers, family members, advocates, clinicians, professional associations, regulatory and funding agencies, private providers, unions, hospitals, clinics, governmental authorities, and third-party payers) are engaging in actions designed to affect the structure and functions of mental health systems. Understanding these actions is critical as mental health systems not only undertake new initiatives but also attempt to assure the maintenance of vital services. Second, in adapting to environmental pressures, proactive behavior is preferable to a reactive and defensive posture since the latter generally results in erosion of resources, prolonged struggles, and eventual disadvantage. Third, turbulence and change create opportunities for the achievement of service system goals. As mental health system managers, planners, and stakeholders grapple with these mounting challenges, increasingly they are recognizing the value of effective strategic planning and action. In fact, the need for strategic planning is greatest in a competitive and/or conflictual context where mental health systems are surrounded by powerful and change-resisting forces (Quinn, Mintzberg, and James, 1988).

Consequently, the practice of mental health system planning is evolving rapidly. In the 1980s, numerous state and county mental health authorities as well as Community Mental Health Centers (CMHCs) have developed a strategic orientation as they plan for, develop, and restructure mental health service systems. This emerging orientation has significantly affected the process and content of mental health planning in the United States.

The change in *process* is from a reliance on formal and analytic methods toward a more incremental, collaborative, situationally determined, and political approach. The purpose is to identify critical issues within and outside the mental health service system and then seek, create, and capitalize on opportunities that lead to the achievement of organizational and service system objectives. The *content* of mental health planning has also changed in the 1980s. Mental health authorities are expanding and improving community-based service systems and targeting at-risk and most-in-need populations. To summarize, these processes and content changes are influencing mental health planning along four dimensions.

1. Service system structure and operations. Contemporary plans, policies, and programs are expanding community-based services as the foundation of public mental health systems. Many state mental health authorities are actively promoting integrated, focused, and responsive community-based service systems through initiatives that seek to

- shift fiscal and work-force resources from inpatient to community services;
- shift from attempting to cure major mental disorders (given the state of our knowledge) to promoting rehabilitation and community integration;
- enhance clients' self-sufficiency, dignity, and participation in treatment planning;
- decentralize authority, responsibility, accountability, and delivery of services; and
- improve the quality and responsiveness of the service system continuum while emphasizing the least restrictive and most clinically appropriate interventions.

Consistent with these goals, Public Law 99–660 currently requires all states to develop and implement plans for improving and expanding comprehensive community-based mental health service systems that particularly target priority populations.

2. Priority populations. In light of policy values and resource constraints, service systems are now targeting people who are most in need and underserved or inappropriately served. County and state mental health authorities are increasingly placing the highest service priority on children with serious emotional disturbances and adults with serious and persistent mental disorders and are encouraging the active involvement of consumers and family members in service planning and delivery. The Child and Adolescent Service System Project (CASSP) and the Community Support Program (CSP) are National Institute of Mental Health (NIMH) initiatives that are leading these national efforts.

3. Funding. Mental health systems are shifting from single-source to multi-source funding and services. This move to broaden the resource base explicitly recognizes the diversity of clients' service needs as well as the importance of interagency cooperation, resource linkage, and shared responsibility in addressing mental health, residential, human service, health, and vocational needs. Public mental health systems in such states as Ohio, Colorado, and Rhode Island are leading the national effort in funding initiatives that increase interagency communication and cooperation, link with and leverage other service delivery systems, and recognize clients' multiple needs and service requirements as well as the benefits of multiple funding sources.

4. Values and vision. The values promoted in contemporary mental health planning include client empowerment, normalization, participatory decision making, community-based services, and least restrictiveness. Diffusion of these values requires the development of relations with consumers, family members, direct service staff, media, local governing bodies, legislators, and other stakeholders. Effective diffusion is being demonstrated by agency activities that broadcast exemplary programs, publicize clients' successes, conduct proactive and preemptive media and public education efforts, and address ambivalence and resistance to progressive service system vision, values, and policies.

Clearly, a strategic orientation is not only highly desirable but often essential for managers, providers, advocates, consumers, and other service system change agents. This chapter offers an integrative planning framework for strategic thinking, planning, and action in public mental health service systems. With some differences of emphasis, the framework and methods are equally applicable to actors and participants at national, state, and substate levels.

DEFINING AND DEMYTHOLOGIZING STRATEGY

According to Bertram Brown (1986), former director of NIMH, strategy results from two conditions: "You have a goal or goals you want to achieve in the foreseeable future for which you have limited resources, and you have to operate in a hostile or competitive environment. Strategic planning is how you harness your resources to reach your goal or goals." James (1984: 11) proposes that "strategy is a set of policies used for the conduct of conflict. . . . Simply defined, strategy is the organized deployment of resources to achieve specific objectives against competition from rival organizations.'' Quinn (1980: 7) asserts that strategies consist of goals, policies, and action sequences to achieve a vision: ''A well-formulated strategy helps to *marshal* and *allocate* an organization's resources into a *unique* and *viable posture* based on its relevant *internal competencies* and *shortcomings*, anticipated *changes in the environment*, and contingent moves by *intelligent opponents*.''

The following concepts build on these definitions. *Strategies* are ways and means to achieve desired ends in a challenging environment. *Strategic planning* is a process for individuals and/or organizations to first envision and then develop and engage in selected actions (i.e., ways and means) to achieve their goals. A *strategic plan* links the mission and vision of individuals and organizations with ways (e.g., programs, activities, maneuvers, initiatives) and means (e.g., policies, mechanisms, and financial, information, and human resources) to achieve goals. Effective strategies link strengths (i.e., organizational and system resources) with opportunities (i.e., cooperative relationships with, and resources in, the environment) to achieve desired aims.

In short, planning seeks to adapt the organization to a challenging environment. The environment may be challenging due to turbulence, ambiguity, opposition, or competition. *Turbulence* may reflect unpredictability, instability, and rapid change among external forces. *Ambiguity* may result from uncertainty, mixed messages, or confusion. *Opposition* may consist of resistance, entrenched power, or inertia. *Competition* may be for resources, attention, credibility, and sufficient priority for the organization's activity, and may occur in regard to populations, service components, the public and private sector, and geographic areas within a state. Competition may also exist between mental health and other disabilities, other health and human service systems, and other social problems. Finally, competition may exist between the value of mental health services and other social values, such as economic prosperity, military strength, and scientific and technological advancement.

In Defense of Strategic Planning

Some mental health providers, planners, and advocates express discomfort or are uneasy about a strategic orientation to mental health system planning. Their objections—to placing program development within a strategic context and to emphasizing competition and the pursuit of advantage—merit response. Strategic planning depends on innovative and empirically established program approaches, but recognizes barriers and resistance to change by forces within and outside mental health systems. Progressive programs are essential but not sufficient to assure optimal improvement and expansion of public mental health services; strategy augments and facilitates program development.

Strategic planning is explicitly concerned about competition even though its basic aim is cooperation and mutual benefit. The intent of strategic action is to achieve the maximum benefit and mutual advantage for all clients, family members, clinicians, and individuals and organizations involved, and its preference is to reframe win-lose dilemmas into win-win opportunities. Nevertheless, a strategic orientation recognizes that service system problems and environmental forces often adversely affect people experiencing mental illness and the services they require. Public mental health issues are frequently the target of strategic maneuvers by environmental actors. Consequently, the importance of a strategic orientation is based on three critical realities.

First, mental health service systems exist in an increasingly competitive environment. At the national level, mental health priorities are caught in a vise of escalating military expenditures and a burgeoning national debt and trade imbalance. Within states, proprietary hospital chains as well as health and human service systems affected by health care deregulation are aggressively competing for scarce mental health resources. Public mental health systems risk being placed at even greater disadvantage as some private sector organizations maneuver to serve less challenging clients and secure available financial resources while public systems are requested to offer what are often better and more economical services.

Second, over two-thirds of our nation's public mental health service resources remain devoted to inpatient treatment while more than 90 percent of persons experiencing serious mental illness live in the community. Research reviews, however, document that adequately funded and appropriately designed community alternatives are more effective as well as generally less expensive than hospitalization (Kiesler, 1982a, 1982b). As one family advocate expresses it, "We must identify and implement means to reduce inpatient funding to 20 to 30 percent of our mental health resources so that the remainder of mental health funds are devoted to mobile crisis teams, crisis homes, case management, and other community support services" (Schneier, 1986). Strategic planning is a systematic approach to address the complexity and controversy of shifting funds and staff from mental hospitals to comprehensive community-based service systems.

Third, and most important, people who experience mental illnesses are disfranchised and devalued in our society. A strategic orientation has been demonstrated to be highly useful in state and local efforts to reverse prejudice and discrimination, and to empower consumers and support their family members.

Debunking Planning Myths

More than merely forecasting desirable results, strategic planning asks such basic questions as "What is the purpose of our organization?" and "In light of our environment, what are our priority goals?" The wide gap between what is forecast and what agencies want to happen or are able to achieve through their operations and resources requires strategic planning (Steiner, 1979). Rather than a blueprint, however, strategic planning offers a compass to guide agencies around obstacles and beyond the horizon as they move toward their vision and the achievement of their mission (Hayes, 1985). Since the future is unknowable, effective planning must be flexible in taking advantage of emerging knowledge of the environment (Quinn, 1982; Steiner, 1979).

Strategic planning does not necessarily include preparation of "massive, detailed, and interrelated sets of plans" (Steiner, 1979: 16). Elaborate and voluminous plans tend to become rapidly obsolete or irrelevant, may protect the status quo, make unrealistic assumptions about the future and environment, and hamper flexible action. Traditional planning that focuses on formulating normative goals for the utilization and supply of services in an idealized context "often becomes bureaucratized, rigid and costly paper-shuffling exercises divorced from the actual decision process" (Quinn, 1980: ix).

Rather than attempt to displace managerial intuition and judgment, an effective planning process applies the creative, intuitive, and flexible thinking and action of successful managers or change agents throughout the organization (Steiner, 1979). In this context, centralization of planning responsibility (within or external to an agency) can hamper strategic action. Effective planning depends on the involvement of key management personnel throughout the organization, and must be integrated with resource deployment and program initiatives. Rather than a collection of functional work plans or an extrapolation of current budgets, effective strategic planning "is truly a systems approach to maneuvering an enterprise over time through the uncharted waters of its changing environment to achieve prescribed aims" (Steiner, 1979: 16).

Planning Cautions

Within this context of critical functions, several cautions should be understood:

1. Strategic planning does not assure organizational success. Even though research has demonstrated that agencies engaging in strategic planning are more likely to be effective, success is also influenced by accidents and errors, exceptionally adroit or inept implementation of initiatives, fortuitous events, and the application of overwhelming strength (Quinn, 1980).

2. Although strategic analysis and planning may be the basis for success, they are at the service of action: they are valuable to the degree they aid managers' efforts to adaptively guide organizations and effectively cope with environmental challenges.

3. A normative planning process (Parrish and Lieberman, 1987) may provide a useful method for facilitating system development or change. Indeed, both the normative and strategic planning processes share a common foundation in the assessment of population needs (see chapter 18 of this volume). The formality of the planning structure and process is what typically distinguishes normative and strategic planning activity. However, Quinn (1980) notes that effective managers often use only those aspects of formal planning that allow them to best pursue their objectives.

4. Planning must not be evaluated on the basis of effort, eloquence, or execution, but rather on effectiveness and efficiency. Analysis and planning are ways and means to achieve organizational and system goals, not ends in themselves.

AN INTEGRATIVE FRAMEWORK FOR STRATEGIC PLANNING

Effective strategic thinking and action may be usefully viewed as a four-phase sequence that is interdependent and iterative. Phase 1 is to *scan* the environment. Phase 2 is to *orient* individuals, the organization, and relevant stakeholders for analysis, planning, and action. Phase 3 is to *commit* individuals and the organization to action: choosing initiatives, integrating initiatives into one or a few coherent and flexible thrusts, galvanizing motivation, and mobilizing resources. Phase 4 is to *act*, first in a preemptive, cooperative, competitive, or indirect manner, and then to solidify gains and/or link back to earlier phases. The acronym for scan, orient, commit, and act is SOCA; the process may be referred to as a SOCA-cycle (see Figure 19–1).

Principles of effective planning and action emerge from research by Wrapp (1984) and Quinn (1982) on the behaviors of successful strategists. Wrapp (1984) has identified five critical skills that strategic managers exhibit. They:

1. Keep open many pipelines of information.
2. Spot opportunities and relationships in the stream of operating problems and decisions.
3. Give the organization a sense of direction with objectives that are open-ended.
4. Concentrate attention and resources on a limited number of significant issues.
5. Identify neutral zones (i.e., areas where competitors or stakeholders are relatively unconcerned about the organization's actions), and then move forward in them.

Skills 1 and 2 scan the organization and environment; skill 3 orients the organization; skill 4 marshals organizational commitment; and skill 5 is a key scanning-to-acting sequence.

Wrapp's findings are consistent with research identifying the styles of effective strategists (Quinn, 1982: 613). Arranged in the SOCA-cycle framework, these are as follows:

Scan: Analyze the external environment "to forecast the forces *most likely* to impinge on [the organization's] future and the probable nature and range of their potential impacts."

Orient: Construct a broad and flexible vision of success.

Commit: Attempt to "build a *resource base* and a *posture* that is so strong and flexible that the enterprise can survive and prosper toward its vision despite all but the most devastating events."

Act: Pursue one or a few initiatives that maximize achieving goals within resource constraints. Also, attempt to place some "side bets" to decrease catastrophic risk and to expand future options.

In analyzing successful change efforts, Quinn (1982: 613–614) discovered that strategists

Figure 19–1
Integrative Framework for Strategic Planning and Action

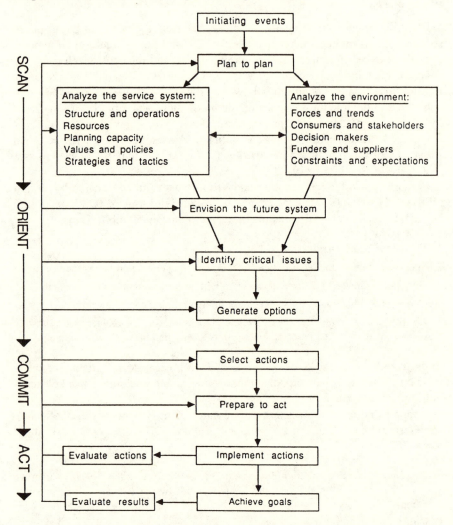

initially worked out in their own minds—and shared with selected colleagues—only a few integrating concepts, principles, or philosophies that would help rationalize and guide [the organization's] overall movements. They proceeded step by step from the early generalities toward later specifics, clarifying the strategy incrementally as events permitted or dictated. In early stages they consciously avoided over-precise statements which might impair the flexibility or imagination needed to exploit new information or opportunities. They constantly reassessed the future, found new congruencies as events unfurled, and blended the organization's skills and resources into new balances of concentration and risk dispersion as external forces and internal potentials intersected to suggest better, but never perfect, alignments. The process was dynamic with neither a real beginning or end.

Quinn's (1982: 618) research findings also counter the common perception ''that in large organizations one can realistically first formulate a detailed overall strategy, announce it, and then proceed to implement it. Much more subtle, interrelated, continuous evolutionary processes tend to dominate strategy development . . . .''

Several implications follow from this planning framework:

1. A SOCA-cycle may be as discrete and small scale as a verbal interchange that induces desirable change, or as expansive as a comprehensive plan to transform a mental health system from a facility to community-based orientation.
2. A SOCA-cycle may encompass improvisational approaches (e.g., ''small wins,'' described below), indirect maneuvers (Hart, 1967), and formal plans (Steiner, 1979).
3. As orientation and commitment skills become sufficiently developed, managers and planners may move smoothly and rapidly from scanning to action.
4. The SOCA-cycle highlights activities and conditions generally associated with successful implementation: effective action may occur without each preparatory phase, but each should be considered in a planning process.
5. A useful means to diagnose the lack of program impact is to examine the SOCA-cycle in reverse, evaluating action, commitment, orientation, and scanning phases.
6. The SOCA-cycle is a ''scanning-to-acting'' sequence through which various initiatives can converge or be clustered for a synergistic impact.
7. Individuals or organizations able to move through the SOCA-cycle rapidly, flexibly, skillfully, and incisively thereby gain advantage over resource-superior forces that either resist change or engage in countermoves. Consequently, mastery of the SOCA-cycle strengthens the capacity of managers, planners, and advocates to induce and guide constructive service system change in a challenging environment.

CASE STUDY ONE: A SOCA-CYCLE ANALYSIS OF STRATEGIES FOR EXPANDING COMMUNITY SUPPORT PROGRAMS

Community Support Programs (CSPs) for individuals experiencing serious and long-term mental disabilities have often been referred to as public mental health's ''best kept secret.'' No other treatment or rehabilitation approach with as much demonstrated clinical efficacy and relevance to mental health system improvement is so little recognized or understood outside the public mental health field. Community Support Programs assertively engage in outreach to persons experiencing serious mental illness with coordinated residential, rehabilitation, medication, vocational, case management, crisis stabilization, and other therapeutic and natural support services. CSPs have significantly advanced the state of the art for delivering biomedical and psychosocial rehabilitation services to individuals with the most challenging clinical disorders. Since 1977, the National Institute of Mental Health has funded CSP planning efforts in every state (see, also, chapter 12 of this volume).

Beyond their clinical efficacy, CSPs can serve as a strategic pivot to constructively influence or transform the structure and functioning of mental health systems. CSP philosophy and practice are grounded in strategic principles and actions: coalition building, consensus development, empowerment of disfranchised persons, orchestration of small wins and bold strokes (described below), optimistic attitudes toward service system challenges, proactive orientation toward the environment, flexibility, hustle, value-driven action, power sharing among allies, and commitment to an ambitious vision. Further, from an agency and service system perspective, expanding CSPs is a highly valuable strategy to address changing and emerging client needs (e.g., homeless mentally ill persons or young and seriously disabled persons), respond to concerns about involuntary civil commitment, prevent future excess inpatient facility capacity, provide managers greater flexibility and creative options when serving other underserved populations, and enhance the quality of life, self-sufficiency, and community integration of persons experiencing serious and persistent mental illness.

The historical emergence of CSPs in Wisconsin as a cost-effective alternative to inpatient treatment may be understood within a strategic planning and action perspective. The following account integrates the strategic sequence presented by Quinn (1980: 160, 161) with the SOCA-cycle.

Background to Service System Reform

The Wisconsin mental health system was transformed in the 1970s from a reliance on inpatient care to the development of a comprehensive community-based service system. Four activities guided and propelled the change. First, the state, with a population approaching five million, has reduced its inpatient capacity from over 13,000 public psychiatric beds in the 1960s to 1,000 public beds presently. The planning effort to divest underused and unneeded inpatient beds involved hundreds of state and local staff and advocates.

Second, a revised mental health statute merged and decentralized service responsibility and authority by establishing local mental health boards responsible to offer or assure the availability of a full array of community and inpatient services. Henceforth, local programs received state inpatient funding as well as admission authority, thereby having financial incentives to minimize inpatient treatment to a clinically appropriate level. According to Dr. Leonard Stein, a CSP pioneer, and Dr. Leonard Ganser, the Wisconsin mental health commissioner during that period, the major effect has been

to place responsibility for developing and coordinating mental health services on one county agency and to provide funding whereby the dollar follows the patient . . . [I]f a county uses inpatient facilities extensively, there is little money left for community programming, owing to the high cost of hospital care. In contrast, if a county chooses to develop comprehensive community services to help stabilize its CMI [chronically mentally ill] population, then it can use saved inpatient dollars to do so. (Stein and Ganser, 1983: 27, 28)

Third, changes in Wisconsin's Involuntary Civil Commitment law restricted involuntary commitment of mentally ill persons refusing treatment to those who were dangerous to themselves or others, thereby limiting unwarranted inpatient admissions and further empowering local mental health agencies. These three changes provided the context for the most significant service system development, the creation and eventual statewide establishment of Community Support Programs. Wisconsin's pioneering CSP effort began when doctors Mary Ann Test, Leonard Stein, and Arnold Marx at Mendota State Hospital investigated the then controversial idea that people with severe mental disabilities could successfully receive treatment in communities (Stein and Test, 1985). Through NIMH-funded research in the early 1970s, the Program for Assertive Community Treatment (PACT) demonstrated the effectiveness, improved quality of life, and cost savings of community treatment of people experiencing serious and persistent mental disabilities.

Scan—*Probe competitors' strengths and weaknesses.* Wisconsin CSP pioneers realized that inpatient services were financially and politically entrenched and reflected the prevailing treatment wisdom. However, inpatient services also were expensive, sometimes iatrogenic, and unable to sufficiently prepare individuals for postrelease success. CSP pioneers also engaged in an incisive clinical and ecological analysis of the conditions promoting community tenure and causes of recidivism among the target population, which led to the development of creative community support services and systems.

Orient—*Require competitors to stretch their commitments.* Inpatient services were unable to demonstrate competitive advantage on the multiple dimensions of client quality of life, economy, integration of clients into the community, decrease in readmissions, decentralization of service delivery, and services that were flexible, individualized, and relevant to postrelease adaptation. Conversely, CSP innovators could devise interventions likely to prove superior in several of these areas.

Commit—*Concentrate resources.* CSP innovators integrated and packaged innovative psychosocial and biomedical interventions in a flexible outreach mode most likely to be responsive to and accepted by clients.

Act (Initial)—*Apply strengths against competitors' weaknesses.* Implementation of research and demonstration efforts highlighted significant CSP advantages in comparison to traditional hospital-based approaches.

Act (Initial)—*Convincingly succeed in a selected segment of the competitors' territory.* Demonstrated successes with particular clients, agencies, and communities answered the basic question of whether comprehensive community-based treatment could be more economical and therapeutically effective than institutional treatment.

Act (Subsequent)—*Build a bridgehead in the competitive territory.* Subsequent actions of the initial CSP were to pursue fiscal survival and political acceptance, address and adapt to facility countermoves, and refine and enlarge their knowledge and skill base.

Act (Subsequent)—*Regroup and expand to gain success in a wider field.* Subsequent competitive gains included widespread local CSP dissemination, achievement of state mental health agency support, adaptation of the CSP approach and knowledge to other disabilities, and adoption of the CSP initiative at the state level and by the National Institute of Mental Health.

This review of the strategic campaign waged in Wisconsin is not intended to suggest that community and inpatient services are inherently in conflict: comprehensive community-based mental health service systems continue to utilize a minimal level of cost-effective, responsive inpatient services. The challenge to managers, planners, providers, and advocates is to assure that CSP and inpatient treatment are singularly effective and mutually beneficial. However, a common occurrence is a funding imbalance that gives priority to inpatient systems while the vast majority of persons experiencing serious mental illness reside in the community and CSPs lack sufficient financial and policy support. Addressing this programmatic and fiscal disparity consequently is a critical action area that requires a variety of competitive and cooperative strategies.

PROCESS OF STRATEGIC PLANNING AND ACTION

Having outlined the SOCA-cycle and its application in analyzing the development of CSPs in Wisconsin, I now present the process of strategic planning in greater detail.

Scan

The definition of scan is not only to survey the environment broadly and quickly but also to inspect closely. Both activities are appropriate for stimulating and informing planning and action; generally, the broad view identifies issues that then merit focused attention. A widely used method for synthesizing information about the environment and the organization is to conduct a WOTS-up analysis: *W*eaknesses of the organization, *O*pportunities and *T*hreats in the environment, and *S*trengths of the organization. A WOTS-up analysis is to identify weaknesses and threats in order to manage or avoid them, and to consider actions that match agency strengths with environmental opportunities.

Individuals and organizations appropriately begin the process with a *plan to plan*. This commitment to a planning orientation and ongoing function recognizes the importance of attending to environmental and future issues despite and because of the press of events and demands. This readiness facilitates analysis of the organization service system, and its environment. Service system analysis focuses on several facets: structure and dynamics; whether human and financial resources are sufficient and appropriately distributed; skills and orientation of existing planning functions; and the service system's values and policies as well as strategies and tactics for improvement and expansion. Likewise, environmental analysis has multiple aspects: demographic, economic, political, social, and service forces and trends; values and views of consumers, family members, and other stakeholders; styles and capacity of decision makers (e.g., legislators, courts, referral agencies) that influence the service system; service funders (e.g., legislatures, insurers, and local government) and suppliers (see Figure 19–2 supply side); and service system constraints and expectations imposed by external forces.

Since systematic, penetrating assessment of the environment is as crucial as it is neglected, some of Webber and Peters's (1983) environmental assessment techniques may be useful:

1. Engage in a multilevel analysis: worldwide, national, industrywide, regional, state, and local.
2. Distinguish between controllable and uncontrollable trends and events. The former call for preventive measures; the latter require contingency thinking. Attempts to influence uncontrollable situations waste valuable planning resources.
3. Search for changes in underlying conditions.
4. Identify early signals of opportunities and threats.
5. Develop alternative approaches for coping with future uncertainty.

Porter's (1979) competitive analysis framework, which is adapted in Figure 19–2, is highly useful for understanding the forces within and outside mental health systems. Porter identifies five forces that influence any service industry: rivalry among existing corporations, negotiation with primary and secondary consumers, negotiation with service suppliers, addressing market share threats from potential entrants to the industry, and dealing with alternatives to the industry that offer a superior value to consumers. The evolution of industries is frequently based on the development of superior alternatives, as witnessed by movie theatres being outflanked in succession by television, cable movies, and video cassette recorders. In the mental health industry, inpatient services have now been outflanked by Community Support Systems and other community-based alternatives (Kiesler, 1982a, 1982b). The strategic challenge is to influence systematically the industry's entry, exit, and mobility barriers. Specifically, methods and mechanisms may be devised to channel services to community treatment in lieu of, or prior to, possible inpatient services; prevent inappropriate expansion of inpatient capacity; shift staff and funds from hospital to community treatment; and identify alternative uses for unnecessary inpatient capacity.

Practical approaches for analyzing the organization and environment are through discussion among the top management team, interviews of team man-

Figure 19–2
Strategies for Increasing Barriers to Inpatient Services and Developing Superior Alternatives

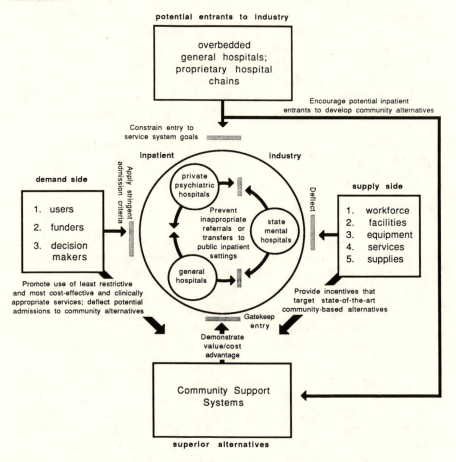

agers, or an off-site retreat among key managers to review organizational strategy and conduct a strategic audit of the agency.

A specific application of the SOCA-cycle framework is occurring within the Washington State Mental Health Division (Peterson et al., 1987). The division has involved consumers, family members, and local mental health agency staff in mental health system planning by requesting participants to *scan* the environment, *orient* their organizations, and *commit* themselves to key strategic initiatives. Environmental scanning in Washington State entails assessing local service trends and needs, gathering input from constituents and stakeholders, and identifying opportunities, threats, and neutral zones. The orient and commit phases are described in greater detail in the respective sections below.

Orient

Orientation links scanning with commitment to action. Orienting activity thus identifies purpose, synthesizes issues identified through scanning, and generates options for actions.

Constructive vision and values as well as workable policies and realistic goals are essential for effective planning and action. For instance, planners may advance a vision of the service system's structure, roles, and functions, in terms of such assertions as:

- community-based treatment is the foundation of mental health service delivery—portal of entry, triage, and arena for most services;
- in the heart of the system, CSPs are not only therapeutically efficacious but also may serve as a vehicle for allocating inpatient and community resources; and
- inpatient treatment functions are a critical backup to be used selectively and when well-developed community resources are insufficient.

From analysis of purpose, the organization, and the environment, issues may be extracted that guide planning and action. A strategic issue may be thought of as "a problem generator: resolve it or fix it, and you get rid of a bunch of problems" (McMillan, 1978: 44).

In Washington State, orienting is an ongoing process for generating and analyzing service improvement options. First, participants have envisioned the ideal future of the mental health system through a statement of philosophy developed with broad input from consumers, family members, and providers. Then, in light of environmental and organizational issues, they identify areas for service system improvement such as unmet service needs, improvements in service coordination, and administration. They then analyze each proposed improvement according to its service system priority, clarity, potential for multicounty collaboration, degree of support or opposition, and resource requirements.

Commit

In a study of postmortems of organizations' strategic planning failures (Day, 1986), the most common shortcoming cited was lack of rigorous debate at critical phases of strategy formulation. An effective strategy capitalizes on environmental trends and creates an enduring advantage; is based on realistic assumptions and accurate information; can be achieved with available resources; is internally consistent; is acceptable to the operating managers who will be responsible for implementation; is flexible enough to respond to unexpected developments; and will create client, program, and system value within acceptable risk limits. Day concludes: "Strategies that do not meet these criteria are unlikely to succeed. No champion will be willing to step forward and galvanize operating managers into action, and no director will award it total support. Such strategies are especially vulnerable to the actions of competitors with a strong commitment to their own well-reasoned strategy" (Day, 1986: 68). In Washington, selection of service system improvement actions is based on a set of well-considered criteria: actions that are of highest priority *and* have the greatest likelihood of success.

Managers must also decide between several avenues of action—cooperation versus competition; "bold strokes" versus "small wins"; and attrition versus indirect maneuvers.

Cooperation versus competition. A fundamental decision for selecting strategic initiatives is whether to cooperate or compete. A helpful way to consider the choice is to decide whether the mental health agency and the other stakeholders (e.g., affected work force, unions, professional organizations, consumers, families, legislators, and public) are at an advantage or disadvantage in dealing with the particular issue. Each combination of advantage and disadvantage suggests alternative actions.

1. Mutual advantage. Cooperation or collaboration in situations of mutual advantage can lead to major gains in achieving desirable goals. Unquestionably, service system enhancement is most assured when cooperative approaches are identified and pursued. Quinn (1980: 119) emphasizes that successful strategists not only "coopt or neutralize serious opposition . . . or find zones of indifference where the proposition would not be disastrously opposed," but they also seek win-win situations "that would activate all important players positively in their own self-interest." Filley (1975) and Fisher and Ury (1981) offer excellent guidance on construing competitive and conflictual situations as opportunities to cooperate and collaborate. In fact, a valuable use of strategy in general is to reconstrue asymmetrical and win-lose situations as opportunities of mutual advantage. Nevertheless, many issues and problems confronting mental health agencies and systems are essentially zero-sum situations; that is, one actor's gain is another's loss.

2. Organizational advantage in regard to competitors. The most useful approaches are to engage in cooperation and bring stakeholders into a mutually advantageous arrangement, or to achieve advantage through decisive actions that are least likely to provoke retaliation and include the possibility for future cooperation.

3. Organizational disadvantage in regard to competitors. In the competition for adequate funding, sufficient work force, citizen acceptance and attention, or legislative support, it is painfully obvious that other health, public safety, and social values often have superior backing. Consequently, the quintessential strategic challenge for mental health advocates is reversing this asymmetry so that mental health initiatives achieve sustainable advantage. Gaining advantage in regard to politically stronger competitors may be facilitated by the action guidelines and other approaches described below.

4. Mutual disadvantage. Regrettably, many issues decompose into mutual losses. Examples abound: funding and management-labor stalemates between community versus facility services; involuntary civil commitment law debates; internecine battles among professional groups, and between core professionals and other mental health workers; rivalry for support among various disabilities; rivalry between the private and public sector; and struggles between health and mental health care systems. If issues cannot be construed as other than no-win situations, the wisest policy is to assiduously avoid struggles of attrition that may degenerate into deadlock and distract the agency and system from pursuing opportunities for gain.

"Small wins" versus "bold strokes." Small wins are "controllable opportunities" of modest size where people can act quickly, visibly, and successfully (Weick, 1984: 43–44). Weick persuasively argues for a "small wins" approach when confronting apparently intractable system resistance and obstacles to change. Quinn (1982: 620) supports Weick's arguments: "Beginning moves are often handled as mere tactical adjustments in the enterprise's existing posture and as such they encounter little opposition. . . . Such programs allow the guiding executive to maintain the enterprise's on-going strengths while shifting momentum—at the margin—toward new needs."

Feinberg and Levenstein (1984: 23) offer a rationale for the small-win approach: "In the final analysis there are only two strategies for progress in any human activity: (a) striving for the bold stroke, which may mean going for broke, or (b) playing for small increments that eventually add up." Situations appropriate for pursuing small wins include (1) when long-range goals are being sought; (2) when circumstances allow for incrementalism; and (3) when problems are likely to be repetitive. Following are Feinberg and Levenstein's small-win tactics:

1. Notice details ignored by others. Specific causes of clients "falling through the cracks" and of agencies failing to engage challenging clients can lead to more responsive and effective services.

2. Add a new ingredient. Examples include linking familiar functions that have been dissociated in the past and joining a new element with an old one.

3. Rearrange components. Sort out critical factors and examine the effects of changing each. Reverse the chain of cause and effect.

4. Focus on the unusual. An example is analyzing complaints to generate ideas for developing policies.

5. Go beyond the paper chase. Reports, plans, and memoranda at best only mirror reality; consequently, planners and administrators must visit the scene of the action.

As a Wisconsin CSP leader asserts, "Every time we work with one county and its Community Support Program to effectively deal with one very difficult client who is currently in a facility placement, we improve the mental health system. We get our foot in the door to show them what's possible'' (Carpenter, 1984). In fact, most mental health system planning is the pursuit of small wins while taking and making opportunities for bold strokes. Bold strokes are attempts to make quantum leaps. Successful bold moves have high payoffs, but also may mobilize opposition, involve significant risks, or produce backlash. Opportunities or threats, however, may be so great that bold strokes are the most reasonable or advisable course of action. As a result, Stockdill (1987) argues for *opportunistic incrementalism*, relying on small wins (i.e., incrementalism) and then attempting opportunistic bold moves when encountering major environmental opportunities and threats.

Attrition versus indirect maneuvers. Powerful and large bureaucracies dealing with comparatively weaker stakeholders often attempt to gain advantage through attrition of the lesser's resources. When mental health agencies find themselves waging uphill struggles to achieve program goals, an indirect maneuver approach is thus preferable. One of the most serious errors in implementation is to directly confront change resisting and powerful competitors and stakeholders. Examples include pursuit of major increases in insurance coverage for mental health services despite well-organized insurer resistance, announcing intent to close mental hospitals, and confronting other disability interests regarding the reallocation of scarce resources. Such direct moves trigger strenuous resistance and enmesh the opponent in a struggle of attrition that degenerates into losses and distraction. Consequently, organizations are more likely to succeed when they deftly slip around Maginot lines rather than fling their scarce resources at the sources of resistance.

As managers decide the degree to which their initiatives will be competitive, small-win, and indirect, they set the context for motivating key actors, mobilizing resources, and acting. The following guidelines may aid in the ongoing process. Effective managers, planners, and change agents are likely to select a few focused and integrated initiatives with open-ended and/or alternative objectives. Quinn's research (1980: 162–163) discovered that successful strategists moved forward incrementally with a few thrusts which give them

cohesion, balance, and focus. Some thrusts are temporary; others are carried through to the end of the strategy. Some cost more per unit gain than others. Yet resources must be *allocated in patterns* that provide sufficient resources for each thrust to succeed regardless of the relative cost/gain ratio. And organizational units must be coordinated and actions controlled to support the intended thrust pattern or else the total strategy will fail.

In addition, by selecting actions that offer alternative or open-ended objectives and tactical targets, opponents are put on the horns of a dilemma regarding which objectives will be pursued. This not only increases the likelihood of being able to gain at least one objective, but also facilitates subsequent efforts to gain additional goals or advantages upon achieving the first (Hart, 1967). Managers also benefit by allocating the minimum necessary resources to achieve secondary goals (Quinn, 1980) and by expressing their initiatives as positive messages that encourage cooperation, or at least neutrality, from competitors and opponents.

With major thrusts selected, it is highly useful to broaden and strengthen the coalition among relevant stakeholders with regard to impending action. Within the organization, it is equally important to develop a consensus among key managers and planners regarding what to do and how to proceed. A major responsibility of top managers is to promote staff commitment to the selected initiatives; managers can then assign and establish leadership and responsibility for each initiative. Quinn (1982: 623) describes the process: "As each thrust comes into focus, strategic managers ensure that some individual(s) feel responsible for its execution. Plans are locked into programs or budgets, and control and reward systems are aligned to reflect intended strategic emphases." In mental health agencies, top managers can further solidify commitment by shortening communication lines between themselves and their key initiatives, using informal information processes to monitor the initiatives, and engaging in symbolic as well as tangible activities that declare organizational support for the initiatives. As a final step leading to action, managers should marshal organizational resources into a strong, flexible posture (Quinn: 1980, 1982).

Act

The fulfillment of strategic planning is effective action leading to desired results. Initiative development and implementation blur as preparation merges into action. Further, implementation consists of actions and reactions since initiatives usually provoke countermoves by opponents and competitors.

Mental health system actions combine content (i.e., what to do) with process (i.e., how to act). Most mental health planning and system change literature focus on substance (see, for instance, Broskowski, O'Brien, and Prevost, 1982; Goplerud, Walfish, and Apsey, 1983; Kane, 1982; Lackey, Stockdill, and Goodrick, 1985; Pardes and Stockdill, 1984). Consequently, it is useful to consider substance and process as forming a matrix with the following process guidelines as column headings, while content initiatives (e.g., CSP, crisis beds, prevention and early intervention) form rows. Thus, managers and planners select program actions and facilitate their successful implementation through relevant process guidelines.

Another critical distinction is between initial and subsequent actions (Hart, 1967). To achieve strategic success, two major problems must be solved: how to create a competitive advantage and then how to capitalize on it. One precedes and the other follows the specific initiative. Individuals and organizations gain advantage by creating or taking an opportunity; they significantly enhance their impact by capitalizing on the second opportunity that occurs before competitors regroup and respond.

Guidelines for initial actions

1. Preempt competitors (MacMillan, 1982, 1984). In a competitive struggle, acting only after others have seized the initiative leads to reactive, defensive, and often ineffectual countermoves. Individuals and organizations that are first to analyze the competitive environment realistically may engage in preemptive actions to gain advantage over more powerful and resource-rich, but less skilled, competitors.

2. Concentrate resources and apply organizational strengths against competitors' weaknesses (Hart, 1967).

3. Pursue avenues that are likely to provoke the least resistance. Specifically, identify and advance in neutral zones (Wrapp, 1984).

4. Within value constraints, use speed, surprise, or unpredictability to maneuver past unprepared and unsuspecting competitors or opponents having superior force (Hart, 1967).

5. Place "side-bets" (i.e., secondary actions) to (a) reduce catastrophic risk and (b) expand future options (Quinn, 1982).

6. Encourage flexible execution (Harrigan, 1985), and engage in actions that can adapt to changing and unpredictable circumstances.

Guidelines for subsequent actions

1. Maintain the initiative to influence the course of events, and capitalize on momentum. Attempt to keep competitors off balance with regard to what additional actions may occur. Seek and seize unfolding opportunities.

2. Consolidate gains into a critical mass, and expand future efforts into neutral zones or other areas where success is likely.

3. Be prepared to concede select positions or aspects of initiatives. Not only does this facilitate interaction between the organization (or service system) and its environment, but it also reflects the wisdom of initially pursuing more than the amount of gain is desired.

4. Address relationships with other stakeholders. Where possible, encourage collaboration. If competitive advantage has been achieved in regard to competitors, engage in conciliatory actions that lessen the likelihood of unnecessary competitive or retaliatory action. If further competition is necessary, review the course of action in order to devise novel actions for future engagement (Hart, 1967).

5. Along with or contingent upon action, evaluate impact, effectiveness, and efficiency. Evaluation may suggest continuation of actions and/or identify further initiatives that capitalize on agency momentum and broaden the base of success. Evaluation systematically retraces the phases of a SOCA-cycle: *refine, revise*, or *redirect* actions; *review* plans and *reconsider* decisions; *reorient* in regard to issues, policies, and options; and *reanalyze* the organization and environment. Thus, evaluation triggers iteration of the SOCA-cycle, contributing to its ongoing flow and adaptive evolution.

CASE STUDY TWO: WISCONSIN'S INVOLUNTARY CIVIL COMMITMENT DEBATE

How the Wisconsin Office of Mental Health (OMH) preemptively reframed the nondangerous involuntary civil commitment debate offers a final case study of the SOCA-cycle. Since the mid–1970s, Wisconsin has had a stringent involuntary civil commitment law (Goodrick, 1984). While local judicial systems have interpreted and administered the statute with varying degrees of strictness, involuntary civil commitment of mentally ill individuals who refuse treatment has required demonstration, through omission or commission, of behavior dangerous to self or others. The perennial debate about the strictness of the law's criteria has generated articulate and polarizing arguments by mental health professionals and by family members on both sides of the issue.

Scan

The OMH director and staff engaged in an informal analysis of the situation that produced several findings. The growing chorus of complaints by some family members and mental health professionals regarding the statute was likely to lead to the introduction of a legislative proposal for a nondangerous commitment criterion whose fate would be decided by legislative vote and ultimately by court decision. Local mental health agencies having strong CSPs and constructive relations with law enforcement agencies and courts asserted that the existing statute was sound and should not be changed. Also, some efforts to establish a nondangerous criterion could be construed as an end run to fund financially strained inpatient units, undermine community treatment, and reinstitutionalize Wisconsin's community-based mental health system. Specifically, petitioners would be able to force court-ordered involuntary inpatient care of treatment-refusing clients, and local mental health agencies would in some instances have to pay with funds they more appropriately could use for community-based treatment and outreach services to these persons.

Orient

These concerns precipitated a meeting chaired by OMH personnel with other state agency staff and legal and consumer advocates who represented broad constituencies. The meeting led to clarification and consensus of values and purpose: protection of the public mental health system while promoting increased responsiveness; protection of civil liberties of psychotic individuals who refuse treatment but are not dangerous; and promotion of creative attempts to engage such individuals therapeutically. Through discussion of environmental threats and opportunities, resources, possible action scenarios, and potential counter-moves, a set of options emerged. The key ingredient was to reframe the issue: rather than react defensively to alleged or apparent commitment problems, the group asserted that the salient issues were insufficient fiscal resources, uneven responsiveness of local mental health agencies, lack of petitioner knowledge for negotiating the commitment process, and lack of coordination between the mental health and judicial systems.

Commit

Meeting participants agreed on the importance of unity among local mental health providers, legal advocates, consumer advocates, and the OMH; this coalition would address commitment problems by pursuing the goals expressed through reframing. The participants decided to share the proposed option package with their colleagues, adopt a proactive stance with leadership by the OMH to be shared with other responsible parties, and engage in selective preemptive actions.

Act

The first action was preemptive. A policy paper circulated to over 1,000 advocates, providers, private practitioners, and family members redefined the issue by articulating the policy orientation of the OMH with backing of its administratively superordinate department, presenting constructive options, and creating a fresh agenda for subsequent discussion. Open meetings chaired by the OMH director offered interested persons the opportunity to express their views. The meetings grew increasingly large and sometimes were the forum for acrimonious debate, but they also provided a vehicle for exploring alternatives to a nondangerous criterion and set the stage for subsequent actions. Open-meeting participants requested that the OMH conduct a statewide survey of the prevalence and dynamics of the problem, which became an eighteen-month process, thereby delaying precipitous introduction of nondangerous commitment criterion legislation. Momentum grew as OMH staff delivered speeches to professional associations and consumer groups elaborating on the reframed perspective and action agenda. A manual was developed to be used by families and other interested persons for pursuing involuntary civil commitments. The coalition of the OMH, statewide association of local mental health providers, consumers, legal advocates, and others resulted not only in successful lobbying for a 20 percent state funding increase of CSPs but also in the nation's first statute mandating CSPs in every local mental health system. While some proponents of nondangerous commitment claimed that the issue of CSP development and commitment law change were unrelated, the approach linking them was persuasive to sufficient providers, advocates, and legislators to achieve the strategic goals.

CONCLUSION

Mental health systems exist in an environment where stakeholders are demonstrating sophistication and influence in shaping events that contribute to or may interfere with mental health service goals. In light of this challenge, strategic concepts and approaches are available for mental health system managers, planners, and advocates to refine and apply. The value of incisive environmental analysis followed by opportunity-oriented strategic planning and action is increasing dramatically, and will certainly accelerate in the future. Advocates for progressive mental health systems recognize that change is inevitable, and can in fact be capitalized on to achieve mental health service goals. Skill in strategic thinking and behaving in conjunction with the growing knowledge base about effective actions can be invaluable for individuals and organizations committed to improving public mental health services.

ACKNOWLEDGMENT

An earlier version of this chapter appeared as David Goodrick, *Health Planner's Guide to Mental Health System Strategic Planning*. Washington, D.C.: Alpha Center, 1986.

REFERENCES

Broskowski, A., O'Brien, G. M. St. L., and Prevost, J. 1982. Interorganizational Strategies for Survival: Looking Ahead to 1990. *Administration in Mental Health* 9: 198–210.

Brown, B. S. 1986. Claiming the Unclaimed Children: Developing Systems of Care for Severely Emotionally Disturbed Children and Youth. Presentation at the Child and Adolescent Service System Project. Boulder, Colo., July.

Carpenter, E. 1984. Personal Communication.

Day, G. 1986. Tough Questions for Developing Strategies. *Journal of Business Strategy* 6 (Winter): 60–68.

Feinberg, M., and Levenstein, A. 1984. Developing and Making the Most of the Slight Edge. *Wall Street Journal*, July 9, p. 23.

Filley, A. 1975. *Interpersonal Conflict Resolution*. Glenview, Ill.: Scott Foresman.

Fisher, R., and Ury, W. 1981. *Getting to Yes: Negotiating Agreement without Giving In*. Boston: Houghton Mifflin.

Goodrick, D. 1984. Survival of Public Inpatient Mental Health Systems: Strategies for Constructive Change. *NASMHPD State Report*, National Association of State Mental Health Program Directors, Alexandria, Va., July 25.

Goodrick, D. 1987. *A Strategic Plan for Advancing the National Community Support Program Initiative*. Submitted to the National Institute of Mental Health by the National Technical Assistance Center for Mental Health Planning, COSMOS Corporation, Washington, D.C., November.

Goplerud, E., Walfish, S., and Apsey, M. O. 1983. Surviving Cutbacks in Community Mental Health: Seventy-Seven Action Strategies. *Community Mental Health Journal* 19: 62–76.

Harrigan, K. R. 1985. *Strategic Flexibility*. Lexington, Mass.: Lexington Books.

Hart, B.H.L. 1967. *Strategy*. New York: New American Library.

Hayes, R. H. 1985. Strategic Planning—Forward in Reverse? *Harvard Business Review* 63 (November-December): 111–119.

Isenberg, D. J. 1987. The Tactics of Strategic Opportunism. *Harvard Business Review* 65 (March-April): 92–97.

James, B. G. 1984. *Business War Games*. Middlesex, England: Penguin Books.

Kane, T. 1982. Reorganization Following Drastic Limitations of Resources. *Administration in Mental Health* 9: 191–197.

Kiesler, C. 1982a. Mental Hospitals and Alternative Care: Noninstitutionalization as Potential Public Policy for Mental Patients. *American Psychologist* 37: 349–360.

Kiesler, C. 1982b. Public and Professional Myths about Mental Hospitalization: An Empirical Reassessment of Policy-Related Beliefs. *American Psychologist* 37: 1323–1339.

Lackey, G. L., Stockdill, J., and Goodrick, D. 1985. *Alternative Mental Health Resources in the United States*. Rockville, Md.: National Institute of Mental Health, Division of Education and Service Systems Liaison.

MacMillan, I. C. 1982. Seizing Competitive Initiative. *The Journal of Business Strategy* 2: 43–57.

MacMillan, I. C. 1984. Preemptive Strategies. In *Handbook of Business Strategy*, ed. W. Guth. New York: Warren, Gorham, and Lamont.

MacMillan, N. 1978. *Planning for Survival: A Handbook for Hospital Trustees*. Chicago: American Hospital Association.

Pardes, H., and Stockdill, J. 1984. Survival Strategies for Community Mental Health Services in the 1980s. *Hospital and Community Psychiatry* 35: 127–132.

Parrish, J., and Lieberman, M. 1987. *Toward a Model Plan for a Comprehensive, Community-Based Mental Health System*. Rockville, Md.: National Institute of Mental Health, Division of Education and Service Systems Liaison.

Peterson, P., Hoppler, J., Hidano, E., Westgard, R., Daniels, L., and Goodrick, D. 1987. *Washington State's Innovative Approach for Promoting State and Local Mental Health Strategic Planning*. National Technical Assistance Center for Mental Health Planning, COSMOS Corporation, Washington, D.C., March.

Porter, M. 1979. How Competitive Forces Shape Strategy. *Harvard Business Review* 57 (March-April): 137–145.

Porter, M. 1980. *Competitive Strategy: Techniques for Analyzing Industries and Competitors*. New York: Free Press.

Quinn, J. B. 1980. *Strategies for Change: Logical Incrementalism*. Homewood, Ill.: Richard D. Irwin.

Quinn, J. B. 1982. Managing Strategies Incrementally. *OMEGA: The International Journal of Management Science* 10: 613–627.

Quinn, J. B., Mintzberg, H., and James, R. M. 1988. *The Strategy Process: Concepts, Contexts, and Cases*. Englewood Cliffs, N. J.: Prentice-Hall.

Schneier, M. 1986. Personal Communication.

Stein, L., and Ganser, L. 1983. Wisconsin's System for Funding Mental Health Services. In *Unified Mental Health Systems: Utopia Unrealized*, ed. J. Talbott. *New Directions for Mental Health Services*, No. 18. San Francisco: Jossey-Bass.

Stein, L., and Test, M. A., eds. 1985. *The Training in Community Living Model: A*

Decade of Experience. New Directions for Mental Health Services, No. 26. San Francisco: Jossey-Bass.

Steiner, G. A. 1979. *Strategic Planning: What Every Manager Must Know*. New York: Free Press.

Stockdill, J. 1987. Strategic Planning and the Use of Incremental Opportunism. Paper presented at the Washington State Conference for Promoting State and Local Mental Health Strategic Planning, Seattle, Wash., March 5.

Webber, J. B., and Peters, J. P. 1983. *Strategic Thinking: New Frontier for Hospital Management*. Chicago: American Hospital Publishing.

Weick, K. 1984. Small Wins: Redefining the Scale of Social Problems. *American Psychologist* 39: 40–49.

Wrapp, H. E. 1984. Good Managers Don't Make Policy Decisions. *Harvard Business Review* 62 (July-August): 18–31.

Part 7
Enduring Problems and Opportunities

20

Toward the Year 2000 in U.S. Mental Health Policymaking and Administration

DAVID MECHANIC

In the decades following World War II, a strong coalition emerged emphasizing environmental factors as prominent contributors to mental illness and championing the importance of substituting new patterns of community care for the traditional reliance on public mental hospitals for the seriously mentally ill. In the period from approximately 1955 to 1975, this coalition vastly influenced public policy toward the mentally ill and shaped the federal role in mental health policy (Mechanic, 1980; Grob, 1987).

Those associated with this movement often assumed that mental illness was a simple continuum from mild to severe dysfunction in contrast to a heterogeneous collection of unrelated disorders, that early intervention could prevent serious mental disorder, that population dynamics and the population at risk were unchanging, and that use of mental health resources for outpatient psychiatric care was always more cost-effective than hospital care. These were all testable assumptions, but they were mostly accepted on faith (Mechanic, 1980). In the 1960s the rhetoric of community care developed a momentum of its own, importantly shaping agendas and debates on mental health policy, and broadly influencing the thinking of intellectual elites, public policy makers, and the general public (Grob, 1987). In the process many dedicated professionals and reformers lost touch with the heterogeneity of mental health problems and the tough realities of designing and implementing effective programs appropriate for the most seriously mentally ill.

Mental health policy, particularly as it pertains to serious and chronic mental illness, is badly served by much of the social and preventive care ideology that attained dominance and is still commonly espoused. The excesses of ideology, and particularly naive notions about labeling and normalization processes, provided a target for critics of deinstitutionalization who focus on exaggerated claims and obvious failures of community care, proclaim the intent of deinstitutionalization as naive and counterproductive, and argue for the reestablishment of an enlarged mental hospital sector. Neither type of advocacy serves the needs of the mentally ill well nor contributes to a well-informed public.

Beginning with a critical overview of changes in the mental health system over the past thirty years and some of the dogmas accompanying them, the purpose of this chapter is to identify directions for the further development and improvement of public mental health care in the United States through the remainder of this century.

REVIEWING THE PAST

Mental health professionals have the impression that service systems are relatively impervious to change, that traditional institutions resist innovations, and that the entire mental health sector is exceedingly slow in responding to obvious need. At a gut level most professionals and concerned lay persons readily endorse these sentiments despite the lack of any reference point or criterion. What they mean, perhaps, is that the services fall short of what they deem desirable, or that the priorities for allocation are inequitable, but by any criterion the mental health sector has experienced an extraordinary degree of ferment, an enormous growth in size, and a virtual revolution in structure in a period of only thirty years (Mechanic, 1980).

A variety of forces dramatically reshaped the mental health services system and the location of care. These included the growing burden on state mental health budgets of institutionalizing the chronically mentally ill; the widespread use of psychotropic drugs that alleviated some of the most troublesome symptoms of schizophrenic patients; the professional attack on the large public mental hospital and its role in the development of secondary disabilities associated with institutional tenure; and a vigorous civil liberties movement on behalf of the rights of the mentally ill. These influences encouraged the release of many long-term patients from public mental hospitals and shorter periods of stay for newly admitted patients. But most chronic mental patients are highly disabled and unable to support themselves. The introduction of Medicare and Medicaid in 1966 and the growth of Social Security Disability Insurance (SSDI) and Supplemental Security Income (SSI) allowed the retention of patients in community settings or alternative institutions such as nursing homes that expanded rapidly with federal support.

Transformation of the Mental Health Sector

In 1955 the number of episodes treated in mental health facilities was 1.7 million, and the vast majority occurred in public mental hospitals. Inpatients in public mental hospitals peaked at 559,000 at this time, and services available in outpatient settings were limited severely by the ability to pay. By the middle 1980s inpatients in public mental hospitals fell to 115,000, and general hospitals became the major site of acute psychiatric care. In 1984 there were almost 1.7 million discharges from short-stay hospitals with a primary diagnosis of mental illness, and an average length of stay of approximately twelve days (Dennison, 1985). The elderly demented as well as many elderly mentally ill are now in nursing homes; estimates made on the basis of the 1977 Nursing Home Survey total some 668,000 patients with mental illness or dementia (Goldman, Feder, and Scanlon, 1986). In short, there was a dramatic reorganization of inpatient psychiatric care, a major change in the distribution of patients among sites of care, and a transformation of the pattern of hospitalization for acute psychiatric illness. None of these changes suggests the elimination of important disparities by socioeconomic status, race, and ethnicity, although public programs significantly improved access among disadvantaged groups.

As a consequence of reductions in the populations of public mental hospitals, and the transfer of many hopeless chronic patients to nursing homes, the public mental hospital was in many instances transformed from a custodial institution to an active treatment unit. The professional-patient and staff-patient ratios improved enormously, and active treatment and rehabilitation programs were developed to a point where in many instances there was little resemblance between the hospital as it had once been and as it is now. It is, of course, difficult to describe conditions in the United States because each state maintains its own mental health system and there is great diversity in the availability of facilities, funding patterns, and relative emphasis put on different aspects of care. But, by 1982, the typical state mental hospital had 529 inpatients and 807 employees, with average expenses per patient of more than $31,000 per year. Between 1970 and 1982 the average number of patients per employee was reduced from 1.7 to .7, and the average expenditure per patient increased from $4,359 to $12,500 in constant 1970 dollars (Dolan, 1986).

Even more impressive has been the overall growth of the mental health sector. In 1980 mental illness was the third most expensive category of disorder, accounting for more than $20 billion of health care expenditures (U.S. Department of Health and Human Services, 1983). This level of expenditure has been made possible by the growth of mental health coverage in both public and private health insurance programs. The Bureau of Labor Statistics "Level of Benefits Survey" shows considerable depth of inpatient mental health coverage among employees studied in firms above a minimum size (Brady, Sharfstein, and Muszynski, 1986). In 1984 almost all (99 percent) had inpatient psychiatric coverage, and about half had it on the same basis as any other illness. Ninety-six percent had outpatient coverage, but only 7 percent on the same basis as other illnesses. Most common restrictions were dollar limits and coinsurance levels (typically 50 percent). Increased coverage has contributed to the purchase of millions in additional services. The Institute of Social Research at the University of Michigan surveyed the U.S. population in 1957 and 1976 using many of the same questions. Over the twenty-year period, use of professional help for psychological problems increased from 14 to 26 percent, although the levels of well-being in the population were approximately the same (Kulka, Veroff, and Douvan, 1979).

As one would expect, the greatly increased capacity to pay for services and their provision are linked to a dramatic increase in mental health manpower of every type. In 1947 there were only 4,700 psychiatrists in the United States, and only 23,000 mental health professionals in psychiatry, clinical psychology, social work, and psychiatric nursing; by 1977 their numbers had increased to 121,000, with large increases continuing to the present in clinical psychology, social work, and other disciplines oriented to psychotherapy (Mechanic, 1980). The National Medical Care Utilization and Expenditure Survey (NMCUES) found that psychiatrists and psychologists each had approximately one-quarter of mental health visits, approximately 40 percent were to other providers in office settings (social workers, nurses, counselors, etc.), and about one-tenth occurred in mental health clinics, outpatient departments, and emergency rooms (Taube, Kessler, and Feuerberg, 1984). Mental health has become a large and diversified sector.

Deinstitutionalization and Drugs

Psychiatric writers commonly focus on the widespread introduction of neuroleptic drugs in the mid–1950s, but in doing so, they generally neglect the critical state of psychiatric hospitals in the decade after the war. Federal aid to the states for mental health services decreased during the Korean War, and the Hoover Commission in 1955 criticized the abruptness of the reduction of such federal support. States were acutely aware of their financial and personnel limitations, and were seeking a way of joining the then optimistic spirit emerging in the mental health field.

The widespread introduction of neuroleptic drugs in the 1950s was an important tool, then, but not the cause of deinstitutionalization. Psychoactive drugs were extraordinarily helpful in blunting patients' most bizarre symptoms and giving professionals, administrators, family members, and the community more confidence that patients' most troublesome and frightening symptoms could be contained. They facilitated unlocking hospital wards, allowed more patient movement within the hospital, and aided discharge to the community. There are documented instances in some localities of such changes without the use of antipsychotic drugs (Scull, 1977), but it is unlikely that significant reductions in hospital populations, facilitated by a combination of social forces, could have been sustained without drugs.

An avoidable failure was the unwillingness to recognize the devastating side effects of the drugs for some patients when those effects first became evident. Had we been more sensitive to the effects and to ways of limiting them by regulating dose and regimen, we might have avoided some of the negative responses to psychoactive medication (Estroff, 1981). Growing awareness of extrapyramidal motor reactions, tardive dyskinesia, and other adverse drug effects, while impressing us again with the tradeoffs and costs involved in management of chronic psychosis (Kane and Smith, 1982), does not refute the continuing importance of medication. But it makes evident the crucial responsibility for high-quality drug monitoring and management.

The phenothiazines were particularly welcomed in large public hospitals that were overcrowded and understaffed and in which hospital personnel lacked confidence in their ability to manage patients or to communicate to families or the community that such patients were controllable. The drugs changed attitudes and encouraged flexibility, but the reduction of public hospital populations proceeded only very slowly, approximately 1.5 percent per year between 1955 and 1965.

Cost Shifting and the Nursing Home Alternative

With the introduction of Medicaid and the expansion of other social programs in the middle 1960s, deinstitutionalization rapidly accelerated, with populations dropping an average of about 6 percent a year between 1965 and 1980 (Gronfein, 1985). Medicare and Medicaid stimulated the rapid expansion of nursing home beds, which provided a custodial alternative for elderly patients with dementias and a new option for some younger psychotic patients as well. But although the newly available nursing home beds provided the alternatives, the driving force was the economic advantages for the states by transferring obligations from their own mental health budgets to federal programs.

As this process grew apace, there was little constructive examination of whether nursing homes truly provided care that was better than or even comparable to the services available in mental hospitals, however deficient. The crowded and understaffed public mental hospitals were often highly regimented and impersonal. But they had mental health staff and varying mental health program elements, at least for their more acutely ill patients. In contrast, nursing homes typically had few or no medical or mental health professional staff, patients were commonly oversedated to ease management problems, and there were limited opportunities for activity (Stotsky, 1970; Vladeck, 1980; and Linn et al., 1985). Comparable conditions existed in many community residences for the mentally ill (Lamb, 1979). Yet one fact we learned well in the treatment of chronic illness is that inactivity leads to additional disabilities not inherent in the underlying illness, disabilities that can be limited by effective management (Wing, 1978).

In comparison with states' opportunities to shift costs, concerns about quality of care played little part in this major transition to nursing homes. The motives for this shift were of course complex and were influenced by dominant mental health ideologies, the desire to improve acute care in mental hospitals, growing civil liberties litigation on behalf of the mentally ill, and ingenuity in garnering all available financial resources. As the supply of nursing home beds becomes more constrained because of the growing numbers of disabled elderly, it will be increasingly difficult to place publicly supported chronic mental patients even in this inadequate housing alternative. Identifying and financing appropriate housing for the chronic mentally ill, consistent with rehabilitation needs, continues to be one of the most pressing issues for the years ahead.

Reform and Treatment Ideologies

Antihospital ideologies. If cost shifting was the major benefit in patient relocation, the change was greatly facilitated by the antihospital movement, aided and abetted by the social science community (Scull, 1977). The movement had a scientific basis for its ideology, particularly research demonstrating secondary disabilities associated with custodial hospital care and inactivity. But in condemning the mental hospital, the antihospital movement made no distinction between good and bad hospitals, nor did it recognize that any patients might benefit from asylum (Scull, 1977).

The attack on the hospital rested on the assumption that community-based services would be developed, which in retrospect was a naive view. The availability of SSDI and SSI allowed patients to remain in the community, but the then-emerging community mental health centers, despite the rhetoric used in their support, did little to assist deinstitutionalized patients, nor did they welcome them as clients. In short, until fairly recently the major federal initiative in community mental health care had little to do with the increasing numbers of chronic mental patients in the community (Gronfein, 1985).

Communities did not welcome the deinstitutionalized patient, but it was also a time of legal activism and of increasing focus on the civil liberties of the mentally ill (see chapter 15 in this volume). Civil commitment was characterized by substantial abuses and thus was a main target for civil liberties litigation (Ennis, 1972; Miller, 1976). The legal rights movement contributed a great deal to the civil liberties of the mentally ill, many of whom were harmless and in no personal danger.

But in the process of legal change it became difficult to take custody over patients who were harmful enough to themselves or others to need involuntary intervention. As a consequence of major changes in commitment procedures and their interpretation by the psychiatric community and by many judges, it became more difficult to protect patients and the community during serious psychotic episodes. Many mentally impaired patients unsuitable for civil commitment but involved in law violations were then, and are now, increasingly dealt with through the criminal justice system (Lamb and Grant, 1982).

Dominance of psychodynamics. The 1960s were also a period in which psychodynamic conceptions dominated many major psychiatric teaching centers and the mental health professions in general. The period was characterized by facile psychodynamic interpretations that blamed families, particularly parents, for disorders ranging from autism to schizophrenia.

There was a distinct failure to separate family responses that contributed to mental disorder from those that were efforts to adapt to the disruptive adversity of having a seriously impaired family member. Families were typically excluded from the treatment process and were often made to feel responsible for the patient's disabilities. There was an extraordinary failure to mobilize the experience and the personal commitment that many families had developed in dealing with serious mental illness, or in helping to relieve their burdens. Even now the value of building on family resources is not adequately appreciated, and not uncommonly is depreciated, despite controlled studies demonstrating how family supportive interventions can reduce exacerbation of symptoms and readmissions for schizophrenic patients (Falloon et al., 1985; Leff et al., 1982).

The idealism of community care. The community mental health movement was a blend of idealism, optimism, opportunism, and naïveté. It was particularly naive in the assumption that community tenure had any necessary relationship to community integration (Segal and Aviram, 1978). It failed to anticipate the extent to which patients could be lost in the community, in unsupervised living settings or simply without homes, and the degree to which they could be isolated from social contact and human services and even victimized (Talbott, 1985). But despite its failures, the community mental health movement vastly improved living options for mental patients, and many patients lead more satisfying lives than they did in the past.

The ideology and practice of deinstitutionalization were vague and involved opposing ideas (Bachrach, 1976). The concept covered such significantly different outcomes as independent living, return to families, sheltered community residence, or transfer to nursing homes. And at times there was little connection between professional ideology and advocacy and the realities of admission and transfer policies. A variety of studies, for example, found little relationship between the establishment of community mental health centers and the reduction of public mental hospital populations, suggesting that they were parallel if not independent processes (Gronfein, 1985).

Psychiatry as a profession has been slow to respond to the challenge of community care as reflected in its movement away from hospital practice, chronic populations, and the public sector (Grob, 1983). The profession began as a hospital-based specialty and achieved some success in the use of moral treatment (Bockoven, 1972). But by the early 1900s the aging of the population, the growing numbers of patients with paresis and dementia for whom no alternative institutional care was available, and the large proportion of chronic patients made the hospital less attractive for professional practice.

The shift to outpatient psychiatry in the decades preceding World War II reflected the ethos of the times as well as new preventive mental health ideologies. By the 1950s the popular acceptance of psychodynamic ideas and their influence in psychiatric training, as well as fee-for-service medicine and its embodiment in health insurance, supported the resulting system of private psychiatric practice. States were strained by the burden of financing care for the growing numbers of patients in public hospitals, and conditions had deteriorated. Psychiatry directed its attention primarily to middle-class patients with limited disorders and problems in living.

As psychiatry now moves closer to biomedical concerns, it seems evident that despite its important medical and organizational leadership in the care of the chronically mentally ill, many of the services chronic patients need are not medical. Providing such services efficiently will depend on the effective organization of nurses, social workers, psychologists, and other mental health professionals.

THE CONTEMPORARY CONTEXT

Even using conservative measures, unmet mental health needs persist, and they are enormous (Shapiro et al., 1984; Leaf et al., 1985). If one accepts broad definitions of such needs, then it is evident that no conceivable society is likely to meet them. But the evidence shows that a majority of individuals even with major mental illness have received no mental health care of any kind during the prior six months. In order to address the policy challenges presented by this situation, we must first define clearly the most critical needs and priorities as well as the generic functions of mental health service systems.

Composition of the Seriously Mentally Ill Population

Deinstitutionalization has been a rallying cry for those advocating community care and a target of their critics. Because the term is used imprecisely and is not clearly tied to particular patient populations or relocation sites (Bachrach, 1976), it has little empirical utility. Deinstitutionalization is viewed as a source of many current problems and has a certain currency in the ideological debate, but the debate is more a source of heat than light.

Even prior to 1955, most inpatients in public mental hospitals returned to the community. In any given year the net releases and deaths—the typical way of tracking inpatient occupancy—almost equaled the rate of new admissions. In 1950, for example, there were 152,000 admissions, 100,000 releases, and 41,000 deaths. The longer a patient remained in the hospital, the less the likelihood of release, but a significant proportion of new admissions returned to the community within a few months. Beginning in 1956 net releases and deaths exceeded new admissions but only by 7,952 individuals. It wasn't until 1970 that net releases (excluding deaths) actually exceeded the number of new admissions during the year (President's Commission on Mental Health, 1978: 94). Moreover, in any given year the vast majority of patients leaving were those who were admitted relatively recently.

These simple data indicate that the deinstitutionalized population is a heterogeneous collection of varying patient cohorts. Many would have been returned to the community in the absence of policy change, and common references to the deinstitutionalized seem to refer to clients who have never been part of the long-term mental hospital population at all. While, in theory, these population processes can be explicated, much of the relevant empirical work has not been attempted. It is not fully clear who among the "deinstitutionalized population" would have been the long-stay patients in earlier eras.

Public mental hospital populations were reduced by deaths, return of a residual group of long-term care patients to nursing homes or other community settings, substantial reductions of the average length of stay among newly admitted patients (median, twenty-three days in 1980), and by more stringent admission criteria. Of public hospital patients resident in 1955, a large proportion either have since died or have been relocated to nursing homes. The current large population of nursing home patients with diagnoses of mental illness or dementia includes transfers from mental hospitals, but probably most came to nursing homes directly from the community. Kiesler and Sibulkin (1987) estimate that as many as half of the elderly discharged from mental hospitals in the post–1964 years came to nursing homes. Nursing homes played a significant role for relocation of the elderly mentally ill, but a small role for younger patients. In 1977 only about 5,500 patients under age forty-five and primarily with mental illness were residing in nursing homes (Goldman, Feder, and Scanlon, 1986).

General discussion of deinstitutionalization appears often to refer to the original hospitalized cohorts, but, in fact, the populations that alarm the community are later cohorts, most of whom have never been long-stay patients and some of whom never had a psychiatric admission at all. As mental health services organization has changed, acute psychoses are treated typically with short inpatient admissions in community general hospitals and in reconstituted public mental hospitals. Most such patients have had entirely different histories with the mental health system than earlier cohorts, relying less on inpatient care and more on community services. Some proportion of these patients would have been long-term residents of mental hospitals in an earlier era.

The amount of serious mental illness in the population, with schizophrenia as the prototype, depends on both the rate of incidence and the size of the population at risk. Much of the increasingly evident problem of serious mental illness in the community is not due to deinstitutionalization, or even to changes in the way psychiatric hospitalization is used, but more to shifts in the demography of the population with large subgroups at ages with highest risk of incidence. Kramer (1977) predicted these problems more than a decade ago simply by projecting demographic trends. The misattribution of the source of changes to deinstitutionalization, vaguely defined, encourages serious errors in policymaking. Unless the society was prepared to maintain a massive public hospital system, or alternative institutions, for new occurrences of mental illness, the problem would have been evident in communities regardless of what we did.

Long-term care in aging provides an analogy. The demand for service is substantially a product of the growth of the elderly population, the increased prevalence of the oldest-old subgroup with high risks of functional disability, and the delay of mortality. Despite enormously increased nursing home beds at large national expense, providing for 1.5 million residents, the numbers of disabled elderly in the community far outnumber those in nursing homes. Except for those most incapacitated, there is no real alternative to community care. A similar logic pertains to the criminal justice system. As the subgroups of youth at high risk of criminal activity and arrest in the population swelled, we substantially increased prison capacity. Such capacity, however, could not keep up with the increase in offenders, and in many localities only the most serious and persistent offenders are jailed, and many convicts are released early because of prison overcrowding.

A population of major concern to the mental health system, and to the community, are young schizophrenics and other seriously disturbed youth, who are aware of their civil liberties and hostile or indifferent to psychiatric ideologies. They frequently are uncooperative with the types of treatment made available to them, and their mental illnesses are commonly complicated by abuse of drugs and alcohol. They mix with other street people, constitute a significant minority of the homeless population, and at various points in their life trajectories are hospitalized, jailed, or live on the streets (Lamb and Grant, 1982; Lamb, 1984). The problems are compounded by the fact that the age groups at highest risk have increasing numbers of minority and disadvantaged youth that connect the stigma of mental illness with the social difficulties associated with color and disadvantage. This population poses difficult problems of appropriate treatment and requires approaches for establishing contact and trust that are very different from the conventional office-based mental health services. Blaming deinstitutionalization for these problems is wrongheaded since most of these patients are not appropriate clients for long-term institutional care. The barriers to designing acceptable care are not constructively addressed by simple distinctions between hospital versus community services. In contrast, they will depend on carefully developed strategies of community care.

Necessary Functions of Community Mental Health Systems

Viable systems of community mental health services for the seriously mentally ill must take three important facts into account. First, the population is diverse, encompassing individuals with different disorders and needs, varying types of disabilities and capacities, and at different points in their illness trajectories. Second, service planning must take place in a context where it is difficult to predict the prognosis of patients over a long period of time. In the case of schizophrenia, for example, a significant proportion of patients do reasonably well over the long term, while others have frequent exacerbations and increasing chronicity and disability. It is clear from a number of studies, however, that schizophrenia does not result in inevitable deterioration and incapacity (Harding et al., 1986; Bleuler, 1978; Ciompi, 1980; Clausen, Pfeffer, and Huffine, 1982; Huber, Gross, and Scheuttler, 1979). Third, the problems associated with illness are often significantly compounded by the disadvantages of poverty and racism.

Hospitals have certain advantages in treating the most seriously disabled mental patients needing a high intensity of service, just as the nursing home serves a comparable advantage for the most incapacitated elderly, who may be disoriented, incontinent, and difficult to control. Many of the difficulties in the care of highly disabled clients relate to loss of control in community care relative to the control that hospitals typically have in performing treatment and custodial functions. The community is deficient in supplying many needs we take for granted in hospitals: housing, basic medical care, and opportunities for social participation. Also, maintaining contact over time, monitoring medication compliance, and encouraging regular routines, typical of hospital care, are no small tasks in the decentralized settings of present community care. And opportunities for persuasion to achieve conformity to reasonable bounds of behavior, what sociologists refer to as social control, is more difficult to exercise in community care, particularly for many young patients who reject the legitimacy of psychiatric concepts and treatment, than in the more coercive context of a total institution, however benevolent it may be.

In the process of deinstitutionalization the psychiatric hospital was devalued, and little effort was made to differentiate good from poor inpatient programs. There is some segment of the patient population for whom refuge is the most practical and humane solution (Gudeman and Shore, 1984) and perhaps necessary to protect the community as well. But community care for most patients is the desired approach, not only because it is impractical and expensive to hospitalize most of the seriously mentally ill for a lengthy period, but also because it is more consistent with patients' preferences and important values relevant to personal autonomy, independence, and minimal restriction. The vigorous civil liberties activities of the 1960s that reformed civil commitment procedures and created a variety of new patient rights increased sensitivity to the implications of restricting personal choice and introduced significant improvements in the use of coercive interventions. Criteria for involuntary hospitalization, use of isolation and other punishments, and the opportunity to impose unwanted treatments have been narrowed, consistent with modern concepts of civil liberties. Moreover, the vast majority of seriously mentally ill prefer deprivations in the community to coercion, however well intentioned. Whenever patients are asked about their preferences, the vast majority prefer treatment in the community. Appropriate models can be developed to provide care and rehabilitation, superior to most hospitals (Kiesler, 1982; Stein and Test, 1978), but the necessary tasks are neither easy nor as inexpensive as some advocates suggest (Weisbrod, Test, and Stein, 1980). If we are to avoid re-creating large mental hospital systems, an alternative increasingly advocated by observers frustrated with the failures of community care, much developmental effort in communities is essential. We will examine these developmental strategies later.

The expansion of the mental health sector obscures the important issue of the equitable distribution of mental health dollars. Hard data on resources spent on those most seriously mentally ill and incapacitated are almost impossible to obtain, but the indications are that some subgroups of the most seriously mentally ill may have less access to essential services than ever before. These deficiencies result from underfunding of chronic care, the failure to shift funding from traditional to new types of programs, and the limited insurance coverage among the most needy population. The homeless mentally ill, now found in significant numbers in every large city of our nation, convey both the magnitude of the challenge and the diversity of needs that must be met to suitably respond to the multifaceted character of long-term mental illness (Lamb, 1984). The homeless are but the tip of the iceberg. The severely mentally ill remain a substantially neglected population.

KEY ISSUES IN MENTAL HEALTH POLICYMAKING AND ADMINISTRATION

Fortunately a consensus about appropriate care for the chronically mentally ill is emerging. There is broad agreement that chronic mental illness must be addressed through a perspective based on rehabilitation and education and that the challenge is to preserve function and limit disability. There is also wide recognition that patients' needs in the community have not been met, along with awareness of models of care that allow successful management of the disruptive and publicly disturbing behavior associated with psychotic illness (Stein and Test, 1978). It seems clear that for most patients the presence of a well-managed community mental health delivery system can facilitate a reasonable pattern of adjustment, and developing such systems is a course preferable to institutional care (Gudeman and Shore, 1984; Kiesler, 1982).

Points of Leverage

Understanding clearly how deinstitutionalization occurred provides clues to the types of social policies that shape the services system and offer possible points of leverage. Most mental health professionals are insular in their concerns and have focused on relatively small categorical grant programs and their conversion to block grants, neglecting the much larger state and federal arenas that drive the system: state mental health budgeting and financing mechanisms, and federal programs such as Medicaid and Social Security. This failure to focus on the major points of leverage has resulted in neglect of the most likely possibilities for reform.

Refunding state mental health budget priorities. Mental illness has been a state responsibility and constitutes a major part of each of the fifty state budgets. States have invested heavily in their mental institutions, and with reduction of public inpatients many states significantly have improved their hospitals and treatment and rehabilitation programs. The vast majority of seriously mentally ill are in the community, but most states continue to be focused institutionally because of their commitments to maintain hospital improvements in a context of increased court scrutiny, because of the pressures of hospital employees and communities that depend on the financing of hospitals, and because states are reluctant to take on large, new community obligations within a context of fiscal constraint. In 1981 two-thirds of state expenditures continued to support state hospitals although the proportion varied from more than 90 percent in such states as Georgia, Iowa, and Mississippi, to a minority of expenditures in California and Wisconsin (National Institute of Mental Health, 1985). In the latter instances, there are strong state incentives for local government to seek alternatives to inpatient care. In Wisconsin, mental health financing encourages managed care and tradeoffs between community and inpatient care (Stein and Ganser, 1983).

The problem of getting services to follow the patient is inherently more difficult in states having well-established hospital systems, communities economically dependent on hospitals, and well-organized and unionized employees. Such systems require transition strategies that allow funds to follow the patient on a graduated basis, that guarantee the stability of the hospital system over some period of time, and that facilitate working closely with unions and employees in programs of scheduled attrition and retraining to the extent that is feasible. Concomitantly, structures need to be developed for diversion of inappropriate admissions to community programs and for intensive discharge planning commencing soon after a patient is admitted to a state hospital.

Because of the barriers in many states to a community-based system, phasing in such programs may initially require enhanced funding to build community care structures while maintaining some redundant hospital support. To the extent that such financing allows the initiation of a more rational financial process, it is a wise long-term investment, although it may require considerable persuasion before state legislatures, facing resource constraints, see the wisdom of this course.

At the federal level, the two major welfare changes that affected mental health were the Medicaid program and the expansion of disability coverage. Disability coverage had the dual function of providing community subsistence but also automatically including recipients under public health insurance programs. These supports are vital to the future of the public mental health system. Unfortunately, those who made policy in these areas have little awareness or knowledge of serious mental illness, and the impact of these initiatives on the mentally ill is a by-product of other health policy concerns. The mental health sector has not related meaningfully to the formulation of many of these important policies and their administrative implementation.

Improving disability determination. The disability program, as it affects the mentally ill, is instructive. Based on a concept of permanent and total disability, eligibility criteria are believed to reinforce a sense of personal defeat and to be a disincentive to rehabilitation. Many mental health professionals feel ambivalent in encouraging clients to enter the disability system. Viable community care, however, depends on such support since many severely mentally ill cannot maintain employment, or are too disoriented, or behave too bizarrely to be acceptable to employers. By the mid–1970s there had been a major expansion of numbers of disabled persons receiving disability insurance, among whom the mentally ill were a major subgroup. The growth in these costs led to the 1980 amendments to the Social Security Act in which Congress required the review of all awards at least every three years. These reviews resulted in the loss of benefits among large numbers of the severely mentally ill and, subsequently, to much litigation in the federal courts. It became apparent that the application of existing disability criteria seriously underestimated the incapacities of many chronic patients to work in a sustained way, and stripped significant numbers of their benefits. Subsequently, new psychiatric criteria based on an integrated functional assessment were developed that have supported the reinstatement of many patients excised from the disability roll.

Disability determinations require considerable discretion on the part of the Social Security Administration (SSA), and success in gaining eligibility depends in no small way on how the claim is constructed, how appropriate medical and psychiatric information is obtained, and how persistent the potential recipient is. There are several levels of review, and administrative law judges (ALJs) who hear appeals for the SSA reverse denials in approximately half of the cases they review (Mashaw, 1983). Seriously mentally ill persons often have difficulty making an appropriate application for disability, presenting their needs in a way that increases probable success, or understanding their options when faced with denial. Because of the large numbers of mentally ill denied benefits in recent years, mental health workers and other advocates have taken an aggressive role in pursuing appeals at both the ALJ level and in the federal courts.

Expeditious attainment of disability benefits is important in order to stabilize the chronic patients' life situations and plan appropriate care. Barriers include the common delays in awarding benefits and the contradictory eligibility criteria for such benefits and access to vocational rehabilitation services. We need a better way of providing the chronic patient essential subsistence so as not to discourage rehabilitation. In some localities, mental health personnel and state agencies administering disability determinations have government workers located in mental health service facilities to make the disability filing process more simple and accessible. But if the potential of this system is to be better realized, the disability system must be linked to stronger incentives for rehabilitation.

This requires reconciling contradictory assumptions and eligibility requirements in these program areas.

The need for Medicaid reform. The key to effective community care systems is reimbursement and the financial incentives that shape service provision. The Medicaid program is vital to the long-term mentally ill, the vast majority of whom are poor and depend on the public system. It constitutes the largest potential source of federal funding for reconstituting our system of public mental health care. Medicaid accounted for expenditures of $991 million in state and county mental hospitals in 1983 (Redick et al., 1986), primarily for the population under the age of twenty-one and over the age of sixty-four. In 1980 Medicaid was the expected principal source of payment for 1.9 million inpatient days in nonfederal general hospitals and private psychiatric hospitals (estimated from National Institute of Mental Health, 1985: 46). Because of the fragmentation of service organizations, in the typical system of community services there is little ability to track mentally ill clients. The chronic patients having an exacerbation of symptoms come in or are brought to emergency rooms where they are seen by physicians unfamiliar with them, and who choose hospitalization because of the insecurities that uncertainty provokes. In a well-organized community program many of these admissions could be prevented and the patient referred to more appropriate care. About two-thirds of Medicaid mental-illness bed days relate to the chronic population; more effective use of these expenditures could contribute much to revitalizing public mental health services.

Reforming Medicaid in this context is particularly complex in light of the wide range of mental health benefits across states. Several short-term options can be pursued, however. Demonstrations are now being planned that facilitate the pooling of expected inpatient and outpatient Medicaid contributions under the control of a single public entity that establishes systems of managed care for a defined population of public patients. Waivers will not only permit the responsible entity to balance community and outpatient care, and psychiatric and social service, but, even more important, could allow a sufficient resource base to construct the necessary components of service into a system. There are technical barriers involving assessing and sharing risk, and arriving at a realistic basis for estimating federal contributions, particularly in the present context where many patients are not receiving even minimal services. Such an approach, however, offers a strategy for a coherent way of managing one of the most difficult and disorganized arenas of care for seriously impaired persons.

Managing Care for the Severely Mentally Ill

Effective community care for the most seriously disabled patients requires performance of many of the same functions as the mental hospital, ranging from assuring appropriate shelter to managing serious medical and psychiatric problems. To do so in the community context requires some influence over areas of responsibility involving different sectors (housing, medical care, social services, welfare) and varying levels of government. To re-create these functions outside the hospital without the control over resources that hospitals typically have is a formidable challenge and one that has to be assessed in relation to the political culture and legal and professional environments of varying localities. Performance of the task requires a sense of mission, clear definition of responsibility, and an understanding of the longitudinal challenge. The system is overwhelmed by difficult patients who need long-term management and persistent efforts for modest results. The responsible organization must have the financial and organizational capacity to provide the necessary services directly or through contract. Especially difficult areas include housing and case management. Each deserves some discussion.

The problem of housing. The homeless have become a growing problem in our nation's large cities. Estimates of the size of the population vary a great deal, with a range from a quarter of a million to three million. Among the explanations suggested for the increased homeless population are a changing employment market and increased joblessness, the loss of low-rent housing in cities with conversion of housing stock, redevelopment and gentrification in inner-city neighborhoods, the erosion of the safety net for the poverty population, and the deinstitutionalization of the mentally ill. Many of the homeless have profound mental health needs, but the notion that deinstitutionalization caused homelessness is a gross misconception. Individual studies differ in criteria for judging mental illness among the homeless, but existing evidence suggests that as many as one-third to two-fifths of the homeless suffer from significant mental impairments, and that this is a population of immense medical and mental health need (Lamb, 1984; Rossi et al., 1987). These problems are exacerbated and, in some cases, may be in consequence of lack of adequate shelter. The homeless mentally ill are simply the most visible of much larger populations that are not only inadequately housed but are not receiving the medical and mental health services they need (Lamb and Grant, 1982). In every large city, local mental health services lack access to housing they require to organize care effectively for the patients they serve. Mental health agencies in large cities control limited housing placements, have only superficial relations with public housing authorities, and almost all report housing needs for the severely mentally ill that substantially exceed availability. In many instances, housing placements constitute as little as 5 to 10 percent of estimated need.

In recent years cities have encountered vigorous resistance to the siting of group facilities for the chronic mental population as well as other stigmatized groups. This has seriously limited the neighborhoods in which group homes can be located, often resulting in concentration of such facilities in marginal and transitional neighborhoods. Many cities have come to see scattered-site housing as a pragmatic response to community concern. They justify this strategy in terms of promoting patient independence, which may be appropriate for some but not many others. Communities need viable plans for developing a range of housing from group homes and supervised apartments to independent living.

There is room for different views on the appropriate mix, but it is unlikely that any limited option could serve a population as heterogeneous as this one.

Housing for the mentally ill, as one component of a much larger housing problem, exemplifies the gap between needs and reality. Housing is an integral part of a coherent community care approach, but while many chronically mentally ill are eligible for housing assistance, they get little attention from city and county housing authorities, who have little understanding of their special needs, and, in any case, face profound problems of identifying available housing stock to meet pressing demands from many groups. Progress in this area depends on enlarged appropriate housing sites and collaboration between the mental health services and public housing authorities. Cooperation makes possible joint ventures and relationships with nonprofit developers to stimulate housing opportunities appropriate to the severely mentally ill. These arrangements can be made more acceptable if the responsible mental health entity provides support services and emergency response systems for landlords. Initiatives for developing housing opportunities within organized mental health systems, as in the recent program by the Robert Wood Johnson Foundation and the U.S. Department of Housing and Urban Development that is discussed below, are a critical need (Aiken, Somers, and Shore, 1986). But in the final analysis, while improvements are possible within current constraints, effective solutions will depend on the willingness of government at all levels to face the crisis in low-income housing and take meaningful steps to remedy the displacement of the poor from housing opportunities in many of our large cities.

Case management. As communities view the challenge of developing appropriate care for the most disabled, they embrace the case management concept. The concept has varied meanings in different contexts, but case management has a long tradition in social work, where the case worker helped identify and mobilize a variety of community services on behalf of a client. Many of the case management approaches used in social work for decades, such as street teams, crisis intervention, and brokering community services, are being adopted particularly in relation to the new young chronic patients and the homeless mentally ill who are less inclined toward traditional service approaches.

Case management is loosely thought of as a solution to a wide variety of difficult problems. But the responsibilities it is expected to bear are alarming in the context of the realities of system disorganization and the types of personnel given these tasks. Thinking about case management in the more restricted medical context, the case manager is the primary care physician who serves as the doctor of first contact, provides the necessary continuing care and supervision, and makes appropriate referral for specialized medical and other services. The integrity of this role requires high-level and broad-scope clinical judgment, linkage with the needed specialized services, and authority with other doctors and professionals and with the patient. What is more important, it requires the authority under reimbursement programs or existing financial arrangements to provide or prescribe necessary services (Lewis, Fein, and Mechanic, 1976).

Case management with the chronically mentally ill population is inherently more complex. It not only requires appreciation of general medical and psychiatric needs and care, but sophistication about such varied issues as housing, disability and welfare benefits, psychosocial rehabilitation, sheltered and competitive work programs, and issues relating to the legal and criminal justice systems. In some systems of care, the case manager functions as a therapist as well as a broker of services; in others the case manager helps define and marshal the necessary services but has no direct therapeutic relation to the client. The scope of case management functions, the typical caseload, the level of expected training and experience, and the authority of the case manager vary enormously both within and among systems of care. Indeed, the concept is used so broadly as to have no specific meaning at all.

While the concept of the case manager has intuitive appeal, it remains unclear whether it is appropriate or realistic to assign such varied and complex functions to individuals in contrast to more complex teams or subsystems of care. First, there must be a clear definition of continuing responsibility; few professionals other than physicians have traditionally taken such roles. Second, given the diverse and complex functions necessary, specialization is more likely to lead to effective service. Third, case management of these patients is clearly a longitudinal process, but the half life of case managers is short, and attrition is high. Case managers typically have neither the training and experience, control over resources, or professional standing to command resources from other organizations or even to be persuasive with them. Thus, case management to be effective must be embedded in an organizational plan that defines clearly who is responsible and accountable for the care of the most highly disabled patients, that has in place the necessary service elements to provide the full spectrum of needed services, and that can coordinate and control diverse resources that flow into the system so that balanced decisions can be made about the expenditure of limited resources.

Organizational Barriers

In the hospital we take shelter, activity, and basic medical supervision for granted, but each poses serious challenges for community programs of care. The closed character of hospitals allows staff to monitor patient activities carefully, to ensure medication regulation and compliance, and to induce appropriate behavior through a system of rewards. In the community, each of these areas becomes problematic and presents organizational challenges. Even approximations of these responsibilities require a level of organization and coordination absent in most community mental health service programs. Scarce resources, fragmentation of funding and service elements, lack of clear definitions of responsibility, and poorly developed career structures for the mental health professions in community care pose significant obstacles.

The absence of a clear focus of responsibility and authority. In most of the nation's urban areas, responsibility for serving the mentally ill is fragmented among varying levels of government and categorical service agencies. There is typically little coordination among governmental sectors and providers of service, resulting in inefficiencies, duplication, poor use of resources, and failure to serve clients in need. Public mental hospital units, funded and administered by the state or county, may be poorly or not at all linked with outpatient psychiatric care or psychosocial services. Admission to and discharge from inpatient units often occurs without relation to an ongoing system of community services, or careful long-term planning of patients' needs. Agencies serving the homeless, the substance abuser, or the retarded maintain separate service systems, making it particularly difficult to help patients with multiple problems, and inpatient care under Medicaid and local medical assistance programs often function independently of outpatient care or psychosocial rehabilitation services in the community.

The precise shape of the necessary administrative structures remains unclear; different structures will fit varying political, legal, and service delivery environments. While establishment of mental health authorities implies centralization, an administrative authority could promote local diversity and program innovation. Concentration, however, can lead to less flexibility, innovation, and public support. In one city, for example, the director of a functioning authority for most of the chronic patients in that community made the strategic decision not to take over a number of smaller agencies serving some of these patients. The rationale was that each of these agencies had an enthusiastic board who served as advocate for improved care and such advocacy outweighed the advantages of his taking direct control over these agencies.

There are a variety of models for nonprofit and public authorities in such areas as transit systems, freeways, and redevelopment efforts (Walsh and Leigland, 1986). Unlike authorities that can raise capital through income-producing potential, the idea of a mental health authority comes closer to state educational authorities intended to operate with more flexibility than typical government bureaucracies. The ideal is not always realized, and these agencies do develop their own bureaucratic cultures.

The relative merits of organizing mental health services through government agencies, special boards designated by statute, nonprofit voluntary groups, or some hybrid of these forms remain unclear. Nor is it obvious to what degree such entities should be direct-service providers as well as planning, financing, and administrative bodies, or whether they should restrict themselves to limited administrative and regulatory functions in relation to contracting agencies. These assessments cannot be made in the abstract but must be weighed in relation to the organization and effectiveness of existing service providers, statutory requirements, and the political culture of the locality. In theory, performance contracting and the competition it implies seem advantageous to publicly organized services, but in practice the funders often become dependent on their contractees and may have few real options (Dorwart, Schlesinger, and Police, 1986).

In 1985 the Robert Wood Johnson Foundation, in collaboration with the U.S. Department of Housing and Urban Development, established a $100 million program for communitywide projects aimed at consolidating and expanding services for the chronically mentally ill. As part of the program the Social Security Administration brings SSA caseworkers into mental health settings to help grantees improve the disability determination process. The program, funds projects in eight of the sixty largest urban centers, seeking to develop mental health authorities, and the projects are expected to provide a wide spectrum of services including health, social services, and housing. The program should provide an excellent opportunity to learn a great deal more about the potentialities and difficulties of organizing and coordinating fragmented services for relatively large populations.

The specific strategy for governance is perhaps less crucial than the message that the mental health public sector is being revitalized. Public mental health services are in low repute among professionals, many patients, and the general public. They have typically become excessively bureaucratic, self-protective, risk-aversive, and have provided little incentive for innovation. Yet, there is little likelihood that the complex needs of the chronic mental patient will be met by the private sector. Public mental health services require greater control over resources and flexibility in operation if they are to engage the attention and energies of outstanding administrators, psychiatrists, and other mental health personnel. By engaging the interest of professional communities, university training programs, and the larger public, the isolation of public-sector services can be reduced. Reasonable career structures for mental health professionals in the public sector can be developed with more opportunity to enhance the professional training and continuing education of those who work in public mental health. But achieving this will require the development of a strong and more independent entity than is now evident in most state mental health systems.

Appropriate Mix of Health Personnel

Psychiatry is one of the few medical specialties anticipated to be in relatively short supply in the future. In recent years we have seen less interest in psychiatry among medical students and residents, and those choosing psychiatric careers are more oriented to biological psychiatry than to community care or rehabilitation. Few psychiatrists seem enthusiastic about working with the chronically mentally ill. Sophisticated drug management is essential for appropriate care of most psychiatric illness and to avoid the dangers of serious side effects associated with psychotropic drugs, but psychiatrists might more realistically function in this area as consultants to practitioners organizing chronic care than as primary caretakers. There clearly seems to be an appropriate role for a new nursing specialty, the psychiatric nurse practitioner.

Psychiatric nurse practitioners can be an invaluable resource in staffing a variety of institutional facilities, outpatient services, and community care programs for the mentally ill (Mechanic, 1982). While psychologists and social workers also have essential roles to play, the appropriately trained nurse practitioner is potentially in a strategic position. Nurses bring to this role a long tradition in socioemotional and supportive aspects of care and some familiarity with medication monitoring and pharmacological issues. Also, nurses are increasingly conversant with behavior modification techniques and supportive group therapies. The close association between nursing and medicine ensures credibility with physicians and patients in the area of medication administration and monitoring, and psychiatric nurse practitioners can also serve as effective "boundary practitioners" for many patients who resist treatment within the psychiatric sector but more readily accept general medical and nursing assistance. A major problem even among chronic patients is their resistance to psychiatric conceptualizations of their distress and behavior. Nurses with enhanced mental health capabilities could play an important leadership role. Since nurse practitioners and nurse specialists have comparable roles in other areas of patient care, the necessary adjustments and role transitions would not be insurmountable.

In reality, nurses and other nonpsychiatric personnel have provided most of the available care for chronic patients. However, their formal training has not fully prepared them for the tasks they perform. The psychiatric nurse practitioner, for example, should receive more intensive training in psychopharmacology and, with improved training, could prescribe a limited range of psychotropic drugs using approved protocols. While this would require legislative changes, nurse practitioners in other areas already have such responsibility and authority, for example, pediatric nurse practitioners. Also, more intensive training should include a broader understanding of the complex range of social programs and financial entitlements that are central to maintaining mental patients in the community. Such nurses, in short, must learn to be effective case managers as part of their role.

MENTAL HEALTH ADVOCACY

The increased involvement of families of the severely mentally ill through the National Alliance for the Mentally Ill and other organizations is leading to a forceful constituency. Severe mental illness constitutes one of the nation's most serious health care problems, but support for appropriate services and research is substantially less than in the case of other categorical disease entities that have had strong, persistent, and effective political constituencies. Mental illness interests have been less persuasive politically for many reasons, but inability to unite their advocacy groups and the reluctance of influential family members to speak openly about the devastating impact of these problems and to lobby have been major deficiencies. With the organization of the alliance and coalition building among varying interest groups, prominent persons more commonly acknowledge mental illness in their families and lobby aggressively for greater government investment in services and mental health research. Health care financing is in substantial part a political activity, and the mentally ill will only get their share when they can use the political process as effectively as those representing cancer, heart disease, and Alzheimer's disease.

Mental illness continues to suffer from discriminatory treatment in public as well as private health insurance. Such programs as Medicare, affecting not only the elderly but also the younger disabled population, have coinsurance and maximum benefit limitations that ration mental health services more than any other care for diseases of comparable magnitude. Medicaid, in many state programs, provides little or no mental health coverage, and even in the most generous states, benefits are relatively limited. Similarly, private health insurance, even in the largest firms, has more limits on coverage for mental conditions than others, and often outpatient benefits involve extremely high coinsurance (Brady, Sharfstein, and Muszynski, 1986). Under nonprofit insurance programs, mentally disabled dependent children may fail to receive coverage comparable to that available to physically disabled dependent children (Rubin, 1987).

An important motive for limits on mental health coverage is cost containment, but this does not explain the special status of mental health benefits. The traditional responsibility of state government, and the deep prejudice toward disorders of the mind, probably play some role, but it is also apparent that major health policymakers know less and care less about mental illness than many other major morbidities. Gaining equity in the current cost-conscious context is difficult, but this could be a continuing point of pressure for mental health advocacy groups.

Insurance reform remains a long-term objective, but a more focused and acute problem is the underfinancing of the public mental health sector. Most chronic mental patients inevitably end up in the public sector when personal resources are depleted and limited insurance coverage, if there is any, is exhausted. These patients depend, thus, on the generosity of state and local mental health funding, and the quality of Medicaid coverage. The federal government has removed itself from the mental health services arena, arguing it is a state responsibility. Perhaps the most likely route to federal assistance will come as greater pressures build to seek federal relief for the growing uninsured population that now numbers 37 million people. Addressing needs of the chronic patient thus inevitably requires forceful advocacy, close attention to the organization of public-sector services and public financing, more generally, and opportunities to build coalitions with other interested constituencies.

CONCLUSION

The problems commonly attributed to deinstitutionalization are more complex than the debate suggests, reflecting important changes in the nation's demography, concepts of civil liberties, social welfare, and in financing and providing medical services more generally. Ample evidence exists that structures can be developed to provide appropriate community care for most mental patients (Stein and Test, 1980a, 1980b; Falloon et al., 1984, 1985; New South Wales, Department of Health, 1983; Kiesler and Sibulkin, 1987; Leff et al., 1982). Success of important components of essential programs has been demonstrated in many settings (Fairweather et al., 1969; Stein and Test, 1978; Tessler and Goldman, 1982), but they rarely all come together in a single community. An effectively constituted public entity with the ability to direct substantial resources would allow linking components essential for maintenance of function and rehabilitation into a responsible alternative to long-term or episodic hospital care. The approach is a logical one, especially in light of contemporary cost-containment pressures on the health care system as a whole and in a context of tightening eligibility within many categorical programs on which the chronic patient depends. The course is not fully clear, and there is much uncertainty about the future. Existing evidence and experience suggest, however, that we have the capacity to do far more than at present, even within the limited means available.

ACKNOWLEDGMENTS

This chapter incorporates material by the author that previously appeared in the following articles: "Mental Health and Social Policy: Initiatives for the 1980s," *Health Affairs* (1985) 4: 75–88 (Copyright © 1985 by David Mechanic); "The Challenge of Chronic Mental Illness: A Retrospective and Prospective View," *Hospital and Community Psychiatry* (1986) 37: 891–896; and "Correcting Misconceptions in Mental Health Policy: Strategies for Improved Care of the Seriously Mentally Ill," *Milbank Quarterly* (1987) 65: 203–228. Permission to reprint was received from the publishers, *Health Affairs, Hospital and Community Psychiatry*, and the Milbank Memorial Fund.

REFERENCES

Aiken, L. H., Somers, S. A., and Shore, M. F. 1986. Private Foundations in Health Affairs: A Case Study of the Development of a National Initiative for the Chronically Mentally Ill. *American Psychologist* 41: 1290–1295.

Bachrach, L. L., 1976. *Deinstitutionalization: An Analytical Review and Sociological Perspective*. DHEW Publication No. (ADM) 76–351. Washington, D.C.: U.S. Government Printing Office.

Bleuler, M. 1978. *The Schizophrenic Disorders: Long-term Patient and Family Studies*. New Haven: Yale University Press.

Bockoven, J. S. 1972. *Moral Treatment in Community Mental Health*. New York: Springer.

Brady, J., Sharfstein, S. S., and Muszynski, I. L., Jr. 1986. Trends in Private Insurance Coverage for Mental Illness. *American Journal of Psychiatry* 143: 1276–1279.

Brown, G. W., Birley, J.L.T., and Wing, J. K. 1972. Influence of Family Life on the Course of Schizophrenic Disorders: A Replication. *British Journal of Psychiatry* 121: 241–258.

Brown, G. W., Monck, E. M., Carstairs, G. M., and Wing, J. K. 1972. Influence of Family Life on the Course of Schizophrenic Disorders: A Replication. *British Journal of Psychiatry* 121: 55–58.

Caplan, G. 1964. *Principles of Preventive Psychiatry*. New York: Basic Books.

Ciompi, L. 1980. Natural History of Schizophrenia in the Long Term. *British Journal of Psychiatry* 136: 413–420.

Clausen, J. A., Pfeffer, N. A., and Huffine, C. L. 1982. Help-seeking in Severe Mental Illness. In *Symptoms, Illness Behavior, and Help-Seeking*, ed. D. Mechanic. New Brunswick: Rutgers University Press.

Davis, A., Pasamanick, B., and Dinitz, S. 1974. *Schizophrenics in the New Custodial Community: Five Years after the Experiment*. Columbus: Ohio State University Press.

Dennison, C. F. 1985. *1984 Summary: National Discharge Survey*. Vital and Health Statistics 112. Hyattsville, Md.: National Center for Health Statistics.

Dolan, L. W. 1986. *Recent Trends in the Evolution of State Psychiatric Hospital Systems*. New Brunswick: Rutgers-Princeton Program in Mental Health Research.

Dorwart, R. A., Schlesinger, M., and Police, R. T. 1986. The Promise and Pitfalls of Purchase-of-Service Contracts. *Hospital and Community Psychiatry* 37: 875–878.

Ennis, B. 1972. *Prisoners of Psychiatry: Mental Patients, Psychiatrists, and the Law*. New York: Harcourt Brace Jovanovich.

Estroff, S. 1981. *Making It Crazy: An Ethnography of Psychiatric Clients in an American Community*. Berkeley: University of California Press.

Fairweather, G. W. 1978. The Development, Evaluation, and Diffusion of Rehabilitative Programs: A Social Change Process. In *Alternatives to Mental Hospital Treatment*, eds. L. I. Stein and M. A. Test. New York: Plenum.

Fairweather, G. W., Sanders, D. H., Maynard, H., and Cressler, D. L. 1969. *Community Life for the Mentally Ill: An Alternative to Institutional Care*. Chicago: Aldine.

Falloon, I.R.H., Boyd, J. L., McGill, C. W., Williamson, M., Razoni, J., Moss, H. B., Gilderman, A. M., and Simpson, G. M. 1982. Family Management in the Prevention of Exacerbations of Schizophrenia: A Controlled Study. *New England Journal of Medicine* 306: 1437–1440.

Falloon, I.R.H., Boyd, J. L., McGill, C. W., Williamson, M., Razoni, J., Moss, H. B., Gilderman, A. M., and Simpson, G. M. 1984. *Family Care of Schizophrenia*. New York: Guilford Press.

Falloon, I.R.H., Boyd, J. L., McGill, C. W., Williamson, M., Razoni, J., Moss, H. B., Gilderman, A. M., and Simpson, G. M. 1985. Family Management in the Prevention of Morbidity of Schizophrenia: Clinical Outcomes of a Two-year Study. *Archives of General Psychiatry* 42: 887–896.

Goffman, E. 1961. *Asylums: Essays on the Social Situation of Mental Patients and Other Inmates*. New York: Doubleday.

Goldman, H. H., Feder, J., and Scanlon, W. 1986. Chronic Mental Patients in Nursing Homes: Re-examining Data from the National Nursing Home Survey. *Hospital and Community Psychiatry* 37: 269–272.

Goldman, H. H., Gattozzi, A. A., and Taube, C. A. 1981. Defining and Counting the Chronically Mentally Ill. *Hospital and Community Psychiatry* 32: 21–27.

Greenley, J. R. 1972. The Psychiatric Patient's Family and Length of Hospitalization. *Journal of Health and Social Behavior* 13: 25–37.

Grob, G. N. 1983. *Mental Illness and American Society: 1875–1940*. Princeton, N.J.: Princeton University Press.

Grob, G. N. 1987. The Forging of Mental Health Policy in America: World War II to New Frontier. *Journal of the History of Medicine and Allied Sciences* 42: 410–446.

Gronfein, W. 1984. Rhetoric and Reality in Mental Health Policy: The Case of the State Hospitals. New Brunswick: Rutgers-Princeton Program in Mental Health Research.

Gronfein, W. 1985. Incentives and Intentions in Mental Health Policy: A Comparison of the Medicaid and Community Mental Health Programs. *Journal of Health and Social Behavior* 26: 192–206.

Gudeman, J. E., and Shore, M. F. 1984. Beyond Deinstitutionalization: A New Class of Facilities for the Mentally Ill. *New England Journal of Medicine* 311: 832–836.

Harding, C. M., Brooks, G. W., Ashikaga, T., Strauss, J. S., and Breier, A. 1986. *The Vermont Longitudinal Study, II: Long Term Outcome for DSM-III Schizophrenia.* New Haven: Department of Psychiatry, Yale University School of Medicine.

Huber, G., Gross, G., and Scheuttler, R. 1979. *Schizophrenia.* Berlin: Springer.

Kane, J. M., and Smith, J. M. 1982. Tardive Dyskinesia: Prevalence and Risk Factors, 1959–1979. *Archives of General Psychiatry* 39: 473–481.

Kiesler, C. A. 1982. Mental Hospitals and Alternative Care. *American Psychologist* 37: 349–360.

Kiesler, C. A., and Sibulkin, A. E. 1983. Proportion of Inpatient Days for Mental Disorders: 1969–1978. *Hospital and Community Psychiatry* 34: 606–611.

Kiesler, C. A., and Sibulkin, A. E. 1987. *Mental Hospitals: Myths and Facts about a National Crisis.* Beverly Hills: Sage.

Kramer, M. 1977. *Psychiatric Services and the Changing Institutional Scene.* Washington, D.C.: U.S. Department of Health, Education, and Welfare.

Kulka, R. A., Veroff, J., and Douvan, E. 1979. Social Class and the Use of Professional Help for Personal Problems: 1957 and 1976. *Journal of Health and Social Behavior* 20: 2–17.

Lamb, H. R. 1979. The New Asylums in the Community. *Archives of General Psychiatry* 36: 129–134.

Lamb, H. R., ed. 1984. *The Homeless Mentally Ill: A Task Force Report of the American Psychiatric Association.* Washington, D.C.: American Psychiatric Association.

Lamb, H. R., and Grant, R. W. 1982. The Mentally Ill in an Urban County Jail. *Archives of General Psychiatry* 30: 17–22.

Leaf, P., Livingston, M. M., Holzer, E. E., and Myers, J. K. 1985. Contact with Health Professionals for the Treatment of Psychiatric and Emotional Problems. *Medical Care* 23: 1322–1337.

Leff, J., Kuipers, R., Berkowitz, R., Eberlein-Vries, R., and Sturgeon, D. 1982. A Controlled Trial of Social Intervention in the Families of Schizophrenic Patients. *British Journal of Psychiatry* 141: 121–134.

Leighton, A. 1967. Is Social Environment a Cause of Psychiatric Disorder? In *Psychiatric Epidemiology and Mental Health Planning*, eds. R. R. Monoroe, G. D. Klee, and E. B. Brody. Washington, D.C.: American Psychiatric Association.

Lewis, C., Fein, R., and Mechanic, D. 1976. *A Right to Health: The Problem of Access to Primary Medical Care.* New York: Wiley-Interscience.

Linn, M. W., Gurel, L., Williford, W. O, Overall, J., Gurland, B., Laughlin, P., and Barchiesi, A. 1985. Nursing Home Care as an Alternative to Psychiatric Hospitalization. *Archives of General Psychiatry* 42: 544–551.

Mashaw, J. L. 1983. *Bureaucratic Justice: Managing Social Security Disability Claims.* New Haven: Yale University Press.

Mechanic, D. 1979. *Future Issues in Health Care: Social Policy and the Rationing of Medical Services*. New York: Free Press.

Mechanic, D. 1980. *Mental Health and Social Policy*. 2nd ed. Englewood Cliffs, N.J.: Prentice-Hall.

Mechanic, D. 1982. Nursing and Mental Health Care: Expanding Future Possibilities for Nursing Services. In *Nursing in the 1980s—Crises, Opportunities, Challenges*, ed. L. Aiken. Philadelphia: Lippincott.

Mechanic, D. 1985. Mental Health and Social Policy: Initiatives for the 1980s. *Health Affairs* 4: 75–88.

Miller, K. S. 1976. *Managing Madness: The Case against Civil Commitment*. New York: Free Press.

National Institute of Mental Health. 1985. *Mental Health, United States, 1985*. DHHS Publication No. (ADM) 85–1378. Washington, D.C.: U.S. Government Printing Office.

New South Wales, Department of Health. 1983. *Psychiatric Hospital Versus Community Treatment: A Controlled Study*. Sydney.

Pasamanick, B., Scarpitti, F. F., and Dinitz, F. R. 1967. *Schizophrenics in the Community: An Experimental Study in the Prevention of Hospitalization*. New York: Appleton-Century-Crofts.

Polak, P. 1978. A Comprehensive System of Alternatives to Psychiatric Hospitalization. In *Alternatives to Mental Hospital Treatment*, eds. L. I. Stein and M. A. Test. New York: Plenum.

President's Commission on Mental Health. 1978. *Report of the Task Force on the Nature and Scope of the Problems*, Vol. 2. Washington, D.C.: U. S Government Printing Office.

Redick, R. W., Witkin, M. J., Atay, J. E., and Manderscheid, R. W. 1986. *Specialty Mental Health Organizations, United States, 1983–84*. Rockville, Md.: National Institute of Mental Health.

Robins, L. N., Helzer, J. E., Weissman, M. M., Orvaschel, H., Gruenberg, E., Burke, J. D., Jr., and Regier, D. A. 1984. Lifetime Prevalence of Specific Psychiatric Disorders in Three Sites. *Archives of General Psychiatry* 41: 949–958.

Rossi, P. H., Wright, J. D., Fisher, G. A., and Willis, G. 1987. The Urban Homeless: Estimating Composition and Size. *Science* 235: 1336–1341.

Rubin, J. 1987. Mental Illness and Discrimination in Insurance Coverage. In *Advances in Health Economics and Health Service Research*, eds. T. McGuire and R. Scheffler. Greenwich, Conn.: JAI Press.

Schwartz, G., and Goldfinger, S. 1981. The New Chronic Patient: Clinical Characteristics of an Emerging Subgroup. *Hospital and Community Psychiatry* 32: 470–474.

Scull, A. 1977. *Decarceration: Community Treatment and the Deviant*. Englewood Cliffs, N.J.: Prentice-Hall.

Segal, S. P., and Aviram, U. 1978. *The Mentally Ill in Community-Based Sheltered Care: A Study of Community Care and Social Integration*. New York: Wiley-Interscience.

Shapiro, S., Skinner, E. A., Kramer, M., Steinwachs, D. M., and Regier, D. A. 1984. Measuring Need for Mental Health Services in a General Population. *Medical Care* 23: 1033–1043.

Sheets, J., Prevost, J., and Reihman, J. 1982. Young Adult Chronic Patients: Three Hypothesized Sub-groups. *Hospital and Community Psychiatry* 33: 197–202.

Shepherd, G. 1984. *Institutional Care and Rehabilitation*. New York: Longman.
Stein, L. I., and Ganser, L. J. 1983. Wisconsin's System for Funding Mental Health Services. In Unified Mental Health Systems: Utopia Unrealized, ed. J. Talbott. *New Directions for Mental Health Services*, No. 18. San Francisco: Jossey-Bass.
Stein, L. I., and Test, M. A., eds. 1978. *Alternatives to Mental Hospital Treatment*. New York: Plenum.
Stein, L. I., and Test, M. A., eds. 1980a. Alternatives to Mental Hospital Treatment, I: Conceptual Model Treatment Program and Clinical Evaluation. *Archives of General Psychiatry* 37: 392–397.
Stein, L. I., and Test, M. A., eds. 1980b. Alternatives to Mental Hospital Treatment, III: Social Cost. *Archives of General Psychiatry* 37: 409–412.
Stotsky, B. A. 1970. *The Nursing Home and the Aged Psychiatric Patient*. New York: Appleton-Century-Crofts.
Szasz, T. S. 1963. *Law, Liberty, and Psychiatry: An Inquiry into the Social Uses of Mental Health Practices*. New York: Macmillan.
Talbott, J. A. 1985. The Fate of the Public Psychiatric System. *Hospital and Community Psychiatry* 36: 46–50.
Taube, C., Kessler, L., and Feuerberg, M. 1984. Utilization and Expenditures for Ambulatory Medical Care during 1980. *National Medical Care Utilization and Expenditure Survey Data Report 5*. Washington, D.C.: U.S. Department of Health and Human Services.
Tessler, R., and Goldman, H. 1982. *The Chronically Mentally Ill: Assessing Community Support Programs*. Cambridge, Mass.: Ballinger.
Turner, J., and Tenhoor, W. J. 1978. The NIMH Community Support Program: Pilot Approach to a Needed Social Reform. *Schizophrenia Bulletin* 4: 319–344.
U.S. Department of Health and Human Services. 1983. *Health, United States*. Hyattsville, Md.: National Center for Health Statistics.
Vaughn, E. E., and Leff, J. P. 1976. The Influence of Family and Social Factors on the Course of Psychiatric Illness: A Comparison of Schizophrenic and Depressed Neurotic Patients. *British Journal of Psychiatry* 129: 125–137.
Vladeck, B. 1980. *Unloving Care: The Nursing Home Tragedy*. New York: Basic Books.
Walsh, A., and Leigland, J. 1986. *Public Authorities for Mental Health Programs*. Washington, D.C.: Institute for Public Administration.
Watts, F. N., and Bennett, D. H., eds. 1983. *Theory and Practice of Psychiatric Rehabilitation*. New York: Wiley.
Weisbrod, B. A., Test, M. A., and Stein, L. I. 1980. Alternatives to Mental Hospital Treatment, II: Economic Benefit-Cost Analysis. *Archives of General Psychiatry* 37: 400–402.
Wing, J. K. 1978. *Reasoning about Madness*. Oxford: Oxford University Press.
Wing, J. K., and Brown, G. W. 1970. *Institutionalism and Schizophrenia: A Comparative Study of Three Mental Hospitals, 1960–1968*. Cambridge: Cambridge University Press.

A Guide to Sources

Following each chapter in this volume is an extensive list of scholarly sources relevant to the specialized subject matter of that chapter. No attempt will be made here to review this large body of multidisciplinary literature. Instead, the purpose of this bibliographic essay is to provide a brief guide to important generalist works of mental health policy analysis.

There are a number of books that examine mental health policy developments in the post–World War II period. Henry A. Foley and Steven S. Sharfstein's *Madness and Government: Who Cares for the Mentally Ill?* (Washington, D.C.: American Psychiatric Press, 1983) describes the enactment and implementation of the national community mental health centers program. Both authors are former federal administrators, and their stated intent, following cuts in mental health programs by the Reagan administration, is to advocate on behalf of a stronger involvement by the national government. Murray Levine's *The History and Politics of Community Mental Health* (New York: Oxford University Press, 1981) deals with much the same material at somewhat greater length and with an added emphasis on legal issues. In *Community Mental Health: A General Introduction* (Monterey, Calif.: Brooks/Cole, 1977), Bernard L. Bloom also traces the legislative history of the community mental health movement preliminary to considering such concepts as preventive services, crisis intervention, and community needs assessment. Both the books by Bloom and by Foley and

Sharfstein include useful appendix sections reprinting primary government documents—special presidential messages and pieces of legislation—pertinent to national mental health policy.

An erudite work that draws simultaneously on the perspectives of public policy analysis and medical sociology is David Mechanic's *Mental Health and Social Policy*, 3rd ed. (Englewood Cliffs, N.J.: Prentice-Hall, 1989). Philip K. Armour's *The Cycles of Social Reform: Mental Health Policy Making in the United States, England, and Sweden* (Washington, D.C.: University Press of America, 1981) takes a sociological and comparative perspective on mental health reform movements. Three edited volumes—Saul Feldman's *The Administration of Mental Health Services*, 2nd ed. (Springfield, Ill.: Charles C. Thomas, 1980); Stuart E. Golann and Carl Eisdorfer's *Handbook of Community Mental Health* (New York: Appleton-Century-Crofts, 1972); and Herbert C. Schulberg and Marie Killilea's *The Modern Practice of Community Mental Health* (San Francisco, Calif.: Jossey-Bass, 1982)—all contain useful descriptive and analytic material on the national community mental health program, among many other topics covered.

Too numerous to enumerate exhaustively here, the periodical literature also includes many noteworthy contributions to our understanding of community mental health and deinstitutionalization as public policies. See, especially, Ellen L. Bassuk and Samuel Gerson, "Deinstitutionalization and Mental Health Services," *Scientific American* 238 (February 1978): 46–53; Richard Rumer, "Community Mental Health Centers: Politics and Therapy," *Journal of Health Politics, Policy and Law* 2 (Winter 1978): 531–559; and Mary R. Merwin and Frank M. Ochberg, "The Long Voyage: Policies for Progress in Mental Health," *Health Affairs* 2 (Winter 1983): 96–127. The fall 1979 issue of *Milbank Memorial Fund Quarterly* (vol. 57) is devoted in its entirety to the subject of deinstitutionalization in the United States and Great Britain and contains several thoughtful papers. A revealing empirical analysis of the impact of federal policy on deinstitutionalization patterns in the states is provided by William Gronfein in "Incentives and Intentions in Mental Health Policy: A Comparison of the Medicaid and Community Mental Health Programs," *Journal of Health and Social Behavior* 26 (September 1985): 192–206. Contrary to conventional wisdom, Gronfein finds that the former program, while not primarily a mental health initiative, has been the more influential.

Several books address America's community mental health policy in the context of a larger theoretical framework. A progressive, or mainstream liberal, approach is found in Henry A. Foley's *Community Mental Health Legislation: The Formative Process* (Lexington, Mass.: D.C. Heath, 1975), which emphasizes the "oligopolistic" leadership role and humanitarian intent of an elite cadre of federal officials, congressmen, and activist reformers. Revisionist interpretations have been offered by scholars writing within a neo-Marxist political-economy tradition. Important works of this genre, which address the interaction between mental health programs and capitalist institutions and market processes, include Phil Brown's *The Transfer of Care: Psychiatric Deinstitutionalization and Its Aftermath* (London: Routledge & Kegan Paul, 1985), and Andrew Scull's *Decarceration: Community Treatment and the Deviant—A Radical View*, 2nd ed. (New Brunswick, N.J.: Rutgers University Press, 1984). David Ingleby's edited volume, *Critical Psychiatry: The Politics of Mental Health* (New York: Pantheon Books, 1980), presents a similar perspective but makes greater use of psychological concepts and includes case studies of selected Western nations in addition to the United States. For an alternative view that emphasizes the formative impact of shifting social attitudes and beliefs on policymaking for mental health and other social welfare problems, see David A. Rochefort, *American Social Welfare Policy: Dynamics of Formulation and Change* (Boulder, Colo.: Westview Press, 1986). Paul Lerman's *Deinstitutionalization and the Welfare State* (New Brunswick, N.J.: Rutgers University Press, 1982) presents a valuable cross-problem analysis of deinstitutionalization trends in mental health and other policy areas such as delinquency and developmental disability, relating them all to the expansion of the modern American welfare state.

The bulk of the work cited above represents the contributions of sociologists, psychiatrists, psychologists, and social work scholars. Given the close relationship between the discipline of political science and the field of policy studies generally, surprisingly few political scientists have been drawn to mental health policy analysis. A notable exception not yet mentioned is Eugene Bardach, whose *The Skill Factor in Politics: Repealing the Mental Commitment Laws in California* (Berkeley, Calif.: University of California Press, 1972) provides a detailed account of mental health politics in California that led to the passage of the influential Lanterman-Petris-Short Act in 1967. A second book by the same author, *The Implementation Game: What Happens After a Bill Becomes a Law* (Cambridge, Mass.: The MIT Press, 1977), analyzes problems that occurred when officials and administrators undertook to put this California law into effect. Important insights are generated into both the operation of local mental health programs and the theoretical study of public policy implementation. Although quite dated now, two other works focusing on the political process of mental health policymaking are *The Politics of Mental Health* (New York: Columbia University Press, 1968) by Robert H. Connery and associates, and *Mental Health and Retardation Politics: The Mind Lobbies in Congress* (New York: Praeger, 1975) by Daniel A. Felicetti. A real need exists for in-depth research of this kind into national and state mental health politics during the decade of the 1980s, a period of new interest-group formations and intergovernmental relations.

Mental health was also formerly a neglected area of historical writing, but a flurry of scholarly works in the past couple of decades have dramatically altered this situation. Albert Deutsch's *The Mentally Ill in America*, 2nd ed. (New York: Columbia University Press, 1949) predates this movement and helped stimulate it. Deutsch, a journalist by profession, sometimes verges on sensationalism in addressing the mental health system's abuses, while he is insufficiently critical of the record of American mental health reform and the activities of psychiatric professionals. Nonetheless, impressive in scope and learning, Deutsch's work is generally regarded as a classic. Norman Dain's *Concepts of Insanity in the United States, 1789–1865* (New Brunswick, N.J.: Rutgers University Press, 1964) was among the first of a collection of more analytically sophisticated monographs produced by professional historians. Dain later published a biography of National Committee for Mental Hygiene founder Clifford Beers— *Clifford W. Beers: Advocate for the Insane* (Pittsburgh: University of Pittsburgh Press, 1980)—that carefully sets out the social context in which the mental hygiene movement took root. David J. Rothman traces the development of American mental health policies and practices up to the Progressive era in two volumes, *The Discovery of the Asylum: Social Order and Disorder in the New Republic* (Boston: Little, Brown, 1971) and *Conscience and Convenience: The Asylum and Its Alternatives in Progressive America* (Boston: Little, Brown, 1980). Rothman's attempt to relate mental health policy developments with concurrent public action against such problems as poverty and juvenile delinquency yields engaging historical interpretations, yet it diffuses somewhat the treatment given to mental health issues and their sources and implications.

Preeminent among historians of U.S. mental health policy is Gerald N. Grob, whose first study, *The State and the Mentally Ill: A History of Worcester State Hospital in Massachusetts, 1830–1920* (Chapel Hill, N.C.: University of North Carolina Press, 1966), looked at changing features of public mental health care over the nineteenth century as reflected in one vanguard state institution. Grob subsequently turned his attention to a broad-ranging three-volume history of American mental health care of which the first two volumes have now been published, entitled *Mental Institutions in America: Social Policy to 1875* (New York: The Free Press, 1973), and *Mental Illness and American Society, 1875– 1940* (Princeton, N.J.: Princeton University Press, 1983). Widely praised as models of careful historical scholarship, both books are invaluable sources for persons interested in this topic. Other recent historical studies that merit mention include Richard W. Fox, *So Far Disordered in Mind: Insanity in California, 1870–1930* (Berkeley, Calif.: University of California Press, 1979); Leland V. Bell, *Treating the Mentally Ill: From Colonial Times to the Present* (New York: Praeger, 1980); Nancy J. Tomes, *A Generous Confidence: Thomas Story Kirkbride and the Art of Asylum Building, 1840–1883* (Cambridge: Cambridge University Press, 1984); Elliot S. Valenstein, *Great and Desperate Cures: The Rise and Decline of Psychosurgery and Other Radical Treatments for Mental Illness* (New York: Basic Books, 1986); and Mary Ann Jimenez, *Changing Faces of Madness: Early American Attitudes and Treatment of the Insane* (Hanover, N. H.: University Press of New England, 1987).

A recent handful of edited volumes help to illuminate the myriad issues that surround the organization and financing of services within the contemporary mental health system. Though repetitious in places, W. Richard Scott and Bruce L. Black's *The Organization of Mental Health Services: Societal and Community Systems* (Beverly Hills, Calif.: Sage, 1986) does a good job of examining service coordination problems. David Mechanic's *Improving Mental Health Services: What the Social Sciences Can Tell Us, New Directions for Mental Health Services*, No. 36 (San Francisco, Jossey-Bass, 1987) concentrates attention on the chronically mentally ill and the service delivery problems they experience, as well as related legal and policy issues. A special issue of the journal *American Behavioral Scientist* [30 (November/December 1986)], edited by Robert F. Rich, is concerned with recent trends toward administrative decentralization and growing state influence in U.S. mental health policy. More general in focus though far from comprehensive are Morton O. Wagenfeld, Paul V. Lemkau, and Blair Justice (eds.), *Public Mental Health: Perspectives and Prospects* (Beverly Hills, Calif.: Sage, 1982); and Leonard J. Duhl and Nicholas A. Cummings (eds.), *The Future of Mental Health Services: Coping with Crisis* (New York: Springer, 1987).

The best summary of statistical information and analysis concerning mental hospitals in the contemporary era is Charles A. Kiesler and Amy Sibulkin's *Mental Hospitalization: Myths and Facts about a National Crisis* (Newbury Park, Calif.: Sage, 1987). Originally prepared as a report for the U.S. Office of Technology and Assessment, Leonard Saxe and associates' *Children's Mental Health: Problems and Services* (Durham, N.C.: Duke University Press, 1987) is a concise yet fairly encompassing investigation of children's mental health needs. The phenomenon of homelessness, while certainly more than just a problem affecting mentally ill persons, has become a powerful symbol for the shortcomings of the contemporary deinstitutionalization movement. For analysis and commentary on this subject, see E. Fuller Torrey, *Nowhere to Go: The Tragic Odyssey of the Homeless Mentally Ill* (New York: Harper & Row, 1988); H. R. Lamb (ed.), *The Homeless Mentally Ill* (Washington, D.C.: American Psychiatric Press, 1984); and Michael J. Dear and Jennifer R. Wolch, *Landscapes of Despair: From Deinstitutionalization to Homelessness* (Princeton, N.J.: Princeton University Press, 1987).

Finally, a refreshing nonacademic treatment of the subject of chronic mental illness and the challenges it poses for service system development is Susan Sheehan's *Is There No Place on Earth for Me?* (Boston: Houghton Mifflin, 1982). Sheehan, a gifted journalist, carefully relates the life story of one chronically schizophrenic patient she calls "Sylvia Frumkin." The book, which won the Pulitzer Prize, succeeds so well because it tells a richly detailed personal story while also managing to incorporate statistics and scholarly research and theories pertinent to modern psychiatric practice and policy. A perceptive analysis of the book with special attention to its lessons for mental health policymakers is found in Ann E. Moran, Ruth I. Freedman, and Steven S. Sharfstein, "The Journey of Sylvia Frumkin: A Case Study for Policymakers," *Hospital and Community Psychiatry* 35 (September 1984): 887–893.

Author Index

Abbott, E. S., 106
Abramson, L. N., 55
Abt Associates, 198, 205, 211
Acosta, E., 444
Adams, G. L., 137
Adams, N., 316
Advisory Commission on Intergovern-
    mental Relations, 145, 147
Agranoff, R., 145
Ahr, P. R., 158
Aiken, L. H., 12, 14, 167, 493
Alan Guttmacher Institute, 412, 424
Albee, G. G., 403, 406, 426
Albert, M. B., 204
Alford, R., 185
Allen, D. B., 201
Allen, L., 406, 423
Alloy, L., 55
Altman, L., 357, 358
American Bar Association, 372
American Law Institute, 372

American Medical Association, 349
American Psychiatric Association, 46, 51
Andranovich, G., 301
Andreasen, N. C., 55
Anthony, W. A., 248
Appel, J. W., 108
Appelbaum, P. S., 330, 334, 375, 376,
    377, 378, 379
Apsey, M. O., 467
Apte, R. Z., 247
Arce, A., 70
Archer, J., 137, 316
Arey, S. S., 54, 75
Armour, P. K., 174, 175, 176, 178
Ashbaugh, J. W., 67
Astrachan, B. M., 206
Atay, J., 326
Austin, M. J., 163
Aviram, U., 239, 242, 243, 244, 245,
    249, 250, 251, 259, 260, 483
Ayd, F. J., Jr., 111

Babigian, H. M., 136
Bachman, J. G., 417, 420
Bachrach, K. M., 440, 442, 443
Bachrach, L. L., 44, 67, 70, 71, 137,
    200, 238, 274, 295, 311, 321, 329,
    330, 331, 333, 334, 483, 484
Badger, L., 76, 77
Baekeland, F., 201
Bahl, R., 435
Bailey, P., 106
Baker, F., 219, 220
Balch, F., 203, 219
Baldwin, W. H., 425
Bales, J., 378, 379
Ball, F. L. J., 301
Baltes, M. M., 284
Bandy, P., 418, 419
Banziger, G., 281, 443
Bardach, E., 176
Barfield, C. E., 16, 143, 144, 145, 147,
    148
Barker, L. F., 103, 106
Barnes, F. F., 277, 278, 281
Barnett, R. C., 59
Barrett, A. M., 104
Barrett, S. A., 267
Barrow, S., 304, 305
Barter, J., 329, 330
Barth, R. P., 413
Barton, E., 284
Barton, W., 329, 330
Baruch, G. G., 59
Baskett, G. T., 108
Bass, R. D., 136, 197, 199, 200, 203,
    206, 207, 208, 212
Bassuk, E. L., 68, 136, 137, 270, 304,
    307, 316, 388
Baumohl, J., 239, 240, 256, 260
Baxter, E., 305
Bean, L. L., 403
Beard, J. H., 249
Beck, P., 284
Beers, C. W., 105, 178
Beigel, A., 80, 137, 154, 158, 206
Beiser, M., 71
Belknap, I., 109
Bell, L. V., 90, 105, 108
Bell, R. A., 437

Bell, R. Q., 409
Bergner, L. P., 209
Berkman, L. F., 72
Bernstein, J., 219
Berube, M., 183
Beshai, N., 438
Betts, J., 239
Bickel, H., 71
Bigelow, D. A., 218
Bingham, A. T., 106
Blackwell, B., 111
Blain, D., 111
Blaustein, M., 258
Blazer, D., 79, 282
Bleuler, M., 487
Bloom, B. L., 133, 134, 211, 406, 407,
    421, 424, 443
Blout, W. R., 417
Blunt, B. E., 435, 439
Bock, A. V., 107
Bockoven, J. S., 98, 483
Bok, D. C., 381
Bond, E. D., 106, 107
Bonn, E. M., 111
Bonner, B. L., 445
Bonnie, R. J., 369
Bonsteel, R. M., 108
Bootzin, R. R., 271, 273, 278, 279
Borus, J. F., 205
Botvin, G., 419, 420
Boutilier, C., 444
Bovbjerg, R. R., 273
Bowlyow, E., 285
Boyd, J. H., 70
Boydell, K., 443
Braceland, F. J., 108
Bradshaw, J., 436
Brady, J., 351, 352, 479, 498
Braff, J., 373
Brakel, S. J., 363, 380
Brand, J. L., 109
Braun, P., 68, 252
Briggs, L. V., 107
Brill, H., 111
Britt, D. W., 423
Brockway, J. M., 437, 438
Brodsky, G., 218
Bromet, E., 70, 71, 74

Brook, B. D., 254
Brooks, A., 363
Broskowski, A., 163, 164, 213, 467
Brown, B. S., 12, 154, 442, 451
Brown, P., 10, 123, 135, 137, 311, 321
Brown, S., 106
Brownell, A., 57
Buck, J. A., 154, 197
Bucknill, J. C., 100
Burnam, M. A., 77
Burnham, J. C., 103
Burns, J. M., 126
Burt, M. R., 159, 160, 161, 166, 412, 425
Butcher, J. N., 408
Butler, R. N., 286

Caffey, E. M., 245
Cagle, L. T., 437, 440, 441, 443
Cahalan, D., 78, 79
Caldwell, R. A., 408
California Commission on Health and the Economy, 238, 239
Callahan, J. J., Jr., 14, 154
Callahan, L., 371, 372, 373
Cameron, J. M., 127, 136
Campbell, C. M., 104, 106
Cannon, M. S., 198, 200
Caplan, G., 129, 406, 407
Caplan, R., 96, 100, 102, 312
Card, J., 412
Carlson, E. T., 92, 93
Carpenter, E., 466
Carter, D. B., 210, 211
Catalano, R., 60
Caton, C. L. M., 69
Caudill, W., 109
Caulfield, S. C., 244, 250, 255
Cazares, P. R., 210, 211
Center for Health Studies, 202
Chacko, R. J., 137
Chale, M. F., 93
Chandler, M. J., 409
Checker, A., 325, 328
Chelimsky, E., 145
Cheney, C. O., 107
Chidester, L., 108
Chilman, C. S., 425

Chu, F. B., 215, 316, 388
Ciarlo, J. A., 208, 215, 217, 218, 219, 226, 440
Cibulka, J. G., 208
Ciompi, L., 487
Cisin, I., 78, 79
Clarke, G. J., 252
Clausen, J. A., 181, 487
Clauser, S. B., 267, 272
Cleary, P. D., 58, 59, 60
Cloward, R. A., 127
Cobb, R. W., 5
Cockerham, W. C., 35
Cohen, B. F., 248
Cohen, G. D., 283, 348
Cohen, I. M., 111
Cohen, M. R., 248
Cohen, S., 57
Cole, J. O., 225
Collins, C., 357
Community Mental Health Project, 213
Comptroller General of the United States, 208
Conaway, L., 201
Connery, R. H., 12, 123, 130, 154
Cook, E. W., 154, 157, 158, 160, 161, 162, 163, 164
Cook, R., 419
Cook, T. D., 218
Cooper, B., 71
Cornely, P., 74
Costello, E., 75
Coughlin, R. M., 174, 176, 186
Cousineau, M. R., 70
Covington, M. V., 418
Cowen, E. L., 405, 408, 409
Cox, G. B., 217
Craig, T., 329
Crandell, D. L., 51
Crossley, H., 78, 79
Crowell, B. A., 79
Cummings, E., 403
Cunningham, R. J., 103
Cuvelier, F., 246

Dain, N., 91, 93, 95, 105, 314
Daniels, S., 378
Davies, J. D., 95, 107

Davis, C., 218
Davis, M., 348
Dawes, R. M., 217
Day, G., 464
Dear, M., 260
Dembo, R., 417
Dennis, D. L., 296, 298, 321, 334
Deutsch, A., 90, 97, 109, 178, 179, 181
Dewey, R. S., 102
Dickey, B., 15, 17
Dill, A. E. P., 15
Dingman, P., 329, 330
Dinkle, J., 209
Ditmar, N., 245, 258, 279
Dohner, V. A., 419
Dohrenwend, B. P., 48, 49, 50, 51, 53,
    54, 56, 74, 423, 440, 442
Dohrenwend, B. S., 49, 54, 56, 440,
    442
Doidge, J. R., 207
Dolan, L. W., 479
Donovan, E., 136
Dooley, D., 60
Doolittle, F. C., 143, 148, 155, 156, 167
Doris, J., 424
Dorwart, R. A., 495
Douvan, E., 480
Dowell, D., 212, 226
Downs, A., 13
Dressler, W. W., 76, 77
Drude, K., 220, 438, 441
Dubey, S. N., 155, 156, 157, 158, 160
Dubin, W. R., 217
Duhl, L., 129
Dunham, H. W., 49, 54, 242, 443
Dunn, M., 108
Dynes, J. B., 108

Earle, P., 98, 99
Earnest, E., 103
Eaton, L., 93
Eaton, W. W., 54, 70, 409
Eckstein, H., 175
Edwards, D. W., 56, 205, 217, 220
Edwards, L. G., 164
Eggert, G. M., 258
Eisdorfer, C., 283
Elder, C. D., 5

Elliott, D. F., 277
Ellis, R. H., 219
Elpers, J. R., 247, 249, 260, 334
Emch, M., 107
Emerson, R. M., 251
Endicott, J., 46
Ennis, E., 482
Essex, D., 219
Estes, C. L., 161, 162, 163, 164, 166
Estroff, S., 481
Everett, B., 425
Everett, F. L., 445
Eysaman, C. O., 244, 250

Faden, V. B., 208
Fairweather, G. W., 254, 499
Faletti, M. V., 282
Falloon, I. R. H., 483, 499
Faris, R. E. L., 49, 54, 242, 443
Feder, J., 277, 485
Federspiel, C. F., 280
Feeley, M., 376
Fein, C., 493
Feinberg, M., 465
Feldman, S., 8, 9, 196
Felicetti, D. A., 124
Felix, R. H., 109, 111, 131
Fennell, E. B., 440
Fergus, E., 220
Feuerberg, M., 480
Fiese, B., 409
Fiester, A. R., 218, 219, 220
Filley, A., 464
Fillmore, K., 78
Fine, T., 158
Fischer, J., 75
Fisher, B., 106
Fisher, R., 464
Flaherty, E. W., 208, 219
Flay, B. R., 418
Fleming, M., 301
Flinn, D., 357
Flomenhaft, K., 199
Flora, P., 176
Flynn, T. C., 203, 220
Foley, H. A., 11, 14, 16, 123, 125, 131,
    133, 134, 135, 140, 146, 175, 179,
    181, 311, 312

Folkman, S., 57
Foos, D., 443
Ford, K., 412
Ford, W. E., 438
Forman, B. D., 163
Forsythe, A. B., 80
Fort, D. J., 219, 220
Foster, F. M., 219
Fottler, M. D., 281
Fox, J., 219
Fox, P. D., 267, 272
Fox, P. J. 162, 166
Frank, R. G., 3, 10, 11, 12, 35, 166,
    220, 342, 345, 356, 349, 352
Franklin, J. L., 279
Freedman, A. M., 55, 112
Freeman, H. E., 111
French, L. M., 72
Freud, S., 54
Friedman, M. J., 442
Frisman, L., 357, 358
Fry, W. R., 285
Fulton, J. P., 371, 373

Ganser, L., 334, 458, 459, 489
Gapin, C., 102
Gattozzi, A. A., 244
Gaylin, W., 25
George, L. K., 79
German, P. S., 278
Gerson, S., 136, 137, 270, 316, 388
Gesell, A., 106
Gifford, G. E., Jr., 103
Gilchrist, L. D., 413, 417, 418
Gitteil, M., 183
Glass, G., 216
Glasscote, R. M., 211, 247, 249, 260,
    278
Glasser, J., 257
Glover, R., 390
Glueck, B., 106
Goertzel, V., 255, 329
Goffman, E., 275
Goldberg, I. D., 24, 391
Goldfarb, A., 277
Golding, S. L., 375
Goldman, H. H., 3, 15, 71, 205, 206,
    208, 244, 277, 299, 307, 311, 312,

316, 320, 321, 329, 330, 332, 334,
    335, 342, 346, 348, 349, 350, 354,
    355, 356, 360, 387, 485, 499
Goldmeier, J., 248
Goldsmith, H., 440
Goldstein, A. S., 371
Goldstein, J., 437, 438, 439, 440, 441,
    443, 445
Goldstein, J. M., 69
Goldston, S. E., 209
Goleman, D., 34
Golightley, M., 69
Gomez, E., 137
Goodhart, D., 437, 438, 439, 440, 441,
    443, 445
Goodman, R. R., 370
Goodrick, D., 467, 469, 471
Goodstein, L. D., 378
Goplerud, E. N., 163, 164, 467
Gordon, G. C., 260
Gordon, R. S., 406, 410, 411
Gore, S., 59
Gormally, J., 414
Gorman, M., 109, 181
Gorman, P., 154
Gorodezky, M. J., 163
Gough, I., 179
Gould, M. S., 74
Gove, W., 59
Gralnick, A., 284, 329
Grange, K. M., 92
Grant, R. W., 483, 486, 492
Graves, S. C., 440
Gray, J. P., 99
Gray, L., 197
Greenberg, J. A., 418
Greenblatt, M., 109, 110, 111, 247
Greenspan, S. I., 440
Geerkin, M., 59
Grey, C., 136
Griffiths, B., 80
Grissom, E., 100
Grob, G. N., 4, 5, 94, 95, 98, 104, 135,
    174, 177, 246, 312, 313, 314, 315,
    477, 483
Gronfein, W., 24, 25, 482, 483
Gross, G., 487
Grove, W., 59

Gruenberg, E. M., 137, 314, 316, 320
Gruenberg, L., 244
Gudeman, J. E., 17, 247, 249, 260, 488
Gurel, L., 281
Gutheil, T., 375, 376, 377, 378, 379

Haas, L. J., 107
Hagan, B. J., 163
Hagedorn, H., 437, 438, 440
Hailey, A. M., 185
Hale, G. E., 145, 147
Hale, N. G., 103
Hall, G. B., 441
Hall, M. J., 281
Hall, T., 369
Hamberg, J., 295
Hammond, W. A., 102
Harding, C. M., 68, 487
Harding, P. S., 79
Hare, E., 70
Harper, M. S., 280, 284
Harrigan, K. R., 468
Harrington, C., 272, 273
Harris, P., 444
Harrison, M. J. G., 284
Hart, B. H. L., 457, 467, 468
Hartstone, E., 329
Haskins, B., 198, 211
Hatfield, A., 334
Hauber, F. A., 243
Havassy, B. E., 301
Hawke, D. F., 92
Hawkins, G., 363
Hawley, T. T., 260
Hay, J. R., 175
Hayes, R. H., 453
Heagy, T. C., 10, 11
Health Care Finance Administration, 283
Healy, W., 105
Heclo, H., 175
Heidenheimer, A. J., 176
Heinan, E. M., 136
Heitler, J. B., 442
Heller, K., 57
Helzer, J. E., 52
Henderson, A. S., 73
Henry, G. W., 107
Hersch, C., 6

Hersen, M., 212
Hiday, V., 370
Hill, L. B., 107
Hinkle, B., 103
Hoare, G., 163
Hobbs, N., 422
Hoch, P. H., 108
Hodges, W. F., 424
Hoge, S. K., 377, 378
Holahan, J., 273
Holcomb, W. R., 158
Holland, J. A., 107
Holmes, T. H., 56
Holzer, E. E., 54, 75, 79, 439
Hopkins, R., 213
Hopper, K., 295, 305
Horgan, C. M., 24
Horizon Institute, 220
Hornstra, R. K., 204
Horwitz, A., 59
Hough, R. L., 422, 423
Howard, A., 175
Huber, G., 487
Hudson, C. G., 155, 156, 157, 158, 160
Huffine, C. L., 487
Hunt, C. W., 107
Hunter, R. J., 91
Hunter, T. S., 280
Hustead, E., 343, 353

Igra, A., 256
Ingelsman, F., 245
Intergovernmental Health Policy Project, 301

Jacobs, J. H., 137
Jackson, R. L., 60
James, B. G., 451
James, R. M., 450
James, W. L., 281
Jarrett, M. C., 104, 105
Jarvis, E., 98
Jason, L. A., 418
Jerrell, J. M., 161, 162, 163, 164, 165, 199, 206, 211, 390, 391, 392, 393, 394, 395, 398, 399
Jerrell, S. L., 164, 395
Jimenez, M. A., 94

Johnson, D. L., 416
Johnson, E., 240
Johnson, K., 412
Johnston, L. D., 417, 420
Joint Commission on Mental Illness and
    Health, 125, 126, 312
Jones, C. O., 4, 6
Jones, K., 69, 174, 178
Jones, S. J., 282
Jones, T., 212

Kahn, A. J., 436
Kahn, J. R., 413
Kalinowsky, O. B., 108
Kamerow, D. B., 79
Kamlet, M. S., 3, 10, 11, 12, 35, 166,
    345
Kane, J. M., 274, 481
Kane, R. A., 282
Kane, R. L., 281, 282
Kane, T., 467
Kanter, R. M., 183
Kantner, J. F., 412, 424
Kaplan, A., 381
Kaplan, D. M., 199
Kaplan, H. I., 55
Karlen, A. L., 408
Karno, M., 77
Kashgarian, M., 280
Katon, W., 278
Kavka, J., 92
Keilitz, I., 369, 371, 372, 373
Kellert, S., 136
Kelly, J. G., 403
Kennedy, J. F., 112, 130
Kessel, M., 244, 250, 255
Kessler, M., 54, 352, 480
Kessler, M., 403
Kessler, R. C., 54, 57, 58, 59, 60, 75
Kety, S. S., 55
Kiesler, C. A., 16, 199, 237, 252, 453,
    461, 485, 488, 499
Kim, S., 420
Kindred, J. J., 106
Kindwall, J. A., 107
Kirchner, J., 219
Kirk, S. A., 136, 137
Kirlin, J., 127

Kirshner, M. D., 260, 333
Kittrie, N. N., 101
Klee, G. D., 443
Klerman, G. L., 54, 311, 335, 391, 440
Klett, C. J., 245
Koch, H., 267
Kohlberg, L., 409
Kohn, M. L., 57
Konan, M., 202, 204
Kopeloff, N., 107
Koran, L. M., 23, 24, 25, 32, 33, 34,
    443
Koss, M. P., 408
Kovacs, M., 73
Kramer, M., 185, 274, 278, 333
Kraus, R. T., 284
Kruzich, J. M., 282
Kuhn, T., 175
Kulka, R. A., 136, 480
Kuntz, N. R., 268, 271
Kusserow, R. P., 242

Lackey, G. L., 467
La Crosse, J., 409
Ladner, S., 298
Lamb, H. R., 137, 238, 249, 255, 274,
    329, 481, 486, 488, 492
Landman, J. T., 217
Landsberg, G., 163, 220
Landy, D., 247
Langer, E. J., 284
Langner, T., 50, 51
Langsley, D. G., 199, 205, 206
Lansky, D., 78
Larsen, J. K., 161, 162, 163, 164, 165,
    199, 206, 211, 390, 391, 392, 393,
    394, 395, 398, 399
Laska, G., 329
Lauriet, A., 304
Lave, J., 356
Lazarus, R. S., 57
Leaf, P. J., 35, 76, 78
Lebowitz, B., 73
Lee, D. T., 246
Leff, J., 70, 483, 499
Lehman, A., 358
Leiby, J., 4, 178
Leighton, A. H., 8

Leighton, D. C., 50, 54
Leigland, J., 495
Lemke, S., 282
Lempinen, E. W., 256
Lerman, P., 137
Levenstein, A., 465
Levey, S., 282
Levin, B., 357
Levine, D. S., 195, 214
Levine, I. S., 71, 293, 297, 301, 307
Levine, M., 10, 11, 135, 138
Levine, M. S., 206
Levinson, D. J., 109
Levy, L., 443
Lewis, R., 493
Lezak, A. D., 71, 307
Lieberman, M. A., 282, 454
Lief, A., 104
Lindeman, C., 281
Linn, B. S., 281
Linn, M. W., 69, 245, 247, 252, 260,
    279, 281, 282, 283
Lippman, W., 364
Lipset, S. M., 183
Liptzin, B., 282
Little, N. F., 93
Liu, K., 281
Locke, B. Z., 3
Logan, B. M., 156, 157, 158, 160, 161,
    162, 163, 164
Loh, W. D., 381
Longest, J., 202, 204
Looney, J. G., 17
Lord, J. R., 106
Lorion, R. P., 201, 403, 405, 408, 409,
    411, 421
Lounsbury, J. W., 389
Lovell, A., 304, 305
Lowi, T., 176, 179
Lowry, J. V., 109
Lueger, R. J., 212
Luft, L. L., 220
Lundwall, L., 201
Lutterman, T., 151, 390

Macdonald, D. I., 79
Macht, L. B., 136
MacMurray, V. D., 209

Manderscheid, R. W., 3, 67, 324, 335
Mangione, T., 59
Mannino, R., 248
Manton, K. G., 281
Mark, V. H., 227, 284
Marmor, T. R., 10, 11, 182
Marquette, U., 212
Marsden, C. D., 284
Marshall, H. E., 97
Martin, J., 378
Martin, M., 295
Mashaw, J. L., 490
Massad, P. M., 435, 439, 444
Matthews, S. M., 252
Matza, D., 176, 177
Maxwell, J. S., 413
May, P., 77
Mayer, C., 371, 372, 373
Mazade, N. A., 159, 390
McCoin, J. M., 242
McGovern, C. M., 97
McGovern, M. P., 17
McGuire, T., 349, 354
McLeod, J. D., 59
McMahon, T., 357
McMillan, I. C., 463, 468
McNeel, B. H., 108
McRae, J. A., 59, 60
Mechanic, D., 8, 12, 14, 59, 60, 128,
    136, 167, 267, 268, 273, 275, 477,
    478, 493, 497
Mednick, S. A., 55
Meerloo, J. A., 111
Meinhardt, K., 443
Melick, C. F., 244, 250
Mellinger, G. D., 78
Meloy, J. R., 375
Melton, G., 202
Menaghan, E. G., 57
Mendel, W., 329
Menn, A., 252, 260
Menninger, W. C., 108
Mental Disability Law Reporter, 252
Merves, E. S., 57
Merwin, M. R., 24
Midanik, L., 78
Milazzo-Sayre, L. J., 74
Miller, H., 239

Miller, K. S., 482
Miller, M. B., 277
Miller, R., 329, 330, 333
Miller, W. R., 55
Millon, T., 55
Mills, A. B., 98
Mills, C. W., 4
Mintzberg, H., 450
Mirowsky, J., 54, 56, 59, 60
Mitchell, C. C., 164
Mitchell, S. W., 103
Mollica, R. F., 137
Moltzen, S., 285
Monahan, J., 329, 381
Montgomery, J., 354
Moore, D. N., 399, 439
Moore, K., 412, 425
Moore, M. S., 371
Moore, W. J., 151
Moos, R., 256, 282
Moran, R., 371
Morgan, J. A., Jr., 12, 154
Morganthau, T., 36
Moroney, R. M., 268, 271
Morris, N., 363
Morris, R., 285
Morrison, L. J., 215
Morrissey, J. P., 136, 137, 246, 296, 298, 299, 307, 311, 312, 317, 320, 321, 329, 330, 333, 334, 335, 387
Morse, G., 298
Morton, T. G., 91
Morton, T. L., 16
Mortimer, J. A., 72
Moses, J., 281
Mosher, J. M., 104
Mosher, L. R., 252, 260
Moyles, E. W., 255, 256, 260
Moynihan, D. P., 176, 182
Mueller, D. P., 56
Mulkern, V., 305
Munger, R., 203
Munroe, R., 55
Murphy, G. E., 77
Murphy, J. M., 237
Murphy, M. B., 245
Murray, M. M., 418
Murrell, S. A., 437, 438

Musto, D. F., 211, 312
Muszynski, I., 343, 344, 349, 351, 352, 356, 357, 479, 498
Myers, J. K., 53, 79, 403

Naierman, N., 198, 211, 389
Nathan, P. E., 78
Nathan, R. P., 143, 145, 148, 155, 156, 167
National Association for the Protection of the Insane and the Prevention of Insanity, 102
National Association of Mental Health Program Directors, 36
National Center for State Courts, 367, 368
National Council of Community Mental Health Centers, 161, 163
National Institute of Aging Task Force, 284
National Institute of Mental Health, 24, 25, 26, 27, 29, 30, 31, 32, 33, 34, 35, 36, 38, 39, 199, 201, 202, 204, 210, 211, 212, 214, 299, 489, 491
Neal, J., 201
Neighbors, H. W., 54, 75
Neigher, W. D., 218
Nelson, R., 220
Nelson, R. H., 209
Neugebauer, R., 72
Newer, B., 107
Newman, D. E., 220
New South Wales Department of Health, 499
Newton, P. M., 210, 211
Nichols, C. W., 285
Nisbet, R., 183
Nunn, P. L. S., 55

O'Brien, G. M. St. L., 467
Ochberg, F. M., 24
Okin, R. L., 160, 161, 162, 163, 165, 166, 327, 328
Ojemann, R. H., 209
Olds, D., 415
Olsen, K., 208, 219
O'Malley, M., 107
O'Malley, P. M., 417, 420

Orzech, M. J., 284
Overholser, W., 97, 110
Owen, W. L., 217
Ozarin, 208, 212

Palley, M. L., 145, 147
Palmer, K. T., 143
Palmer, R. R., 177
Parad, H. J., 211
Paradis, B. A., 17
Pardes, H., 467
Parrish, J., 454
Parry, J., 363, 367, 377, 380
Paschall, N., 219
Patterson, J. T., 175
Patti, R. J., 163
Patton, R. E., 111
Paulson, R. I., 17
Paykel, E. S., 56
Pearlin, L. I., 57, 58, 59, 60
Pepper, B., 68, 69, 214, 260, 330, 331, 333, 334
Perlmutter, F. D., 210, 213
Peters, B. G., 4, 5
Peters, J. P., 461
Peterson, G. E., 155, 156, 157, 158
Peterson, P., 462
Peterson, R. S., 163
Pfeffer, N. A., 487
Pierson, D. E., 415, 416
Pincus, H. A., 79
Pinel, P., 92, 93, 177
Pittman, K. J., 159, 160, 161, 166
Piven, F. F., 127
Police, T. T., 495
Polit, D. F., 413
Pollack, B., 418
Pollock, H. M., 107, 108
Pond, M. A., 154
Pomp, H. C., 17
Porter, M., 461
Pratt, G. K., 106
President, P. A., 418, 419
President's Commission on Mental Health, 24, 139, 184, 202, 403, 404, 485
Pressman, J., 176
Prevost, J., 69, 467

Price, R. H., 54, 57, 58, 409, 410, 421
Price, W. S., and Associates, 198, 199, 205, 216
Prince, M., 103
Pumphrey, R. E., 105

Quen, J., 314
Quinn, J. B., 450, 452, 454, 455, 457, 458, 464, 465, 466, 467, 468

Rabkin, J. G., 56, 217
Rachlin, S., 329
Rahe, R. H., 56
Radloff, L., 59, 60
Ramey, C., 415, 416
Ranney, M. H., 98
Rapoport, D., 377
Raschko, R., 213
Raskind, M. A., 277, 278, 281
Ray, W. A., 280
Reade, C., 100
Redick, R. W., 201, 202, 321, 326, 491
Redlich, F., 136
Redlich, F. C., 49, 54, 403
Regier, D. A., 3, 24, 53, 128, 207, 237, 391
Reiff, S., 80
Reihman, J., 69
Reynolds, P., 239
Rhodes, J. E., 418
Rich, R. F., 7, 14, 16, 165
Richman, A., 444
Rickel, A. U., 406
Ricks, D., 409
Reissman, E., 217
Rinkel, M., 111
Rivers, W. H. R., 106
Robbins, L., 439
Robert Wood Johnson Foundation, 15
Roberts, R., 357
Robertson, M. J., 70
Robins, E., 46, 50, 51, 52
Robins, L. N., 72, 77
Robins, L. S., 145
Robinson, G., 198, 211
Robinson, M., 69

Robischer, J., 320, 330
Rochefort, D. A., 4, 6, 7, 8, 11, 12, 13, 136, 156, 157, 158, 160, 161, 162, 163, 164
Rochford, E. B., 251
Rodin, J., 284
Roesch, R., 375
Rog, D., 302
Rogers, C. W., 207
Rook, K., 60
Rose, S., 316
Rosen, B. M., 204, 207, 440
Rosenbaum, S., 412
Rosenblum, S., 301
Rosenfeld, A. H., 278
Rosenfield, S., 50, 54, 59, 60
Rosenkrantz, B. G., 98
Rosenstein, M., 200, 203, 210, 212, 322, 323, 324, 329, 335
Rosenthal, D., 55
Ross, C. E., 54, 56, 59, 60
Ross, R., 103
Rossi, P. H., 492
Roth, D., 298
Roth, L. H., 377
Rothman, D. J., 94, 107, 174, 177, 178, 312, 313
Rotter, J. B., 57
Roush, S., 281
Rovner, B. W., 277, 278
Rowitz, L., 443
Royse, D., 438, 441
Rubin, J., 15, 16, 215, 272, 498
Rubin, L., 304
Rupp, A., 356
Rush, B., 92
Russell, W. L., 105
Rutter, M., 74, 75
Ryglewicz, H., 68, 69, 214, 260, 330, 331, 333
Sabatier, P., 435, 439
Sabin, 277, 284
Sackler, A. M., 108
Sadock, B. J., 55
Sahakian, B. J., 55
Sahakian, W. S., 55
Sales, B. D., 435, 439, 444
Salkever, D., 356

Salmon, T. W., 105, 106
Salzman, C., 280
Salzman, K., 220
Sameroff, A. J., 409
Sampson, L. M., 220
Sandall, H., 260
Sanford, N., 403
Santos, E. H., 101
Sarason, S., 424
Savino, M. T., 98
Scales, P., 425
Scanlon, W., 277, 485
Schaffner, W., 280
Scherl, D. J., 136
Scheuttler, R., 487
Sachinke, S. P., 413, 414, 417, 418
Schlesinger, A. J., Jr., 175
Schlesinger, M., 495
Schmidt, L. J., 267, 279
Schmittdiel, C. J., 438
Schneck, J. M., 103
Schneier, M., 453
Schooler, C., 57, 58
Schulberg, H., 70, 71
Schulte, P., 437, 438
Schulz, C., 70
Schulz, J. H., 272
Schuman, L. M., 72
Schwab, J. J., 75, 437, 440
Schwab, S. I., 106
Schwartz, M., 109
Schwartz, S., 209
Schweinhart, L. J., 416
Scott, R. R., 203
Scull, A., 313, 480, 482
Scully, D., 207
Segal, S. P., 239, 240, 243, 244, 245, 249, 250, 251, 255, 256, 259, 260, 483
Seliger, J., 202
Seligman, M. E. P., 55, 57
Seltzer, M. M., 241, 244
Selye, H., 56
Selznick, P., 333
Shadish, W. R., 218, 271, 273, 278, 279
Shadoan, R., 238
Shah, S., 363, 365, 369, 372, 380

Shapiro, R., 329
Shapiro, S., 71, 237, 278, 484
Sharfstein, S. S., 11, 14, 15, 16, 23, 24, 25, 32, 33, 34, 133, 134, 135, 140, 146, 166, 175, 176, 179, 181, 204, 275, 311, 312, 342, 344, 346, 348, 349, 351, 352, 354, 355, 356, 440, 479, 498
Shaw, L., 251
Sheets, J., 69
Sheridan, E., 213
Shershow, J. C., 97
Sherwood, C. C., 241, 244, 283
Sherwood, S., 244
Shields, E., 107
Shifren, I., 293, 299, 300, 301
Shore, M. F., 14, 17, 248, 329, 488, 493
Shryock, R. 92
Shumaker, S. A., 57
Sibulkin, A. E., 485, 499
Sicherman, B., 105, 312, 314
Siegel, A. P., 206
Silver, A. A., 408
Simmons, O. G., 111
Simms, L. M., 282
Simons, L. S., 220, 437, 439, 443
Simpson, W. H., 209
Sirrocco, A., 267
Skinner, A., 334, 342, 356
Slaikeu, K. A., 408
Slem, C. M., 443
Smith, C. J., 200
Smith, H. L., 281
Smith, J. M., 274, 481
Smith, M., 216
Smith, R. K., 443
Smith, S. S., 410, 421
Snow, D. L., 210, 211
Snyder, L. H., 284
Sobel, J. L., 418
Socio-Technical Systems Associates, 212
Solomon, G., 219
Solomon, N. C., 111
Somers, S. A., 493
Somerville, P. D., 76
Southard, E. E., 104, 106

Spaniol, L., 296
Spar, J. E., 251, 257
Spence, R., 205
Spitzer, R., 46
Spitzka, E. C., 102
Srole, L., 50, 54, 403
Stainbrook, E., 101
Stan, J., 239
Stanfield, R. L., 144
Stanton, A., 109
Stapp, J., 33
Starling, G., 436
Steadman, H. J., 329, 372, 373, 374
Stein, E. M., 282
Stein, L. I., 252, 301, 334, 458–59, 488, 498, 499
Stein, S., 281, 282
Steiner, G. A., 453, 454, 457
Steinwachs, D., 356
Stern, M. S., 136
Stewart, R., 436, 438
Stockdill, J. W., 12, 154, 200, 297, 466, 467
Stockman, D., 186
Stotsky, B. A., 270, 281, 282, 283, 481
Stotsky, B. S., 270, 281
Straw, R. B., 252
Strikland, A. J., 386
Struening, E. L., 56, 217
Sue, S., 201
Surber, R. W., 159, 160, 161, 162
Surles, R., 159
Surles, R. C., 7, 159
Swan, J. H., 162, 166
Swazey, J. P., 110, 180
Swift, C. F., 210, 211
Swindle, R., 57

Talbott, J. A., 7, 8, 15, 137, 273, 275, 329, 331, 335, 483
Taube, C. A., 24, 198, 200, 203, 207, 208, 244, 267, 316, 322, 323, 324, 329, 332, 348, 349, 350, 354, 391, 480
Taylor, S. M., 260
Tcheng-Laroche, F., 245
Teeter, R. B., 277

TenHoor, W. J., 71, 138, 293, 301
Teplin, L., 213
Tessler, R., 330, 499
Test, M. A., 252, 301, 488, 499
Therrien, M. E., 137
Thoits, P. A., 56, 57, 60
Thom, D., 108
Tomes, N. J., 94, 96
Thompson, A. A., 386
Thompson, F. J., 156, 166
Thompson, J., 322, 323, 324, 325, 328, 329
Tibshirani, R., 443
Tobin, S. S., 282
Toff, G. E., 161
Torrey, E. F., 55
Tortu, S., 419
Trainor, I., 443
Trattner, W. I., 178
Trotter, S., 215, 316, 388
Truitt, R. P., 106
Trute, B., 260
Tudor, J., 59
Tuke, S., 93
Turner, J. C., 71, 138, 293, 299, 300, 301
Tweed, D., 202, 204

Udell, B., 204
Ulbrich, P., 59, 60
Ury, W., 464
U.S. Conference of Mayors, 295
U.S. Congress, Office of Technology Assessment, 75, 162
U.S. Department of Health and Human Services, 3, 153, 158, 283, 295, 297, 303
U.S. Department of Health, Education, and Welfare, 269
U.S. General Accounting Office, 14, 135, 136, 137, 144, 148, 156, 157, 158, 277
U.S. Department of Housing and Urban Development, 15, 295, 303

Vladeck, B . C., 268, 281
VandenBos, G. R., 33
Van Putten, T., 251, 257

Vaughn, C., 70
Vayda, A. M., 210, 213
Veith, I., 103
Vergare, M., 70
Veroff, J., 136, 480
Viek, C., 258
Vinovskis, M. A., 98, 424
Visotsky, H. M., 167
Vitug, A. J., 277, 284

Wagenfeld, M. O., 137
Walfish, S., 163, 164, 467
Walker, L., 381
Walsh, A., 495
Walsh, J., 209
Walter, R. D., 103
Walters, R. B., 180
Warheit, G. J., 54, 75, 437, 439, 440
Washburn, S., 199, 217
Wasserman, D. B., 199, 389
Watson, W. H., 283
Webber, J. B., 461
Weick, K., 465
Weikart, D. P., 416
Weiner, B., 363, 380
Weiner, R. S., 199
Weiner-Pomerantz, R., 199, 389
Weisbrod, B. A., 252, 488
Weiss, K. J., 217
Weissman, M. M., 51, 54, 72, 74, 79, 440
West, A. N., 442
Westman, J. C., 421, 424
Wethington, E., 59
Wexler, D. B., 365, 373, 374, 376–77
Wheaton, B., 57, 60
White, W. A., 106
Wildavsky, A., 167, 176
Wilder, J. F., 244, 250, 255
Wilensky, H. L., 174, 176, 179, 187
Williams, R. H., 109
Williams, W. H., 91
Wills, T. A., 57
Wilner, G. G., 195, 214
Wilson, N. Z., 219
Windle, C., 136, 196, 197, 200, 201, 203, 204, 206, 207, 208, 212, 219

Wing, J. K., 185, 314, 482
Winslow, W. W., 20, 207, 223
Wise, L., 412
Witkin, M. J., 207, 325, 326, 328, 335
Witman, D. A., 10
Wittels, F., 92
Wittman, D. A., 11
Wolfe, T., 210
Wolin, S. S., 183
Wood, J. B., 161, 163, 164
Woods, E. A., 92
Wortman, C. B., 54, 57, 58
Woy, R. J., 159, 199, 389
Wrapp, H. E., 455, 467
Wright, F., 109
Wu, I., 201
Wunsch-Hitzig, R., 74

Wutchiett, R., 444
Wykle, M. H., 281

Yarvis, R. M., 56, 205, 217
Yates, B. T., 440
Yoder, K. K., 282
Youket, P., 285

Zaske, D., 280
Zautra, A., 437, 438, 439, 440, 441, 442, 443, 445
Zawadski, R. T., 285
Zelnik, M., 412, 424
Zinn, H. K., 201
Zinober, J. W., 209
Zins, J., 213
Zipple, A., 296
Zusman, J., 403

Subject Index

Abortion, 425
Access of Monroe County, N.Y., 285
Acquired immune deficiency syndrome
  (AIDS), 190
Action for Mental Health (1961), 111–12,
  125, 274. *See also* Joint Commission
  on Mental Illness and Health
Adolescent Family Life Program, 424
Adolescent Health, Services, and Preg-
  nancy Prevention and Care Act of 1978
  (Public Law 95–626), 424
Adolescents: increased public mental
  health services for, 391–92; prevention
  of pregnancy among, 412–14, 424–25;
  prevention of substance abuse among,
  417–20; severely mentally ill, 486. *See
  also* Children
Advisory Commission on Intergovernmental Relations (ACIR), 146
Affective psychosis, prevalence of, 53
Alcohol, Drug Abuse, and Mental Health
  Administration (ADAMHA), 10, 404

Alcohol, Drug Abuse and Mental Health
  Amendments of 1984 (Public Law 98–
  509), 151
Alcohol, Drug Abuse, and Mental Health
  block grant, 14
—and the Alcohol Abuse, Drug Abuse,
  and Mental Health Amendments of
  1984, 151
—apportionment of, 149
—design of, 144, 148–49
—dilemma of emphasis on chronically
  mentally ill, 166
—fiscal 1988 distribution by state, 152–
  53
—funding levels of, 149–51; as proportion of total spending for substance
  abuse and mental health services, 151,
  153
—impact on community mental health
  centers, 154, 155–56, 158–67 (*See
  also* Community mental health centers,
  impact of Alcohol, Drug, and Mental

Health block grant on; Mental health administration, within community mental health centers)

—impact on use of nursing homes as mental health facilities, 275

—impact on state mental health systems, 154–58 (*See also* State mental health systems, and Alcohol, Drug Abuse, and Mental Health block grant)

Alcoholic and Narcotic Addict Rehabilitation Amendments of 1968 (Public Law 90–574), 133

Alcoholism, prevalence of, 53, 78–79. *See also* Substance abuse disorders

Alliance for the Mentally Ill, 10. *See also* National Alliance for the Mentally Ill

Alternatives Approach program (for drug prevention education), 419

Alzheimer's disease, 72, 190, 272, 284, 498; modification in Medicare benefits for, 348

American Bar Association (ABA) Appreciation test for criminal responsibility, 372

American Federation of State, County, and Municipal Employees (AFSCME), 10, 185

American Journal of Insanity, 97, 180

American Law Institute (ALI) test for criminal responsibility, 372

American Medical Association (AMA): influence on Community Mental Health Centers Act of 1963, 130–31; influence on Community Mental Health Centers Amendments of 1965, 132

American Psychiatric Association (APA), classification of mental disorders, 10. *See Diagnostic and Statistical Manual of Mental Disorders*, 3rd edition; *Diagnostic and Statistical Manual of Mental Disorders*, 3rd edition, revised

American Psychological Association (APA), 10; Task Force on Prevention, 210

American Public Health Association (APHA), 406

Anti-Drug Abuse Act of 1986 (Public Law 99–570), 151

Antihospital movement, 482–83. *See also* Community mental health movement; Deinstitutionalization

Antisocial personality disorder, 48; prevalence of, 53

Aristotle, 371

Association of Medical Superintendents of American Institutions for the Insane (AMSAII), 97

Asylums. *See* History of mental hospitals; Mental hospitals, historical development

Autism, in children, 74

Balanced Budget and Emergency Deficit Control Act of 1985 (Gramm-Rudman-Hollings Act, Public Law 99–177), 151, 275–76

Baltimore Epidemiologic Catchment Area Study (1985), 298

Barrett, Albert M., 104

Beautiful Babies Right From the Start program, 422

Beers, Clifford, W., 105, 314; *A Mind That Found Itself* (1908), 178, 314

Behavior Screening Questionnaire, 73–74

Bettelheim, Bruno, 109

Block grants: definition of, 144–45, 146–47; evaluation studies of early block grants, 147; and relationship to history of federal grants system, 145–47; use of block grants in Reagan administration, 147–48. *See also* Alcohol, Drug Abuse, and Mental Health block grant

Blue Cross and Blue Shield, 349, 351, 354

Board-and-care facilities, 239, 247, 248, 256—57. *See also* Community residential care

Braceland, Francis, 123

British Mental Aftercare Association of Released Psychiatric Patients, 247

Brookline Early Education Project (to prevent maternal and child health problems), 415

Bucknill, John C., 100

Bureau of Labor Statistics (BLS) Levels of Benefits Survey, 351–52, 479

Callahan, James, J., Jr., 14
Capitation, 15, 356–58; for high-risk groups, 358. *See also* Financing of mental health care
Carolina Early Intervention Program (to prevent developmental problems in children), 415–16
Carter, President Jimmy, 184–85; and Mental Health Systems Act of 1980, 139–40, 186, 275; and President's Commission on Mental Health, 138–39, 275
Carter, Rosalynn, and President's Commission on Mental Health, 139–40, 184
Case management, 14–15, 392, 493–94. *See also* Community Support Program
Center for Epidemiologic Studies Depression Scale (CES-D), 51
Charitable Organization Societies, 268
Children. *See also* Adolescents
—and community mental health center services, 162, 202
—mental disorder in: autism, 74; correlates of, 74–75; prevalence of, 73–74
—prevention of mental disorders in, 408, 414–17
—service utilization of, 75
Chlorpromazine (CPZ), 110
Chronically mentally ill
—and Alcohol, Drug Abuse, and Mental Health block grant, 158, 161–62, 166
—and community mental health centers, 137–38, 161–62, 165, 166, 206–7, 223–224
—definition of, 3, 67–68 (*See also* Schizophrenia)
—and health insurance, 353, 354–55
—increased services for, 7, 391–92
—managing community care for, 491–92; case management, 493–94; problem of housing, 492–93
—and nonpsychiatric personnel, 497
—number of, 3, 8, 67
—and policymaking, 13–17, 185, 239–40, 486–88
—and public mental hospitals, 329
—service utilization of, 70–71

—types of: discharged long-term patients, 68–69; homeless mentally ill, 70 (*See also* Homeless mentally ill); young adult chronic patients, 69
Cohen, Wilbur, 187
"Columbus complex," 177
Community Mental Health Act (New York, 1954), 111
Community mental health centers (CMHCs). *See also* Community mental health movement —administration of (*see* Mental health administration)
—changing staffing patterns of, 35
—evaluation of: awareness and accessibility of services, 203–4; citizen participation in, 208–9; client satisfaction, 219–20; coordination of services, 212–14; cost of services, 214–15, 225; effect on admissions rates to state hospitals, 207–8; effect on inappropriate hospitalization, 208; effectiveness of services, 216–18; efficiency problems, 216; fiscal viability, 199–200; identification of goals, 196, 220–22, 385–88; increased services, 197–98; increased specialized services, 198; maintenance of community approach, 198–99; needs assessment, 224–25; prevention of mental disorders, 209–11, 224, 420–421; quality assurance, 220; services for children, 202; services for high-need populations, 204–5; services for minorities, 201, 222–23; services for the elderly, 202; services for rural clients, 202–3; services for the poor, 200–201; services for the severely and chronically mentally ill, 205–7, 223–224
—funding of, 132–34, 135, 136, 138, 199–200
—impact of Alcohol, Drug Abuse, and Mental Health block grant on, 149, 154, 157, 165–67 (*See also* Mental health administration); geographic variability, 166; loss of state funding, 155–56; management and administration, 163–64; movement towards "business model," 163–64, 385; programmatic

effect, 159; revenue effects, 159–61; service patterns, 161–63; service patterns for chronically mentally ill, 161–62, 165, 166, 391–92; staffing developments, 164–65, 394
—number of, 25
Community Mental Health Centers (CMHC) Act of 1963 (Public Law 88–164), 6, 23, 24, 112, 130–31, 159, 183, 274, 316, 387–88
—amendments to: Alcoholic and Narcotic Addiction Rehabilitation Amendments of 1968 (Public Law 90–574), 133; Community Mental Health Centers Amendments of 1970 (Public Law 91–211), 133; Comprehensive Drug Abuse Prevention and Control Act of 1970 (Public Law 91–513), 133; Health Programs Extension Act of 1973 (Public Law 93–45), 134; Health Revenue Sharing and Health Services Act of 1975 (Public Law 94–63), 134, 138, 198, 200, 202, 205, 209, 218, 225, 388; Mental Health Amendments of 1967 (Public Law 90–31), 132–33; 1965 amendments (Public Law 89–105), 132, 183, 388
—Community Support Program (CSP) and, 138, 388; influence of National Institute of Mental Health on, 131 (*See also* Mental Health Systems Act of 1980)
Communtiy Mental Health Journal, 209, 389
Community mental health movement, 6, 11, 14, 104, 195–96. *See also* Community mental health centers
—and chronically mentally ill, 137–38
—development of: during post-war era, 122–25; during Kennedy administration, 125–27; during Nixon administration, 137; during Carter administration, 138–40; during Reagan administration, 140
—effect on public attitudes toward mental health, 136
—fragmentation of services, 136–38, 494–95

—ideology of, 127–29, 483–84
—influence of National Institute of Mental Health on, 124
—need for organization, 494–96
—origins of, 111—12
—role of psychiatry, 137, 483–84
Community residential care
—as an alternative to community care, 254–56
—as an alternative to hospitalization, 252–54
—characteristics of, 241–42
—client characteristics of, 244–45
—models of: as a developmental context, 239–40; as a residential system of custody, 239; as a treatment continuum, 238–39
—need for, 237–38, 492–93
—number and population of, 242–44
—problems of: community resistance, 260, 492; economic viability, 257–58; service ambiguity, 257–58
—services provided by, 258–59
—and the severely mentally ill, 492–93
—types of: board-and-care homes, 239, 247, 248, 249–50, 256–57; family care homes, 245–47, 249–50; halfway houses, 247–48, 249–50; psychopathology of residents, 250–51; psychosocial rehabilitation facilities (PRFs), 248; relationship to community, 249–50; satellite house programs, 248–49; variations of cost among, 251–52, 253
Community Support Program (CSP), 138, 275, 293–94, 299–300, 457–58
—case study of Community Support Program efforts in Wisconsin, 458–60
—functions of, 300
—mental health treatment and rehabilitation, 302–3
—outreach, 301
—service delivery for homeless mentally ill; case management, 301–2; continuum of residential assistance, 303: long-term housing, 304–5; shelters and drop-in centers, 303–4; transitional housing, 304
—staff training for, 305

Community Support System (CSS), 223–24, 299, 307. *See also* Community Support Program

Comprehensive Drug Abuse Prevention and Control Act of 1970 (Public Law 91–513), 133

Comprehensive State Mental Health Planning Act of 1986 (Public Law 99–660), 305–6, 450

Council of State and Territorial Mental Health Authorities, 124

Deinstitutionalization, 274, 391, 482, 483; "benign phase" of, 316–17, 320; demographic trends, 485–86; and drugs, 480–81; history of, 484; and homeless mentally ill, 297–98; and nursing homes, 485; "radical phase" of, 320–21; rate of, 24, 28, 317, 318–19, 481. *See also* Community mental health movement; Mental hospitals, public

Deutsch, Albert, *The Shame of the States* (1948), 181

Diagnosis-related groups (DRGs), 16, 349. *See also* Financing of mental health care; Health insurance; Medicare

Diagnostic and Statistical Manual of Mental Disorders, 3rd edition (DSM-III, 1980), 51

Diagnostic and Statistical Manual of Mental Disorders, 3rd edition, revised (DSM-III-R, 1987), 46, 48

Diagnostic Interview Schedule (DIS), 51–52

Disability programs for the mentally ill, 490–91

Dix, Dorothea, 5, 96, 174, 178, 179, 190, 275, 313

Drug abuse/dependence, among minorities, 77–78. *See also* Substance abuse disorders

Drug therapy, 110–11, 480–81, 496; influence of National Institute of Mental Health on, 124. *See also* Phenothiazines; Psychopharmacology; Psychotropic medications

Drummond, Edward, 371

Dusky v. United States (1960), and the Dusky test for competency to stand trial, 374–75

Earle, Pliny, 98–99

Eastern Lunatic Asylum (Virginia), 91, 177

Elderly
—and community mental health center services, 162, 201–2
—dementia in: cause of, 72; correlates of, 72–73; definition of, 71–72; prevalence of, 72
—service utilization of, 73 (*see also* Nursing homes, as mental health facilities)

Electric convulsive therapy (ECT), 108

Elizabethan Poor Law (1601), 90, 174, 177

Emergency Jobs Appropriation Act of 1983 (Public Law 98–8), 150–51

Epidemiological Catchment Area (ECA) studies
—prevalence rates of mental disorders, 52–54, 70–71; among minorities, 76–78
—substance abusers' service utilization, 80

Etiology of mental disorder: behavioral model, 55; biological model, 55–56; psychoanalytic model, 54–55; stressful life events model, 56–61 (*see also* Stressful life events)

Extended care facilities (ECFs), 271

Ewalt, Jack, 123

Fairweather Lodge experiment, 254–55

Families, and mental disorder, 483

Family care for the mentally ill, 245, 247. *See also* Community residential care

Family Planning Services and Population Research Act of 1970 (Public Law 91–572), 424

Felix, Robert, H., 111, 123, 124, 130, 182

Financing of mental health care. *See also* Capitation; Health insurance; Health

maintenance organizations; Medicaid; Medicare; Mental health care expenditures; Mental health care revenues; Preferred provider organizations; Social Security Disability Insurance; Supplemental Security Income
—cost shifting and nursing homes, 481–82
—costs of mental health care, 345
—equity in, 346
—fee-for-service payment, 341–42, 351
—future of, 358–60; refunding state mental health budget priorities, 489–90
—historical development of, 341–43
—parity in, 348–49
—problems of, 15
—sources of, 345–46, 347
Fogarty, Representative John, 185
Ford, President Gerald, and CMHC program, 134, 184
Fort Logan Mental Health Center (Colorado), 254
Fountain House (New York City), 248, 249
Franklin, Benjamin, 91
Freud, Anna, 109
Freud, Sigmund. *See* Etiology of mental disorder, psychoanalytic model

Ganser, Dr. Leonard, 458
Geel, Belguim, adult family care program for mentally ill in, 246
General Accounting Office (GAO)
—impact of reviews of community mental health centers program, 184
—study of Alcohol, Drug Abuse, and Mental Health block grant funding trends and state implementation, 15–155
Goddard Riverside outreach program for homeless mentally ill, 304–5
Gorman, Mike, 124, 181
Gramm-Rudman Act. *See* Balanced Budget and Emergency Deficit Control Act of 1985
Gramm-Rudman-Hollings Act. *See* Balanced Budget and Emergency Deficit Control Act of 1985

Gray, John P., 99
Griesinger, Wilhelm, 99
Group for the Advancement of Psychiatry (GAP), 122–23, 181
"Guidelines for Involuntary Civil Commitment" (1986), 367–68, 369–70

Halfway houses, 247–48. *See also* Community residential care
Hall, G. Stanley, 103
Health insurance. *See also* Financing of mental health care; Medicaid; Medicare
—cost containment and utilization control, efforts in, 349–50, 355, 498
—costs of mental health care, 345
—current coverage of mental health care benefits: gaps in, 354–55; growth in, 479–80; mandated mental health benefits, 353–54; in private insurance, 351–52; in public insurance, 352–53;
—discriminatory treatment of mental disorders by, 343, 498
—equity in, 346
—history of and mental health care, 342–43
—impact of policies on community mental health centers, 199
—for inpatient mental health care, 30
—parity in, 348—49
—reasons for inadequate mental health benefits in, 343–45: adverse selection, 344–45; moral hazard, 344
—retroactive reimbursement versus prospective payment, 355
Health maintenance organizations (HMOs), 355; for mental health problems, 15–16, 356–57
Health Programs Extension Act of 1973 (Public Law 93–45), 134
Health Revenue Sharing and Mental Health Services Act of 1975 (Public Law 94–63), 134, 138, 200, 202, 205, 209, 218, 225, 388
Healy, William, 105
Henry Phipps Psychiatric Clinic, 103–4
High Scope/Perry Preschool Program (to prevent developmental problems in children), 416

Hill, Senator Lister, 185
Hill-Burton Act. *See* Hospital Survey and
  Construction Act of 1946
Hinckley, John, 371
History of mental health care. *See also*
  Mental hospitals
—development in United States: community mental health movement, 111–12
  (*see also* Community mental health
  movement); during the Enlightenment,
  92–93; during the Progressive era,
  102–6; effect of World War II on,
  108–9, 122–23; in colonial America,
  90–91; mental hygiene movement,
  105–6, 314–15; moral treatment approach, 93, 313–14; public asylum
  movement, 94–97
—drug therapy, 110–11
—hydrotherapy, 107
—and mental health policymaking, 174–
  75, 177–78
—overview of, 4–7, 89–90, 112–13,
  312–13
—psychotherapy, 103
—shock treatment, 108
—social class bias of, 93, 94, 95, 98
—and somaticism, 92, 99–100
—the rest cure, 103
—use of restraints, 91, 100
History of mental hospitals. *See also* History of mental health care; Mental hospitals, public
—development: origin as asylums, 90–
  91, 313–14; in colonial America, 91–
  93; during the public asylum movement, 94–97; during the Depression,
  107–8; during World War II, 108–9;
  and community mental health movement, 111
—development of psychiatric wards in
  general hospitals, 104
—development of university psychopathic
  hospitals, 104, 107
—effects of overcrowding, 98
—effects of tranquilizing drugs on, 110
—investigations of abuse and neglect in,
  101–2, 109
—overview of, 89–90, 479

—and staff of, 101
—therapies in, 107
Homeless mentally ill, 70, 185, 189,
  293–94, 488
—causes of homelessness in, 296–98
—and Community Support Program,
  300–305, 307 (*see also* Community
  Support Program)
—definition of homelessness, 294
—demographics of, 295–96
—federal assistance for, 305–6; Comprehensive State Mental Health Planning
  Act, 305–6; Stewart B. McKinney
  Homeless Assistance Act, 305, 306
—need for housing of, 306, 492–93
—number of homeless, 294–95
—as proportion of total homeless population, 295–96
—research findings on, 298–99
Hoover Commission, 480
Hopkins Symptom Checklist Depression
  Scale, 77
Hospital Survey and Construction Act of
  1946 (Hill-Burton Act, Public Law 79–
  725), 269
Houston Parent-Child Development Project (to prevent developmental problems
  in children), 416

Incidence of mental disorder, definition
  of, 48. *See also* Prevalence of mental
  disorder, definition of; Psychiatric epidemiology
Inpatient care
—admission rates: demographic differences, 27–29; diagnostic differences,
  29–30; payment-based differences, 30;
  state differences, 27
—bed capacity, 25–27
—changes in during 1980s, 393
—in community mental health centers,
  199
—days of care, 26
—types of treatment, 30
Institute of Social Research (University of
  Michigan), 480
Institutional mental health care: decline

in, 24; history of, 5. *See also* History
   of mental hospitals; Mental hospitals
Institutions of mental disease (IMDs),
   273, 353
Intermediate care facilties (ICFs), 271,
   272
Involuntary civil commitment, 366–68; as
   outpatient, 368–70; in Wisconsin, 459,
   469–70

James, William, 103, 314
Jarrett, Mary C., 104
Johnson, PResident Lyndon, 132; use of
   block grants, 146
Joint Commission on Mental Illness and
   Health, 24, 111–12, 182, 274, 315–16

Kennedy, President John F., 112, 125–
   26, 129–30, 182–83
Kennedy, Senator Edward M., 184–85
Kerr-Mills Bill of 1960 (Public Law 86–
   778), 269–70
Keys Amendment to Social Security Act,
   242
Kirkbride, Thomas S., 96

Langner Scale, 50–51. *See also* Midtown
   Manhattan Study
Lanterman-Petris-Short Act (California,
   1967), 188, 238, 274
Lasker, Mary, 124, 181
Level of Benefits Survey, 351–52, 479
Life Skills Training program (for prevent-
   ing substance abuse), 419

Malpractice in mental health care, 378–
   80
Mann, Horace, 177
Marine Hospital Service (MHS), 178
Marx, Dr. Arnold, 459
Mather, Cotton, 90
McKinney Act. *See* Stewart B. Mc-
   Kinney Homeless Assistance Act of
   1987
Medicaid, 16, 24, 320, 343, 478, 481;
   and abortion, 425; current coverage of
   mental health benefits, 352–53; dis-
   criminatory treatment of mental illness

by, 498; during the 1980s, 159, 161;
   establishment of Title XIX, 270; and
   the Miller Amendment, 271; and the
   Moss Amendments, 270–71; need for
   reform of, 491; and Public Law 92–
   603, 271–72; and public mental hospitals, 332
Medicare, 16, 24, 320, 343, 355, 478,
   481; current coverage of mental health
   benefits, 352–53; discriminatory treatment of mental illness by, 498; during
   the 1980s, 272–73; establishment of
   Title XVIII, 270; and parity of coverage, 348; Prospective Payment System
   (PPS), 349, 350, 353, 355–56; and
   Public Law 92–603, 272–72; and public mental hospitals, 332–33. *See also*
   Diagnosis-related groups; Medicare
   Catastrophic Coverage Act of 1988
Medicare Catastrophic Coverage Act of
   1988 (Public Law 100–36), 272
Mendota State Hospital (Wisconsin), 459
Menniger, William, 122–23
Mental disorder. *See also* Etiology of
   mental disorder; Pyschiatric epidemiology
—definition of, 8
—incidence of, 48; as affected by preventive interventions, 409, 411
—major categories of, 46–48
—measurement of: early prevalence studies, 48–49; treated rates, 49–50; by
   community surveys, 50–52
—prevalence of: as affected by preventive interventions, 407–8, 409, 411;
   Epidemiological Catchment Area Studies, 52–54; population differences, 54
—prevention of, 403–6 (*see also* Mental
   health care, preventive services in)
Mental health administration
—the context of the 1960s and 1970s,
   387–88; Community Mental Health
   Centers Act and amendments, 387–88
   (*see also* Community Mental Health
   Centers Act of 1963)
—issues of the 1960s, 1970s, 388–89
—the context of the 1980s, 389–91; creation of Alcohol, Drug Abuse, and

Mental Health block grant, 389–91 (*see also* Alcohol, Drug Abuse, and Mental Health block grant); growth of community-based services, 391
—developments in administration in the 1980s: business strategies, 395–96; catchment area concept, 397; citizen participation, 396; governing boards, 396; increased competition, 397; service diversification, 397–98
—developments in service provision in the 1980s, 391–95, 398–400; cutbacks in services, 393–94; growth of services to selected target populations, 391–92; quality issues, 394–95; staffing changes, 394; transformation of inpatient services, 393
—environmental fit of organization, 386–87
—operating fit of organization, 386–87
—points of leverage in, 488–89; appropriate mix of health personnel, 496–97; improving disability determination, 490–91; Medicaid reform, 491; ; organizational barriers in, 494–96; refunding state mental health budget priorities, 489–90
—for the severely mentally ill, 491–94; case management, 493–94; housing problems, 492–93
Mental health advocacy: insurance reform, 498; need for organization, 497–98; underfinancing of public mental health sector, 498
Mental Health Association (MHA), 10
Mental health care, general trends in, 23–25, 479–80. *See also* Deinstitutionalization; Inpatient care; Institutional mental health care; Mental health care, preventive services in; Mental health facilities; Mental hospitals; Outpatient care
Mental health care, preventive services in, 403–4, 425–26. *See also* Community mental health centers, evaluation of prevention of mental disorders; Mental disorder, prevention of; *and specific prevention programs by name*

—for avoidance of adolescent pregnancy, 412–14, 424–25
—cutbacks in during 1980s, 393
—definition of a positive preventive outcome, 404–6
—funding problems of, 420–21
—Gordon's prevention typology, 410–11; and benefit-cost estimates, 411–12
—public health typology of, 406–7; categories of preventable mental disorders in, 406; primary prevention, 406, 409–10; secondary prevention, 407–9; tertiary prevention, 407
—for reducing developmental delay in children from high-risk families, 414–17
—risk assessment in, 422–24
—and social reform, 424–25
—for substance abuse, 417–20
—target populations of, 421–22
Mental health care expenditures, 15, 35–39, 345, 479
Mental health care policy. *See also* Community Mental Health Centers Act; Mental health law; *and other legislative enactments*
—benefits and objectives of, 9
—and civil liberties of mentally ill, 188–89, 487
—cyclical development of, 13, 175–78
—deinstitutionalization, 316–21
—effect of budget cuts on, 13–14 (*see also* Alcohol, Drug Abuse, and Mental Health block grant; Mental health administration, the context of the 1980s)
—effect of ideology, 477–78; antihospital ideologies, 482; psychodynamic conceptions, 483
—effect of lobbying on, 187–88, 497–98
—effect of public opinion on, 11
—emergence of, 4–7
—fragmented policy structures, 12
—future direction of: improving disability determination, 490–91; need for Medicaid reform, 491; refunding state mental health budget priorities, 489–90
—and the homeless, 189

—and housing, 492–93

—impact of prominent health issues on, 190

—interests concerned with, 10–11

—intergovernmental relations, 12 14, 16, 126 (*see also* Alcohol, Drug Abuse, and Mental Health block grant)

—and multiple service systems, 11–12, 167

—nature of problem addressed by, 8–9

—necessary functions of community mental health systems, 486–88

—post-World War II mental health reform, 180–82; and community care, 183–85; and the federal bureaucracy, 182: impact of interest groups on, 185; and the presidency, 182–83

—public-private relationship, 12

—and the prison system, 189–90

—rediscovery of categorical subpopulations, 185

—shift from state hospital-based to community-based care, 24, 39–40 (*see also* Community mental health movement)

—social insurance vs. categorical spending programs, 186–87

—sociopolitical, institutional, and ideological elements of reform, 179–80

—trends of 1980s and 1990s: ascendance of financing, 15–16; ascendance of management, 13–15; federal reorientation, 16; reassessment and renewal, 16–17

—and the welfare state, 174

Mental health care politics: during Carter administration, 138; and the community mental health centers program, 183–84; during Kennedy administration, 126–27, 182–83; during Nixon administration, 137; during Reagan administration, 140, 143–44; organization of interests, 10–11, 185; public opinion, 11

Mental health care revenues, 36, 38–39, 345–46, 347

Mental Health Demographic Profile System (MHDPS), 440–41

Mental health facilities, 22–23. *See also* Community mental health centers; Community residential care; Mental hospitals; Nursing homes, as mental health facilities

Mental health law. *See also* Mental Health Law Project

—advocacy during 1960s and 1970s, 364–65, 482–83, 487

—competency to stand trial, 374–77; Dusky test, 374–75; "sunshine chronic," 375–76

—emergence of mental health law, 363–64

—insanity defense, 371–74; American Bar Association (ABA) Appreciation test, 372; American Law Institute (ALI) test, 372; "irresistible impulse test," 372; McNaughtan test, 371–72, 373

—involuntary civil commitment, 366–68

—malpractice liability, 378—80

—outpatient involuntary civil commitment, 368–70

—shifts in approach, 364–65, 380–81

—treatment refusal, 377–78

Mental Health Law Project, 10, 363

Mental health personnel: need for appropriate mix of, 496–97; trends in, 33–35, 480; types of, 32–33. *See also* Nurses, in mental health care; Psychiatric nurse practitioners; Psychiatric social workers; Psychiatrists; Psychologists

Mental Health Study Act of 1955 (Public Law 84–182), 24, 111, 125, 315

Mental Health Systems Act of 1980 (Public Law 96–398), 138, 139–40, 165, 184–85, 186–87, 203, 225, 275, 404

Mental hospitals. *See also* Inpatient care; Institutional mental health care

—historical development, 89–113 (*see also* History of mental hospitals)

—private: expenditures for, 36; number of, 25; revenues for, 38

—public, 24, 311–12: capacity and volume of, 321–22; changes in, 479; debate over, 326–30;

deinstitutionalization, 316–17, 320–21; expenditures for, 36; finances of, 326, 327, 328, 332–33; future problems of, 332–34; future role of, 330–31; mental hygiene and the psychopathic hospital, 314–15; moral treatment and the asylum, 313–14; number of, 25, 321; patient characteristics of, 322–24; population of, 316, 317, 318–19; reform cycles, 312–13; revenues for, 38; staffing of, 325, 328; types of treatment at, 325–26

Mental illness, term adopted, 106. *See* Mental disorder

Mental Retardation Facilities and Community Mental Health Centers Act of 1963. *See* Community Mental Health Centers Act of 1963

Meyer, Adolf, 103–4, 314

Midtown Manhattan Study, 50. *See also* Langner Scale

Miller Amendment (Public Law 90–248), 271

Mills, C. Wright, 4

Minorities
—mental disorder in, 75; correlates of, 77–78; prevalence of, 76–77; suicide rates of, 76–77, 78
—service utilization of, 78, 201, 222–23

Mitchell, S. Weir, 103

Mood disorders, 46

Moral treatment, 5, 94–97, 177–78, 313

Moran, Donald W., 143

Mosher, J. Montgomery, 104

Moss, Senator Frank, 271

Moss Amendments, 270–71

Myerson, Abraham, 109

National Alliance for the Mentally Ill (NAMI), 187, 225, 334, 497

National Association for the Protection of the Insane and the Prevention of Insanity (NAPIPI), 101–2

National Association of State Mental Health Program Directors (NASMHPD), 10

National Coalition for the Homeless, 306

National Committee Against Mental Illness, 125, 181

National Committee for Mental Hygiene, 105, 106, 178, 314

National Council of Community Mental Health Centers (NCCMHC), 10

National Institute of Mental Health (NIMH), 10; Community Support Program, 299–306 (*see also* Community Support Program); creation of, 6, 10, 178, 181, 315; early work of, 123–25, 182; influence on community mental health movement, 124, 131

National Long-Term Care Channeling Project, 285

National Medical Care Utilization and Expenditure Survey (NMCUES), 480

National Mental Health Act of 1946 (Public Law 79–487), 109, 123, 181

National Nursing Home Survey of 1977, 276–77, 278, 282

National Plan for the Chronically Mentally Ill. *See Toward A National Plan for the Chronically Mentally Ill*

Needs assessment techniques, for mental health services, 435–36, 444–45
—combined approaches, 441–44; to address attrition, 441, 445 (note 1); to assist in staff planning, 441–42; and empirical relationship between social indicators and service utilization, 442–44; to examine geographic and demographic accountability 442; and identification of unmet need, 442, 445 (note 2); to plan treatment process, 442
—definition of, 436; types of need, 436
—future research directions, 444
—social indicator, 437–38, 440–41; heightened interest in, 440; Mental Health Demographic Profile System (MHDPS), 440–41; problems of, 441
—techniques: community forum, 437; key informant, 436–37; rates-under-treatment, 437–440
—usefulness to policymakers, 435, 444–45

Network Against Psychiatric Assault (NAPA), 187

Neurotic disorders, prevalence of, 53
New York City Shelter Study (1986), 298
Nixon, President Richard M.: and community mental health centers movement, 133–34, 137, 184; and general revenue sharing, 146; and nursing home care, 271–72
Nurses, in mental health care, 33, 496–97; and the Moss Amendments, 271; number of, 34. *See also* Psychiatric nurse practitioners
Nursing homes, as mental health facilities, 240, 267–68, 481–82
—alternatives to, 283–85
—effect of Medicaid and Medicare on, 270, 272–73, 481
—effect of Miller Amendment on, 271
—effect of Moss Amendments on, 270–71
—effect of Public Law 92–603 on, 271–72
—effect of Social Security on, 268–69
—factors contributing to use of: Alcohol, Drug Abuse and Mental Health block grant, 275; deinstitutionalization, 274, 485; psychotropic medications, 273–74; social and political climate, 275
—historical development of, 268
—and the Hill-Burton Act, 269
—improving psychiatric care in, 280–83
—and the Kerr-Mills Bill, 269–70
—number and population of, 267
—outcomes of psychiatric patients in: inappropriate drug use, 280; lowered functional level, 279; undetected mental disorders, 278–79
—prevalence of mental illness in, 276–78

Occupational therapy, 107
O'Connor v. Donaldson, 188, 274
Okin, Robert, 327
Old Age and Survivors Insurance (OASI), 268
Old Age Assistance (OAA), 268
Older Americans Act, 285
Ombudsman program (for drug abuse prevention), 419
Omnibus Budget Reconciliation Act of

1981 (OBRA, Public Law 97–35), 140, 143–44, 186, 353, 389; and Alcohol, Drug Abuse, and Mental Health block grant, 149, 151; and Medicaid, 159; and Medicare, 272
Omnibus Budget Reconciliation Act of 1987 (OBRA, Public Law 100–203), 272, 284, 286, 353
Outpatient care, 23, 24; changes in during the 1980s, 392–93; demographic differences, 31; effect of community mental health centers on available services, 197–98; state differences, 31–32; types of programs and facilities, 31

Packard, Elizabeth, 100–101
Patient care episodes, defined, 40 n.1. *See also* Inpatient care; Outpatient care
Peel, Sir Robert, 471
Pennsylvania Hospital, 91
Personality disorders, 48; prevalence of, 53
Phenothiazines, 481. *See also* Drug therapy; Psychopharmacology; Psychotropic medications
Pierce, President Franklin, 174–75
Pinel, Philippe, 92
Planning. *See* Strategic Planning, mental health systems
Preferred provider organizations (PPOs), 355, 356–58
Prenatal/Early Infancy Project (to prevent maternal and child health problems), 415
President's Commission on Mental Health (1977), 138–39, 184, 202, 275, 404
President's Interagency Task Force on Mental Health, 129–30
Prevalence of mental disorder, definition of, 48. *See also* Incidence of mental disorder; Psychiatric epidemiology
Preventive intervention research centers (PIRC), 404
Preventive services. *See* Mental health care, preventive services in
Primary Mental Health Project (as mental health prevention service via early intervention), 408

Prisons, mentally ill in, 189–90
Professional Standards Review Organizations (PSROs), 271
Program for Assertive Community Treatment (PACT), 459
Project Redirection (for problem of adolescent pregnancy), 413
Prospective Payment System (PPS). *See* Diagnosis-related groups; Medicare
Psychiatric epidemiology. *See also* Children; Chronically mentally ill; Elderly; Etiology of mental disorder; Mental disorder; Minorities; Substance abuse disorders
—definition of, 45
—methods of measurement: community surveys, 50–52; prevalence studies, 48–49; treated rates, 49–50
—prevalence rates, 52–54; class differences, 54; race differences, 54; sex differences, 54
Psychiatric Epidemiology Research Interview (PERI), 51
"Psychiatric ghettos," 185
Psychiatric health facilities (PHFs), 285
Psychiatric nurse practitioners, 496–97. *See also* Nurses, in mental health care
Psychiatric social workers, 32–33; number of, 34; origin of, 104
Psychiatrists, 32; geographic distribution of, 33; and malpractice, 378; number of, 33, 34, 496
Psychiatry, role of during World War II, 50
Psychoanalytic theory, and the community mental health movement, 128; effect of psychodynamics on mental health professions, 483
Psychologists, 32; and malpractice, 378–79; number of, 33, 34
Psychopharmacology: origins of, 110; and psychiatric nurse practitioners, 496–97. *See also* Drug therapy; Phenothiazines; Psychotropic medications
Psychosocial rehabilitation facilities (PRFs), 248. *See also* Community residential care
Psychotropic medications, 480–81; and declining interest in psychiatry, 496; used in nursing homes, 273–74. *See also* Drug therapy; Phenothiazines; Psychopharmacology
Public Law 92–603. *See title of enactment for other public laws*; and nursing homes, 271–72.
Public mental hospitals. *See Mental hospitals*

Quarterway house, 247–48

R.A.J. v. Miller, 189
Reade, Charles, 100
Reagan, President Ronald, 140, 404; and creation of block grants to reform intergovernmental relations, 143, 147–48, 157–58, 186
Rehabilitation Act of 1973 (Public Law 93–112), 202
"Report on the National Conference on Graduate CMHCs" (1980), 199
Residential care. *See* Community residential care
Robert Wood Johnson Foundation, 493, 496
Ruiz v. Estelle, 189
Rush, Benjamin, 92
Rutland Corner House, 247

Salmon, Thomas, W., 106
Satellite housing for mentally ill, 248–49. *See also* Community residential care
Schedule of Affective Disorders and Schizophrenia (SADS), 52
Schizophrenia, 46–48; community mental health center utilization by schizophrenics, 205–6; correlates of, 70; prevalence studies of, 53; problems of care for young chronic schizophrenics, 47, 69, 486
Schweicker, Senator Richard, 185
Search and Teach program (to identify kindergarten children with reading problems), 408
Sex education, 425. *See also* Adolescents, prevention of pregnancy among
Shannon, James, 124

Shock treatment, 108

Single Audit Act of 1984 (Public Law 98–502), 157

Skilled nursing facilities (SNFs), 271, 272

SOCA (scan, orient, commit, and act) cycle of, 455–57; application within Washington State Mental Health Division, 462–63, 464; case study of Community Support Programs in Wisconsin, 458–60; case study of Wisconsin's involuntary civil commitment debate, 469–70

—scan: by use of WOTS-UP analysis, 460; competitive analysis framework, 461, 462; definition of, 460; environmental assessment techniques, 461; service system analysis, 460–61

—orient, 463

—commit: attrition vs. indirect maneuvers, 466; cooperation vs. competition, 464–65; importance of debate in process, 463–64; initiatives in implementation, 466–67

—act: combination of contect with process, 467; initial and subsequent actions, 467–68

Social Security Act, 186, 268–69 and disability determination for the mentally ill, 490–91

Social Security Administration (SSA), 490, 496

Social Security Amendments of 1967, 270–71

Social Security Disability Insurance (SSDI), 16, 24, 332, 478, 482, 490–91; under Reagan administration, 159

Social workers, 32–33; number of, 34

Society of Friends, and mental health care, 92–93

Solomon, Harry C., and reforms to Boston Psychopathic Hospital, 109

Specialty mental health organizations, defined, 40 n.1. See also Mental health facilities

State Care Act (New York, 1890), 315

State Lunatic Hospital (Massachusetts), 94

State mental health agencies (SMHAs): expenditures of, 36, 37–38; revenue sources of, 39, 151

State mental health systems. See also Mental hospitals, public; State mental health agencies

—and Alcohol, Drug Abuse, and Mental Health block grant: allocation decisions, 157–58; management performance, 156–57; program priorities, 158; replacement of lost federal funds, 154–56

—variation in, 36, 37–38, 39, 166

Stein, Dr. Leonard, 458–59

Stewart B. McKinney Homeless Assistance Act of 1987 (Public Law 100–77), 305, 306

Stirling County Study, 50

Strategic planning, mental health systems

—cautions, 454

—and community-based services, 450

—defense of, 452–53

—definition of, 451–52; debunking of planning myths, 453–54

—need for, 449–51, 452–53, 471; changing service systems, 450; new funding initiatives, 451; serving priority populations, 451; values, 451

Stressful life events

—chronic stress model, 58

—needed future research, 60–61

—overview of stress model, 56–58; role of personal resources in, 57–58; role of social support in, 56–57

—and prevention services, 423–24

—social class and sex differences, 58–60

Subcommittee on Long-Term Care of the Senate Special Committee on Aging, 271

Substance abuse disorders: correlates of, 79–80; among the homeless, 305; prevalence of, 53, 78–79, 420; prevention services for, 417–20; utilization patterns, 80

Supplemental Security Income (SSI), 16, 24

Tax Equity and Fiscal Responsibility Act of 1982 (Public Law 97–248), 353
Test, Dr. Mary Ann, 459
Three-quarterway house, 247–48
Title XX of Social Security Act, 285
Toward A National Plan for the Chronically Mentally Ill (1980), 275, 283
Transinstitutionalization, 321. See also Nursing homes, as mental health facilities
Tuke, William, 92–93

U.S. Census, 443
U.S. Children's Bureau, 178
U.S. Department of Health and Human Services (DHHS), and Alcohol, Drug Abuse, and Mental Health block grant, 148
U.S. Department of Housing and Urban Development (HUD), 392, 493, 496
U.S. Public Health Service (PHS), 178, 181
Urban Institute, survey of Alcohol, Drug Abuse, and Mental Health: block grant spending and state implementation, 155

Veterans Administration, 246–47

Washington State Mental Health Division, use of SOCA-cycle analysis by, 462–63, 464
Waxman, Representative Henry, 184–85
Welfare state, history of, 174–75
White House Conference on Aging (1971), 271, 276
White House Conference on Children (1909), 178
Wisconsin mental health system: case study of expansion of Community Support Programs in, 458–60, 465–66; debate over involuntary civil commitment, 469–70
Wisconsin Office of Mental Health (OMH), 469–70
Woodward, Samuel, 94–95, 97
Wyatt v. Stickney, 188, 274

Yolles, Stanley, 132, 183

About the Editor and Contributors

LARUE ALLEN, Ph.D., is Associate Professor in the University of Maryland's Clinical/Community Psychology Program. She received her A.B. from Harvard in 1972 and her doctorate from Yale in 1980. She is on the editorial boards of the *Journal of Pediatric Psychology*, the *Journal of Community Psychology*, and the *Journal of Child Clinical Psychology*. Her research focuses on risk factors in adolescent development, the influence of ethnicity and gender on socioemotional development in children and adolescents, and humor responsiveness as a measure of adaptive behavior in children.

PHILIP K. ARMOUR, Ph.D., is Associate Professor of Sociology and Political Economy at the University of Texas at Dallas. Besides serving on the Texas Indigent Health Care Task Force and coauthoring a forthcoming evaluation of the politics and impact of these health care reforms, Armour has recently published (with Linda Lloyd) the findings of a social epidemiological study of teenage suicide in Texas. He is currently collaborating on an analysis of cross-national welfare policies and politics in advanced societies with Richard M. Coughlin.

LELAND V. BELL, Ph.D., is Professor and Chairman of the History Department at Central State University in Wilberforce, Ohio. He is the author of several publications, including *Treating The Mentally Ill* (1980) and (with Peter L. Tyor) *Caring for the Retarded in America: A History* (1984). He is currently engaged in a project dealing with mental illness in West Africa.

BARRIE E. BLUNT, Ph.D., is Associate Professor in the Public Administration program at the University of Maine. His research has focused on mental health policy, empirical methodology, and administrative theory.

EVELYN J. BROMET, Ph.D., is Professor of Psychiatry and Behavioral Science and of Preventive Medicine at the State University of New York at Stony Brook. She holds a doctorate in epidemiology from Yale University and has published in the areas of schizophrenia, alcoholism, occupational mental health, and stress research.

JAMES M. CAMERON, Ph.D., is Assistant Professor in the School of Public Administration at the University of Southern California. He has held faculty positions at the Center for Health Studies at Yale University and the School of Public Health at the University of California, Los Angeles. In addition to research in mental health policy, he has conducted studies aimed at the development and application of medical case-mix classification systems, the cost of graduate medical education, and problems of access to care for the poor. His current research interests include an appraisal of alternative health care financing arrangements.

JAMES A. CIARLO, Ph.D., is Director of the Mental Health Systems Evaluation Project and Research Professor of Psychology at the University of Denver. From 1968 to 1976 he was Director of Research and Evaluation for the Northwest Denver Community Mental Health Center, a part of the Denver Department of Health and Hospitals. He earned his doctorate in Social Relations at Harvard University, with a specialty in Clinical Psychology. He currently teaches, consults, and directs research in mental health program evaluation and utilization of evaluation. He was co-editor of the *Community Mental Health Journal* from 1978 to 1981.

DAVID A. DOWELL, Ph.D., is Professor of Psychology at California State University, Long Beach. He was trained in community psychology and program evaluation at the University of Tennessee. He has published evaluation research reports on rehabilitation of juvenile delinquents and adult female offenders, basic skills education for adolescents, validity of student evaluation of university instruction, mental health services in Madrid, Spain, and board and care facilities for the long-term mentally ill. Currently he is working in the area of homelessness, having recently completed a needs assessment of the homeless population in Long Beach, which is in the greater Los Angeles area, often called the "homeless capital of the USA."

HOWARD H. GOLDMAN, M.D., M.P.H., Ph.D., is a research psychiatrist who directs the Mental Health Policy Studies Program at the University of Maryland School of Medicine, where he is Associate Professor of Psychiatry. Goldman is Principal Investigator of the National Evaluation of the Robert Wood Johnson Foundation's Program for the Chronically Mentally Ill. Goldman also holds a faculty appointment as Research Associate in the Center for Health Services Research and Development at the School of Hygiene and Public Health at Johns Hopkins University, and is Co-Principal Investigator there of the Center for Organization and Financing of Care for the Severely Mentally Ill, sponsored by the National Institute of Mental Health. In addition, he continues to serve as a consultant in mental health financing policy to the NIMH, where he was an Assistant Director from 1983 to 1985.

DAVID GOODRICK, Ph.D., established and directs the National Institute of Mental Health-funded National Technical Assistance Center for Mental Health Planning at the COSMOS Corporation, Washington, D.C. Former Director of the Wisconsin Office of Mental Health, Goodrick has twenty years of clinical, strategic planning, and management experience in public mental health systems. As Associate Director of the Alpha Center from 1985 to 1987, he directed a project sponsored by the NIMH offering strategic planning training to managers and planners in state mental health agencies. He has consulted with states and counties throughout the United States in their efforts to develop comprehensive community-based mental health systems.

LORETTA K. HAGGARD, B.A., is Assistant Coordinator of the National Institute of Mental Health Program for the Homeless Mentally Ill. She received her bachelor's degree from Princeton University's Woodrow Wilson School of Public and International Affairs in 1986. Prior to joining the federal government, Haggard served as a consultant to the NIMH. She plans a career in law and psychiatric social work.

JEANETTE M. JERRELL, Ph.D., is Director of Evaluation and Research at the Santa Clara County Bureau of Mental Health in San Jose, California. She has conducted research on administrative and service changes in mental health organizations and currently is performing services evaluation research on programs for the chronically mentally ill and severely disabled adolescents.

S. LEE JERRELL, Ph.D., is Director of Graduate Programs and Associate Professor of Management and Organization at San Jose State University School of Business. He conducts research on the formulation of effective business strategy for industries undergoing rapid change, including health care.

INGO KEILITZ, Ph.D., is founding Director of the Institute on Mental Disability and the Law, an arm of the National Center for State Courts, and a lecturer in mental health law at the Marshall-Wythe School of Law, College of William and Mary. He has directed numerous national projects of the institute including, from 1981 to the present, the Involuntary Civil Commitment Project, a multiyear effort funded by the MacArthur Foundation and a consortium of local foundations that is aimed at improving the adult civil commitment process throughout the country. He has previously held professorships in psychology at Creighton University and in special education at the University of Missouri, as well as other research and clinical positions. He received his doctorate in experimental psychology from Kansas State University in 1971. He is the author of a book, numerous monographs, and over fifty articles on mental disability and the law, special education, psychology, and program evaluation.

PAMELA KOTLER, Ph.D., is Project Manager of the Mental Health and Social Welfare Research Group, University of California, Berkeley.

IRENE SHIFREN LEVINE, Ph.D., is Associate Director of the Division of Education and Service Systems Liaison, National Institute of Mental Health. In that capacity, she has directed NIMH's Program for the Homeless Mentally Ill for the past five years and has coordinated Public Health Service initiatives for the homeless population with mental health problems, alcoholism, or drug abuse problems. Between 1978 and 1980, Levine helped to launch the NIMH Community Support Program, a program of grants to states for community-based mental health and support services for severely mentally ill individuals. Levine is trained as a clinical psychologist; prior to joining the federal government, she worked as both a clinician and an administrator in state and local programs serving the severely mentally ill.

MARGARET W. LINN, Ph.D., is Director of Social Science Research, Veterans Administration Medical Center, Miami, Florida, and Professor with the University of Miami Department of Psychiatry. She has published numerous studies on mental health, nursing homes, and the aged.

BRUCE M. LOGAN, Ph.D., is Director, Systems Procurement and Planning, Massachusetts Department of Public Welfare, where he was formerly Assistant Budget Director for Administration. His research interests and publications center on public policy analysis, including the human services, public management, and Irish politics.

RAYMOND P. LORION, Ph.D., is Professor of Psychology and Director of the Clinical/Community Psychology Program at the University of Maryland at College Park. He received his doctorate in 1972 from the University of Rochester and has served as a faculty member at the University of Rochester, Temple University, and the University of Tennessee. Between 1982 and 1984, he served as Visiting Scientist to the Center for Prevention Research at the National Institute of Mental Health. He was Acting Associate Administrator for Prevention at the Alcohol, Drug Abuse, and Mental Health Administration from 1983 to 1984 and remains a senior policy consultant to that agency. He is the author or coauthor of ten books and approximately sixty articles and chapters.

PHILLIP M. MASSAD, Ph.D., is Clinical Research Psychologist at the Veterans Medical Administration in White River Junction, Vermont. He is the director of a research grant concerning the interaction between psychiatric and medical utilization and psychotherapeutic outcome. In addition, he is active in clinical practice.

DAVID MECHANIC, Ph.D., is Director of the Institute for Health, Health Care Policy, and Aging Research, University Professor, and the René Dubos Professor of Behavioral Sciences at Rutgers University. He was formerly Dean of the Faculty of Arts and Sciences in New Brunswick. He is the author of numerous books and other publications on health policy and health services research, including *Mental Health and Social Policy* (3rd ed., 1989); *From Advocacy to Allocation: The Evolving American Health Care System* (1986); *Future Issues in Health Care: Social Policy and the Rationing of Medical Services* (1979); and *Medical Sociology* (2nd ed., 1978). Mechanic is a former member of the National Advisory Council on Aging, National Institutes of Health, and Chairman of the Council's Program Committee. He is a member of the Institute of Medicine of the National Academy of Sciences, and former Chair of the Section on Social, Economic, and Political Sciences of the American Association for the Advancement of Science.

JOSEPH P. MORRISSEY, Ph.D., is Associate Professor of Social and Administrative Medicine and Deputy Director, Health Services Research Center, University of North Carolina at Chapel Hill. Formerly he directed the Evaluation Research Unit for the New York State Office of Mental Health, served as a Research Sociologist in the Division of Biometry and Epidemiology at the National Institute of Mental Health, and held teaching positions at SUNY-Albany, Brandeis, and Clark universities. He has published widely on the sociology of mental hospitalization, mental health service delivery, criminal justice and mental health issues, and on interorganizational analysis of mental health service systems.

FREDERIC G. REAMER, Ph.D., is Professor in the School of Social Work, Rhode Island College. His research interests include mental health, public welfare, criminal justice, and professional ethics. Reamer is the author of *Ethical Dilemmas in Social Service* (2nd ed., 1989) and (with Charles Shireman) *Rehabilitating Juvenile Justice* (1986).

M. SUSAN RIDGELY, M.S.W., is a Research Associate in Psychiatry in the Mental Health Policy Studies Program and has a faculty appointment in the

Department of Psychiatry at the University of Maryland School of Medicine. She has been involved in mental health services and policy analysis concerning the chronically mentally ill since she began her clinical work at a community mental health center in the late 1970s. Ridgely has also served as the national mental health policy analyst for the American Federation of State, County, and Municipal Employees and as Assistant Director for Public Policy of the National Mental Health Association. Currently she is part of the national evaluation team for the Robert Wood Johnson Foundation's Program for the Chronically Mentally Ill and a consultant to the state of Maryland on the organization and financing of mental health services.

DAVID A. ROCHEFORT, Ph.D., is Associate Professor in Political Science and Public Administration at Northeastern University. He teaches courses in health policy and politics, American social welfare policy, policy analysis, and research methods. Rochefort is a former National Institute of Mental Health postdoctoral fellow in the Rutgers-Princeton Program in Mental Health Research and the author of *American Social Welfare Policy: Dynamics of Formulation and Change* (1986). He has served as a policy consultant and planning specialist for government agencies in the states of Rhode Island, Massachusetts, and New Jersey.

SARAH ROSENFIELD, Ph.D., is Assistant Professor in the Department of Sociology and a member of the Institute for Health, Health Care Policy, and Aging Research at Rutgers University. Her research interests are sex differences in psychiatric disorders, labeling theory of mental illness, and services for the chronically mentally ill.

HERBERT C. SCHULBERG, Ph.D., is Professor of Psychiatry and Psychology at the University of Pittsburgh. He holds a doctorate in clinical psychology from Columbia University Teachers College and an M.S.Hgy. from the Harvard School of Public Health. He has published in a variety of areas, including mental health evaluation research, depression in primary medical care patients, and mental health policy.

STEVEN P. SEGAL, Ph.D., is Professor of Social Welfare and Director of the Mental Health and Social Welfare Research Group, University of California, Berkeley, where he codirects the National Institute of Mental Health pre/post-doctoral training program in the organization and financing of mental health services at the Schools of Public Health and Social Welfare. Segal is also Principal Investigator of the Institute of Scientific Analysis in Berkeley.

SHAYNA STEIN, Ph.D., is Social Science Researcher with the Veterans Administration Medical Center, Miami, Florida, and Assistant Professor with the University of Miami Department of Psychiatry. She has published in geriatrics, focusing on the elderly in nursing homes and in the community.